Spinal Cord Medicine

Spinal Cord Medicine

Edited by Peter Ponce

hayle
medical

New York

Hayle Medical,
750 Third Avenue, 9ᵗʰ Floor,
New York, NY 10017, USA

Visit us on the World Wide Web at:
www.haylemedical.com

ISBN: 978-1-63241-520-2

Cataloging-in-Publication Data

Spinal cord medicine / edited by Peter Ponce.
    p. cm.
Includes bibliographical references and index.
ISBN 978-1-63241-520-2
1. Spinal cord--Wounds and injuries. 2. Spinal cord--Diseases. I. Ponce, Peter.
RC400 .S65 2018
616.83--dc23

Table of Contents

Preface

In my initial years as a student, I used to run to the library at every possible instance to grab a book and learn something new. Books were my primary source of knowledge and I would not have come such a long way without all that I learnt from them. Thus, when I was approached to edit this book; I became understandably nostalgic. It was an absolute honor to be considered worthy of guiding the current generation as well as those to come. I put all my knowledge and hard work into making this book most beneficial for its readers.

Spinal cord injuries affect the spinal cord causing damage that may be temporary or permanent. Total loss of muscle function, paralysis, paraplegia and other processes such as respiratory rate and pupillary response are some of the outcomes of spinal cord injuries. This book elucidates the concepts and innovative models around prospective developments with respect to spinal cord injury medicine. Those with an interest in this field would find this book helpful.

I wish to thank my publisher for supporting me at every step. I would also like to thank all the authors who have contributed their researches in this book. I hope this book will be a valuable contribution to the progress of the field.

Editor

Delayed Administration of a Bio-Engineered Zinc-Finger VEGF-A Gene Therapy Is Neuroprotective and Attenuates Allodynia Following Traumatic Spinal Cord Injury

Sarah A. Figley[1,2], Yang Liu[1], Spyridon K. Karadimas[1,2], Kajana Satkunendrarajah[1], Peter Fettes[1], S. Kaye Spratt[3], Gary Lee[3], Dale Ando[3], Richard Surosky[3], Martin Giedlin[2], Michael G. Fehlings[1,2,4]*

1 Department of Genetics and Development, Toronto Western Research Institute, and Spinal Program, Krembil Neuroscience Centre, University Health Network, Toronto, Ontario, Canada, 2 Institute of Medical Sciences, University of Toronto, Toronto, Ontario, Canada, 3 Department of Therapeutic Development, Sangamo BioSciences, Pt. Richmond, California, United States of America, 4 Department of Surgery, University of Toronto, Toronto, Ontario, Canada

Abstract

Following spinal cord injury (SCI) there are drastic changes that occur in the spinal microvasculature, including ischemia, hemorrhage, endothelial cell death and blood-spinal cord barrier disruption. Vascular endothelial growth factor-A (VEGF-A) is a pleiotropic factor recognized for its pro-angiogenic properties; however, VEGF has recently been shown to provide neuroprotection. We hypothesized that delivery of AdV-ZFP-VEGF – an adenovirally delivered bio-engineered zinc-finger transcription factor that promotes endogenous VEGF-A expression – would result in angiogenesis, neuroprotection and functional recovery following SCI. This novel VEGF gene therapy induces the endogenous production of multiple VEGF-A isoforms; a critical factor for proper vascular development and repair. Briefly, female Wistar rats – under cyclosporin immunosuppression – received a 35 g clip-compression injury and were administered AdV-ZFP-VEGF or AdV-eGFP at 24 hours post-SCI. qRT-PCR and Western Blot analysis of VEGF-A mRNA and protein, showed significant increases in VEGF-A expression in AdV-ZFP-VEGF treated animals ($p<0.001$ and $p<0.05$, respectively). Analysis of NF200, TUNEL, and RECA-1 indicated that AdV-ZFP-VEGF increased axonal preservation ($p<0.05$), reduced cell death ($p<0.01$), and increased blood vessels ($p<0.01$), respectively. Moreover, AdV-ZFP-VEGF resulted in a 10% increase in blood vessel proliferation ($p<0.001$). Catwalk™ analysis showed AdV-ZFP-VEGF treatment dramatically improves hindlimb weight support ($p<0.05$) and increases hindlimb swing speed ($p<0.02$) when compared to control animals. Finally, AdV-ZFP-VEGF administration provided a significant reduction in allodynia ($p<0.01$). Overall, the results of this study indicate that AdV-ZFP-VEGF administration can be delivered in a clinically relevant time-window following SCI (24 hours) and provide significant molecular and functional benefits.

Editor: Hatem E. Sabaawy, Rutgers-Robert wood Johnson Medical School, United States of America

Funding: This study was supported by Sangamo BioSciences and the Krembil Chair in Neural Repair and Regeneration (held by Dr. Michael G. Fehlings). The funders had no role in data collection, data analysis, or decision to publish; however, they did participate in some aspects of study design and reviewed the manuscript prior to publication.

Competing Interests: The personnel associated with Sangamo Biosciences, Inc. – Kaye Spratt, Gary Lee, Dale Ando, Richard Surosky and Martin Giedlin – fully disclose a conflict of interest related to this research. Each individual is an employee of Sangamo Biosciences, Inc. and receives either a salary and/or ownership interest (stock, stock options, patent or other intellectual property). Sarah Figley, Yang Liu, Spyridon Karadimas and Michael Fehlings disclose that research support (receipt of therapeutics, supplies and equipment) was provided by Sangamo Biosciences, Inc. for the experiments conducted in this manuscript.

* E-mail: michael.fehlings@uhn.on.ca

Introduction

In North America, it is estimated that approximately 1.5 million individuals are currently living with SCI, with over 12,000 traumatic SCI cases occurring each year [1]. Spinal cord injury is divided into two events, to separate the physical and the cellular pathologies. The primary injury, is associated with the initial mechanical trauma that the cord undergoes, whereas the secondary injury refers to the physiological cascade that propagates from 1 minute to 6 months following the initial injury [2]. Although the primary injury is responsible for triggering all of the downstream events, it is widely accepted that the processes that take place in the "secondary injury" phase are predominantly responsible for a significant portion of the damage and degeneration that is associated with SCI, including inflammation,

ischemia, lipid peroxidation, production of free radicals, disruption of ion channels, necrosis and programmed cell death [3–5]. Moreover, radical alterations to the spinal microvascular architecture and function occur following SCI and contribute to the secondary injury. Reduction in blood flow, hemorrhage, systemic hypotension, loss of microcirculation, disruption of the blood-spinal cord barrier (BSCB) and loss of structural organization, ultimately enhance the cellular damage post-injury [2,6]. Despite the fact that these secondary events are responsible for the majority of the damage associated with SCI, many of these pathways alternatively provide an opportunity to target with therapeutic interventions.

Recently, research has given much attention to therapies designed at repairing or minimizing vascular damage following injury. Angiogenic factors, such as vascular endothelial growth factor (VEGF)-A, are known to promote the proliferation of endothelial cells and initiate angiogenesis [7]. Emerging evidence suggests that VEGF-A (which will be referred to as VEGF) also has neurotrophic, neuroprotective, and neuroproliferative effects [8]. VEGF is a homodimeric glycoprotein that is expressed as multiple splice variants encoded by a single gene; however, VEGF signals as a homo- or heterodimer via VEGF receptors (VEGFRs) [9]. The predominant isoforms in the central nervous system are $VEGF_{121}$, $VEGF_{165}$ and $VEGF_{189}$. Studies have demonstrated that VEGF and its receptors are upregulated during and after hypoxic/ischemic injury to the brain and spinal cord, which suggests that VEGF likely plays a neuroprotective (or beneficial) role in these pathophysiological processes.

Perhaps the most devastating outcomes of spinal cord injury are paralysis and neuropathic pain. Paralysis is caused by damaged axons and neurons in motor pathways at or above the level of injury. Many models of SCI have been used to model the physical deficits post-injury, and thoracic injuries are among the best-characterized for the targets loss of hindlimb function. Motor impairment following SCI results from damage to and/or loss of both upper and lower motor neurons. Injury to first and second order spinothalamic neurons, or first order neurons from the medial lemniscus pathway, interrupts sensory information processing *at* and *below* the level of injury and prevents normal signal transmission to the brain. Miscommunication in sensory pathways can result in severe complications for patients suffering from SCI. Development of neuropathic pain occurs in many patients, and although the exact mechanism is unknown, it is hypothesized that it is caused by misguided axonal sprouting or abnormal sodium channel excitability in sensory neurons [10].

Previously described approaches using VEGF have relied on the introduction of a single splice isoform of VEGF-A ($VEGF_{165}$), which may not result in optimal neuroprotective or angiogenic effects. In this study, we utilize novel ZFP-VEGF technology – a viral vector encoding a zinc-finger transcription factor protein (ZFP), which activates endogenous VEGF-A expression to produce multiple splice isoforms of VEGF – which has previously demonstrated induced expression of VEGF-A protein, increase vascular counts and significant functional recovery following SCI [11]. Although we have already shown beneficial effects of AdV-ZFP-VEGF when administered immediately following SCI as a proof-of-concept, the current study aims to investigate a clinically-relevant administration of AdV-ZFP-VEGF by *delaying* administration by 24 hours post-SCI.

Materials and Methods

All animal experiments were conducted with approval from the Animal Care Committee, University Health Network (Toronto, Canada).

Viral Vector Constructs

The VEGF-A-activating ZFP and controls were provided in viral vectors by Sangamo BioSciences (Pt. Richmond, CA) and have been previously described [12,13]. The VEGF-A-activating ZFP (32E-p65) – referred to as AdV-ZFP-VEGF – is a 378 amino acid multi-domain protein that is composed of three functional regions: (1) the nuclear localization signal (NLS) of the large T-antigen of SV40, (2) a designed 3-finger zinc-fingered protein (32E) that binds to a 9 base-pair target DNA sequence (GGGGGTGAC) present in the human VEGF-A promoter region and (3) the transactivation domain from the p65 subunit of human NFκB, which is identical to VZ+434, subcloned into

pVAX1 (Invitrogen, San Diego, CA) with expression driven by the human cytomegalovirus (CMV) promoter. Adenoviral (Ad5-32Ep65 or Ad5- eGFP) vectors, referred to as AdV-ZFP-VEGF and AdV-eGFP, respectively, were packaged by transfecting T-REx-293 cells (Invitrogen, San Diego, CA). T-REx-293 cells in ten-stack cell factories were inoculated with Ad vectors at a multiplicity of infection (MOI) of 50 to 100 particles per cell. When adenoviral mediated cytopathy effect (CPE) was observed, cells were harvested and lysed by three cycles of freezing and thawing. Crude lysates were clarified by centrifugation, and 293 cells were seeded at 4×10^7 PFU and grown 3 days prior to transfection. The calcium phosphate method was used for transfection. Infectious titers of the Ad vectors were quantified using the Adeno-X Rapid Titer kit (Clontech, Mountain View, CA).

SCI and Intraspinal Microinjection

Animals were subject to a compressive spinal cord injury using a modified aneurysm clip, which has been extensively characterized by our laboratory and previously described [14]. Briefly, adult female Wistar rats (250–300 g; Charles River, Montreal, Canada) were deeply anesthetized using 4% isoflurane, and were sedated for the remainder of the surgery under 2% isoflurane. Animals received a two-level laminectomy of mid-thoracic vertebral segments T6–T7. A modified clip calibrated to a closing force of 35 g was applied extradurally to the cord for 1 minute and then removed. The animals were divided into four groups in a randomized and "blinded" manner, (1) Sham control group (laminectomy only – no SCI), (2) Non-injected injured control group (laminectomy and SCI – no injection), (3) AdV -ZFP-VEGF treatment group, and (4) AdV-eGFP control group. Using a stereotaxic frame and glass capillary needle (tip diameter 60 μm) connected to a Hamilton microsyringe, a total of 5×10^8 viral plaque forming units (PFU) were injected into the dorsal spinal cord 24 hours post-SCI. Four 2.5 μl (10 μl total) intraspinal injections were made bilaterally at 2 mm rostral and caudal of the injury site. The injection rate is 0.60 μl/min and when the injection was completed, the capillary needle was left in the cord for at least 1 min to allow diffusion of the virus from the injection site and to prevent back-flow. The incision was closed in layers using standard silk sutures and animals were given a single dose of buprenorphine (0.05 mg/kg). Animals were allowed to recover in their cage under a heat-lamp and, subsequently, were housed in a temperature-controlled warm room (26°C) with free access to food and water. Animals were given buprenorphine (0.05 mg/kg) every 12 hours for 48 hours following surgery, and their bladders were manually voided three times daily. A subcutaneous injection of 10 mg/kg of cyclosporin A was administered daily starting 24 hours prior to the SCI until the end of the experiments for immunosuppression.

Western Blotting

Following deep inhalation anesthetic, animals (n = 4–5/group) were sacrificed at five or ten days post-SCI and a 5 mm length of the spinal cord centered at the injury site was extracted. Samples were mechanically homogenized in 400 μl of homogenization buffer (0.1 M Tris, 0.5 M EDTA, 0.1% SDS, 1 M DTT solution, 100 mM PMSF, 1.7 mg/ml aprotinin, 1 mM pepstatin, 10 mM leupeptin) and centrifuged at 15,000 rpm for 10 minutes at 4°C. Supernatants were extracted and used for western blot analysis, where 20 μg of protein was loaded into 7.5% or 12% polyacrylamide gels (Bio-Rad, Mississauga, Canada). Membranes were probed with either monoclonal anti-NF200 antibody (1:2000; Sigma, Oakville, Canada), rabbit IgG anti-VEGF-A antibody

(1:100; Santa Cruz Biotechnology, Santa Cruz, CA), or rabbit IgG anti-NFκBp65 (1:1000; Santa Cruz Biotechnology, Santa Cruz, CA). NFκBp65 rabbit polyclonal antibody was used to recognize the p65 activation domain in the ZFP-VEGF treated animals. Primary antibodies were labelled with horseradish peroxidase-conjugated secondary antibodies (goat anti-mouse/rabbit IgG, 1:3000; Jackson Immuno Research Laboratories, West Grove, PA), and bands were imaged using an enhanced chemiluminescence (ECL) detection system (Perkin Elmer, Woodbridge, Canada). Mouse monoclonal, beta-actin (Chemicon International, Inc., Temecula, CA) was immunoblotted as a loading control. Quality One detection software (Bio-Rad Laboratories, Hercules, CA) was used for integrated optical density (OD) analysis.

Histochemistry

Histological Processing. Five or 10 days (n = 4–5/group), or 8 weeks (n = 10/group) post-SCI, following deep inhalation anesthetic, animals were transcardially perfused with 4% paraformaldehyde (PFA) in 0.1 M PBS. Then, the tissues were cryoprotected in 20% sucrose in PBS. A 10 mm length of the spinal cord centered at the injury site was fixed in tissue-embedding medium. The tissue segment was snap frozen on dry ice and sectioned on a cryostat at a thickness of 14 μm. Serial spinal cord sections at 500 μm intervals were stained with myelin-selective pigment luxol fast blue (LFB) and the cellular stain hematoxylin-eosin (HE) to identify the injury epicenter. Tissue sections showing the largest cystic cavity and greatest demyelination were taken to represent the injury epicenter.

Immunohistochemistry. The following primary antibodies were used: mouse anti-NeuN (1:500; Chemicon International, Inc., Temecula, CA) for neurons, mouse anti-GFAP (1:500; Chemicon International, Inc., Temecula, CA) for astrocytes, mouse anti-APC (CC1, 1:100; Calbiochem, San Diego, CA) for oligodendrocytes, and mouse anti-RECA-1 (1:25; Serotec Inc., Raleigh, NC) for endothelial cells. The sections were rinsed three times in PBS after primary antibody incubation and incubated with either fluorescent Alexa 568, 647 or 488 goat anti-mouse/rabbit secondary antibody (1:400; Invitrogen, Burlington, Canada) for 1 hour. The sections were rinsed three times with PBS and cover slipped with Mowiol mounting medium containing DAPI (Vector Laboratories, Inc., Burlingame, CA) to counterstain the nuclei. The images were taken using a Zeiss 510 laser confocal microscope.

Quantification of Blood Vessels. Tissue sections – taken from animals sacrificed 10 days post-SCI – were used for immunofluorescence studies with a monoclonal antibody specific for RECA-1 (Rat Endothelial Cell Antibody). Vessels counts were performed on 4 selected fields (ventral horn, dorsal horn, left and right lateral columns) in each section under 25X magnification (0.14 mm^2). The number of RECA-1-positive vessels was calculated at 2 mm and 4 mm, both rostral and caudal from the epicenter, for each animal.

Quantification of Angiogenesis. Tissue sections – taken from animals sacrificed 5 days post-SCI – were used to quantify angiogenesis following SCI and AdV-ZFP-VEGF administration. Angiogenesis was calculated as vessels co-labelled with RECA-1 and Ki67 (cellular proliferation). Angiogenesis quantification was performed on 4 selected fields (ventral horn, dorsal horn, left and right lateral columns) in each section under 25X magnification (0.14 mm^2). The number of angiogenic vessels was calculated at 1, 2 and 3 mm, both rostral and caudal from the epicenter, for each animal. Rostral and caudal values were pooled for each distance.

Quantification of Apoptosis. An *in situ* terminal-deoxytransferase mediated dUTP nick end-labeling (TUNEL) apoptosis kit (Chemicon International, Inc., Temecula, CA) was used to label apoptotic cells in tissues extracted from animals 5 days post-SCI. TUNEL staining was completed as described in the manufacturer's instructions. The numbers of TUNEL positive nuclei were counted at the epicenter, as well as at 1, 2 and 3 mm (rostral and caudal) from the injury epicenter. In each tissue section, the whole section was counted to include all apoptotic nuclei visible.

Quantification of Neurons. Tissue sections – taken from animals sacrificed 5 days post-SCI – were used for immunofluorescence studies with a monoclonal antibody specific for NeuN (Neuronal Nuclei). Neuron quantification was conducted only in the grey matter under 25X magnification (0.14 mm^2), and all cells were counted. The number of NeuN-positive cells was calculated at 1, 2 and 3 mm, both rostral and caudal from the epicenter, as well as at the epicenter.

Assessment of Tissue Sparing and Cavity Formation. Tissue sparing and cavity formation was analyzed 8 weeks after SCI, at the center of the lesion, 2 mm above and 2 mm below the epicenter. Sections were stained with LFB-HE. The measurements were carried out on coded slides using StereoInvestigator® software (MBF Bioscience, Williston, VT). Cross-sectional residual tissue and cavity areas were normalized with respect to total cross-sectional area and the areas were calculated every 500 μm within the rostrocaudal boundaries of the injury site.

Behavioural Testing

Open-field Locomotor Scoring. Locomotor recovery of the animals (n = 8–10/group) was assessed by two independent observers using the 21 point Basso, Beattie, and Bresnahan (BBB) open field locomotor score [15] from 1 to 8 weeks after SCI. The BBB scale was used to assess hindlimb locomotor recovery including joint movements, stepping ability, coordination, and trunk stability. Testing was done every week on a blinded basis and the duration of each session was 4 min per rat. Scores were averaged across both the right and left hindlimbs to arrive at a final motor recovery score for each week of testing.

Automated Gait Analysis (CatWalk). Gait analysis was performed using the CatWalk system (Noldus Information Technology, Wageningen, Netherlands) as described [16,17]. In short, the system consists of a horizontal glass plate and video capturing equipment placed underneath and connected to a PC. In our work, for correct analysis of the gait adaptations to the chronic compression, after standardization of the crossing speed, the following criteria concerning walkway crossing were used: (1) the rat needed to cross the walkway, without any interruption (2) a minimum of three correct crossings per animal were required. Files were collected and analyzed using the CatWalk program, version 7.1. Individual digital prints were manually labeled by one observer blinded to groups. With the CatWalk, a vast variety of static and dynamic gait parameters can be measured during spontaneous locomotion. In the present study, a blinded examiner generated and analyzed data for the following parameters:

- forelimb stride length (expressed in mm): distance between two consecutive forelimb paw placements
- hindlimb print area – maximal area of the paw print in contact with the detection surface of the CatWalk^{TM} (expressed in mm^2)
- hindlimb print width – the maximal distance spanning the medial and lateral contact points of the paw (expressed in mm)
- hindlimb print length – the maximal distance spanning the cranial and caudal contact points of the paw (expressed in mm)

- hindlimb swing speed (expressed in pixels/sec): is the speed of the paw during the swing phase (the duration of no paw contact with the glass plate during a step cycle).

Acclimation and training to the walking apparatus were performed as described by Gensel *et al.* [18]. Since Catwalk quantifies weight support and stepping, only a sub-set of animals exhibiting weight support (BBB scores >9) were used in the CatWalk experiments (n = 5/group). Most AdV-eGFP animals did not reach BBB scores >9; however, animals for this group were subject to CatWalk^{TM} analysis to provide consistency in our experiments.

Mechanical Allodynia. At-level mechanical allodynia was determined at 4 weeks and 8 weeks post-SCI using 2 g and 4 g von Frey monofilaments as previously described [19]. Animals were acclimatized for 30 minutes in an isolated room for 30 minutes prior to pain testing. The von Frey monofilament was applied to the dorsal skin surrounding the incision/injury site 10 times and animals' behavioural response to each was recorded. An adverse response to the application of the monofilament (determined in advance of experiments) included vocalization, licking, biting and immediate movement to the other side of the cage. The proportion of rats to exhibit allodynia in each group is reported, and an increased number of responses was associated with the development of at-level mechanical allodynia. Below-level mechanical allodynia was determined by quantifying the pain threshold of the hindpaws. Animals were placed in stance on a raised grid, allowing von Frey filaments to be applied to the plantar surface of the hindpaw. Increasing monofilaments were used (2, 4, 8, 10, 16, 21, and 26 g) until the animal displayed an adverse response (as described above). The weight of the von Frey filament that elicited the response was recorded as the pain threshold value, with lower threshold values indicating increased sensitivity to mechanical stimuli (and perhaps the development of mechanical allodynia). Finally, below-level thermal allodynia was assessed using the tail flick method. A 50°C thermal stimulus was applied to the distal portion of the animals' tail by a Tail Flick Analgesia Meter (IITC Inc. Life Science, Woodland Hills, California, USA), and the time for the animal to remove its tail from the stimulus was recorded. The latency time is graphed for each treatment group, and decreased latency times were associated with the development of thermal allodynia.

Electrophysiology

Motor Evoked Potentials. Motor evoked potential recordings (MEPs): In addition to the behavioural assessements, MEPs were recorded *in vivo* to assess the physiological integrity of spinal cord. This approach has been extensively used in our laboratory in rodent models of SCI. *In vivo* recordings of motor evoked potentials were recorded from the each of the treatment and control groups at 8 weeks post-injury (n = 6/group). For MEPs, rats were under light isoflurane anaesthesia (<1%), and recordings were obtained from hindlimb biceps femoris muscle. Stainless steel subdermal needle electrodes were inserted into the muscle. Recordings were acquired using Keypoint Portable (Dantec Biomed, Denmark). A reference electrode was placed under the skin between the recording and stimulating electrodes. Stimulation was applied to the midline of the cervical spinal cord using a silver ball electrode (0.13 Hz; 0.1 ms; 2 mA; 200 sweeps). The interlaminar ligaments were removed and a small amount of bone was removed from the vertebra (not a full laminectomy, just enough to create a space for the electrode to reach the cervical cord). The amplitude was determined by the difference between the positive peak and negative peak. Latency was calculated as the time from the start of the stimulus artifact to the first prominent peak. For individual rats, the average of peak amplitude and latency was averaged from 200 sweeps and analyses were undertaken by ANOVA.

H-Reflex. The Hoffmann reflex is one of the most studied reflexes in humans and is the electrical analogue of the monosynaptic stretch reflex. The H-reflex is evoked is evoked by low-intensity electrical stimulation of the afferent nerve, rather than a mechanical stretch of the muscle spindle, that results in monosynaptic excitation of alpha-motorneurons. H-reflex can be used as a tool (in combination with other outcome measures) to examine spasticity and short- and long-term plasticity. Recording electrodes were placed two centimeters apart in the mid-calf region and the posterior tibial nerve was stimulated in the popliteal fossa using a 0.1 ms duration square wave pulse at a frequency of 1 Hz. The rats were tested for maximal plantar H-reflex/maximal plantar M-response (H/M) ratios to determine the excitability of the reflex. The recordings were filtered between 10–10000 Hz.

Statistical Analysis

Data were analyzed with SigmaPlot software (Systat Software Inc., San Jose, California, USA). For data that investigated the percentage of cells, the data were subject to an arcsine transformation prior to statistical analysis to attain a more normal distribution. For comparison of groups sampled at various distances from the injury site (TUNEL, RECA-1, NeuN), a two-way analysis of variance (ANOVA) with repeated measures was used, followed by the post-hoc Holm-Sidak test. For comparisons of multiple groups at a single time point (Western blotting, BBB, Catwalk, Electrophysiology), a one-way ANOVA was performed, followed by the post-hoc Holm-Sidak test.

The Holm-Sidak post-hoc was used, as it is recommended as the best multiple comparisons test following an ANOVA [20,21]. The Holm-Sidak test is more sensitive and powerful compared to Bonferroni or Tukey post-hoc tests, therefore it is more likely to detect all significant results and increases the probability of <u>not</u> committing type II errors (reduces the chance of rejecting something that is true).

In all figures, the mean value ± SEM are used to describe the results. Statistical significance was accepted for p values of <0.05.

Results

AdV-ZFP-VEGF Delivery into the Injured Spinal Cord

To evaluate the transduction efficiency of the adenoviral constructs *in vivo*, AdV-eGFP was injected into animals at 24 hours post-SCI. The AdV-eGFP fluorescent signal was detected in both the white and grey matter of the injured spinal cord five days after SCI (Figure 1A). Figures 1B and 1C demonstrate eGFP expression in neurons, astrocytes, endothelial cells and oligodendrocytes, indicating successful adenoviral transduction into each cell type. Further quantification of co-labelled cells showed that AdV vector non-preferentially transduces all cell types (Neurons – 30.0%±3.6%, Oligodendrocytes – 26.9%±4.2%, Astrocytes – 21.4%±2.9%, Endothelial cells – 17.2%±3.3%). Since the AdV-ZFP-VEGF construct contains the p65 subunit of the human NFκB transcription factor as the activation domain [12], we were able to confirm delivery of AdV-ZFP-VEGF by immunoblotting using an NFκB p65 antibody to detect the presence of the transcription factor (Figure 1D). As a positive control, HEK293 cells were transduced with ZFP-VEGF and cell lysates were processed for immunoblotting using the same NFκB p65 antibody (data not shown). These results demonstrate the successful delivery of a localized gene therapy to the injured spinal cord.

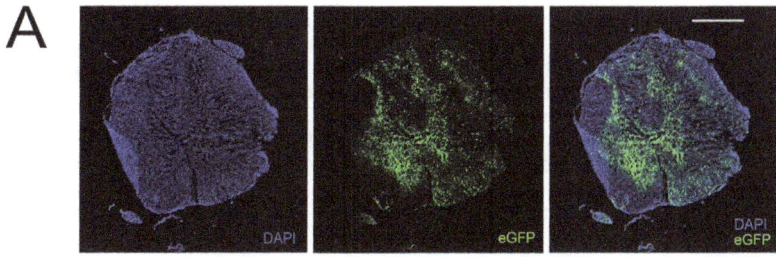

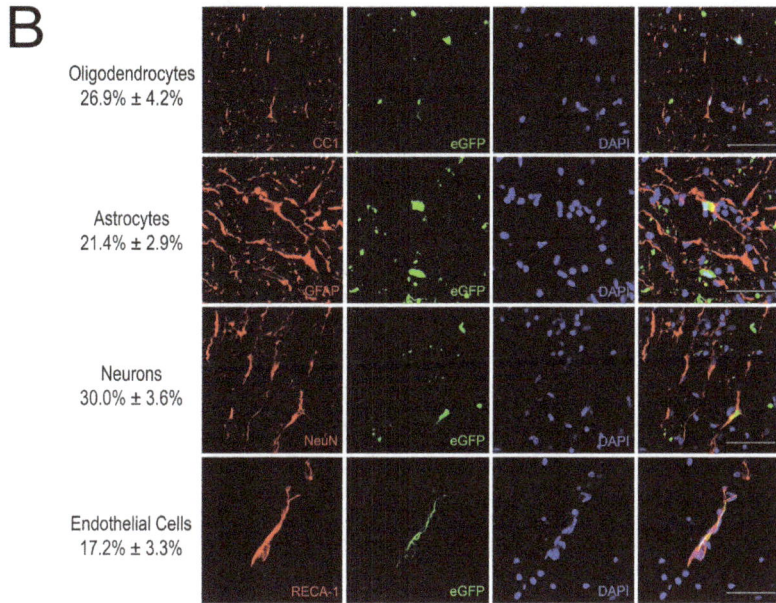

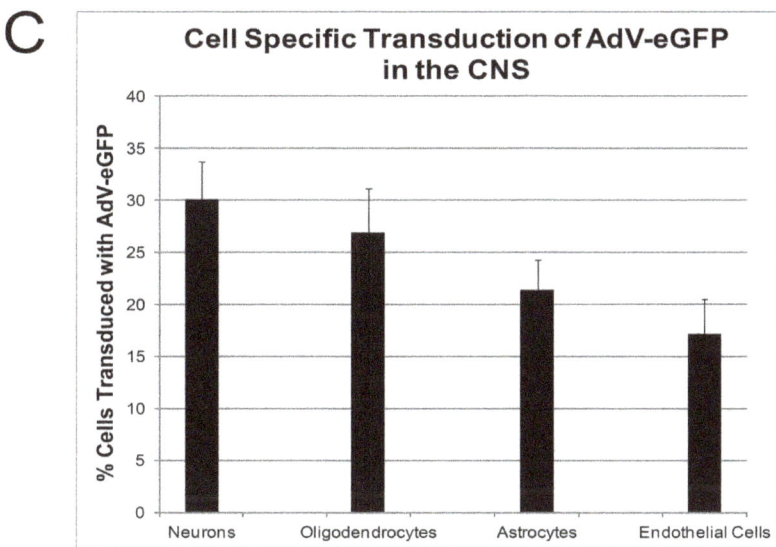

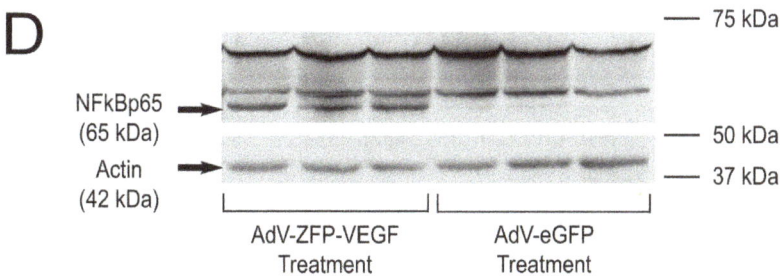

Figure 1. Transduction of AdV-eGFP/AdV-ZFP-VEGF into the spinal cord. (A) Photomicrographs showing a transverse section of rat spinal cord obtained adjacent to the injury site 10 days after spinal cord injury and AdV-eGFP injection. eGFP signal was detected in both the gray matter and white matter. (B) High-power (63X) confocal images show that the AdV-eGFP vector (green) transfected neurons (NeuN), astrocytes (GFAP), oligodendrocytes (CC1) and endothelial cells (RECA-1). Cells have been counter-stained with DAPI (blue) as nuclear marker. (C) Bar graph displays quantification of transduced cell types ± SEM, as identified by the cell-specific markers NeuN, GFAP, RECA-1 and CC1. (D) Evaluation of AdV-ZFP-VEGF gene transfer. Western blot showed that the NFκB p65 rabbit polyclonal antibody recognizes the p65 activation domain in the AdV-ZFP-VEGF treated animals. The higher molecular weight bands are endogenous NFκBp65 fragments, which are also recognized by the antibody; however, these bands are present in both the control and treatment groups. The lower band (arrow) corresponds to the AdV-ZFP-VEGF and was only present in the treated animals. Lower panel shows actin expression as a protein control. Scale bar: 1000 μm for A; 100 μm for B.

VEGF mRNA and protein expression is increased following 24 hour delayed AdV-ZFP-VEGF administration

Animals were sacrificed 5 days post-SCI and mRNA expression levels of three predominant VEGF isoforms found in the CNS – $VEGF_{120}$, $VEGF_{164}$ and $VEGF_{188}$ – were measured by quantitative real-time PCR (qRT-PCR). Figure 2A shows that 24 hour delayed administration of AdV-ZFP-VEGF resulted in significant increases in VEGF mRNA of isoforms 120 ($p < 0.001$), 164 ($p < 0.001$), but not isoform 188, when compared with AdV-eGFP control animals and injured control animals ($n = 4$/sham and injured control; $n = 5$/AdV-ZFP-VEGF and AdV-eGFP). VEGF-A protein expression was assessed at 10 days following SCI by Western blot using anti-VEGF antibodies, which detect the 42 kDa and 21 kDa bands and are recommended for the detection of the 189, 165 and 121 amino acid splice variants of VEGF. In Figures 2B and 3C, we show that the 42 kDa VEGF-dimer protein was significantly increased by approximately 2.5-fold in AdV-ZFP-VEGF treated animals versus AdV-eGFP and injured control groups ($p < 0.02$), and by approximately 1.8-fold in AdV-ZFP-VEGF treated animals compared to sham animals ($p < 0.05$) ($n = 4$/sham, injured control and AdV-eGFP, $n = 5$/AdV-ZFP-VEGF group). Previous studies using AdV-ZFP-VEGF have shown increases in VEGF mRNA and protein levels [11,22–24]. Consistent with these studies, our results confirm that AdV-ZFP-VEGF increases both mRNA and protein levels of VEGF in the spinal cord following 24 hour delayed administration.

Apoptosis is reduced in animals treated with AdV-ZFP-VEGF 24 hours post-SCI

Our laboratory has previously shown that apoptotic cell death occurs as early as 6 hours following SCI and persists until 14 days post injury [25]. To assess the effects of AdV-ZFP-VEGF treatment on apoptotic cell death, *in situ* terminal-deoxy-transferase mediated dUTP nick end-labeling (TUNEL) staining was performed 5 days after injury (Figure 3). TUNEL-positive cells were found evenly distributed through the gray and white matter in the injured spinal cord, with the greatest apoptosis observed near the injury epicenter. TUNEL-stained nuclei were counted at the injury epicenter, and at 1, 2, and 3 mm from the injury epicenter both rostral and caudal to the lesion site, but rostral and caudal values were pooled. Figure 3B shows that AdV-ZFP-VEGF treatment was associated with an overall significant reduction in the number of TUNEL-positive cells rostral and caudal from the injury epicenter, when conducting a two-way ANOVA for distance from the injury epicenter and treatment group (Two-way ANOVA, Holm-Sidak post-hoc; $p < 0.01$; $n = 4$/sham and injured control groups, $n = 5$/AdV-eGFP and AdV-ZFP-VEGF groups).

24 hour delayed AdV-ZFP-VEGF administration provides neuroprotection

Neurofilament protein (NF200), a hallmark protein lost following neurodegeneration, was quantified in the injured region of the cord to assess the neuroprotective effects of AdV-ZFP-VEGF after SCI. Previous research from our laboratory indicated a significant loss of NF200 after SCI [26,27]. As shown in Figure 4, the amount of NF200 protein was significantly increased by approximately 2-fold at 10 days following SCI in animals treated with AdV-ZFP-VEGF versus control animals (Figure 4A and 4B) ($p < 0.05$).

To further assess the neuroprotective effects of AdV-ZFP-VEGF following SCI, we quantified spared neurons 5 days after injury. NeuN, which recognizes neuronal cell bodies, was used to identify neurons in cross-sections of spinal cord tissue. Figures 4C and 4D demonstrate that AdV-ZFP-VEGF treatment results in a significant sparing of neurons spanning the lesion site, when compared to injured control and AdV-eGFP animals (Two-way ANOVA comparing AdV-ZFP-VEGF with other injured animals across all distances from the epicenter, Holm-Sidak post-hoc; $p < 0.02$). AdV-eGFP animals show a significant decrease in NeuN counts compared to injured control animals ($p < 0.01$), and the additional loss of cells is likely attributed to the physical damage caused by the intraspinal injections.

24 hour delayed AdV-ZFP-VEGF administration results in an increased number of vessels and promotes angiogenesis

In order to quantify the vascular response to ZFP-VEGF, we conducted immunostaining with RECA-1, a monoclonal antibody specific for endothelial cells, at 10 days following SCI. The severity of the compression injury resulted in considerable disruption to the spinal cord vasculature at the injury epicentre, thus we were unable to quantify the epicenter accurately. Therefore, we assessed spinal cord tissue sections at 2 mm and 4 mm – both caudal and rostral – from the lesion epicenter (Figure 5A). Figures 5B and 5C show that AdV-ZFP-VEGF administration markedly increases the number of RECA-1-positive vessels both rostral and caudal, when compared to control animals ($p < 0.01$). These results are consistent with previous findings from our laboratory in studies administering AdV-ZFP-VEGF immediately following injury [11].

To investigate some of the potential mechanisms of AdV-ZFP-VEGF action, we examined the effects of 24 hour delayed AdV-ZFP-VEGF administration on endothelial cell proliferation. One of the most characterized roles of VEGF is promoting angiogenesis in both embryonic development and wound healing [28], therefore we aimed to study if AdV-ZFP-VEGF administration would further promote angiogenesis. Tissues co-labeled with RECA-1 and Ki67 at 5 days following SCI indicated that AdV-ZFP-VEGF administration increased angiogenesis by approximately 10% ($p < 0.001$) (Figure 5D and 5E). These results indicate that AdV-ZFP-VEGF administration, which results in an increase in VEGF expression, ultimately promotes angiogenic pathways following SCI. Other research has suggested that VEGF administration results in angiogenesis; however, these studies simply show an increase in the number of vessels present. Here, we demonstrate that VEGF increases endothelial cell proliferation *in*

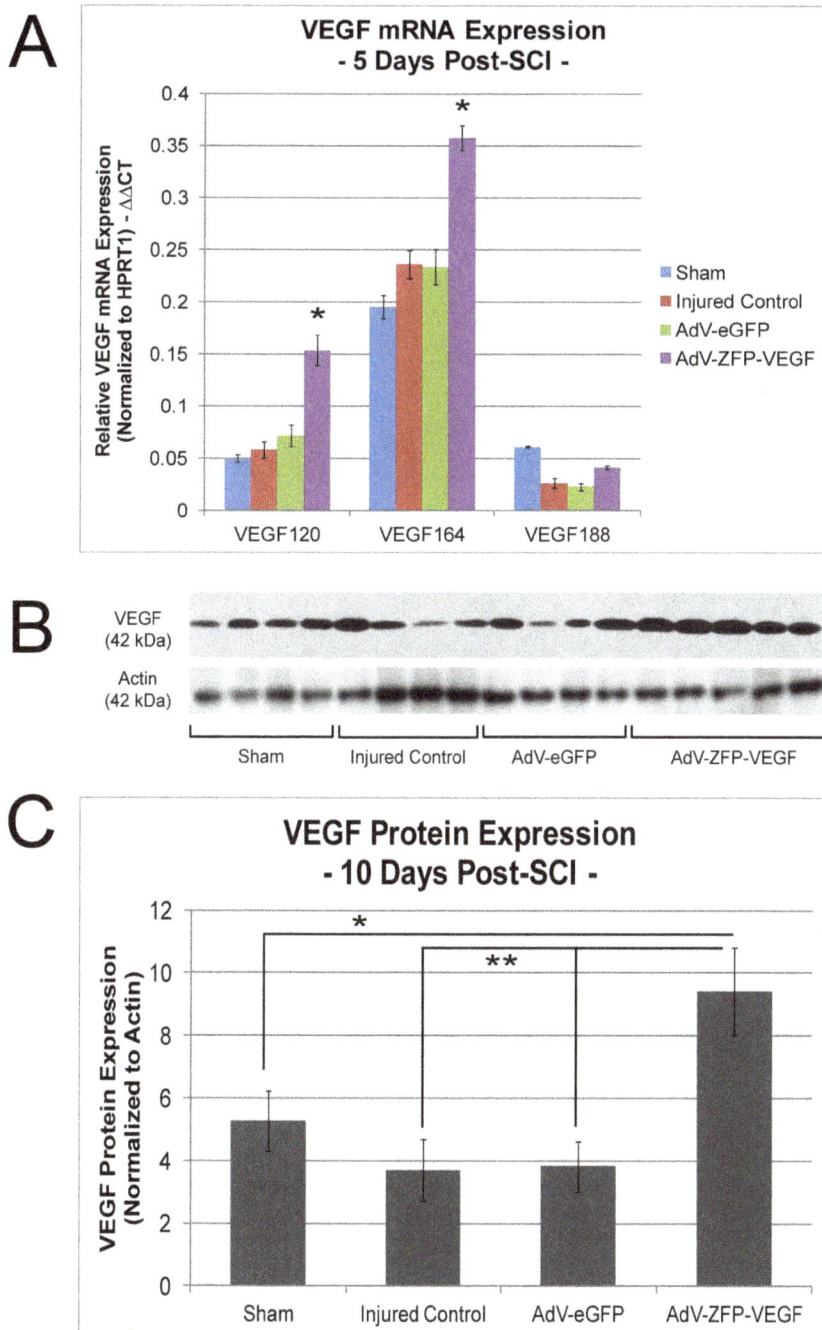

Figure 2. AdV-ZFP-VEGF increases VEGF mRNA and protein. (A) VEGF mRNA levels encoding for $VEGF_{120}$, $VEGF_{164}$ and $VEGF_{188}$ isoforms were measured by quantitative real-time PCR at 5 days post-SCI. The bar graph illustrates that administration of ZFP-VEGF resulted in an increase of VEGF mRNA compared with AdV-eGFP and SCI injured control groups. Relative mRNA levels are expressed as the mean $\pm$ SEM, n = 4/sham and injured control groups, n = 5/AdV-eGFP and AdV-ZFP-VEGF groups. One-way ANOVA (Holm-Sidak post-hoc) was completed individually for each isoform **$p < 0.001$, *$p < 0.01$. (B) Western blot showing administration of AdV-ZFP-VEGF resulted in increased VEGF-A protein levels at 10 days post-SCI, and (C) Quantification shows a significant increase in VEGF-A 42 kD protein in AdV-ZFP-VEGF treated animals compared with control groups. Optical density (OD) of VEGF-A was normalized to actin. Data are presented as mean $\pm$ SEM, n = 4/sham, injured control and AdV-eGFP treated groups and n = 5/AdV-ZFP-VEGF treated group. One-way ANOVA (Holm-Sidak post-hoc) **$p < 0.02$, *$p < 0.05$.

vivo following SCI, and to our knowledge, this is the first study to use a delayed VEGF therapy and demonstrate an increase in vessels, that is likely attributable to angiogenesis.

AdV-ZFP-VEGF results in functional improvement

At the cellular/molecular level, we have observed that AdV-ZFP-VEGF results in beneficial effects. However, in order to assess the viability of any therapy, these effects must be translated into functional gains. In our study, we assessed hindlimb function using

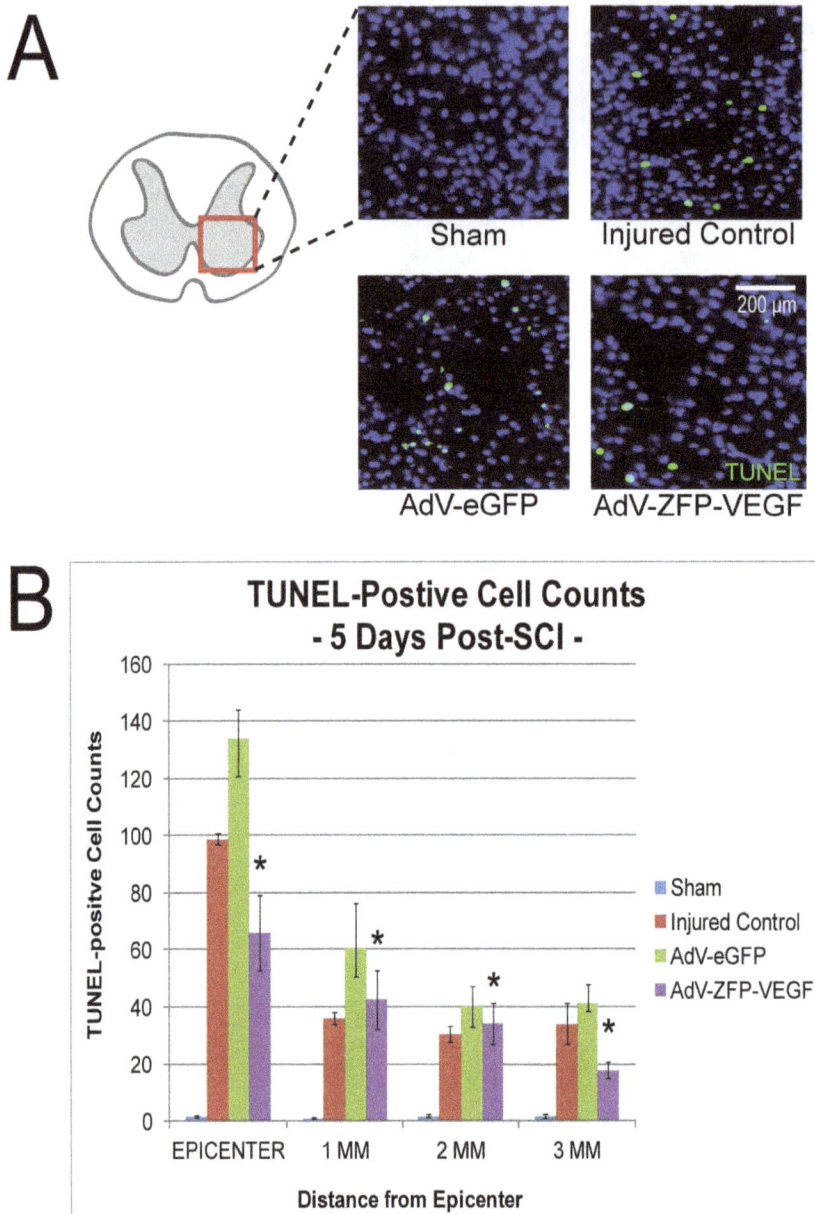

Figure 3. AdV-ZFP-VEGF administration reduces apoptosis after SCI. (A) Representative sections taken 2 mm rostral to the epicenter from animals sacrificed at 5 days post-SCI and tissue processed with TUNEL staining (green); scale 200 μm. An overall reduction of TUNEL-positive cells was observed in the AdV-ZFP-VEGF treated group. Cells have been counter-stained with DAPI (blue) as nuclear marker (B) Bar graph shows quantification of the TUNEL-positive cell counts at 5 days after SCI (pooled values from rostral and caudal counts). There was a significant decrease in TUNEL-positive cells in the AdV-ZFP-VEGF treatment group versus all other injured groups (when compared against other groups and all distances). Values are mean ± SEM, n = 4/sham and injured control groups, n = 5/AdV-eGFP and AdV-ZFP-VEGF groups. Two-way ANOVA (Holm-Sidak post-hoc), *$p < 0.01$.

open-field BBB scoring and Catwalk, between 1-8 weeks following SCI. Analysis of Catwalk data showed that animals treated with AdV-ZFP-VEGF had significantly improved hindlimb weight support ($p < 0.05$) (Figure 6), hindlimb swing speed ($p < 0.02$) (Figure 7), and forelimb stride length ($p < 0.02$) (Figure 7) compared to all other injured control groups. Enhancements in hindlimb weight support and overall gait (hindlimb swing speed, and forelimb stride length) are important changes that may reflect an improved quality of life of individuals suffering with SCI.

AdV-ZFP-VEGF does not result in improved BBB scores

AdV-ZFP-VEGF treated animals did not show improved BBB scores, compared in injured control animals, although they did perform better than AdV-eGFP injected animals ($p < 0.01$) (Figure 8). Significant recovery shown by CatWalk (animals analyzed were a sub-set of animals that achieved >8 for BBB scoring) do not correspond with significantly improved BBB scores between injured control and AdV-ZFP-VEGF animals at 8 weeks post-injury. In the discussion we will provide a more detailed explanation that may validate these findings; however, the treated and AdV-eGFP treated animals immunostained with NeuN at 5 days after SCI; scale 200 μm. A greater number of NeuN-positive cells were observed in animals treated with AdV-ZFP-VEGF. (D) Bar graph shows quantification of the NeuN-positive cell counts at 5 days after SCI. There was a significant preservation of neurons overall in the AdV-ZFP-VEGF group compared to all the other injured groups (two-way ANOVA comparing distance from the epicenter and treatment group). Bar graph shows mean OD values ± SEM. Two-way ANOVA (Holm-Sidak post-hoc), *p<0.02. n = 5/sham, n = 4/injured control, AdV-eGFP and AdV-ZFP-VEGF groups.

discrepancy between BBB and CatWalk data may be due to the more qualitative nature of the BBB, as opposed to the quantitative gait analysis software.

Delayed AdV-ZFP-VEGF administration does not improve motor evoked potentials or H-reflex following SCI

To further examine the functional changes we performed *in vivo* electrophysiology on the hindlimbs of animals at 8 weeks post-SCI. Our data indicate that although AdV-ZFP-VEGF treated animals show an improved gait via CatWalk™ analysis, we did not observe any significant improvements in axonal conduction in the hindlimbs, as assessed by motor evoked potential recordings (Figure 9A and 9B). We also examined the H-reflex (H/M ratios) following SCI as a measure of spasticity, and observed no electrophysiological differences between groups (Figure 9B).

AdV-ZFP-VEGF administration significantly reduces allodynia

A devastating post-injury condition is neuropathic pain, which affects a significant portion of SCI patients [29,30]. In this study we aimed to investigate the development of thermal and mechanical allodynia in AdV-ZFP-VEGF treated animals: hopeful that we would observe no increases in pain unlike the recent report by Nesic *et al.* [31]. Animals were tested for pain at 4 and 8 weeks following SCI, and here we observe that animals receiving AdV-ZFP-VEGF gene therapy have a significant reduction in allodynia, for both at-level and below-level pain, at 8 weeks post-injury (Figure 10). Testing with calibrated von Frey filaments around the lesion site (on the dorsal skin) showed AdV-ZFP-VEGF animals to have a significant reduction in at-level mechanical allodynia (Figure 10A; p<0.005). An increasing application of von Frey filaments to the plantar surface of the hindlimbs demonstrated a marked reduction in below-level alloydnia (Figure 10B), compared to injured control (p<0.05) and AdV-eGFP treated animals (p< 0.005). Furthermore, we examined below-level thermal allodynia (Figure 10C), and observed a significant increase in pain tolerance (increased response time) in animals receiving AdV-ZFP-VEGF (p<0.05).

AdV-ZFP-VEGF treatment results in spared grey matter, but not white matter tissue at 8 weeks post-SCI

Eight weeks after SCI, spinal cord cross-sections were stained serially with LFB-HE. Measurements of tissue sparing were calculated using StereoInvestigator software, and are expressed as the average cross-section area. Spinal cords from AdV-ZFP-VEGF treated rats did not show evidence of white matter tissue sparing compared to control injured animals (Figure 11A); however, AdV-ZFP-VEGF administration exhibited an overall increase in residual grey matter in (sections spanning 2 mm rostral and 2 mm caudal to the injury epicenter) when compared to tissue sections from AdV-GFP and injured control rats (Figure 11B; p<0.001). The grey matter differences observed in the AdV-ZFP-VEGF group are most

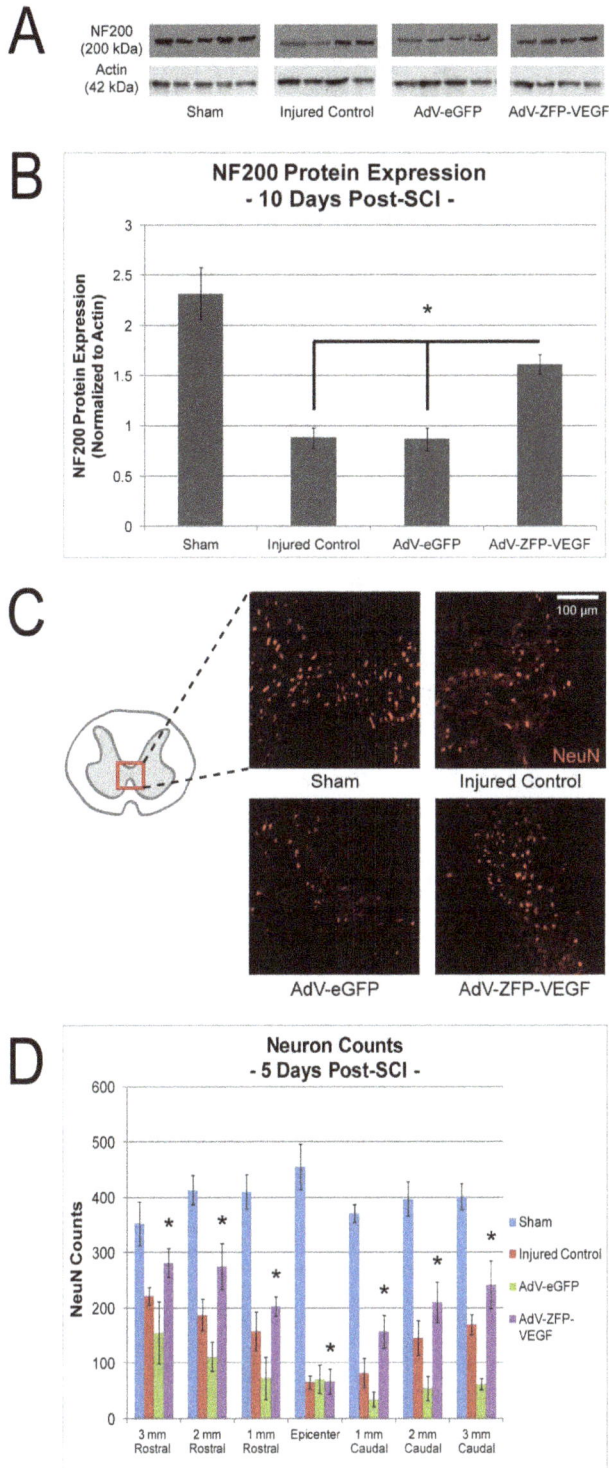

Figure 4. AdV-ZFP-VEGF administration attenuated axonal degradation and increased neuron sparing. (A) Western blot indicates that administration of AdV-ZFP-VEGF resulted in a significant attenuation of NF200 degradation 10 days after injury. Lower panel shows actin protein control. (B) Relative OD value of controls versus AdV-ZFP-VEGF treated animals. Significant NF200 sparing was observed in AdV-ZFP-VEGF-treated animals compared to control groups at 10 days after injury, although all injured groups showed significant NF200 loss following SCI. Optical density of NF200 was normalized to actin. One-way ANOVA (Holm-Sidak post-hoc), *p<0.05. (C) Representative sections taken 2 mm rostral to the epicenter from AdV-ZFP-VEGF

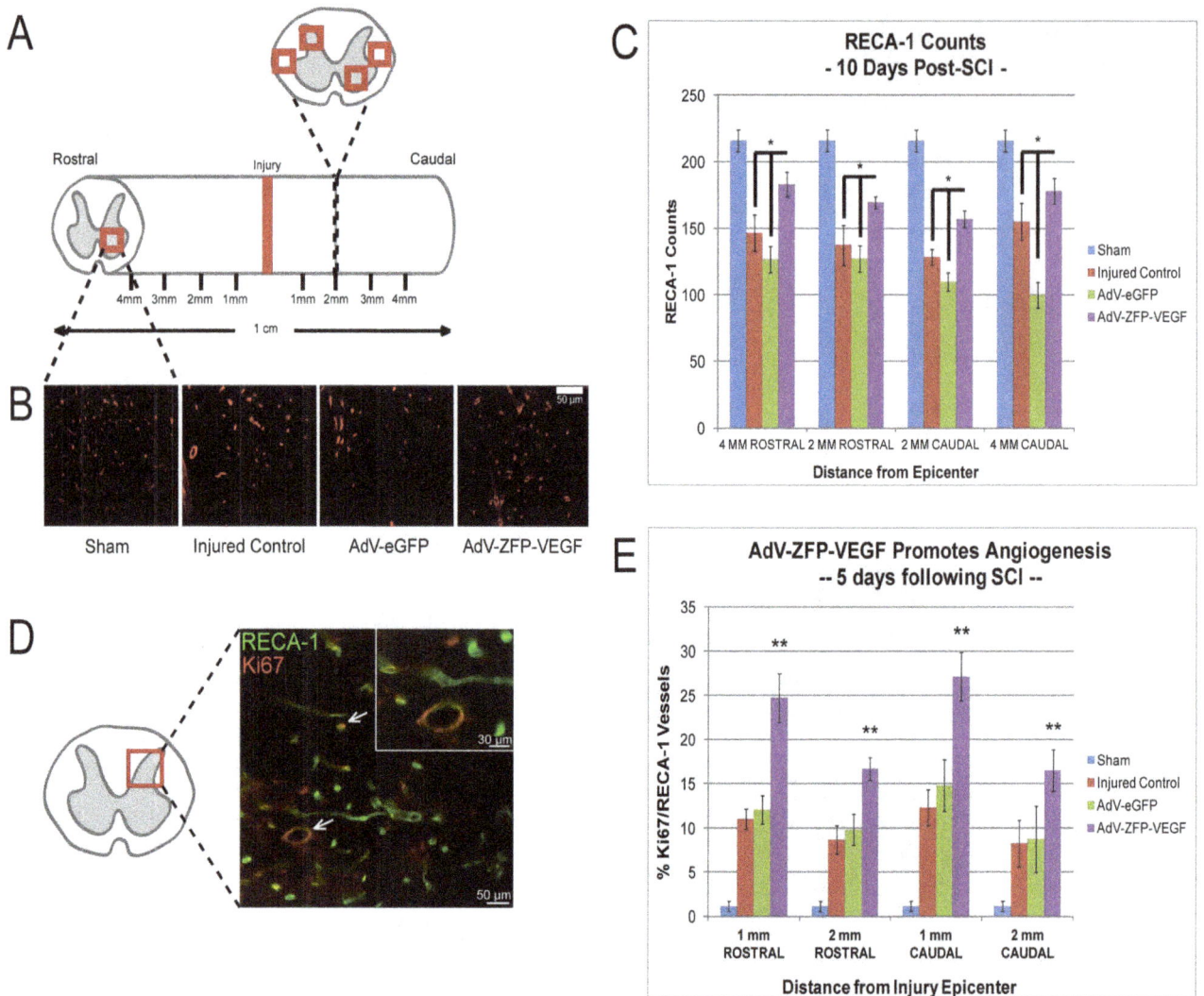

Figure 5. AdV-ZFP-VEGF results in increased vessel counts and angiogenesis. (A) Left panel: Illustration of the area of spinal cord areas used for RECA-1 counting (2 grey matter areas, 2 white matter areas). (B) Representative sections taken 2 mm rostral to the epicenter from a AdV-ZFP-VEGF treated and AdV-eGFP control animal respectively immunostained with RECA-1 at 10 days after SCI; scale 100 μm. An increased number of vessels were observed in the AdV-ZFP-VEGF treated group. (C) Bar graph illustrating the RECA-1 positive cell counts 10 days after SCI. AdV-ZFP-VEGF administration resulted in a significant increase in vascular counts (2 mm and 4 mm away from the epicenter) as compared with the control group. (D) Representative confocal image from an ADV-ZFP-VEGF treated animal at 5 days post-injury. Image was taken at 2 mm rostral from the epicenter, and shows double-labeled cells. Cells were stained for endothelial cells (RECA-1, green) and proliferation (Ki67, red). Scale bar =50 μm (30 μm for magnified panel). (E) Angiogenesis was assessed by quantifying Ki67/RECA-1 co-labeled vessels. Data is presented at the percentage of RECA-1+ vessels that were also Ki67+, with an overall average increase of 10% vascular proliferation observed in the animals receiving AdV-ZFP-VEGF administration. All data are presented as mean ± SEM, and was analyzed by Two-way ANOVA (Holm-Sidak post-hoc). Angiogenesis data were analyzed by performing an arcsine transformation of the values, prior to Two-way ANOVA and post-hoc testing. *$p < 0.01$, **$p < 0.001$. n = 4/sham and injured control groups, n = 5/AdV-eGFP and AdV-ZFP-VEGF groups.

notable in the peri-lesional area (1–2 mm rostral caudal to the epicenter). The epicenter of all injured and treated groups showed significant histological damage, and no differences were observed in tissue sparing at the lesion epicenter between the injured groups. Animals treated with AdV-eGFP show significantly reduced grey matter and white matter compared to injured control and AdV-ZFP-VEGF treated groups. As previously mentioned, we attribute the additional damage to the spinal cord in the AdV-eGFP group to the invasive delivery method of the treatment (intraspinal injections).

Discussion

We have shown that AdV-ZFP-VEGF administration can be delayed 24 hours following spinal cord injury, and still provide beneficial effects. To date, we are the first to use AdV-ZFP-VEGF in a delayed fashion, and one of few studies that have used any form of VEGF therapy at a delayed point post-injury [32,33]. In the current research, we chose to investigate the efficacy of 24 hour delayed AdV-ZFP-VEGF administration, which presents a clinically relevant therapeutic window. This form of gene therapy mimics physiological VEGF production, which should result in the production of all VEGF isoforms in the injured spinal

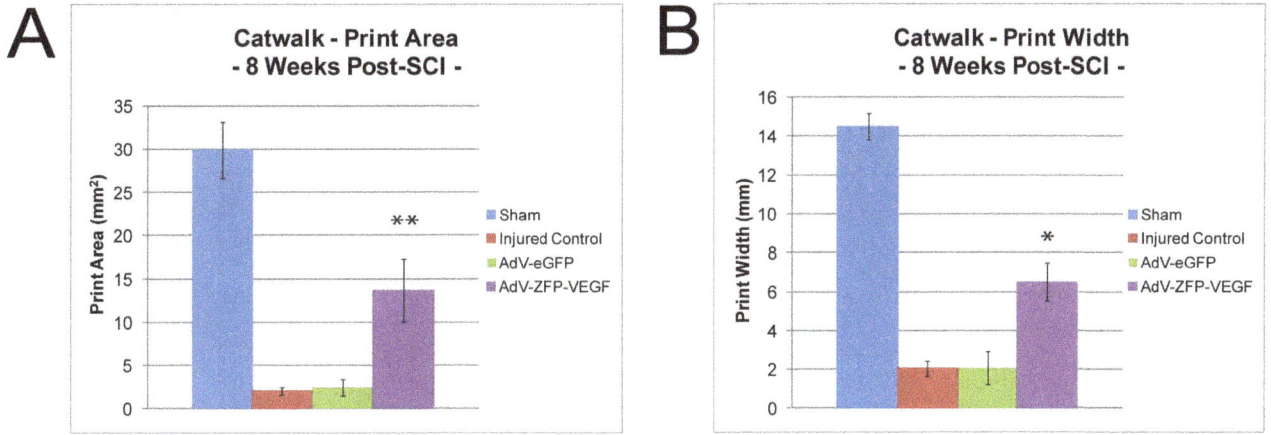

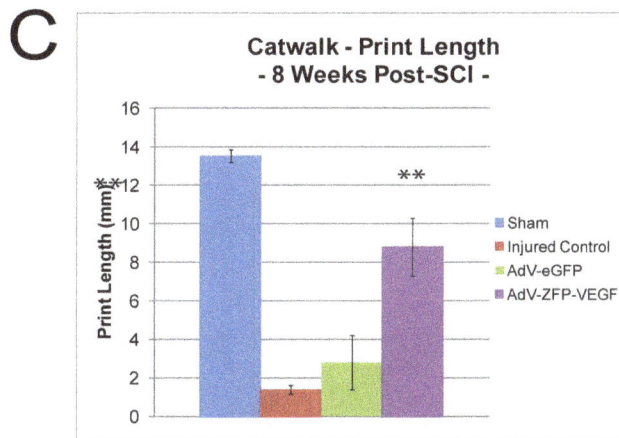

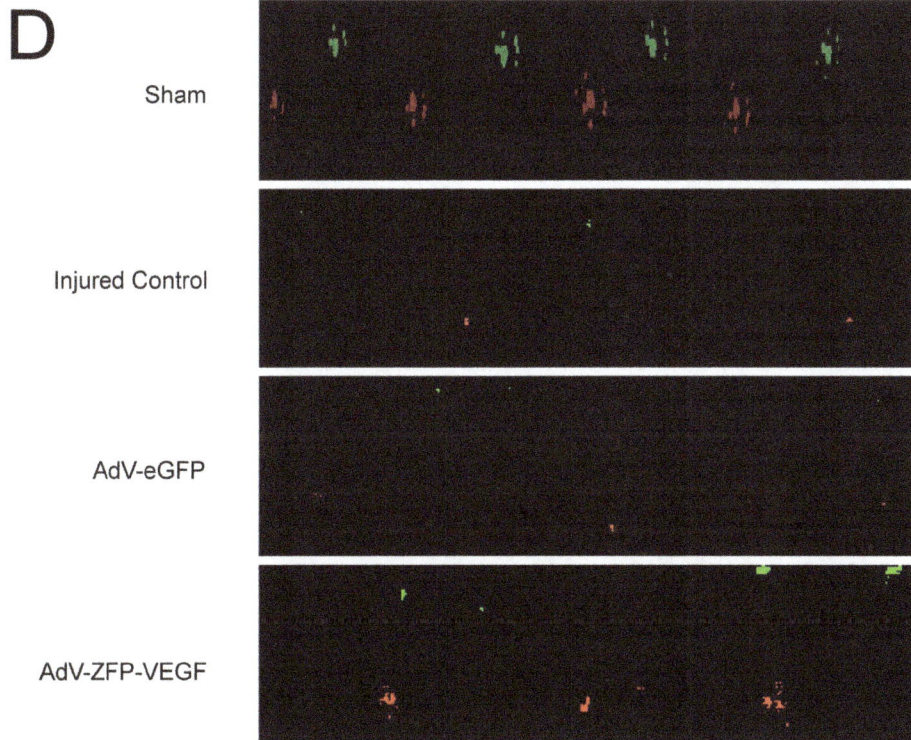

Figure 6. AdV-ZFP-VEGF improves hindlimb weight support. Catwalk gait analysis was used to assess hindlimb weight support. A sub-set of animals (with BBB scores >9) were assessed every week between 4–8 weeks, and each animal performed a standardized Catwalk run. A blinded observer analyzed the data. (A) Paw area: the maximal area of the paw print in contact with the detection surface of the CatWalk (expressed in mm^2), (B) Paw width: the maximal distance spanning the medial and lateral contact points of the paw (expressed in mm), and (C) Paw length: the maximal distance spanning the cranial and caudal contact points of the paw (expressed in mm). (D) Representative images of CatWalk forelimb (green) and hindlimb (red) prints, which were used to quantify the data presented in Figure 6 and Figure 7. Data presented is the mean ± SEM, n = 5/group, at 8 weeks following SCI. One-way ANOVA (Holm-Sidak post-hoc). *p<0.05, **p<0.005.

cord: a necessary component for proper and functional angiogenesis. We observed significant improvements at the cellular and molecular levels, including an increased number of vessels, increased angiogenesis, reduced apoptosis and increased neurons. Additionally, we observed improved functional benefits in animals treated with AdV-ZFP-VEGF, including increased hindlimb weight support and significant reductions in allodynia. Collectively, the data suggest that: (i) administration of AdV-ZFP-VEGF results in an increase in VEGF, which may elicit effects through cell survival and angiogenic mechanisms (ii) AdV-ZFP-VEGF has

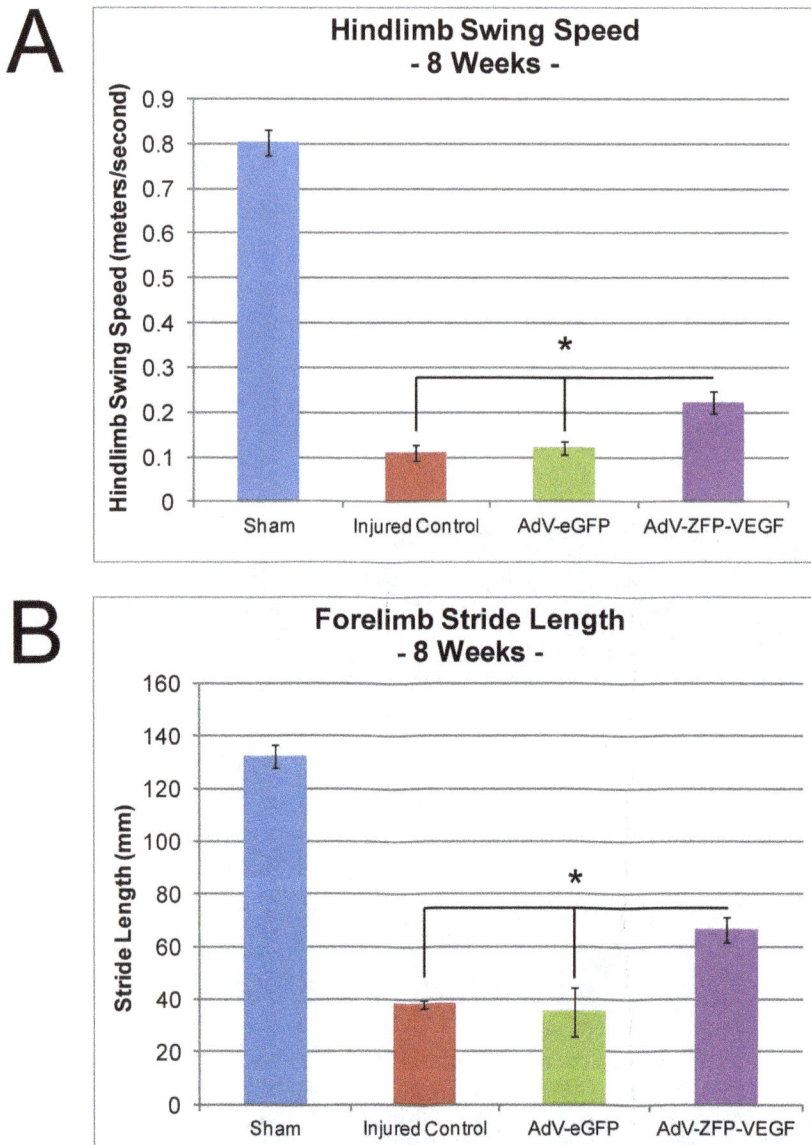

Figure 7. Forelimb and Hindlimb locomotion is improved by AdV-ZFP-VEGF administration. (A) Catwalk gait analysis was used to assess hindlimb swing speed. Animals were assessed every week between 4–8 weeks, and each animal performed a standardized Catwalk run. A blinded observer analyzed the data. Data presented is the mean ± SEM, n = 5/group, at 8 weeks following SCI. One-way ANOVA (Holm-Sidak post-hoc). *p< 0.02. (B) Catwalk gait analysis was used to assess forelimb stride length. Animals were assessed every week between 4–8 weeks, and each animal performed a standardized Catwalk run. A blinded observer analyzed the data. Data presented is the mean ± SEM, n = 5/group, at 8 weeks following SCI. One-way ANOVA (Holm-Sidak post-hoc). *p<0.02.

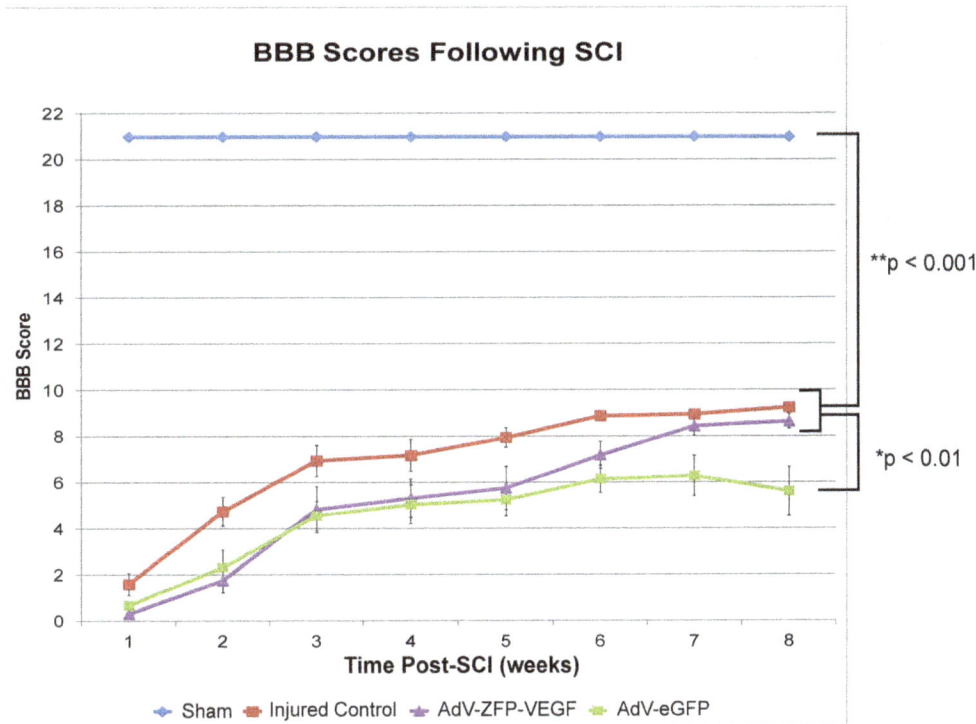

Figure 8. AdV-ZFP-VEGF does not improve open-field walking (BBB) scores following SCI. Open-field locomotion was assessed using the 21-point BBB scale. Animals were assessed weekly for 8 weeks following injury by blinded observers (n = 8/sham and AdV-ZFP-VEGF groups; n = 10/ injured control and AdV-eGFP groups). The left and right limbs were scored individually, but the data presented is the average between left and right hindlimb recovery.

a therapeutic time window following SCI which extends at least until 24 hours following injury, (iii) repairing vascular damage following neurotrauma is an important therapeutic target.

Previously, our lab has shown that immediate administration of AdV-ZFP-VEGF following SCI resulted in neuroprotection, increased vascular counts and improved functional recovery [11]. These promising results encouraged us to investigate a more feasible time-window for clinical intervention: 24 hours post-injury administration of AdV-ZFP-VEGF. Moreover, administration 24 hours following injury aimed to target a few important pathophysiological events post-SCI, particularly vascular damage and apoptosis. In a model of spinal cord contusion, Ling and Liu showed that TUNEL-positive cells are maximally observed at 48 hours following injury in both the grey and white matter [34]. Similarly, Crowe *et al.* demonstrated that maximal apoptosis is observed at 48 hours following contusion injury, with apoptosis identified between 6 hours and 3 weeks [35]. Liu *et al.* showed that following contusion injury TUNEL-positive neurons were observed between 4–24 hours, whereas TUNEL-positive glia were seen between 4 hours and 14 days with maximal numbers observed at 24 hours, although another peak of TUNEL-positive glia were observed at 7 days post-injury [36]. With respect to vascular targets, research suggests that angiogenic therapies should be administered to target endogenous vascular repair, which occurs between 3 and 7 days following injury [6,37]. Therefore, by administrating AdV-ZFP-VEGF 24 hours following injury, we aimed to target and reduce apoptosis as well as enhance vascular regeneration. Our data, showing reduced TUNEL and increased endothelial cell proliferation, suggest that AdV-ZFP-VEGF is in fact capable of both neuroprotection and angiogenesis. Although we have not investigated the detailed mechanisms or signaling

pathways of AdV-ZFP-VEGF *in vivo*, collectively our data provide strong evidence that increasing VEGF following injury may be beneficial and may stimulate cell survival and angiogenic pathways.

Vasculature is a significant target following SCI

SCI results in significant vascular damage, including disruption of spinal cord blood flow, the onset of spinal cord ischemia, hemorrhage, edema and breakdown of the blood-spinal cord barrier (BSCB). These vascular changes encompass many of the earliest pathological processes following SCI, therefore therapies aimed directly at the vascular disruption or the ensuing downstream consequences of vascular injury are highly attractive; hence, we have chosen to address this therapeutic target in our research. In theory, rapid vascular repair following injury will likely result in the most favourable outcomes. Promoting repair and regeneration of vascular structures would mediate ischemia, hemorrhage and further edema by restoring proper blood-flow and stopping leaky vessels. Moreover, restoring the proper structure and function of the BSCB would likely reduce the influx of inflammatory cells into the spinal cord, thereby reducing the damage caused by reactive microglia [38,39]. Recent reports have shown significant correlations between blood vessel density and improvements in recovery following CNS trauma [40–43]. Rescue and regeneration of the microvasculature within the epicenter and penumbra remains largely unexplored, yet may be a promising therapeutic route to facilitate tissue sparing and functional recovery following SCI. It has been shown that substantial trophic support is provided by CNS microvessels [44] and that microvessels are critical for tissue survival [45].

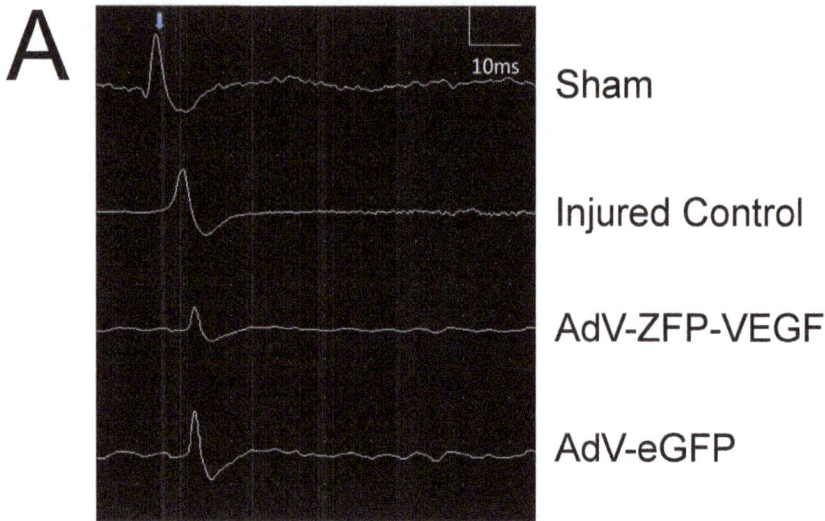

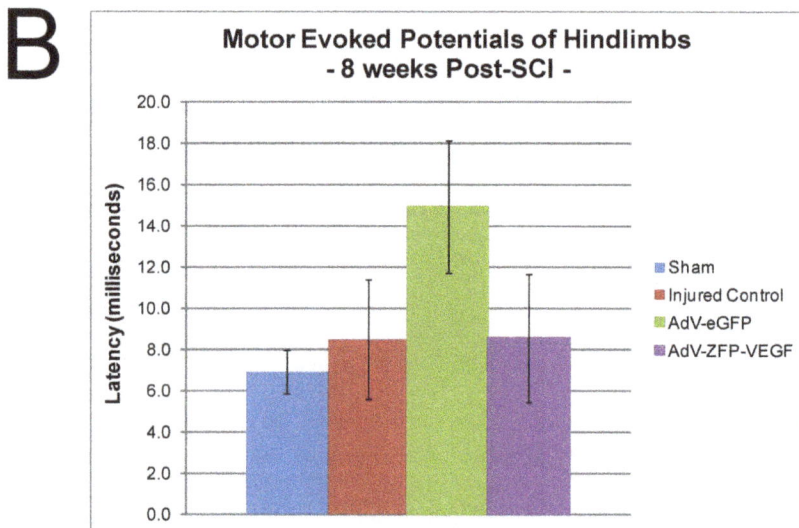

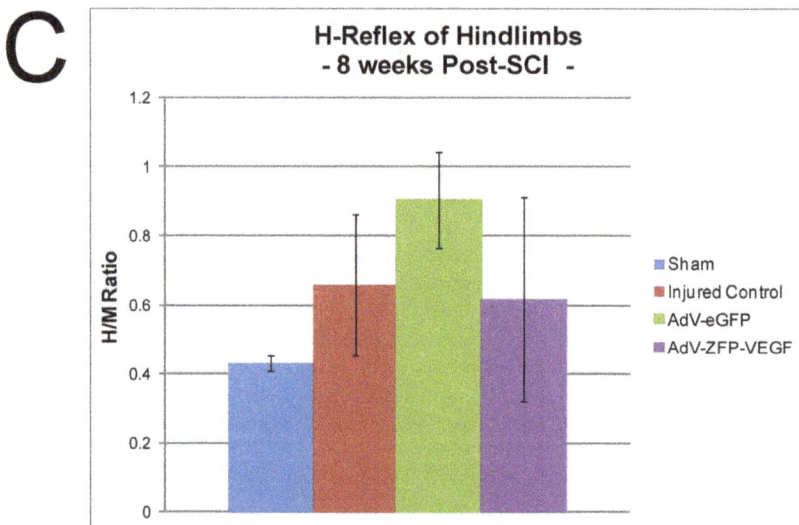

Figure 9. Electrophysiological assessment following AdV-ZFP-VEGF administration. (A) Representative tracings of MEP's recorded from the hindlimb at 8 weeks post-injury. (B) MEP quantification. Recordings were obtained from hindlimb biceps femoris. Stimulation was applied to the midline of the cervical spinal cord (0.13 Hz; 0.1 ms; 2 mA; 200 sweeps). Latency was calculated as the time from the start of the stimulus artifact to

the first prominent peak. AdV-ZFP-VEGF did not result in improved MEP's. (C) H-Reflex quantification. Recording electrodes were placed two centimeters apart in the mid-calf region and the posterior tibial nerve was stimulated in the popliteal fossa using a 0.1 ms duration square wave pulse at a frequency of 1 Hz. The rats were tested for maximal plantar H-reflex/maximal plantar M-response (H/M) ratios to determine the excitability of the reflex. AdV-ZFP-VEGF administration did not significantly alter the H/M ratio. n = 6/group.

VEGF is promising because it targets multiple cellular mechanisms

An immense number of cellular factors are involved in vascular development and repair, and in the pathological processes following SCI, therefore it is often suggested that the best therapy for SCI may involve a combinatorial approach. In the current research, VEGF was specifically selected since it has been shown to support the "neurovascular niche" and appears to play important roles in both vascular and nervous systems: bridging both endogenous systems. Expression of VEGF-R's have been observed in many cell types, including neurons, microglia/macrophages, endothelial cells, smooth muscle cells and astrocytes [46–51]. Through interactions with co-receptors, neuropilins, VEGF is able to influence the function and development of neural cells, which may be a key role for VEGF therapies following neurotrauma [52,53]. Additionally, studies have shown that regenerating axons have a tendency to grow along blood vessels, therefore promoting vascular growth following injury may provide scaffolding for regenerating axons [54,55].

Previous studies using VEGF

In previous research that has used VEGF following SCI, authors have observed varying results. Choi *et al.* used a hypoxia-inducible VEGF-A expression system to treat rats with SCI and observed neuroprotective effects and enhanced VEGF-A expression [56]. Another group used an adenovirus coding for VEGF$_{165}$, delivered via matrigel, in a partial spinal cord transection model. They observed a significant increase in vessel volume and a reduction in the retrograde degeneration of corticospinal tract axons [57]. However, Benton *et al.* [58] reported an exacerbation of lesion size and increased inflammation after the delivery of 2 μg of recombinant VEGF$_{165}$ directly into the contused spinal cord 3 days post SCI. This study highlights several factors which are likely to be critical in the successful application of VEGF-A as a therapy for SCI. The method of VEGF delivery is likely a critical factor. In our study, we injected the ZFP-VEGF adjacent to the injury epicenter as the peri-lesional ischemic penumbra is likely the zone, which would benefit the most from approaches to enhance angiogenesis. Moreover, our delivery technique, using a ZFP-VEGF gene therapy, has the ability to upregulate several isoforms of VEGF-A (specifically we observed an upregulation of the VEGF 120, 164 and 188 isoforms), mimicking endogenous expression. In contrast, most other research has focused on the delivery of a single VEGF isoforms.

Potential pitfalls of VEGF

Although VEGF has many desirable attributes for neuroprotection and vascular repair, it is important to recognize that some of these attributes have the potential to be deleterious and exacerbate damage following SCI. In development or maintenance of vascular structures, VEGF stimulates angiogenesis by signalling matrix-metalloproteinases (MMPs) to breakdown the BSCB and matrix in order to make way for new vascular sprouts. However, following injury, greater amounts of VEGF are released from surrounding cells and vascular remodelling is quickly initiated, which leads to a rapid hyperpermeability of the local vessels. This increase in permeability may contribute to an increased inflammatory response or increased edema following CNS injury. In particular, disruption of the BSCB following injury presents an entry route for inflammatory mediators to enter the CNS without resistance. A previous study reported that VEGF is able to promote monocyte migration *in vitro* and that administration of VEGF therapies may contribute to inflammatory responses following injury [59]. Although we observed no increased inflammatory response in our AdV-ZFP-VEGF animals compared to other injured control groups at 10 days following injury (data not shown), it is possible that VEGF therapies may exacerbate early inflammation.

Disadvantages of intraspinal AdV injections

Although not perfect, direct injection into the spinal cord has some advantages and has been widely used for the delivery of therapeutics and stem cells [60–62]. Firstly, this method allows specific and localized delivery of the ZFP-VEGF gene therapy. We have selected four injections sites directly into the spinal cord, at 1 mm deep into the cord. This depth was selected to administer the vascular therapy close to the highly vascularized grey matter. Injections were administered two-millimeters rostral and caudal to the injury site to target the penumbra of the injury – a site which is more likely to be rescued by a delayed therapeutic intervention compared to the injury epicenter. Additionally, direct injections result in rapid delivery of the therapy, since it is not required to migrate or circulate before reaching the target tissue. In AdV-eGFP treated groups, we observed decreased NeuN counts, increased TUNEL-positive cells, a decrease in RECA-1-positive vessels, and diminished tissue sparing compared to animals which received only a compression injury (injured control group). We hypothesize that these deficits were likely attributed to additional damage caused by the intraspinal injections rather than exacerbated inflammation. Both AdV-eGFP and AdV-ZFP-VEGF groups received cyclosporine-A administration to minimize the inflammatory response, and we have previously shown that there is no difference in inflammation between AdV and control injured groups [11]. AdV-ZFP-VEGF treated animals were able to overcome these additional deficits and still show significant improvement compared to injured control animals, with the exception of white matter sparing. Direct injections (through the dorsal white matter) into the spinal cord may account for the data (Figure 11) that shows reduced white matter sparing for AdV-ZFP-VEGF treated animals compared to injured controls, since the injection likely caused additional physical insult to the spinal cord white matter. The administration of the therapy primarily aimed to rescue the vasculature following SCI, therefore the centrally located grey matter was the initial target and injections were given 1 mm deep into the cord. Although our data (Figure 1) indicate that AdV-ZFP-VEGF is observed in both the grey and white matter, AdV-ZFP-VEGF delivery was perhaps more localized to the deep grey matter tissue, and therefore able to exert the greatest effects on this population of cells (which would be supported by increased neuronal counts and vasculature; Figures 4 and 5, respectively).

In our studies, we believed it was important to include an AdV-eGFP control group to indicate the transduction of the virus *in vivo* (timing and location), and to help elucidate potential adverse effects of administering a gene therapy in an AdV construct. As noted above, the AdV-eGFP control group generally resulted in

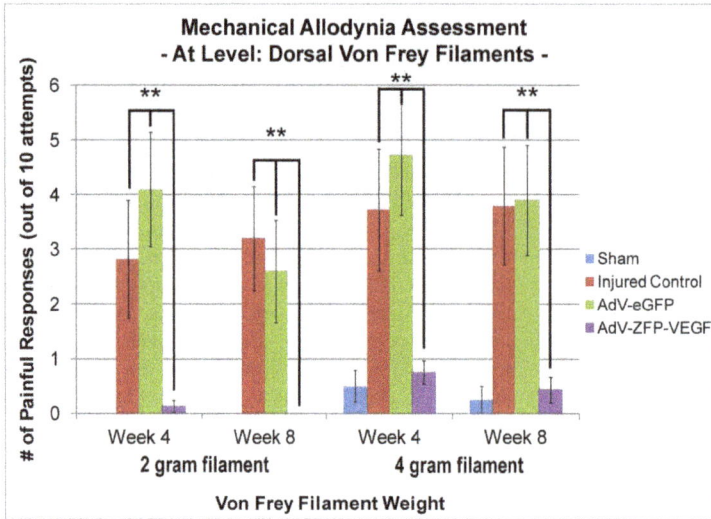

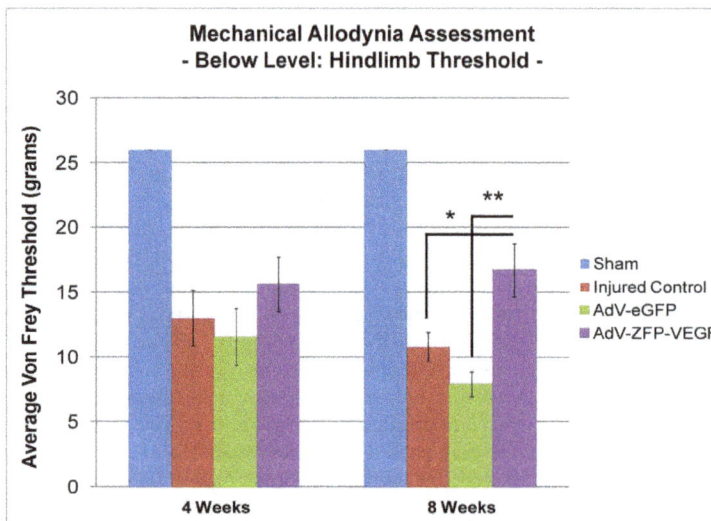

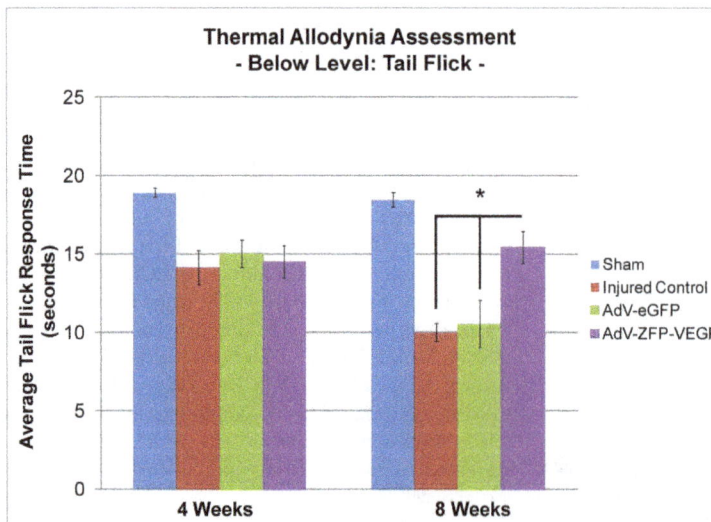

Figure 10. AdV-ZFP-VEGF significantly reduces mechanical and thermal allodynia at 8 weeks post-SCI. Mechanical and thermal allodynia, often used as outcome measures of neuropathic pain, were monitored with von Frey monofilaments and tail-flick tests, respectively. (A) At-level pain. Animals were assessed with 2 g or 4 g von Frey monofilaments around the dorsal incision (above T6–T7 laminectomy and injury). Data are

expressed as the average number of adverse reactions out of 10 applications of the monofilament. There was an overall treatment effect with AdV-ZFP-VEGF using the 2 g and 4 g monofilaments at 4 weeks and 8 weeks post-injury; *p<0.05. (B) Below-level pain. Animals were subject to increasing von Frey filaments (2 g–26 g), and the when they elicited a response, this value was taken as the pain threshold value. Data is reported as the average threshold for each group. AdV-ZFP-VEGF increased hindlimb threshold compared to other injured groups; *p<0.05, **p<0.005. (C) Below-level thermal allodynia. A 50°C thermal stimulus was applied to the distal tip of the tail. The data shown is the average time it took for the animals to withdrawl their tail from the stimulus ("tail flick"). Shorter response times indicate a decreased pain threshold. Animals treated with AdV-ZFP-VEGF showed an increased tolerance/threshold to thermal stimuli at 8 weeks post-injury compared to other injured groups; *p<0.05. Data were analyzed by One-way ANOVA. Error bars represent SEM. n = 8/sham and AdV-ZFP-VEGF groups; n = 10/injured control and AdV-eGFP groups.

poorer outcomes compared to injured animals without injections. Future experiments may choose to include a saline-injected control group to more specifically determine the amount of damage caused by the injection verses the potential inflammatory response of an AdV vector. Moreover, additional studies should aim to investigate alternative delivery methods for AdV-ZFP-VEGF, as VEGF-treated animals may display even greater histological improvements over control animals if AdV-ZFP-VEGF were to be administered in a less invasive manner.

Future studies may also wish to examine the use of alternative viral or non-viral delivery methods. The use of AdV may induce a host inflammatory response, although we attempted to reduce these effects by the use of cyclosporine-A. However, AdV infection may result in an increase in inflammation, and increased inflammation may negatively contribute to the secondary injury. On the contrary, inflammation results in expression of cytokines and activation of matrix metalloproteinases, which ultimately drives angiogenesis and re-vascularization [63]. MMPs de-stablize vascular structures, allowing for vascular remodeling, and expression of pro-inflammatory cytokines actively recruits endothelial cells and promotes endothelial cell proliferation. AdV administration may play a role in inducing re-vascularization; however, our data do not indicate that AdV administration results in any substantial vascular benefits. In fact, we observed AdV-eGFP groups showing reduced vascular proliferation and overall vascular counts (Figure 5).

Assessment of Functional Outcomes

We investigated the effects of 24 hour delayed AdV-ZFP-VEGF on the functional recovery and neuroanatomical preservation following thoracic SCI. In the current study, we used BBB locomotor scoring as well as CatWalk analysis to quantify functional outcomes of AdV-ZFP-VEGF therapy. CatWalk analysis is a relatively new method of assessing functional outcomes; however, the methodology has been widely validated for spinal cord injury models and generates data for many parameters of locomotion, which provides a more in-depth evaluation of functional recovery compared to traditional techniques [17]. CatWalk analysis demonstrated that animals treated with AdV-ZFP-VEGF showed improved locomotion as it was demonstrated by the increased forelimb stride length and the hindlimb swing speed. Interestingly, the animals treated with AdV-ZFP-VEGF exhibited improved hindlimb weight support. No differences were observed by BBB testing or electrophysiological assessment. Moreover, results indicated that AdV-ZFP-VEGF drastically reduced the development of mechanical and thermal allodynia in animals at 8 weeks post-injury. Lastly, results showed that AdV-ZFP-VEGF spared a significant amount of grey matter tissue compared to other injured groups.

The Basso Beattie Bresnahan (BBB) scoring scale to assess hindlimb deficits in thoracic SCI has been, and continues to be the "gold standard" for functional assessment [15]. The scoring system evaluates the hindlimb joint movement and the hind-paw orientation/stepping, provides a general indication of the locomotor capabilities of the animal, and establishes if the animal

can weight-bear. The major shortcomings of the BBB are two-fold. First, although the BBB is to be conducted by blinded observers, the behavioural assessments are still highly subjective to human errors. Secondly – and perhaps the most confounding factor – the BBB is a qualitative system: simply indicating if the animal is competent of defined movements, providing a relatively subjective score of *how much* or *how well* an animal can perform a task (occasional, frequent or consistent). For detecting major functional differences in animals, the BBB scoring scale is highly effective and easy to conduct; however, more subtle differences between treatment groups may not be observed by BBB assessment. Additionally, since the BBB scale is not a linear relationship between the numerical value and the functional gains associated with them, teasing out meaningful results can become a challenge.

In this research, we used both the BBB and the Catwalk gait analysis software to assess functional recovery post-injury. While scoring animals using BBB, subtle differences between animals were noted (some of them moved more normally, and with greater consistency); however, these variations were not strong enough to increase their BBB score. Overall, we observed no differences in BBB scores between groups. On the other hand, Catwalk data indicated that AdV-ZFP-VEGF treated animals have significant improvements in hindlimb weight support, and hindlimb swing speed. It should be emphasized that CatWalk experiments require weight support, and therefore only a sub-set of animals (n = 5) for each group were tested using the Catwalk system. The average BBB scores for the injured control and AdV-ZFP-VEGF animals used for CatWalk experiments were very similar (injured control = 9.5, AdV-ZFP-VEGF = 9.2), whereas the AdV-eGFP animals had poorer BBB scores and the majority of animals did not reach weight-bearing ability (average BBB score = 7.9). Although the BBB is a valid, widely used method of behavioural evaluation, the Catwalk is a more sensitive and quantitative outcome measure, which may reveal understated changes in recovery not observable using the BBB scoring system. From a clinical perspective, improvements in hindlimb weight support and in overall locomotion may have an important impact on the mobility and independence of an injured individual. Interestingly, Catwalk analysis also revealed that AdV-ZFP-VEGF animals showed improved forelimb stride length, suggesting that AdV-ZFP-VEGF could potentially enhance hindlimb-forelimb coordination; although with BBB scores of 9, we did not observe hindlimb-forelimb coordination in any injured animal group. In the histological examination of grey and white matter post-SCI, we did not investigate sparing of specific pathways or specific neuronal phenotypes (i.e. interneurons vs. motor neurons); however, improvements in both hindlimb and forelimb kinetics could suggest that AdV-ZFP-VEGF may spare propriospinal interneurons, which are located at the grey-white matter interface and are involved in coordination of limb movements [64]. Future experiments involving AdV-ZFP-VEGF should aim to investigate the effects of AdV-ZFP-VEGF on interneuron sparing/survival, since these cells have been attributed to regulating central pattern generators (CPGs) and should therefore be of interest for promoting locomotor recovery following SCI.

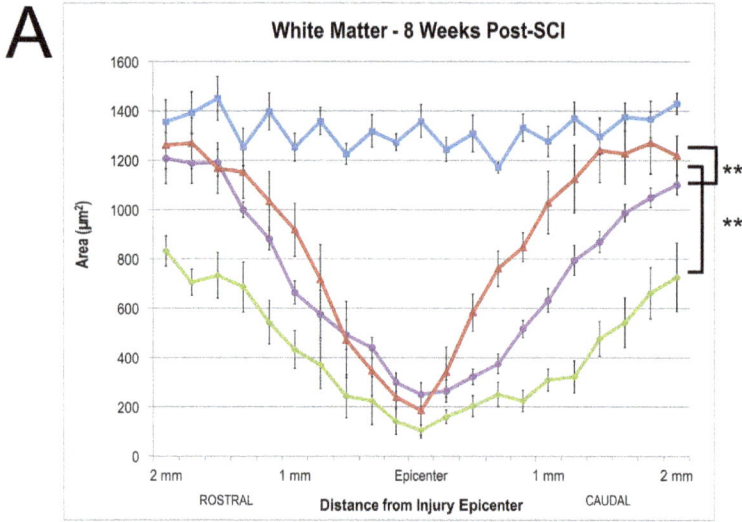

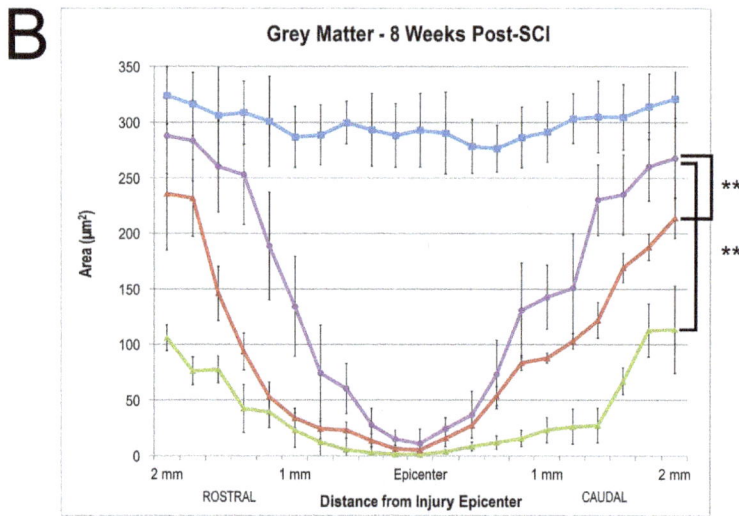

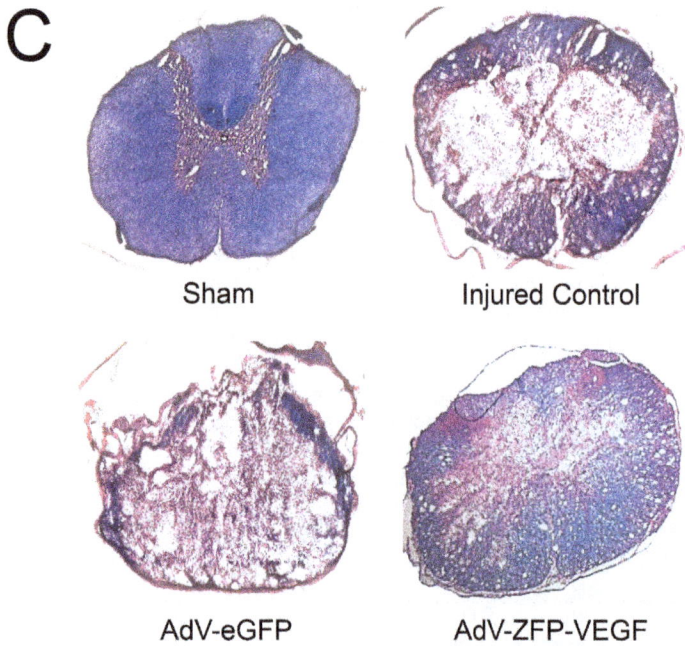

Figure 11. Tissue sparing quantification at 8 weeks post-SCI. (A) Residual white matter quantification. (B) Residual grey matter quantification. AdV-ZFP-VEGF improves spinal cord grey matter preservation. (C) Representative sections are shown from each group. Sections shown are taken 2 mm rostral to the epicenter at 8 weeks after SCI. AdV-ZFP-VEGF treated spinal cord exhibited a larger extent of grey matter spared tissue, but not white matter; **$p < 0.001$. Data are mean $\pm$ SEM values. n = 8/sham and AdV-ZFP-VEGF groups; n = 10/injured control and AdV-eGFP groups.

In compliment to our data showing AdV-ZFP-VEGF spares neurons, in this study we quantified residual tissue at 8 weeks post-SCI and our data show that delayed AdV-ZFP-VEGF administration results in improved grey matter sparing, but not white matter sparing. Taken together, these results suggest that AdV-ZFP-VEGF likely acts by promoting survival of neuronal cell bodies. Additionally, we observe that AdV-eGFP animals show notable decreases in both grey and white matter sparing at 8 weeks post-SCI. We do observe the caudal sections to have even less tissue sparing; however, it is often observed that tissue caudal to a traumatic injury is less preserved due to Wallerian degeneration, axonal disruption and reduced vascular flow. In a previous study, we show that AdV administration (in conjunction with cyclosporine-A) does not result in an increased inflammatory response compared to injured control animals [11]. The functional outcomes observed in our study – improved gait, hindlimb weight support and decreased pain – would be consistent with previous research demonstrating improved function and/or sparing of propriospinal tracts (limb coordination) [65], reticulospinal tracts (locomotion and weight-bearing stepping) [66], and spinothalamic tracts (neuropathic pain) [67,68] following SCI. In our study, we did not investigated the sparing of specific spinal tracts via electrophyisiology or dye-tracing experiments; however, an overall increase in residual grey matter likely contributes to improved pain processing pathways (interneurons) and a decrease in aberrant pain [17,69,70]. Varying studies report that 26-96% of human patients experience neuropathic pain following SCI [30]. Research has identified VEGF as one of the potential factors involved in the development of neuropathic pain; however, it is still unclear if VEGF plays a beneficial or detrimental role. Schratzberger et al., found that intramuscular injections of VEGF improved vascularity, blood flow and peripheral nerve function in a rabbit model of diabetic neuropathy [71]. Since it is believed that diabetic neuropathy is caused from microvascular ischemia, their findings reasonably support the use of VEGF for the treatment of neuropathies. Conversely, Nesic et al. recently showed that VEGF administration into the spinal cord resulted in an increased number of animals displaying neuropathic pain, as well as an increase in myelinated dorsal horn neurons, suggesting that VEGF results in non-specific axonal sprouting [31]. Regardless of whether VEGF therapies result in favourable or damaging outcomes, it is most important for future research to be aware of potential pitfalls of VEGF administration and to consider the

implications they may have on the bench-to-bedside translation of these therapies. Future studies are required to investigate the exact mechanisms of the attenuated allodynia/neuropathic pain observed following AdV-ZFP-VEGF administration.

Conclusions

The present data demonstrate that, similar to the effects seen following immediate administration of AdV-ZFP-VEGF shown by Liu et al., treated animals show increased VEGF mRNA and protein levels, increased vascular counts, increased neuroprotection and reduced apoptosis [11]. Overall, the administration of AdV-ZFP-VEGF shows promise as a therapeutic treatment for SCI, and these findings suggest that AdV-ZFP-VEGF treatment can be delayed up to 24 hours following injury, which presents a feasible time-window for clinical intervention. To the best of our knowledge, we are the first to investigate the delayed administration of AdV-ZFP-VEGF in a model of SCI. Here we observe beneficial effects in a variety of cell populations, and show that these cellular outcomes appear to be translated into improved functional recovery, as well as attenuated allodynia following SCI. Overall, these data suggest that targeting vascular and neuroprotective mechanisms by AdV-ZFP-VEGF administration may be a viable treatment for spinal cord injury. Collectively, this research further supports the use of VEGF as a potential candidate for neurotrauma treatments.

Acknowledgments

The authors would like to express their gratitude to Eunice Cho, Sofia Khan, Ramak Khosravi, Michelle Legasto and Christine Tseng for their help with tissue extraction, tissue processing, immunohistochemistry and cell counting. Thank you to Jared Wilcox and Dr. James Austin for their assistance with data analysis and behavioural techniques. Thank you to Behzad Azad and other members of the Fehlings' lab who assisted with post-operative animal care. The authors thank Philip Gregory and Edward Rebar of Sangamo BioSciences for scientific review.

Author Contributions

Conceived and designed the experiments: SKS GL DA RS MG SAF MGF YL SKK KS. Performed the experiments: SAF YL PF SKS KS. Analyzed the data: SAF YL PF SKK MGF KS. Contributed reagents/materials/analysis tools: SKS GL DA RS MG MGF. Wrote the paper: SAF KS YL SKK MGF.

References

1. Sekhon LH, Fehlings MG (2001) Epidemiology, demographics, and pathophysiology of acute spinal cord injury. Spine 26: S2–S12.
2. Tator CH, Fehlings MG (1991) Review of the secondary injury theory of acute spinal cord trauma with emphasis on vascular mechanisms. J Neurosurg 75: 15–26.
3. Beattie MS (2004) Inflammation and apoptosis: linked therapeutic targets in spinal cord injury. Trends Mol Med 10: 580–583.
4. Fehlings MG, Tator CH, Linden RD (1989) The relationships among the severity of spinal cord injury, motor and somatosensory evoked potentials and spinal cord blood flow. Electroencephalogr Clin Neurophysiol 74: 241–259.
5. Leypold BG, Flanders AE, Schwartz ED, Burns AS (2007) The impact of methylprednisolone on lesion severity following spinal cord injury. Spine 32: 373–378; discussion 379–381.
6. Benton RL, Maddie MA, Minnillo DR, Hagg T, Whittemore SR (2008) Griffonia simplicifolia isolectin B4 identifies a specific subpopulation of angiogenic blood vessels following contusive spinal cord injury in the adult mouse. J Comp Neurol 507: 1031–1052.

7. Shweiki D, Itin A, Soffer D, Keshet E (1992) Vascular endothelial growth factor induced by hypoxia may mediate hypoxia-initiated angiogenesis. Nature 359: 843–845.
8. Greenberg DA, Jin K (2005) From angiogenesis to neuropathology. Nature 438: 954–959.
9. Leung DW, Cachianes G, Kuang WJ, Goeddel DV, Ferrara N (1989) Vascular endothelial growth factor is a secreted angiogenic mitogen. Science 246: 1306–1309.
10. Waxman SG, Cummins TR, Dib-Hajj S, Fjell J, Black JA (1999) Sodium channels, excitability of primary sensory neurons, and the molecular basis of pain. Muscle & Nerve 22: 1177–1187.
11. Liu Y, Figley S, Spratt SK, Lee G, Ando D, et al. (2010) An engineered transcription factor which activates VEGF-A enhances recovery after spinal cord injury. Neurobiology of Disease 37: 384–393.
12. Price SA, Dent C, Duran-Jimenez B, Liang Y, Zhang L, et al. (2006) Gene transfer of an engineered transcription factor promoting expression of VEGF-A protects against experimental diabetic neuropathy. Diabetes 55: 1847–1854.

13. Liu PQ, Rebar EJ, Zhang L, Liu Q, Jamieson AC, et al. (2001) Regulation of an endogenous locus using a panel of designed zinc finger proteins targeted to accessible chromatin regions. Activation of vascular endothelial growth factor A. J Biol Chem 276: 11323–11334.

14. Fehlings MG, Tator CH (1995) The relationships among the severity of spinal cord injury, residual neurological function, axon counts, and counts of retrogradely labeled neurons after experimental spinal cord injury. Exp Neurol 132: 220–228.

15. Basso DM, Beattie MS, Bresnahan JC (1995) A sensitive and reliable locomotor rating scale for open field testing in rats. J Neurotrauma 12: 1–21.

16. Koopmans GC, Deumens R, Honig WM, Hamers FP, Steinbusch HW, et al. (2005) The assessment of locomotor function in spinal cord injured rats: the importance of objective analysis of coordination. J Neurotrauma 22: 214–225.

17. Hamers FP, Koopmans GC, Joosten EA (2006) CatWalk-assisted gait analysis in the assessment of spinal cord injury. J Neurotrauma 23: 537–548.

18. Gensel JC, Tovar CA, Hamers FP, Deibert RJ, Beattie MS, et al. (2006) Behavioral and histological characterization of unilateral cervical spinal cord contusion injury in rats. J Neurotrauma 23: 36–54.

19. Bruce JC, Oatway MA, Weaver LC (2002) Chronic pain after clip-compression injury of the rat spinal cord. Exp Neurol 178: 33–48.

20. Holm S (1979) A simple sequentially rejective multiple test procedure. Scandinavian Journal of Statistics 6: 65–70.

21. Glantz SA (2005) Primer of Biostatistics: McGraw-Hill Companies,Inc. 520 p.

22. Dai Q, Huang J, Klitzman B, Dong C, Goldschmidt-Clermont PJ, et al. (2004) Engineered zinc finger-activating vascular endothelial growth factor transcription factor plasmid DNA induces therapeutic angiogenesis in rabbits with hindlimb ischemia. Circulation 110: 2467–2475.

23. Rebar EJ, Huang Y, Hickey R, Nath AK, Meoli D, et al. (2002) Induction of angiogenesis in a mouse model using engineered transcription factors. Nat Med 8: 1427–1432.

24. Yu J, Lei L, Liang Y, Hinh L, Hickey RP, et al. (2006) An engineered VEGF-activating zinc finger protein transcription factor improves blood flow and limb salvage in advanced-age mice. Faseb J 20: 479–481.

25. Casha S, Yu WR, Fehlings MG (2001) Oligodendroglial apoptosis occurs along degenerating axons and is associated with FAS and p75 expression following spinal cord injury in the rat. Neuroscience 103: 203–218.

26. Schumacher PA, Siman RG, Fehlings MG (2000) Pretreatment with calpain inhibitor CEP-4143 inhibits calpain I activation and cytoskeletal degradation, improves neurological function, and enhances axonal survival after traumatic spinal cord injury. J Neurochem 74: 1646–1655.

27. Karimi-Abdolrezaee S, Eftekharpour E, Fehlings MG (2004) Temporal and spatial patterns of Kv1.1 and Kv1.2 protein and gene expression in spinal cord white matter after acute and chronic spinal cord injury in rats: implications for axonal pathophysiology after neurotrauma. Eur J Neurosci 19: 577–589.

28. Byrne AM, Bouchier-Hayes DJ, Harmey JH (2005) Angiogenic and cell survival functions of Vascular Endothelial Growth Factor (VEGF). Journal of Cellular and Molecular Medicine 9: 777–794.

29. Werhagen L, Budh CN, Hultling C, Molander C (2004) Neuropathic pain after traumatic spinal cord injury—relations to gender, spinal level, completeness, and age at the time of injury. Spinal Cord 42: 665–673.

30. Dijkers M, Bryce T, Zanca J (2009) Prevalence of chronic pain after traumatic spinal cord injury: A systematic review. Journal of Rehabilitation Research & Development 46: 13–30.

31. Nesic O, Sundberg LM, Herrera JJ, Mokkapati VUL, Lee J, et al. (2010) Vascular Endothelial Growth Factor and Spinal Cord Injury Pain. Journal of Neurotrauma 27: 1793–1803.

32. Sun Y, Jin K, Xie L, Childs J, Mao XO, et al. (2003) VEGF-induced neuroprotection, neurogenesis, and angiogenesis after focal cerebral ischemia. The Journal of Clinical Investigation 111: 1843–1851.

33. Widenfalk J, Lipson A, Jubran M, Hofstetter C, Ebendal T, et al. (2003) Vascular endothelial growth factor improves functional outcome and decreases secondary degeneration in experimental spinal cord contusion injury. Neuroscience 120: 951–960.

34. Ling X, Liu D (2007) Temporal and spatial profiles of cell loss after spinal cord injury: Reduction by a metalloporphyrin. Journal of Neuroscience Research 85: 2175–2185.

35. Grossman SD, Rosenberg LJ, Wrathall JR (2001) Temporal-Spatial Pattern of Acute Neuronal and Glial Loss after Spinal Cord Contusion. Experimental Neurology 168: 273–282.

36. Liu XZ, Xu XM, Hu R, Du C, Zhang SX, et al. (1997) Neuronal and Glial Apoptosis after Traumatic Spinal Cord Injury. The Journal of Neuroscience 17: 5395–5406.

37. Loy DN, Crawford CH, Darnall JB, Burke DA, Onifer SM, et al. (2002) Temporal progression of angiogenesis and basal lamina deposition after contusive spinal cord injury in the adult rat. J Comp Neurol 445: 308–324.

38. Kigerl KA, Gensel JC, Ankeny DP, Alexander JK, Donnelly DJ, et al. (2009) Identification of two distinct macrophage subsets with divergent effects causing either neurotoxicity or regeneration in the injured mouse spinal cord. J Neurosci 29: 13435–13444.

39. Mabon PJ, Weaver LC, Dekaban GA (2000) Inhibition of monocyte/macrophage migration to a spinal cord injury site by an antibody to the integrin alphaD: a potential new anti-inflammatory treatment. Exp Neurol 166: 52–64.

40. Glaser J, Gonzalez R, Sadr E, Keirstead HS (2006) Neutralization of the chemokine CXCL10 reduces apoptosis and increases axon sprouting after spinal cord injury. Journal of Neuroscience Research 84: 724–734.

41. Yoshihara T, Ohta M, Itokazu Y, Matsumoto N, Dezawa M, et al. (2007) Neuroprotective Effect of Bone Marrow–Derived Mononuclear Cells Promoting Functional Recovery from Spinal Cord Injury. Journal of Neurotrauma 24: 1026–1036.

42. Kaneko S, Iwanami A, Nakamura M, Kishino A, Kikuchi K, et al. (2006) A selective Sema3A inhibitor enhances regenerative responses and functional recovery of the injured spinal cord. Nature Medicine 12: 1380–1389.

43. Ohab JJ, Fleming S, Blesch A, Carmichael ST (2006) A neurovascular niche for neurogenesis after stroke. Journal of Neuroscience 26: 13007–13016.

44. Raab S, Plate K (2007) Different networks, common growth factors: shared growth factors and receptors of the vascular and the nervous system. Acta Neuropathologica 113: 607–626.

45. Peters KG, De Vries C, Williams LT (1993) Vascular endothelial growth factor receptor expression during embryogenesis and tissue repair suggests a role in endothelial differentiation and blood vessel growth. Proceedings of the National Academy of Sciences 90: 8915–8919.

46. Tsao MN, Li YQ, Lu G, Xu Y, Wong CS (1999) Upregulation of Vascular Endothelial Growth Factor Is Associated with Radiation-Induced Blood-Spinal Cord Barrier Breakdown. Journal of Neuropathology & Experimental Neurology 58: 1051–1060.

47. Skold MK, Gertten CV, Sandbergnordqvist A-C, Mathiesen T, Holmin S (2005) VEGF and VEGF Receptor Expression after Experimental Brain Contusion in Rat. Journal of Neurotrauma 22: 353–367.

48. Jin KL, Mao XO, Nagayama T, Goldsmith PC, Greenberg DA (2000) Induction of vascular endothelial growth factor and hypoxia-inducible factor-1α by global ischemia in rat brain. Neuroscience 99: 577–585.

49. Jin KL, Mao XO, Greenberg DA (2000) Vascular endothelial growth factor: direct neuroprotective effect in in vitro ischemia. Proc Natl Acad Sci U S A 97: 10242–10247.

50. Krum JM, Rosenstein JM (1998) VEGF mRNA and Its Receptor flt-1 Are Expressed in Reactive Astrocytes Following Neural Grafting and Tumor Cell Implantation in the Adult CNS. Experimental Neurology 154: 57–65.

51. Krum JM, Rosenstein JM (1999) Transient Coexpression of Nestin, GFAP, and Vascular Endothelial Growth Factor in Mature Reactive Astroglia Following Neural Grafting or Brain Wounds. Experimental Neurology 160: 348–360.

52. Neufeld G, Kessler O, Herzog Y (2003) The Interaction of Neuropilin-1 and Neuropilin-2 with Tyrosine-Kinase Receptors for VEGF. In: Bagnard D, editor: Springer US. pp. 81–90.

53. Neufeld G, Cohen T, Shraga N, Lange T, Kessler O, et al. (2002) The Neuropilins: Multifunctional Semaphorin and VEGF Receptors that Modulate Axon Guidance and Angiogenesis. Trends in Cardiovascular Medicine 12: 13–19.

54. Bearden SE, Segal SS (2004) Microvessels Promote Motor Nerve Survival and Regeneration Through Local VEGF Release Following Ectopic Reattachment. Microcirculation 11: 633–644.

55. Hobson MI, Green CJ, Terenghi G (2000) VEGF enhances intraneural angiogenesis and improves nerve regeneration after axotomy. Journal of Anatomy 197: 591–605.

56. Choi UH, Ha Y, Huang X, Park SR, Chung J, et al. (2007) Hypoxia-inducible expression of vascular endothelial growth factor for the treatment of spinal cord injury in a rat model. J Neurosurg Spine 7: 54–60.

57. Facchiano F, Fernandez E, Mancarella S, Maira G, Miscusi M, et al. (2002) Promotion of regeneration of corticospinal tract axons in rats with recombinant vascular endothelial growth factor alone and combined with adenovirus coding for this factor. J Neurosurg 97: 161–168.

58. Benton RL, Whittemore SR (2003) VEGF165 therapy exacerbates secondary damage following spinal cord injury. Neurochem Res 28: 1693–1703.

59. Barleon B, Sozzani S, Zhou D, Weich H, Mantovani A, et al. (1996) Migration of human monocytes in response to vascular endothelial growth factor (VEGF) is mediated via the VEGF receptor flt-1. Blood 87: 3336–3343.

60. Karimi-Abdolrezaee S, Eftekharpour E, Wang J, Morshead CM, Fehlings MG (2006) Delayed Transplantation of Adult Neural Precursor Cells Promotes Remyelination and Functional Neurological Recovery after Spinal Cord Injury. The Journal of Neuroscience 26: 3377–3389.

61. Yezierski RP, Liu S, Ruenes GL, Busto R, Dietrich WD (1996) Neuronal Damage Following Intraspinal Injection of a Nitric Oxide Synthase Inhibitor in the Rat. J Cereb Blood Flow Metab 16: 996–1004.

62. Azzouz M, Hottinger A, Paterna J-C, Zurn AD, Aebischer P, et al. (2000) Increased motoneuron survival and improved neuromuscular function in transgenic ALS mice after intraspinal injection of an adeno-associated virus encoding Bcl-2. Human Molecular Genetics 9: 803–811.

63. Naldini A, Carraro F (2005) Role of inflammatory mediators in angiogenesis. Curr Drug Targets Inflamm Allergy 4: 3–8.

64. Flynn JR, Graham BA, Galea MP, Callister RJ (2011) The role of propriospinal interneurons in recovery from spinal cord injury. Neuropharmacology 60: 809–822.

65. Pearse DD, Pereira FC, Marcillo AE, Bates ML, Berrocal YA, et al. (2004) cAMP and Schwann cells promote axonal growth and functional recovery after spinal cord injury. Nature Medicine 10: 610–616.

66. Ballermann M, Fouad K (2006) Spontaneous locomotor recovery in spinal cord injured rats is accompanied by anatomical plasticity of reticulospinal fibers. European Journal of Neuroscience 23: 1988–1996.

67. Defrin R, Ohry A, Blumen N, Urca G (2001) Characterization of chronic pain and somatosensory function in spinal cord injury subjects. Pain 89: 253–263.

68. Österberg A, Boivie J (2010) Central pain in multiple sclerosis – Sensory abnormalities. European Journal of Pain 14: 104–110.

69. Vierck Jr CJ, Siddall P, Yezierski RP (2000) Pain following spinal cord injury: animal models and mechanistic studies. Pain 89: 1–5.

70. Hoheisel U, Scheifer C, Trudrung P, Unger T, Mense S (2003) Pathophysiological activity in rat dorsal horn neurones in segments rostral to a chronic spinal cord injury. Brain Research 974: 134–145.

71. Schratzberger P, Walter DH, Rittig K, Bahlmann FH, Pola R, et al. (2001) Reversal of experimental diabetic neuropathy by VEGF gene transfer. The Journal of Clinical Investigation 107: 1083–1092.

2

Inhibition of GADD34, the Stress-Inducible Regulatory Subunit of the Endoplasmic Reticulum Stress Response, Does Not Enhance Functional Recovery after Spinal Cord Injury

Sujata Saraswat Ohri[1,2], **Ashley Mullins**[1,2], **Michal Hetman**[1,2,3,4], **Scott R. Whittemore**[1,2,4]*

1 Kentucky Spinal Cord Injury Research Center, University of Louisville, Louisville, Kentucky, United States of America, 2 Department of Neurological Surgery, University of Louisville, Louisville, Kentucky, United States of America, 3 Department of Pharmacology & Toxicology, University of Louisville, Louisville, Kentucky, United States of America, 4 Department of Anatomical Sciences & Neurobiology, University of Louisville, Louisville, Kentucky, United States of America

Abstract

Activation of the endoplasmic reticulum stress response (ERSR) is a hallmark of various pathological diseases and/or traumatic injuries. Restoration of ER homeostasis can contribute to improvement in the functional outcome of these diseases. Using genetic and pharmacological inhibition of the PERK-CHOP arm of the ERSR, we recently demonstrated improvements in hindlimb locomotion after spinal cord injury (SCI) and implicated oligodendrocyte survival as a potential mechanism. Here, we investigated the contribution of stress-inducible PPP1R15A/GADD34, an ERSR signaling effector downstream of CHOP that dephosphorylates eIF2α, in the pathogenesis of SCI. We show that although genetic ablation of GADD34 protects oligodendrocyte precursor cells (OPCs) against ER stress-mediated cell death *in vitro* and results in differential ERSR attenuation *in vivo* after SCI, there is no improvement in hindlimb locomotor function. Guanabenz, a FDA approved antihypertensive drug, was recently shown to reduce the burden of misfolded proteins in the ER by directly targeting GADD34. Guanabenz protected OPCs from ER stress-mediated cell death *in vitro* and attenuated the ERSR *in vivo* after SCI. However, guanabenz administration failed to rescue the locomotor deficits after SCI. These data suggest that deletion of GADD34 alone is not sufficient to improve functional recovery after SCI.

Editor: Ken Arai, Massachusetts General Hospital/Harvard Medical School, United States of America

Funding: This study was supported by NS073584, NS054708, RR15576/GM103507, Kentucky Spinal Cord and Head Injury Research Trust, 10-13, Norton Healthcare and the Commonwealth of Kentucky Challenge for Excellence. The funders had no role in study design, data collection and analysis, decision to publish, or preparation of the manuscript.

Competing Interests: The authors have declared that no competing interests exist.

* Email: swhittemore@louisville.edu

Introduction

Spinal cord injury (SCI) is a complex multifactorial pathological condition and strategies to discover new effective therapies remain challenging. Therapeutic intervention has been difficult due to the management of two complex pathological phases following SCI: primary mechanical injury of which some level of cell death and axotomy occurs depending on the severity of the injury, and secondary damage initiated by the primary trauma. Secondary injury mechanisms that include inflammation, hypoxia, excitotoxicity, ischemia and demyelination exacerbate the primary damage [1]. Consequently, rapid cellular necrosis occurs at the injury epicenter with onset of apoptosis that spreads out into the lesion penumbra [2] and contributes to secondary cell death [1,2]. Therapeutic interventions which abrogate secondary cell death mechanisms during the acute phase of SCI are essential for limiting the spread of secondary injury phase and functional deficits after SCI.

While preclinical studies have identified a number of potential neuroprotective agents [3,4], none of these have shown marked therapeutic efficacy in human SCI trials [5,6]. One likely explanation is that multiple pathophysiological mechanisms are being activated simultaneously and current single drug therapies only affect a subset of these. What is hypothetically warranted for optimal therapeutic treatment would be pharmacological therapy that globally targets multiple neuropathological mechanisms in all cell types affected. One such potential target that has proven effective in the acute treatment of SCI is the endoplasmic reticulum (ER) stress response (ERSR).

The ERSR is an evolutionary conserved cellular mechanism that is activated in response to insults that disrupt ER homeostasis [7,8]. It is mediated by three distinct pathways: the protein RNA (PKR)-like kinase (PERK), inositol-requiring protein-1α (IRE-1α) and activating transcription factor-6 (ATF6). Activated PERK phosphorylates the α-subunit of elongation initiation factor 2α (eIF2α) which then results in global inhibition of protein synthesis. Moreover, phosphorylation of eIF2α allows the translation of mRNAs containing short open reading frames in their 5'-untranslated regions, such as activating transcription factor 4 (ATF4). Activated IRE-1α splices the X-box-binding protein 1

(XBP1) mRNA [9] and activates ERSR-specific transcription. Proteolytic processing of ATF6 [10] at the golgi complex also results in distinct expression of ERSR-specific genes. The main objective of the ERSR is cytoprotection by restoring ER homeostasis. However, the ERSR may also activate apoptosis if ER function cannot be timely restored, an event triggered by increased C/EBP homologous protein (CHOP) expression [8].

Dephosphorylation of eIF2α is required to restore protein synthesis after the stress induced attenuation of translation, thereby, terminating stress signaling [11]. Mammalian cells have two eIF2α holophosphatases, each one composed of one PP1 catalytic subunit and either PPP1R15A (growth arrest and DNA damage protein 34 - GADD34) or PPP1R15B (CReP). GADD34 is transcriptionally induced by stress, downstream of ATF4 and CHOP, and its translation escapes the general attenuation of protein synthesis resulting from eIF2α phosphorylation [12]. Thus, GADD34/PPP1R15A is one of the key effectors of negative feedback loop that is induced by stress and subsequently tries to restore homeostasis. Recent studies show that expression of GADD34 sensitizes cells to apoptosis [12,13,14]. Studies using GADD34$^{-/-}$ mice showed diminished oligodendrocyte loss and hypomyelination in experimental autoimmune encephalomyelitis [15] and improved myelination of Schwann cells in model of Charcot-Marie-Tooth IB neuropathy [16].

Independent studies demonstrated the involvement of the ERSR after a moderate contusive SCI in rats [17] and mice [18] or after hemisection SCI in mice [19]. Partial restoration of ER homeostasis using genetic [18], viral [19], or pharmacological [20] interventions showed significant improvement of hindlimb locomotion in these rodent models. Interestingly, our previous studies demonstrated significant upregulation of GADD34 after both moderate and severe SCI [18,21]. Guanabenz, an α2-adrenergic receptor agonist, FDA-approved for the treatment of hypertension, was recently shown to enhance the PERK pathway by selectively inhibiting GADD34-mediated dephosphorylation of eIF2α [22]. Given its FDA-approved status, this study was undertaken to study the therapeutic potential of guanabenz and GADD34 inhibition in modulating the ERSR after SCI.

Materials and Methods

Animals

Wild type C57Bl/6 female mice (6–8 weeks) were obtained from Harlan (Indianapolis, IN). GADD34$^{-/-}$ mice on a 100% C57Bl/6 background were procured from MMRRC (Catalogue No – 30266, Chapel Hill, NC) and bred in-house. Procedures were performed according to the Public Health Service Policy on Humane Care and Use of Laboratory Animals, Guide for the Care and Use of Laboratory Animals (Institute of Laboratory Animal Resources, National Research Council, 1996) and with the approval of the University of Louisville Institutional Animal Care and Use Committee and the Institutional Biosafety Committee.

Isolation of mouse oligodendrocyte precursor cells (mOPCs)

Mouse cortices were dissected from whole brains of wild type and GADD34$^{-/-}$ postnatal day 5–7 pups [23]. Briefly, tissue was dissociated using the Neural Tissue Dissociation Kit (Miltenyi Biotec, Bergisch Gladbach, Germany) according to the manufacturer's instructions. OPC-A media was prepared by adding 2.1 g/L NaHCO$_3$ (Sigma-Aldrich, St. Louis, MO) to DMEM-F12 without HEPES powder (Invitrogen, Carlsbad, CA) and supplemented with N2 supplement (1%), B27 supplement (2%), Penicillin/Streptomycin (1%, all from Invitrogen), BSA (0.01%,

Sigma), 40 ng/ml FGF2 (Millipore, Billerica, MA), and 20 ng/ml PDGFα (Sigma). OPCs were enriched with O4 hybridoma using magnetic cell sorting (MACS) with rat anti-mouse IgM magnetic beads (10% in MACS Buffer). The average yield was 8 −10×10^6 cells/brain with a viability of 85–95%. 9,000–15,000 cells/cm^2 cells were seeded on a PDL/laminin-coated 10 cm tissue culture dish, and incubated at 37°C, 5% CO$_2$ for maintenance.

Tunicamycin treatment, MTT assay

Wild type or GADD34$^{-/-}$-derived mOPCs were seeded in 96-well plates and treated with various concentrations of guanabenz in the presence of tunicamycin (0.01 or 0.025 µg/ml). OPC survival was assayed by measuring the conversion of tetrazolium, MTT (3-(4,5-dimethylthiazol-2-yl)-2,5-diphenyltetrazolium bromide; Sigma) to formazan at a wavelength of 570 nm.

Western Blot Analyses

Protein lysates prepared from WT and GADD34$^{-/-}$-derived mOPCs or 4 mm tissue isolated from sham and injury epicenter of contused spinal cords at 6 hour post-injury in protein lysis solution (20 mM Tris, pH-6.8, 137 mM NaCl, 25 mM B-glycerophosphate, 2 mM NaPPi, 2 mM EDTA, 1 mM Na3VO4, 1% Triton X-100, 10% glycerol, protease inhibitor, 0.5 mM DTT, 1 mM PMSF) were quantified using the BCA Kit (Pierce). Proteins were separated on SDS-PAGE gels and transferred to nitrocellulose membrane (Whatman, Schleicher & Schuell). Membranes were processed and probed with p-eIF2α (Cell Signalling, 1/1000 dilution), eIF2α (Biosource, 1/1000), ATF4 (Santa Cruz Biotechnology, 1/500) and GAPDH (Chemicon, 1/5000) as described previously [20].

RNA Extraction, Reverse Transcriptase PCR

Total RNA was extracted from WT and GADD34$^{-/-}$-derived mOPCs treated with tunicamycin and spinal cord tissue of sham, vehicle- and guanabenz-treated contused wild type (n = 4/group) mice from the injury epicenter (4 mm) using Trizol (Invitrogen, Carlsbad, CA) according to the manufacturer's instructions. The RNA was quantified by UV spectroscopy and RNA integrity was confirmed on an ethidium bromide stained formaldehyde agarose gel. cDNA was synthesized with 500 ng of total RNA using the High Capacity cDNA Synthesis Kit (Applied Biosystems, Foster City, CA) in a 20 µl reaction volume. As controls, mixtures containing all components except the reverse transcriptase enzyme were prepared and treated similarly. All cDNAs and control reactions were diluted 10x with water before using as a template for quantitative real time (qRT)-PCR.

Quantitative PCR Analysis

qRT-PCR was performed using ABI 7900HT Real-time PCR instrument (Applied Biosystems). Briefly, diluted cDNAs were added to Taqman universal PCR master mix (Applied Biosystems) and run in triplicate. Target and reference gene PCR amplification was performed in separate tubes with Assay on Demand™ primers (Applied Biosystems) as follows: ATF4 (Mm00515324_m1), CHOP (Mm01135937_g1), Claudin 11 (Mm00500915_m1) GADD34 (Mm00492555_m1), GFAP (Mm00546086_m1), glutamine synthetase (GS: Mm00725701_s1), GRP78 (Mm01333323_g1), microtubule associated protein 2 (Mtap2: Mm00485230_m1), myelin basic protein (MBP: Mm00521980) neuron-specific enolase (NSE: Mm00468052_m1) Olig2 (Mm01210556_m1) and XBP1 (Mm00457359_m1). The RNA levels were quantified using the ΔΔCT method. Expression values obtained from triplicate runs of

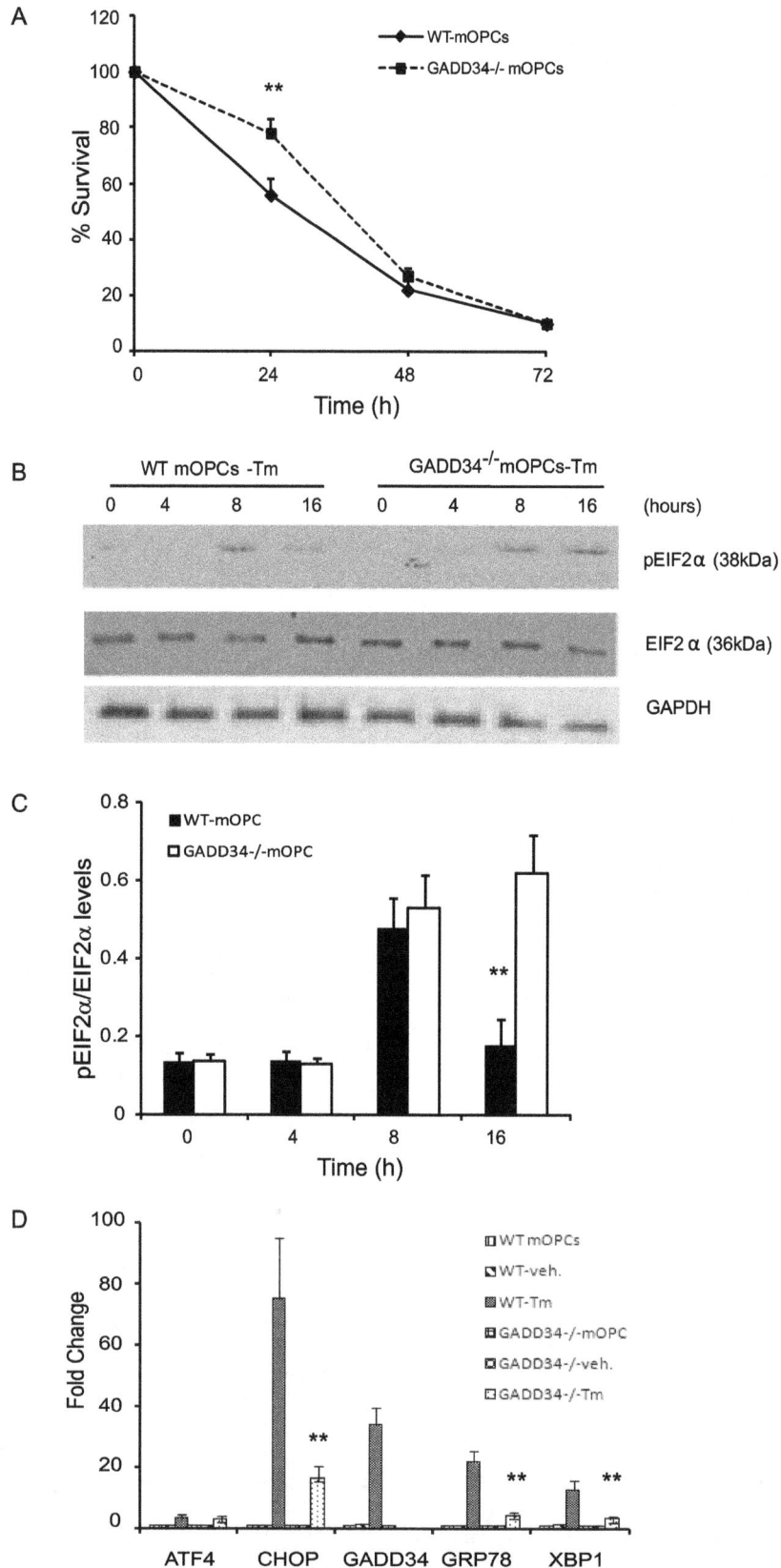

Figure 1. GADD34$^{-/-}$ mOPCS show enhanced survival in response to ER stress. (A) Quantification using MTT assay show increased survival of GADD34$^{-/-}$ mOPCs exposed to tunicamycin (Tm; 0.01 µg/ml) at only 24 hours. (B,C) Western blot shows sustained translational repression in GADD34$^{-/-}$ mOPCs in contrast to WT mOPCs. (D) RT-PCR data shows attenuation in the ERSR in GADD34$^{-/-}$ mOPCs exposed to Tm for 16 hours. Data (A,C,D) are the mean ± SD (n = 4, ** p<0.01).

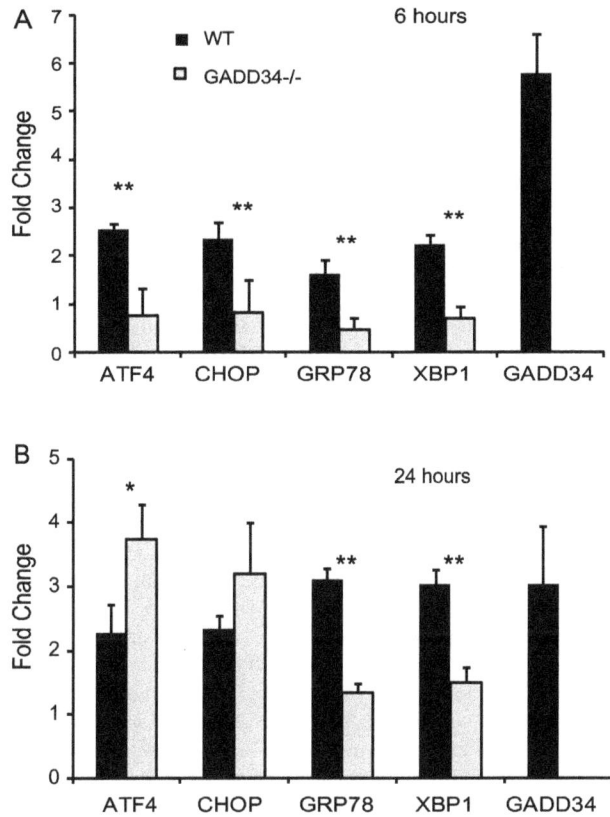

Figure 2. Deletion of GADD34 results in attenuation of the ERSR after SCI. Total RNA was extracted from injury epicenter of WT and GADD34$^{-/-}$ mice at (A) 6 hours and (B) 24 hours-post SCI. Transcript level (normalized to GAPDH) is expressed as fold changes compared with levels in sham controls. Data (A,B) are the mean $\pm$ SD (n = 4, ** p< 0.01).

each cDNA sample were normalized to triplicate value for GAPDH (reference gene) from the same cDNA preparation. Transcript levels are expressed as fold changes compared with respective levels in sham controls.

XBP1 Splicing

qRT-PCR with RT^2 Real-Time SYBR Green Mix (SuperArray Bioscience Corporation) using spliced XBP1 (sense, gagtccgcag-caggtg; antisense, gtgtcagagtccatggga) [24] and GAPDH (sense, ccctcaagattgtcagcctgc; antisense, gtcctcagtgtagcccaggat) primers was performed. The $\Delta\Delta$CT method was used for quantification.

SCI and injections

Mice were anesthetized by an intraperitoneal (IP) injection of 0.4 mg/g body weight Avertin (2,2,2-tribromoethanol in 0.02 ml of 1.25% 2-methyl-2-butanol in saline, Sigma). Lacri-Lube ophthalmic ointment (Allergen, Irvine, CA) was used to prevent drying of eyes and gentamycin (50 mg/kg; Boehringer Ingelheim, St. Joseph, MO) was subcutaneously administered to reduce infection. A laminectomy was done at the T9 vertebrae and moderate contusion injuries (50 kdyn force/400–600 µm displacement) were performed using the IH impactor [25] (Infinite Horizons Inc., Lexington, KY) as described previously [26,27]. Experimental controls included sham animals that received only the T9 laminectomy. Guanabenz (1 mg/kg; in PBS containing 10% FBS and 5% DMSO) or vehicle was administered by an IP

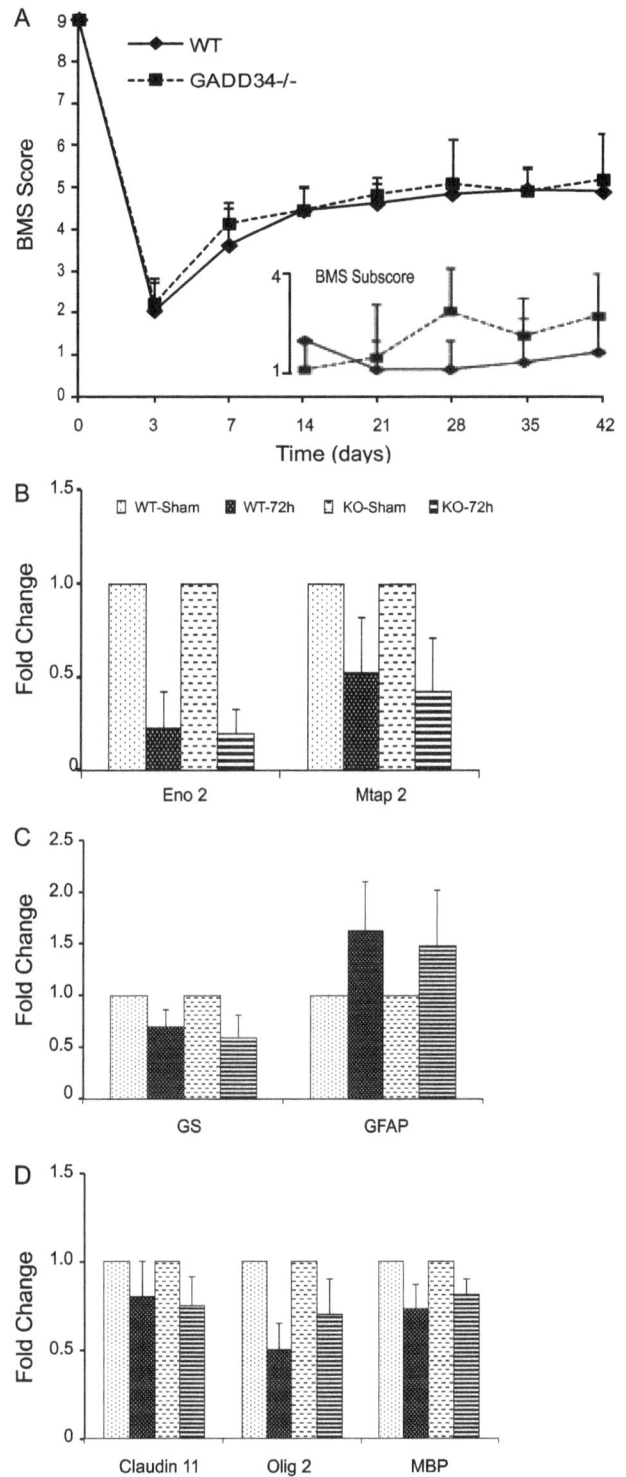

Figure 3. Locomotor assessment in GADD34$^{-/-}$ mice after SCI. (A) BMS locomotor analyses performed weekly following moderate SCI did not reveal any functional recovery in GADD34$^{-/-}$ mice (solid squares) compared to WT mice (solid diamonds). Analysis of BMS subscore post-SCI showed no significant differences in stepping characteristics between the two groups (inset). There is no significant difference in the neuron- (B), astrocyte-(C) and oligodendrocyte-specific (D) transcript levels as indicated between WT and GADD34$^{-/-}$ mice 72 hours post-SCI. Data (A,B) are the mean $\pm$ SD (n = 9).

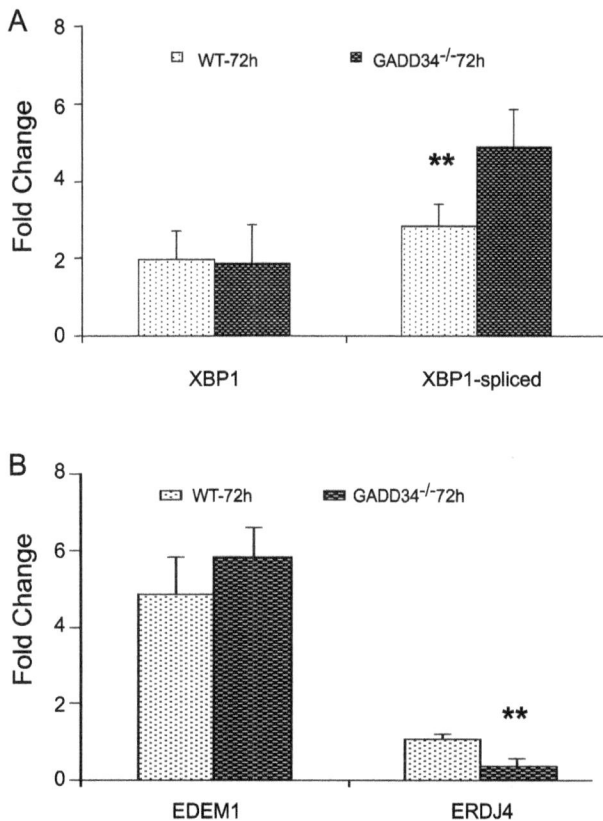

Figure 4. Expression of spliced XBP1 and its downstream target genes. qRT-PCR data shows significant differences in transcript levels of spliced XBP1 (A) and ERDJ4 (B) in GADD34$^{-/-}$ mice compared to WT mice at 72 hours post-SCI.

injection immediately after surgery followed by IP injections for three consecutive days. Post surgery, animals were given 1 cc of sterile saline subcutaneously, 0.1 cc of gentamycin intramuscularly on the day of surgery and 3rd and 5th day post-surgery, and 0.1 cc bupronorphine subcutaneously on the day of surgery and for next 2 days. Animals were placed on a heating pad until full recovery from anesthesia. Postoperative care included manual expression of bladders twice a day for 7–10 days or until spontaneous voiding returned.

Behavioral Assessment

Open field Basso Mouse Scale (BMS) locomotor analyses were performed prior to injury for each animal to determine the baseline scores and weekly following SCI for 6 weeks exactly as defined [28,20]. All raters were trained by Dr. Basso and colleagues at the Ohio State University and were blind to the animal groups.

Statistical Analyses

For functional assessements after injury, a repeated measures analyses of variance (ANOVA) with fixed effects and Bonferroni post hoc t-test was performed to detect differences in BMS score and subscores between the sham and injury groups over the 6 week testing period. Statistical analysis of qRT-PCR data was performed using independent t-test for means with equal or unequal variances or repeated measures ANOVA (one- way or two-way analysis of variance) followed by post-hoc Tukey HSD

test. For all other analyses, independent t-tests for means assuming equal variance were performed.

Results

GADD34$^{-/-}$ mOPCs show a delayed decrease in survival after ER stress

The PPP1R15A/GADD34 complex, a regulatory subunit of protein phosphatase 1, selectively disrupts the stress-induced phosphorylation of eIF2α [29,22]. Our previous studies that showed enhanced functional recovery post-SCI in CHOP$^{-/-}$ mice and suggested oligodendrocyte sparing as a potential mechanism also showed immediate increase in GADD34 transcript levels after moderate SCI [18]. To explore the specific role of GADD34 in OPCs, we first compared the ability of wild type and GADD34$^{-/-}$ mOPCs to survive exposure to ER stress induced by tunicamycin. GADD34$^{-/-}$ mOPCs showed a significant increase in survival only at 24 hours post-treatment (Fig 1A) suggesting acute oligodendrocyte protection. We examined the activation of ERSR in GADD34$^{-/-}$ mOPCs exposed to ER stress. In WT mOPCs, tunicamycin treatment resulted in profound but transient increase of eIF2α phosphorylation. In contrast, GADD34$^{-/-}$ mOPCs showed persistent phosphorylation (Fig 1B,C) and correlated with a decrease in the induction of CHOP, GRP78 and XBP1 transcript levels in response to ER stress (Fig 1D). Together, these data show that GADD34 is one of the key effectors that affects both the translational de-repression and stress-induced gene expression in mOPCs, consistent with earlier studies performed in fibroblasts [29,30,31].

Deletion of GADD34 results in differential ERSR attenuation after SCI

To determine the contribution of GADD34 to SCI pathogenesis, basal levels of ERSR effectors in GADD34$^{-/-}$ mice were compared with wild type mice. The average Ct values of 3.96 vs 3.872 for ATF4, 8.77 vs 8.44 for CHOP, 4.98 vs 5.12 for GRP78 and 6.077 vs 5.78 for XBP1 in GADD34$^{-/-}$ and WT mice respectively, indicated identical basal ERSR in both groups. However, six hours post-SCI, GADD34$^{-/-}$ mice demonstrated a significant reduction in the expression of ATF4, CHOP, GRP78 and XBP1 transcript levels (Fig 2A) indicating an overall attenuation of the ERSR in response to SCI. As the increased survival of GADD34$^{-/-}$ mOPCs was transient, (Fig 1A), we also examined the ERSR at 24 hour post-SCI. The decrease in ATF4 and CHOP transcript levels observed at 6 hours was completely abolished at 24 hours post-SCI, while GRP78 and XBP1 transcript levels remained attenuated (Fig 2B).

We evaluated the role of GADD34 in functional recovery post-SCI. Comparison of the BMS scores between moderately contused WT (n = 9) and GADD34$^{-/-}$ (n = 11) mice revealed no differences. The average BMS score for WT and GADD34$^{-/-}$ animals was 3.61±0.89 and 4.14±0.5 at week 1 and 4.89±0.42 and 5.18±1.08 at week 6, respectively (Fig 3A). Analysis of the BMS subscore also did not show any improvement in the stepping characteristics between WT and GADD34$^{-/-}$ mice (Fig 3A, inset). We next determined the effect of GADD34 deletion on the survival of CNS-resident cells acutely after SCI. There were no significant differences in the neuron- (Fig 3B; NSE and Map2a,b), astrocyte- (Fig 3C; glutamine synthetase and GFAP) and oligodendrocyte-specific (Fig 3D; Claudin 11, Olig2, MBP) transcript levels in GADD34$^{-/-}$ mice compared to WT mice at 72 hours post-SCI and is in contrast to our earlier study done in CHOP$^{-/-}$ mice [18].

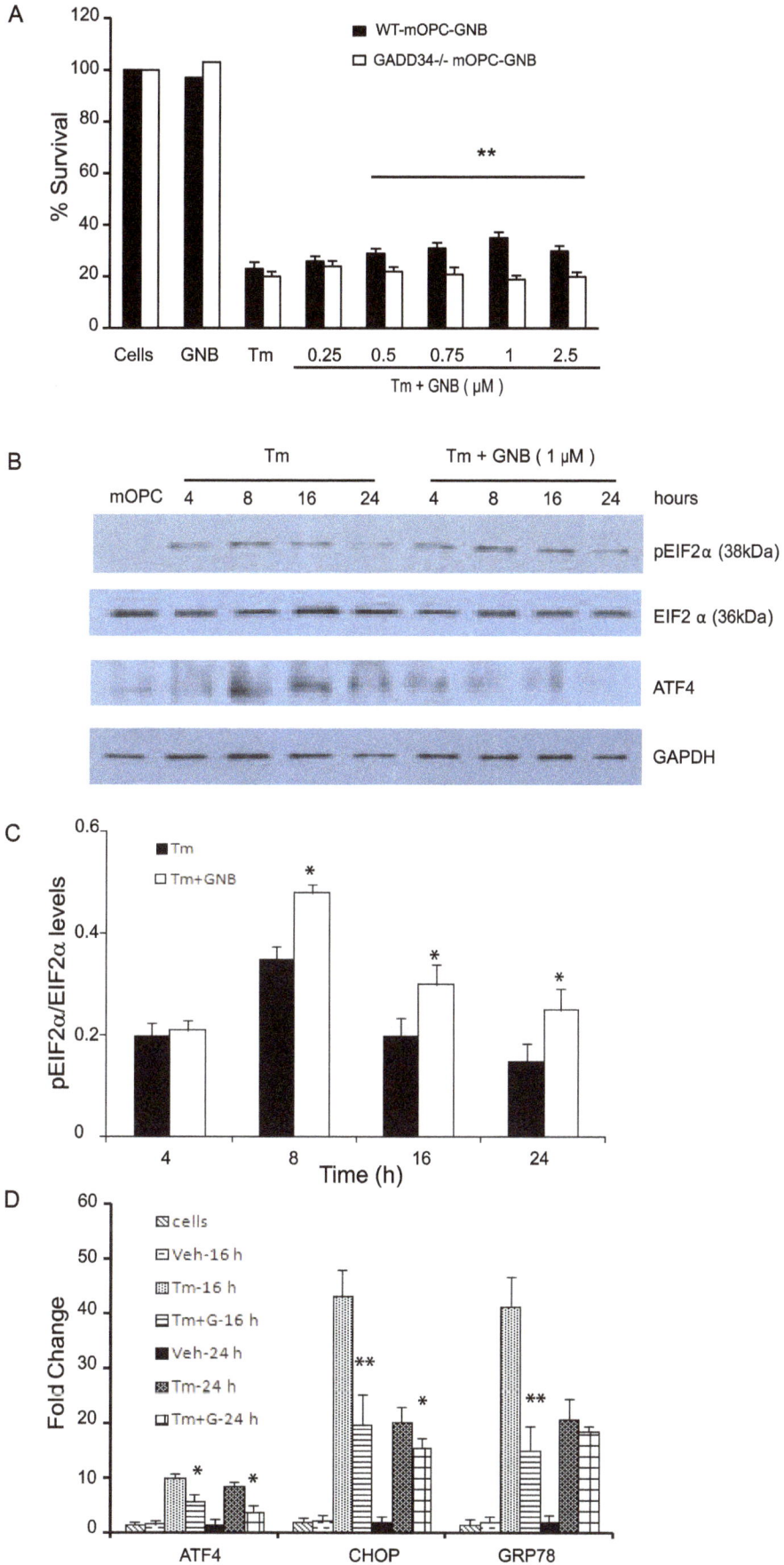

Figure 5. Effect of Guanabenz on WT and GADD34$^{-/-}$ mOPCs. (A) Guanabenz modestly increases survival of WT but not GADD34$^{-/-}$ mOPCs exposed to Tm (0.025 µg/ml) at 24 hours post-treatment assessed by MTT assay. (B,C) Western blot shows that guanabenz delays translational recovery in WT mOPCs treated with Tm. (D) Guanabenz leads to reduction in ATF4, CHOP and GRP78 transcript levels at 16 and 24 hours post-treatment. Data are the mean ± SD (n = 4; *p<0.05, ** p<0.01).

To potentially explain the lack of functional recovery, levels of spliced XBP1 and its downstream target genes were evaluated in WT and GADD34$^{-/-}$ mice 72 hours post-SCI to account for possible compensatory changes. A ~2 fold upregulation of XBP1 mRNA in WT mice is consistent with our previous study [18] and is similar to XBP1 levels in GADD34 $^{-/-}$ mice. Interestingly, transcript level of spliced XBP1 is significantly higher in GADD34$^{-/-}$ mice compared to wild type mice (Fig 4A). In addition, of the two target genes of XBP1 tested (EDEM1 and

ERDJ4) [32], ERDJ4 mRNA level is significantly reduced in GADD34$^{-/-}$ mice (Fig 4B).

Guanabenz modestly promotes the survival of mouse OPCs and delays translational recovery

Guanabenz, an FDA approved antihypertensive drug, was recently identified to display anti-prion activity [33]. It also successfully corrected proteostasis defects by selectively targeting GADD34 and disrupting the stress-induced dephosphorylation of

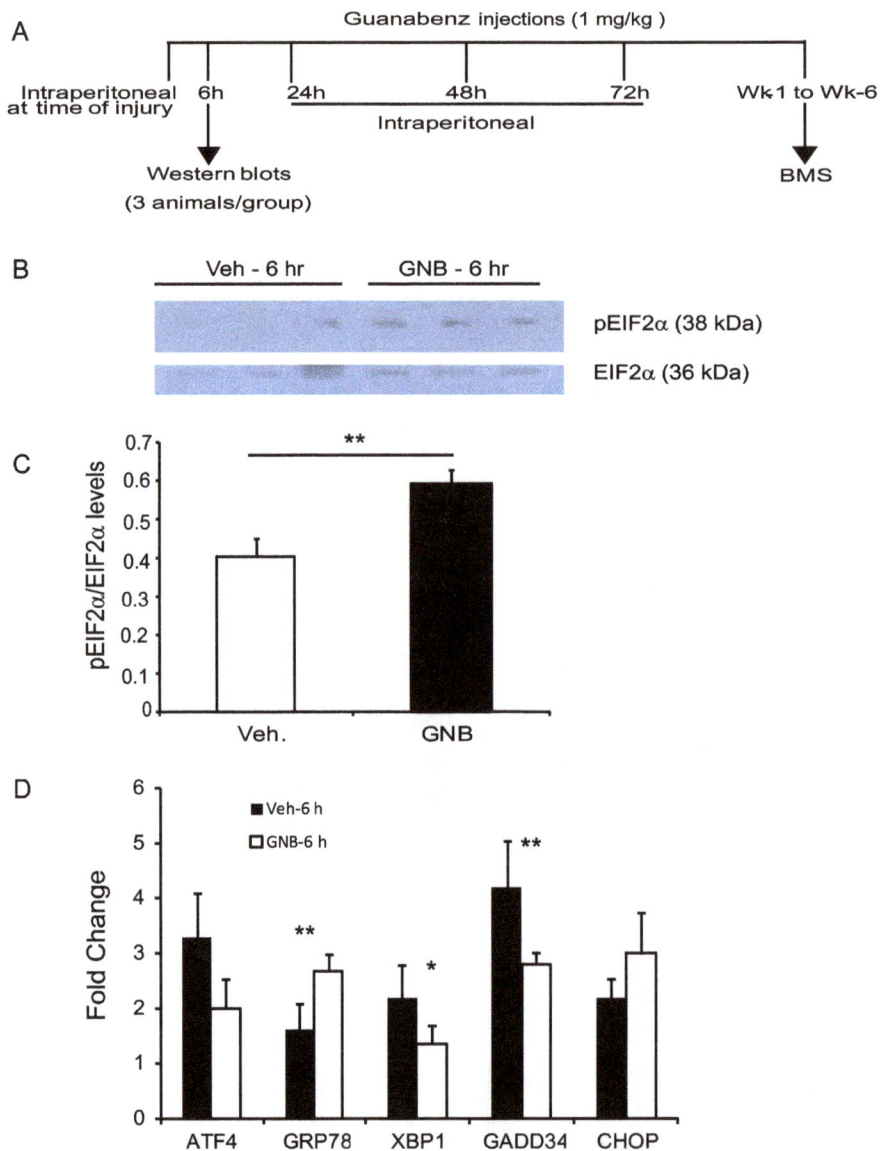

Figure 6. *In vivo* administration of guanabenz results in increased phosphorylation of eIF2α and modulates the key ERSR markers 6 hours post-SCI. (A) Schematic representation of guanabenz injections given at various time points-post SCI. (B,C) Western blots show that guanabenz significantly increases phosphorylated eIF2α levels at the injury epicenter of contused spinal cords. (D) Guanabenz leads to differential modulation in ERSR transcript levels as analyzed by qRT-PCR. Transcript levels are expressed as fold changes compared with respective levels in sham controls. Data are the mean ± SD [n = 3 (B,C); n = 4 (D), * p<0.05, **p<0.01].

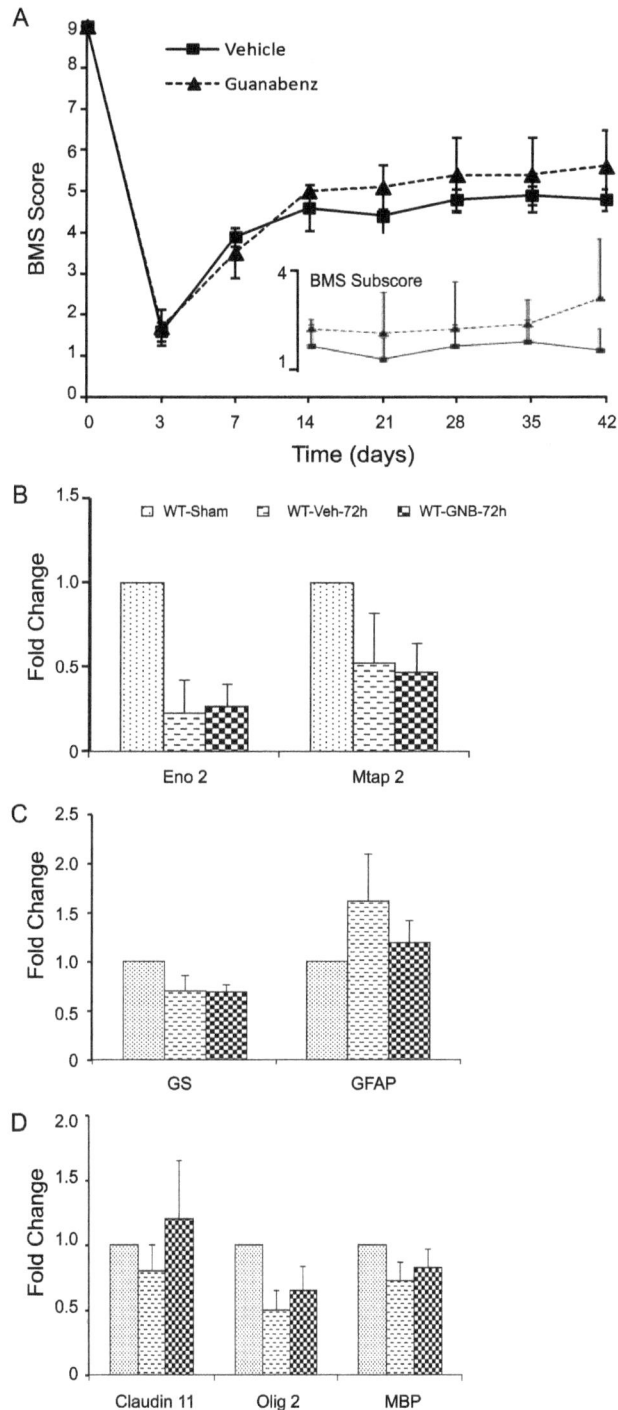

Figure 7. Administration of guanabenz does not enhance hindlimb locomotor function after SCI. (A) Open field BMS locomotor analyses performed weekly did not reveal any significant differences between vehicle- and guanabenz-treated animals. Analysis of BMS subscore also did not show any differences in stepping characteristics between the two groups (inset). Guanabenz treatment does not result in significant differences in the neuron- (B), astrocyte-(C) and oligodendrocyte-specific (D) transcript levels (as indicated) compared to vehicle-treated mice at 72 hours post-SCI. Data (A,B) are the mean ± SD (n = 6).

eIF2α in Hela cells [22]. In wild type mOPCs, guanabenz led to a maximum of 10% enhanced survival in response to cytotoxic ER stress induced by tunicamycin in a dose-dependent manner (Fig 5A). In contrast, GADD34$^{-/-}$ mOPCs did not show any improvement in survival (Fig 5A) indicating that the cytoprotective activity of guanabenz in ER-stressed cells results from its inhibition of GADD34.

To delineate the mechanism(s) involved, the direct effects of guanabenz on stressed mOPCs were determined. Translational attenuation, evidenced by increased eIF2α phosphorylation, 4 hours after addition of tunicamycin, was not changed by guanabenz. However, translational recovery in OPCs treated with tunicamycin was markedly delayed in the presence of guanabenz as determined by evident levels of p-eIF2α at 24 hours (Fig 5B,C). In addition, guanabenz significantly attenuated tunicamycin-induced expression of ATF4, CHOP and GRP78 levels (Fig 5B,D). These data indicate that guanabenz modestly promoted the survival of mOPCs by targeting the PERK-eIF2α pathway of ERSR, consistent with previous data in Hela cells [22].

Guanabenz enhances eIF2α phosphorylation after SCI

To analyze the effects of guanabenz on the PERK-eIF2α pathway in the injured mouse spinal cord, animals were treated with intraperitoneal injection of 1 mg/kg of the drug immediately after injury (Fig 6A). A significant increase in levels of p-eIF2α was seen in guanabenz-treated animals at six hours post-injury (Fig 6B, C) indicating its effectiveness in enhancing this SCI-induced ERSR. Lack of any detectable p-eIF2α levels in the sham samples (Fig 6B) is consistent with our earlier study [18] and confirms the specific activation of ERSR post-SCI at the injury epicenter. Interestingly, while guanabenz significantly attenuated the levels of GADD34 and XBP1 at 6 hours post-injury, there was no significant difference in the ATF4 and CHOP transcript levels between vehicle- and guanabenz-treated animals (Fig 6D). These data demonstrated that guanabenz penetrated the spinal cord tissue *in vivo*, enhanced the PERK-eIF2α signaling and differentially modulated the key ERSR effectors after SCI.

Guanabenz fails to improve functional recovery after SCI

We next examined whether administration of guanabenz that resulted in differential modulation of the ERSR could enhance functional recovery after SCI. Analysis of BMS scores comparing vehicle- and guanabenz-treated animals over a period of six weeks post-injury revealed no significant differences between the two groups. The average BMS score of guanabenz-treated animals was 3.5±0.61 at week 1 which increased to 5.6±0.89 at week 6. Similarly, the average BMS score of vehicle-treated animals was 3.9±0.22 at week 1 which increased modestly to 4.8±0.27 (Fig 7A) at week 6. Analysis of detailed stepping characteristics using BMS subscore also failed to show any significant improvement in locomotion in animals treated with guanabenz (Fig 7-A,inset). Furthermore, guanabenz treatment did not change the levels of neuron- (Fig 7B; NSE and Map2a,b), astrocyte- (Fig 7C; glutamine synthetase and GFAP) and oligodendrocyte-specific (Fig 7D; Claudin 11, Olig2, MBP) transcripts compared to vehicle-treated mice. These data are in contrast to our previous study where a significant increase in neuron- and oligodendrocyte-specific transcripts were observed with salubrinal treatment [22]. Thus, despite being pharmacologically active *in vivo*, guanabenz does not enhance functional recovery six weeks post-SCI.

		GADD34[-/-]	Guanabenz	Salubrinal
Target		GADD34-PP1c	GADD34-PP1c	CReP-PP1c GADD34-PP1c
pEIF2α levels		↑	↑	↑
mRNA levels	ATF4	↓	no diff.	↓
	CHOP	↓	no diff.	↓
	GADD34	—	↓	↓
	GRP78	↓	↑	↓
	XBP1	↓	↓	↓
Functional Recovery		No	No	Yes

Figure 8. Schematic diagram showing the transcriptional and translational comparison and differences between the GADD34[-/-], guanabenz- and salubrinal- treated mice.

Discussion

One of the major acute pathophysiological outcomes after SCI is oligodendrocyte loss both in humans [34,35] and rodents [36]. As white matter sparing is critical to functional recovery after thoracic contusive SCI [37], early pharmacological interventions that could reduce such oligodendrocyte loss might have important functional implications.

Recent studies established that the ERSR is induced in neurons, oligodendrocytes and astrocytes and plays a crucial role in the pathogenesis after SCI [17–20]. The ERSR-associated pro-apoptotic transcriptional regulator, CHOP was specifically upre-gulated in neurons and oligodendrocytes, but not in astrocytes of contused mouse spinal cords [18]. The sensitivity of oligodendro-cytes to ER-stress mediated apoptosis is likely due to their highly developed ER serving the need to produce vast amounts of lipids and proteins for myelin synthesis [38,39,40]. SCI-associated dysregulation of intracellular Ca^{2+} homeostasis is one of the triggers of oligodendrocyte ER stress [41]. Our study using CHOP[-/-] mice demonstrated a complete attenuation of the ERSR, increase in transcript levels of oligodendrocyte-specific MBP and claudin 11 at 72 hours and 6 weeks post-SCI, and a decrease in Olig2+ cells colocalized with cleaved caspase 3 at the injury epicenter and penumbra region [18]. Collectively, these data indicated that CHOP serves as an ERSR specific pro-apoptotic transcription factor in the context of SCI and oligodendrocytes are very sensitive to SCI-induced ER stress [18]. Pharmacological intervention into the PERK/CHOP arm of the ERSR with salubrinal, an inhibitor of the PP1 complex, similarly demonstrated recovery in hindlimb locomotor function [20] suggesting that restoration of ER homeostasis after SCI could be a therapeutically viable approach.

Guanabenz (a FDA-approved drug) was recently identified in a chemical screen of drugs for phase II clinical trials to exhibit anti-prion activity [33]. Importantly, guanabenz selectively inhibited the stress-induced eIF2α holophosphatase by targeting its regulatory subunit (PPP1R15A/GADD34) without affecting the constitutive one (PPP1R15B/CReP) [22]. We previously showed that salu-brinal, which targets both GADD34 and CReP, increased functional recovery after SCI [20]. We expected that guanabenz by selectively targeting the stress-induced GADD34, would similarly result in improved locomotor recovery post-SCI. However, guanabenz administration in vivo did not result in any reduction of locomotor deficits post-SCI. Comparing the effects of salubrinal [20] and guanabenz on SCI (Fig. 8), the simplest explanation would be that CReP is the more important phosphatase in the context of

SCI. More likely, each of these drugs may inhibit non-overlapping PP1 complexes with different spectra of substrates. Therefore, their effects on ERSR and apoptosis may differ. This interpretation is supported by the data showing guanabenz treatment led to attenuation of GADD34 and XBP1 transcript levels only, having no significant effect on ATF4 and CHOP transcript levels. This is in contrast to salubrinal where a complete attenuation of the ERSR was observed [20]. Alternatively, the duration of phospho eIF2α levels that remain after SCI may be crucial. Salubrinal-treated mOPCs showed enhanced protection against tunicamycin and pEIF2α levels returning to basal levels by 16 hours [20] whereas guanabenz-treated mOPCs showed significant higher levels of pEIF2α at 24 hours post-treatment. This delay in translational recovery and subsequent return to cellular homoeostasis in guanabenz-treated mOPCs perhaps is detrimental to their survival. Consistent with this interpretation, it is well known that the resultant survival or cell death outcome of the ERSR is dependent on injury duration and involvement of different components of the ERSR [42]. Finally, the treatment regimen used for in vivo guanabenz administration was based on our previous study [20] and perhaps needs more standardization due to the varied stability and efficiency of the drug in context of SCI. Mice with genetic ablation of GADD34, a direct target of guanabenz, also failed to show any improvement in locomotor outcome. Lack of functional improve-ment coinciding with differential effects on ERSR suggests that the complex interplay of various components of the ERSR pathway is essential for cell survival. Since, GADD34 is an essential component of a negative-feedback loop operating under stress, blocking GADD34 either by pharmacologic or genetic means possibly results in compensatory changes to the ERSR activity that accounts for lack of functional improvement post-SCI.

Acknowledgments

The authors would like to thank Kariena Andres for maintenance of transgenic mice and animal perfusions, Christine Yarberry for help with surgical procedures, Darlene A. Burke for help with statistical analyses, Johnny Morehouse and Jason Beare for BMS analyses and Allison Metz for culturing of mouse oligodendrocyte cells.

Author Contributions

Conceived and designed the experiments: SSO MH SRW. Performed the experiments: SSO AM. Analyzed the data: SSO AM MH SRW. Contributed reagents/materials/analysis tools: MH SRW. Wrote the paper: SSO MH SRW.

References

1. Kwon BK, Tetzlaff W, Grauer Jn, Beiner J, Vaccaro AR (2004) Pathophysiology and pharmacologic treatment of acute spinal cord injury. Spine Journal 4: 451–464.

2. Simon MC, Sharif S, Tan PR, LaPlaca CM (2009) Spinal cord contusion causes acute plasma membrane damage. Journal of Neurotrauma 26: 563–574.

3. Baptiste DC, Fehlings MG (2007) Update on the treatment of spinal cord injury. Progress in Brain Research 161: 217–233.

4. Rowland JW, Hawryluk GW, Kwon B, Fehlings MG (2008) Current status of acute spinal cord injury pathophysiology and emerging therapies: promise on the horizon. Neurosurgery Focus 25 (5): E2.

5. Tator CH (2006) Review of treatment trials in human spinal cord injury: issues, difficulties, and recommendations. Journal of Neurosurgery 59: 957–987.

6. Hurlbert RJ, Hadley MN, Walters BC, Aarabi B, Dhall SS, et al. (2013) Pharmacological therapy for acute spinal cord injury. Neurosurgery 72 (3): 93–105.

7. Schroder M (2008) Endoplasmic reticulum stress responses. Cellular and Molecular Life Sciences 65: 862–894.

8. Tabas I, Ron D (2011) Integrating mechanisms of apoptosis induced by endoplasmic reticulum stress. Nature Cellular Biology 13: 184–190.

9. Yoshida H, Matsui T, Yamamota A, Okada T, Mori Kazatoshi (2001) XBP1 mRNA is induced by ATF6 and spliced by IRE1 in response to ER stress to produce a highly active transcription factor. Cell 107: 881–891.

10. Haze K, Yoshida H, Yanagi H, Yura T, Mori K (1999) Mammalian transcription factor ATF6 is synthesized as a transmembrane protein and activated by proteolysis in response to endoplasmic reticulum stress. Molecular Biology of Cell 10: 3787–3799.

11. Lee YY, Cevallos RC, Jan E (2009) An upstream open reading frame regulates translation of GADD34 during cellular stresses that induce eIF2alpha phosphorylation. Journal of Biological Chemistry 13: 6661–6673.

12. Hollander MC, Zhan Q, Bae I, Fornace AJ Jr (1997) Mammalian GADD34, an apoptosis- and DNA damage-inducible gene. Journal of Biological Chemistry 272 (21): 13731–13737.

13. Adler HT, Chinery R, Wu DY, Kussick SJ, Payne JM, et al. (1999) Leukemic HRX fusion proteins inhibit GADD34-induced apoptosis and associate with the GADD34 and hSNF5/INI1 proteins. Molecular Cell Biology 19: 7050–7060.

14. Marciniak SJ, Yun CY, Oyadomari S, Novoa I, Zhang Y, et al. (2004) CHOP induces death by promoting protein synthesis and oxidation in the stressed endoplasmic reticulum. Genes and Development 18: 3066–3077.

15. Lin W, Kunkler PE, Harding HP, Ron D, Kraig RP, et al. (2008) Enhanced integrated stress response promotes myelinating oligodendrocyte survival in response to interferon-gamma. American Journal of Pathology 173 (5): 1508–1517.

16. D'Antonio M, Musner N, Scapin C, Ungaro D, Carro UD, et al. (2013) Resetting translational homeostasis restores myelination in Charcot-Marie-Tooth disease type 1B mice. Journal of Experimental Medicine 210 (4): 821–38.

17. Penas C, Guzmán MS, Verdú E, Forés J, Navarro X, et al. (2007) Spinal cord injury induces endoplasmic reticulum stress with different cell-type dependent response. Journal of Neurochemistry 102: 1242–1255.

18. Saraswat-Ohri S, Maddie MA, Zhao Y, Qiu MS, Hetman M, et al. (2011) Attenuating the endoplasmic reticulum stress response improves functional recovery after spinal cord injury. Glia 59: 1489–1502.

19. Valenzuela V, Collyer E, Armentano D, Parsons GB, Court FA, et al. (2012) Activation of the unfolded protein response enhances motor recovery after spinal cord injury. Cell Death and Disease 16: e272. doi: 10.1038/cddis.2012.8.

20. Saraswat-Ohri S, Hetman M, Whittemore SR (2013) Restoring endoplasmic reticulum homeostasis improves functional recovery after spinal cord injury. Neurobiology of Disease 58: 29–37.

21. Saraswat-Ohri S, Maddie MA, Zhang Y, Shields CB, Hetman M, et al. (2012) Deletion of the pro-apoptotic endoplasmic reticulum stress response effector CHOP does not result in improved locomotor function after severe contusive spinal cord injury. Journal of Neurotrauma 29: 579–688.

22. Tsaytler P, Harding HP, Ron D, Bertolotti A (2011) Selective inhibition of a regulatory subunit of protein phosphatase 1 restores proteostasis. Science 332: 91–94.

23. Dincman TA, Beare JE, Saraswat-Ohri S, Whittemore SR (2012) Isolation of cortical mouse oligodendrocyte precursor cells. Journal of Neuroscience Methods 30: 219–226.

24. Hirota M, Kitagaki M, Itagaki H, Aiba S (2006) Quantitative measurement of spliced XBP1 mRNA as an indicator of ER stress. Journal of Toxicology Science 31: 149–156.

25. Scheff SW, Rabchevsky AG, Fugaccia I, Main JA, Lumpp JE Jr. (2003) Experimental modeling of spinal cord injury characterization of a force-defined injury device. Journal of Neurotrauma 20: 179–193.

26. Benton RL, Maddie MA, Minnillo DR, Hagg T, Whittemore SR (2008) Griffonia simplicifolia isolectin B4 identifies a specific subpopulation of angiogenic blood vessels following contusive spinal cord injury in the adult mouse. Journal of Comparative Neurology 507 (1): 1031–1052.

27. Han S, Arnold SA, Sithu SD, Mahoney ET, Geralds JT, et al. (2010) Rescuing vasculature with intravenous angiopoietin-1 and $\alpha v\beta 3$ integrin peptide is protective after spinal cord injury. Brain 133: 1026–42.

28. Basso DM, Fisher LC, Anderson AJ, Jakeman LB, McTigue DM, et al. (2006) Basso mouse scale for locomotion detects differences in recovery after spinal cord injury in five common mouse strains. Journal of Neurotrauma 23 (5): 635–659.

29. Novoa I, Zhang Y, Zeng H, Jungreis R, Harding HP, et al. (2003) Stress-induced gene expression requires programmed recovery from translational repression. EMBO Journal 3: 1180–1187.

30. Brush MH, Weiser DC, Shenolikar S (2003) Growth arrest and DNA damage-inducible protein GADD34 targets protein phosphatase 1 alpha to the endoplasmic reticulum and promotes dephosphorylation of the alpha subunit of eukaryotic translation initiation factor 2. Molecular and Cellular Biology 23: 1292–1303.

31. Kojima E, Takeuchi A, Haneda M, Yagi A, Hasegawa T (2003) The function of GADD34 is a recovery from a shutoff of protein synthesis induced by ER stress: elucidation by GADD34-deficient mice. FASEB Journal 17: 1573–1575.

32. Lee A-H, Iwakoshi NN, Glimcher LH (2003) XBP-1 regulates a subset of endoplasmic reticulum resident chaperone genes in the unfolded protein response. Molecular and Cellular Biology 23: 7448–7459.

33. Tribouillard-Tanvier D, Beringue V, Desban N, Gug F Bach S (2008) Antihypertensive drug guanabenz is active in vivo against both yeast and mammalian prions. PLoS one 3: e1981.

34. Emery E, Aldana P, Bunge B, Puckett W, Srinivasan A, et al. (1998) Apoptosis after traumatic spinal cord injury. Journal of Neurosurgery-+ 89: 911–920.

35. Guest JD, Hiester ED, Bunge RP (2005) Demyelination and Schwann cell response adjacent to injury epicenter cavities following chronic human spinal cord injury. Experimental Neurology 192: 384–393.

36. Almad A, Sahinkaya FR, McTique DM (2011) Oligodendrocyte fate after spinal cord injury. Neurotherapeutics 8: 262–273.

37. Magnuson DSK, Trinder TC, Zhang YP, Burke D, Morassutti DJ, et al. (1999) Comparing deficits following excitotoxic and contusion injuries in the thoracic and lumbar spinal cord of the adult rat. Experimental Neurology 156: 191–204.

38. D'Antonio M, Feltri ML, Wrabetz L (2009) Myelin under stress. Journal of Neuroscience Research 87: 3241–3249.

39. Lin W, Popko B (2009) Endoplasmic reticulum stress in disorders of myelinating cells. Nature Neuroscience 12: 379–385.

40. Monk KR, Voas MG, Franzini-Armstrong C, Hakkinen IS, Talbot WS (2013) Mutation of sec63 in zebrafish causes defects in myelinated axons and liver pathology. Disease Models & Mechanisms 6: 135–145.

41. McTigue D, Tripathi RB (2008) The life, death, and replacement of oligodendrocytes in the adult CNS. Journal of Neurochemistry 107: 1–19.

42. Oyadomari S, Mori M (2004) Roles of CHOP/GADD153 in endoplasmic reticulum stress. Cell Death and Differentiation 11: 381–389.

3

Efficacy of a Metalloproteinase Inhibitor in Spinal Cord Injured Dogs

Jonathan M. Levine[1]*, Noah D. Cohen[2], Michael Heller[3], Virginia R. Fajt[4], Gwendolyn J. Levine[5], Sharon C. Kerwin[1], Alpa A. Trivedi[6], Thomas M. Fandel[6], Zena Werb[7], Augusta Modestino[3], Linda J. Noble-Haeusslein[6,8]

1 Department of Small Animal Clinical Sciences, College of Veterinary Medicine and Biomedical Sciences, Texas A&M University, College Station, Texas, United States of America, 2 Department of Large Animal Clinical Sciences, College of Veterinary Medicine and Biomedical Sciences, Texas A&M University, College Station, Texas, United States of America, 3 Department of Bioengineering, University of California San Diego, San Diego, California, United States of America, 4 Department of Veterinary Physiology and Pharmacology, College of Veterinary Medicine and Biomedical Sciences, Texas A&M University, College Station, Texas, United States of America, 5 Department of Veterinary Pathobiology, College of Veterinary Medicine and Biomedical Sciences, Texas A&M University, College Station, Texas, United States of America, 6 Department of Neurological Surgery, University of California San Francisco, San Francisco, California, United States of America, 7 Department of Anatomy, University of California San Francisco, San Francisco, California, United States of America, 8 Department of Physical Therapy and Rehabilitation, University of California San Francisco, San Francisco, California, United States of America

Abstract

Matrix metalloproteinase-9 is elevated within the acutely injured murine spinal cord and blockade of this early proteolytic activity with GM6001, a broad-spectrum matrix metalloproteinase inhibitor, results in improved recovery after spinal cord injury. As matrix metalloproteinase-9 is likewise acutely elevated in dogs with naturally occurring spinal cord injuries, we evaluated efficacy of GM6001 solubilized in dimethyl sulfoxide in this second species. Safety and pharmacokinetic studies were conducted in naïve dogs. After confirming safety, subsequent pharmacokinetic analyses demonstrated that a 100 mg/kg subcutaneous dose of GM6001 resulted in plasma concentrations that peaked shortly after administration and were sustained for at least 4 days at levels that produced robust *in vitro* inhibition of matrix metalloproteinase-9. A randomized, blinded, placebo-controlled study was then conducted to assess efficacy of GM6001 given within 48 hours of spinal cord injury. Dogs were enrolled in 3 groups: GM6001 dissolved in dimethyl sulfoxide (n = 35), dimethyl sulfoxide (n = 37), or saline (n = 41). Matrix metalloproteinase activity was increased in the serum of injured dogs and GM6001 reduced this serum protease activity compared to the other two groups. To assess recovery, dogs were *a priori* stratified into a severely injured group and a mild-to-moderate injured group, using a Modified Frankel Scale. The Texas Spinal Cord Injury Score was then used to assess long-term motor/sensory function. In dogs with severe spinal cord injuries, those treated with saline had a mean motor score of 2 (95% CI 0–4.0) that was significantly (P<0.05; generalized linear model) less than the estimated mean motor score for dogs receiving dimethyl sulfoxide (mean, 5; 95% CI 2.0–8.0) or GM6001 (mean, 5; 95% CI 2.0–8.0). As there was no independent effect of GM6001, we attribute improved neurological outcomes to dimethyl sulfoxide, a pleotropic agent that may target diverse secondary pathogenic events that emerge in the acutely injured cord.

Editor: Hatem E. Sabaawy, Rutgers-Robert wood Johnson Medical School, United States of America

Funding: This study was supported by funds from National Institutes of Health R01NS039278 (Supp)(www.nih.gov) and US Department of Defense SC100140 (http://cdmrp.army.mil/funding/_. Dr. Cohen was supported in part by the Link Equine Research Endowment at Texas A&M University. The funders had no role in study design, data collection and analysis, decision to publish, or preparation of this manuscript.

Competing Interests: The authors have declared that no competing interests exist.

* E-mail: jlevine@cvm.tamu.edu

Introduction

Matrix metalloproteinases (MMPs) are endopeptidases that degrade the extracellular matrix [1]. Several members of the MMP family, including MMP-9 (gelatinase B) and MMP-12, have been implicated in early secondary pathogenesis after spinal cord injury (SCI) [2–4]. These MMPs are released by local cells as well as by infiltrating leukocytes and result in reduced cell-cell adhesion, disruption of the blood-spinal cord barrier, up-regulation of pro-inflammatory cytokines, and demyelination [1,4,5].

Early blockade of MMPs confers neuroprotection after SCI [2,6,7]. Short-term administration of the broad-spectrum MMP inhibitor, GM6001, results in sparing of white matter and improves locomotor function when the drug is given over the first 3 days post-injury [2]. Several lines of evidence suggest that one likely target of GM6001 is MMP-9. This protease is not actively expressed in the uninjured spinal cord and is up-regulated over the first 3 days post-injury, corresponding to the time-course for infiltration of neutrophils [8]. While there are local sources of MMP-9, including glia and endothelial cells, neutrophil depletion studies confirm that these leukocytes are the major source of MMP-9 in the acutely injured cord [7]. As this protease is not complexed with tissue inhibitor of MMP-1, degranulation of neutrophils results in release of activated MMP-9 [9], which then may disrupt the barrier and facilitate transmigration of leukocytes into the injured spinal cord. It thus is not surprising that early administration of GM6001 attenuates the trafficking of neutrophils into the injured spinal cord and stabilizes the blood-spinal cord barrier [2]. There are other members of the MMP family that are also determinants of recovery after SCI including MMP-12 and ADAM-8 (a disintegrin and metalloprotease domain) [3]. Thus, broad inhibitors of MMPs may offer greater benefit than specific inhibitors of these proteases.

In this study, we have used dimethyl sulfoxide (DMSO) in combination with GM6001 [10,11]. While DMSO is commonly used as a vehicle to increase solubility of a drug, it has been reported to have neuroprotective properties in traumatic brain injury and SCI [12,13]. The putative neuroprotective activity of DMSO is thought to arise from its ability to block voltage-sensitive sodium channels and calcium influx into cells, and mitigate opening of ionotropic channels that are activated by glutamate [14].

Few studies have considered a pre-clinical platform involving dogs with naturally occurring SCIs resulting from intervertebral disk herniation (IVDH) [15–17]. This approach mimics pathologic aspects of human SCI including compressive/contusive injuries and a pro-inflammatory response that includes the infiltration of neutrophils and up-regulation of MMP-9 [18–20]. Moreover, these naturally-occurring injuries provide a means for studying therapeutics in the challenging context of varying degrees of injury severity, common in human SCI, but without confounding factors such as anesthetics that are necessary during creation of injury in experimental models.

Here we evaluate the efficacy of GM6001 in dogs with IVDH. Based on a double-blind, randomized, placebo-controlled trial, consisting of 3 groups (GM6001 in DMSO, DMSO alone, or saline) we show enhanced neurological recovery in dogs sustaining severe SCIs when treated acutely with GM6001 solubilized in DMSO or DMSO alone, relative to the saline group. Such findings implicate DMSO in improving neurological recovery, which is consistent with its reported ability to attenuate secondary pathogenic events in various models of neurotrauma [14].

Materials and Methods

Study Design and Inclusion Criteria

A preliminary drug tolerance study was constructed based on Food and Drug Administration guidelines (http://www.fda.gov/AnimalVeterinary/default.htm) and performed in 4 healthy, purpose-bred Beagles. Ten healthy, purpose-bred Beagles were obtained to evaluate pharmacokinetics (PK); this sample size was based on similar animal studies and general recommendations for canine PK investigations [21].

Guidelines for the conduct of SCI trials developed by the International Campaign for Cures of Spinal Cord Injury Paralysis were utilized to assist with the design of a randomized, double-blinded (clinicians and clients were unaware of treatment group), placebo-controlled canine trial including inclusion/exclusion criteria, randomization protocol, data handling, and the a priori definition of outcome metrics and statistical approaches.[22]. Consolidated Standards of Reporting Trials (CONSORT) Statement Guidelines were used to assist with trial performance and data reporting [23,24]. Client-owned dogs with IVDH-associated SCI, admitted to the Texas A&M University Veterinary Medical Teaching Hospital between September 2008 and February 2012, were recruited. The study interval was selected to generate a sample size of >100 dogs, which was considered robust based on previous human phase II and III SCI studies [25,26], animal model studies of SCI using MMP blockers [2], and completed canine SCI studies [27,28]. A formal power calculation was not

performed due to the absence of a phase I canine study examining the effects of GM6001.

Dogs had to meet the following criteria to be included in the clinical trial population: 1) duration of SCI was required to be ≤48 hours; 2) IVDH-associated SCI had to result in non-ambulatory paraparesis or paraplegia at enrollment; 3) IVDH-associated SCI had to be identified between the T8-L6 vertebral articulations and treated via surgical decompression. The exclusion criteria were: 1) concurrent disseminated neoplasia or systemic inflammation; 2) a history of recent breeding/pregnancy; and, 3) glucocorticoid treatment within 7 days of SCI.

The primary outcome of the clinical trial was a validated ordinal SCI score (the Texas Spinal Cord Injury Score [TSCIS]) conducted at 42 days post-injury [29]. The secondary outcome was TSCIS at 3 days after SCI. Dogs were stratified into those with behaviorally severe SCI (absent pelvic limb movement and deep nociception) and those with mild-to-moderate SCI (intact pelvic limb deep nociception with or without movement) at study entry to examine primary and secondary outcomes. This a priori stratification was utilized because a substantially lower proportion of dogs with severe SCI recover independent ambulation at long-term follow-up time-points (approximately 50–60%) in comparison to dogs with mild-to-moderate SCI (approximately 85 to 95%); thus, injury severity might influence the ability to detect treatment-related effects [30–33].

Ethics Statement

All animal procedures were approved by the Texas A&M University Institutional Animal Care and Use Committee (AUP 2007–115; AUP 2011–057; AUP-2011–145) and in the case of client-owned dogs were performed with signed consent. All studies adhered to the National Institutes of Health Guide for the Care and Use of Laboratory Animals.

Drug Preparation, Drug Tolerance, and Pharmacokinetic Procedures

For all canine studies, GM6001 (SAI Advantium, Hyderabad, India) was dissolved in 90% DMSO (Domoso, Fort Dodge Corp, Fort Dodge, IA) at a concentration of 250 mg/mL. The solution was sterilized using a 25-mm syringe filter with 0.22-μm HT Tuffryn membrane (Pall Corporation, East Hills, NY).

Dogs, participating in the drug tolerance study, were acclimatized for 14 days and then randomized as follows: DMSO (at a volume equivalent to that present in a 100 mg/kg GM6001 treatment), 100 mg/kg GM6001, 150 mg/kg GM6001, or 300 mg/kg GM6001 subcutaneously (SC) every 12 hours for 3 days. The doses of GM6001 were selected to exceed those reported previously in a murine model of SCI [2]. A SC route of administration was selected as 1) GM6001 does not remain solubilized in DMSO when exposed to hydrophilic solutions such as blood, prohibiting intravenous delivery and 2) intraperitoneal drug administration is not generally permitted in client-owned dogs at our institution, due to challenges in managing any local drug reactions. Adverse event monitoring was performed for 7 days following the completion of drug administration. All dogs had physical examinations, injection site evaluations, and assessment of food and water intake twice daily. A complete blood count, serum biochemistry profile, urinalysis, and coagulation profile were performed 3 and 7 days following the completion of drug administration. Following the completion of this study, the vehicle and 300 mg/kg GM6001 dogs were euthanized via intravenous administration of 120 mg/kg pentobarbital (Fatal Plus, Vortech Pharmaceuticals, Dearborn, MI). The brain, heart, liver, kidney, lung, intestine, and injection sites were evaluated.

For PK assessments, a single 100 mg/kg SC administration of GM6001 was delivered in 5 dogs with 5 additional dogs receiving a second 100 mg/kg SC of GM6001, 12 hours following the first dose. In dogs with single dosing, serial plasma samples were obtained at 5, 15, and 30 minutes and 1, 2, 3, 6, 12, 24, 36, 48, and 96 hours after GM6001 delivery. In dogs with multiple dosing, blood samples were collected shortly after the second dose, and then at 24, 48, 72, and 96 hours. All samples were stored in a $-80^{o}C$ freezer until analyzed by high performance chromatography (Thermo Electron Co., Waltham, MA) and tandem mass spectroscopy (MDS-Sciex/Applied Biosystems API3000, Concord, ONT) (LC-MS/MS). Concentrations of GM6001 (m/z $389.0\rightarrow356.0$) were determined, using MMP Inhibitor III (m/z $364.0\rightarrow356.0$, Calbiochem, Billerica, MA) as the internal standard. A standard curve was created with blank dog plasma at concentrations 10.0 to 10,204.0 ng/mL, with linear regression and weighting of concentrations ($1/x^2$). After thawing and addition of internal standard (300 µL of 100 ng/mL in 0.5% acetic acid in methanol), plasma samples or standards (100 µL) were centrifuged and reconstituted with 30/70 methanol/10 mM ammonium formate buffer, pH 3.0, for protein precipitation. Supernatant (100 µL) was collected, vortexed, and refrigerated until injection on LC-MS/MS. The mobile phase consisted of 0.1% formic acid in deionized water (A) and acetonitrile/methanol/formic acid (40:60:0.1, v/v/v) (B) with a flow rate of 0.30 mL/minute using a linear gradient starting at 40% B from 0 to 0.01 minutes, to 80% B at 1.5 minutes, to 90% B at 3.5 minutes, to 40% B at 3.6 minutes, with a total run time of 5 minutes.

Randomized, Placebo Controlled Study in Dogs with IVDH-associated SCI

Dogs, enrolled in the clinical trial, had physical and neurological examinations, complete blood count and serum biochemistry profile. Anesthesia was induced with propofol (Rapinovet, Schering-Plough Animal Health Corp, Union, NJ) and maintained with inhalant sevoflurane (SevoFlo, Abbott Laboratories, North Chicago, IL). Diagnostic imaging consisting of myelography, computed tomography (CT), or MRI was performed to identify IVDH. Cerebrospinal fluid (CSF) was collected from the cisterna magna for routine analysis and a 200-µL aliquot was stored at $-80^{o}C$ for determination of MMP-2/MMP-9 activity. Six mL of whole blood were obtained at the time of CSF collection and 3 days following treatment delivery; serum was isolated and frozen at $-80^{o}C$.

Immediately after collection of CSF and blood, dogs were randomized to receive 100 mg/kg GM6001+ DMSO, DMSO, or saline placebo. The dose of both DMSO and saline was 0.4 mL/kg, a volume equivalent to that of 100 mg/kg GM6001+DMSO; this approach was taken to maintain blinding. A randomization sequence was developed prior to the initiation of this trial and randomization was accomplished by blocking the dogs by gender status in a 1:1:1 ratio to each of the treatment groups. Sealed envelopes contained treatment allocations and were delivered to a central location where treatments were formulated by individuals not involved in the assessment of animals. Treatments were covered and marked only with animal identifiers to ensure blinding.

Following surgical decompression, all dogs were recovered in an intensive care unit for 24 hours and during that time were provided post-operative opioid analgesia and bladder evacuation. Physical rehabilitation protocols were standardized for dogs participating in this study. Dogs received thoracic limb and pelvic limb passive range of motion exercises beginning 24 hours post-operatively and until dogs could independently ambulate. Each limb was gently flexed and extended at the carpal, elbow, and hip joints in 3 sets of 10 repetitions, 2 times daily. Supported standing exercises were performed twice daily for 5 minutes by placing a sling immediately cranial to the pelvic limbs and continued until dogs could independently ambulate. Dogs that were non-ambulatory were walked using a sling placed immediately cranial to the pelvic limbs for 5 minutes twice daily. Independently ambulatory dogs were permitted to walk on a leash for 5 minutes 3–4 times per day during hospitalization and were allowed to continue this activity until 42-day re-check. Participating dogs were housed in cages that permitted limited additional activity until 42-day re-check evaluation.

Neurological Assessments

Clinicians responsible for neurologic scoring were blinded to treatment assignments. Two ordinal SCI scores were used to address injury severity at study entry, day 3 post-treatment, and day 42 post-treatment. In both scoring systems, dogs were considered ambulatory if they could spontaneously rise, bear weight, and take at least 10 steps without falling. Dogs that were non-ambulatory had pelvic limb movement evaluated using tail support. Postural responses were evaluated by placing the dorsum of the pes on a non-slick surface while manually supporting the animal and waiting for limb correction. Pelvic limb deep and superficial nociception were evaluated by applying hemostats to a nail-bed or interdigital webbing, respectively and evaluating for the presence of a behavioral or physiological response.

A modified Frankel scale (MFS) was developed to broadly parallel the American Spinal Cord Injury Association Impairment Scale (AIS) [15,29]. Dogs were scored as paraplegic with absent deep nociception (0; equivalent to AIS A), paraplegic with absent superficial nociception (1; equivalent to AIS B), paraplegic with intact nociception (2; equivalent to AIS B), or non-ambulatory with identifiable pelvic limb movement (3; equivalent to AIS C). The MFS was not a primary trial outcome, but instead was used to describe the baseline population (overall and by treatment group) and to stratify the study population for analysis.

The Texas Spinal Cord Injury Score (TSCIS) was used to assess pelvic limb gait, posture and nociception. This is a more refined scale than the MFS [15] with a larger array of sub-categories, including gait assessment that parallels the Basso, Beattie, Bresnahan Scale [34]. The TSCIS gait score ranges from 0 to 6 in each pelvic limb and correlates to the degree of limb protraction and weight bearing. The gait classifications include: no voluntary movement seen when the dog is supported (score = 0); intact limb protraction with no ground clearance (1); intact limb protraction with inconsistent ground clearance (2); intact protraction with ground clearance >75% of steps (3); ambulatory with consistent ground clearance and significant paresis-ataxia that results in occasional falling (4); ambulatory with consistent ground clearance and mild paresis-ataxia that does not result in falling (5); and normal gait (6). Pelvic limb postural responses using the TSCIS were scored in each limb as absent (0), delayed (1, correction occurred >1 second after positioning), and present (2). Nociception was scored in each limb as absent (0), deep nociception only present (1), or both deep and superficial nociception present (2).

Magnetic Resonance Imaging (MRI)

Vertebral column MRI was performed on enrolled dogs, except in cases where animals were evaluated outside of normal operating hours or the scanner was unavailable due to mechanical failure. Between September 2008 and July 2011, a 1.0 T system (Siemens Magnetom, Malvern, PA) was utilized to acquire images; for the remainder of the trial images were generated using a 3.0 T MRI

(Simens Verio, Malvern, PA). Dogs that received MRI had sagittal T2-weighted (T2W) images reviewed by 1 investigator (JML) using commercially available software (eFILM, Merge Healthcare, Chicago, IL) prior to un-blinding. The acquisition parameters for sagittal T2W images generated at 1T and 3T included a repetition time of 3500 ms, echo time of 90 ms, and slice thickness of 2.0 mm. The presence of spinal cord T2W hyperintensity was determined by visually comparing injured parenchyma to surrounding spinal cord. This technique has been used extensively in human and canine MRI studies and produces repeatable results that correlate with behavioral measures of SCI severity and recovery [35,36].

MMP-2/MMP-9 Activity in CSF and Serum

CSF and serum samples (n = 16/treatment group) were randomly selected at the end of the trial by computerized sorting on random numbers. Purpose-bred Beagle dogs (n = 5) were sampled as controls. Serum samples with overt hemolysis were excluded from analysis.

Activity of MMP-2 and MMP-9 in serum and CSF samples was assessed in a blinded manner using a previously developed electrophoretic method [37–39] that included a synthetic peptide (AAPPtec, Louisville, KY) (sequence: Ac-NGDPVGLTAGAGK-NH2), tagged with a fluorophore BODIPY-FL-SE (Invitrogen, Carlsbad, CA). The substrate was mixed with either serum or CSF, with phosphate buffered saline as the negative control. After reacting for 1 hour, aliquots were loaded onto 20% polyacrylamide gels and the samples were electrophoresed. Gels were imaged using a BioDoc-It M-26 transilluminator (UVP, Upland, CA, USA). The image was scanned in a Storm 840 workstation (Molecular Dynamics, Sunnyvale, CA, USA) with ImageQuant v5.2 software and fluorescent signal was quantified using ImageJ (1.440, National Institutes of Health, Bethesda, MD).

To assess ability of GM6001 to inhibit MMP-9, activity (described above) was determined using human recombinant MMP-9 (Sigma, St. Louis, MO) that was serially diluted in DMSO to final concentrations of 0.01 µM to 200 µM. Controls consisted of enzyme and substrate only and substrate and GM6001 only.

Statistical Analyses

Noncompartmental pharmacokinetic analysis was performed (Phoenix WinNonLin 6.3, Pharsight, St. Louis, MO), and estimates of the parameters of T_{max}, C_{max}, $T_{1/2}$, and area AUC_{0-obs} and $AUC_{0-\infty}$ were calculated for the single dose.

Activities of MMP-2/MMP-9 in CSF and serum were compared between healthy control dogs and the dogs with SCI using the Wilcoxon rank-sum test. The Wilcoxon rank-sum test was also used to compare CSF and serum MMP-2/MMP-9 activities between dogs with and without selected characteristics that were potential modifiers of MMP-2/MMP-9 (i.e., age, breed, sex, and markers of disease duration or severity). To compare serum MMP-2/MMP-9 values among treatment groups, the serum MMP-2/MMP-9 activities were converted to ranks, and the ranks were compared using a generalized linear model; multiple pair-wise comparisons between treatments were made using the method of Sidak. Model fit was assessed graphically using diagnostic plots of residuals.

For the clinical trial data, a strategy for analysis of data was developed a priori, including our decision to stratify the population based on SCI severity at admission. Baseline characteristics were compared among the 3 treatment groups to determine whether there was any evidence of differences among groups. Categorical variables were compared using chi-squared analysis and continuous or ordinal variables were compared using Kruskal-Wallis

tests. The primary outcome for the trial was the TSCIS score on day 42. The TSCIS on day 3 was considered a secondary outcome. The association of TSCIS with treatment group and other individual variables was assessed using generalized linear modeling. Individual variables significantly associated with TSCIS were analyzed using multivariable generalized linear modeling using maximum likelihood estimating methods. Multiple comparisons among groups were adjusted using the method of Sidak. Model fit was assessed graphically using diagnostic plots of residuals. Comparisons of proportions among treatments groups (e.g., frequency of adverse events) were made using chi-squared or, when appropriate, Fisher's exact tests. Significance was set at $P < 0.05$ for all analyses. Analyses were performed using S-PLUS statistical software (Version 8.2, TIBCO, Inc., Seattle, WA).

Results

GM6001 is Well Tolerated in Naive Dogs

We first addressed the safety of GM6001 using a dose tolerance study. Four healthy dogs were randomized to receive DMSO vehicle, 100 mg/kg GM6001, 150 mg/kg GM6001, or 300 mg/kg GM6001 SC every 12 hours for 3 days. Following drug delivery, all studied parameters were within normal limits, with the following exceptions: 1) increase in body temperature in all GM6001-treated dogs which peaked 6 days after treatment was completed (Fig. S1); 2) transient decrease in food consumption during the 3 days of drug delivery (mean percentage of food consumed, 64.5% ±12.9%) in comparison to the 3 days following delivery (mean percentage of food consumed, 91.7% ±16.3%); and 3) the presence of subcutaneous nodules at the drug delivery sites that regressed in size following delivery in all animals (Fig. S2). No lesions were detected via necropsy or histopathology in the dog that received vehicle. In the dog receiving 300 mg/kg GM6001 twice daily for 3 days, sites of subcutaneous drug deposition were surrounded by a connective tissue capsule with minimal inflammation; additionally, there was mild bile duct hyperplasia. The absence of substantial adverse events in this tolerance study suggested that GM6001 would have an acceptable safety profile in injured dogs.

GM6001 is Rapidly Detected in Plasma After Subcutaneous Administration

As the PK of GM6001 might differ from that in rodent [40], we determined the PK in normal dogs. GM6001, administered once at 100 mg/kg SC, was detected in plasma at 5 minutes in all dogs, with a mean time to peak concentration (T_{max}) of 0.7 hours (S.D. ±1.3 hours) (Fig. 1). The mean peak concentration (C_{max}) was 1370 ng/mL (S.D. ±361 ng/mL), mean apparent elimination half-life ($T_{1/2}$) was 524 hours (S.D. ±428 hours), and the mean plasma concentration of GM6001 at 96 hours was 80 ng/mL (S.D. ±20 ng/mL). Mean area under the curve (AUC) from time 0 to last observed concentration (AUC_{0-obs}) (16,100 hr*ng/mL ±2981) and mean AUC from time 0 to infinity ($AUC_{0-\infty}$) (58,225 hr*ng/mL ±37,054) resulted in an extrapolated percentage of AUC of 65%. The only notable adverse event was the presence of focal subcutaneous nodules that regressed with time. The GM6001 utilized in the clinical trial had marked in vitro MMP-9 inhibition at concentrations approximating those achieved in dog plasma 96 hours post-drug delivery (Fig. 2). As the objective was to target the acutely injured cord, we selected a single 100 mg/kg SC dose of GM6001 in dogs to achieve plasma drug concentrations which would peak almost immediately after delivery and be sustained at levels sufficient to inhibit MMPs in vitro for at least 96 hours following delivery.

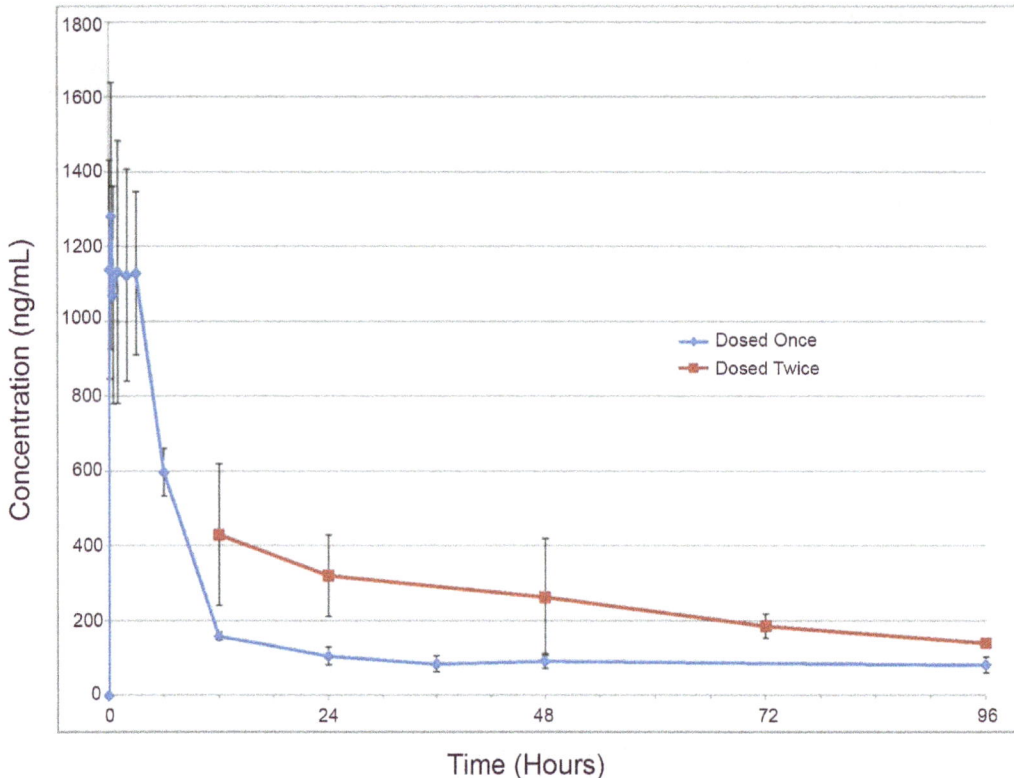

Figure 1. Pharmacokinetics of GM6001 in dogs. Administration of a single 100 mg/kg subcutaneous dose of GM6001 to dogs resulted in the rapid development of peak plasma drug concentrations with drug still detectable 96 hours post-delivery. Administration of a second dose of GM6001 to a sub-group of dogs 12 hours following initial drug delivery resulted in increased plasma drug concentrations at all assessed time points.

Clinical Trial Enrollment

Enrolled dogs were randomized to a saline placebo group (n = 38 dogs), a DMSO group (n = 37), and a GM6001 group (n = 33) (Fig. 3). Three dogs were euthanized prior to discharge from the hospital due to neurologic deterioration and 17 dogs did not return for 42-day follow-up examination. Of critical importance, there were no differences in baseline population characteristics such as breed, gender, or injury level among treatment groups, indicating that confounding based on these parameters was unlikely (Table 1).

Adverse Events in Spinal Cord Injured Dogs

Adverse events were recorded during hospitalization and were classified as fever, gastrointestinal, injection site, urinary, or other (Table S1). A significantly greater number of dogs in the GM6001 group had injection site reactions (45%; 15/33) relative to either the saline control dogs (5%; 2/38) or DMSO dogs (0%; 0/36) (P< 0.0001; Kruskal-Wallis test). These reactions were transient and consisted of focal dermal and subcutaneous swelling.

Increased MRI T2W Signal within the Spinal Cord is Associated with Poor Recovery

Vertebral column MRI was performed on 76/107 dogs enrolled in the clinical trial. In all cases, spinal cord compression associated with IVDH was identified with variable presence of increased T2W signal (27/76 dogs) within the spinal cord (Fig. 4). High spinal cord T2 signal, suggestive of contusion, was significantly more common in dogs with severe SCIs (MFS = 0; 11/13) compared with those with mild-to-moderate SCIs (MFS>0; 16/

63) (P = 0.0001; Fisher's exact test). Dogs with increased T2W spinal cord also had significantly (P<0.0001; generalized linear model) poorer recovery of function 42 days following SCI (estimated TSCIS 9, 95% CI 7–12) compared to dogs with normal spinal cord T2W signal (estimated TSCIS 15, 95% CI 14–17). The presence of compressive SCI with variable presence of T2W hyperintensity in the spinal cord parallels what is found on MRI in humans with traumatic myelopathy, including relationships between function and spinal cord T2 signal [36].

Characterization of Cells in CSF Following Spinal Cord Injury

CSF was acquired immediately prior to drug or placebo delivery in 102/107 (95%) clinical trial dogs; all 5 un-injured control animals also had CSF collected. Total nucleated cell count was significantly (P = 0.0034, Wilcoxon rank-sum test) higher in SCI dogs (median = 3 cells/μL, range 0–71) compared with control dogs (median = 0 cells/μL, range 0–1). Amongst dogs with CSF pleocytosis (total nucleated cell count >5 cells/μL), neutrophils were most frequently identified (median 43%, range 2–89%), followed by mononuclear cells (median 25%, range 6–95%) and lymphocytes (median 18%, range 4–70%). CSF red blood cell count was likewise significantly (P = 0.0022, Wilcoxon rank-sum test) increased in dogs with SCI (median 48 cells/μL, range 0–15,040). Together, these findings support a pro-inflammatory state in the acutely injured canine spinal cord.

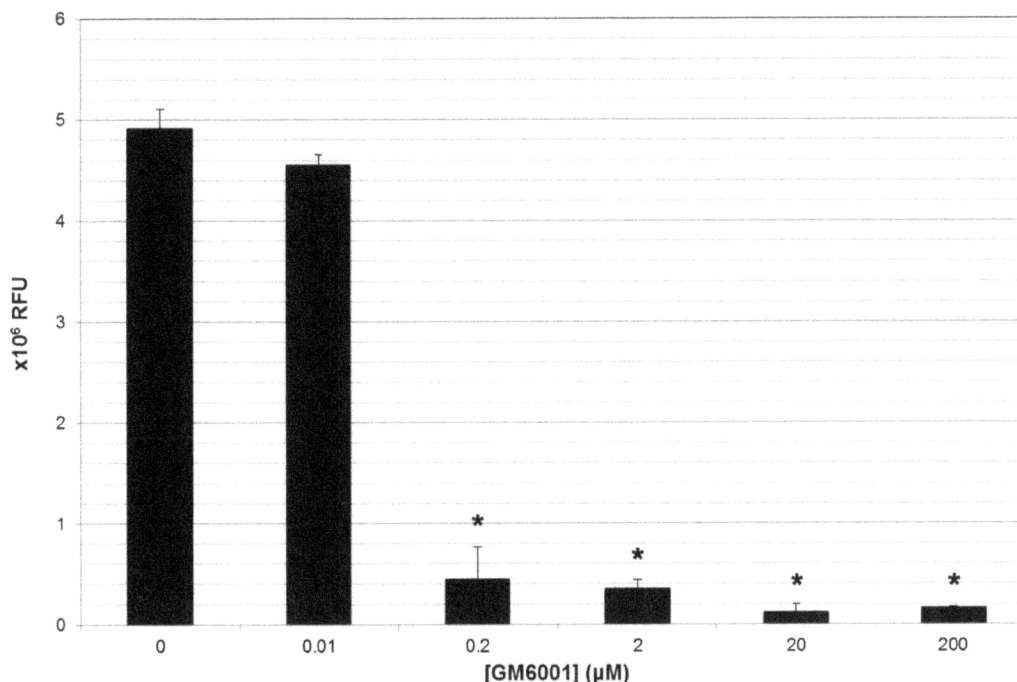

Figure 2. *In vitro* inhibition of MMP-9 by GM6001. Calibrated MMP-9 activity (Log 10^6), as measured by a fluorescent electrophoretic technique, was dramatically attenuated by GM6001 *in vitro* at various concentrations. Plasma concentrations of GM6001, measured 96 hours following a single 100 mg/kg subcutaenous dose (range 0.16−.26 µM or 60–100 ng/mL), approximated those needed *in vitro* to robustly inhibit MMP-9 (0.2 µM or 77 ng/mL). Groups marked with an asterisk (*) had significantly ($P<0.05$) different calibrated MMP-9 activity from reference (no GM6001) using a one tailed Student's t-test.

GM6001 Reduces Gelatinase Activity in Serum of Spinal Cord Injured Dogs

We utilized a fluorescent electrophoretic technique to determine if MMP-2/MMP-9 activity increases in CSF and serum in dogs with SCI and whether activity is reduced after treatment [37–39]. MMP-2/MMP-9 activity in the CSF did not differ between dogs with SCI and control dogs ($P = 0.5011$; Wilcoxon rank-sum test) (Table S2, Fig. S3). Dogs with SCI had significantly ($P = 0.0128$; Wilcoxon rank-sum test) higher serum MMP-2/MMP-9 activity prior to treatment compared with control dogs, but activity did not vary based on clinical factors or MRI features of SCI (Table 2, Fig. 5). Serum MMP-2/MMP-9 activity was significantly ($P<0.05$; generalized linear model) lower in dogs receiving GM6001 3 days following treatment compared to dogs receiving either DSMO or saline (Fig. 6). Thus, these findings confirm the effectiveness of GM6001 in reducing the abnormal elevation of MMP-2/MMP-9 in serum of spinal cord injured dogs.

DMSO Enhances Recovery in Dogs with Severe Spinal Cord Injuries

In dogs with mild-to-moderate SCI (i.e., MFS >0), there was robust recovery of function by 42 days with 64 of 71 (90%) dogs independently walking and 69 of 71 (97%) having intact pelvic limb nociception. Treatment group did not influence 3 or 12 day TSCIS (Fig. 7, Fig. S4). Dogs with mild-to-moderate SCI had significantly higher 42-day TSCIS (mean 15; 95% CI 12–18) compared to those with severe SCI (mean 7; 95% CI 4–9) ($P< 0.0010$; generalized linear model).

In dogs with severe SCI (i.e., MFS = 0), those receiving either DMSO or GM6001 had significantly ($P<0.05$; generalized linear model) more robust functional recovery compared with those receiving saline placebo (Fig. 7) at 42 days. Sub-components of the 42-day TSCIS were examined in dogs with severe SCI to better capture the influence of treatment on motor, sensory, and postural recovery. Sensory and postural scores did not differ significantly between treatment groups. Dogs receiving saline had an estimated mean motor score of 2 (95% CI 0–4.0) (suggesting absent to minimal pelvic limb movement with tail support) that was significantly ($P<0.05$; generalized linear model) less than the estimated mean motor score for dogs receiving DMSO (mean, 5; 95% CI 2.0–8.0) or GM6001 (mean, 5; 95% CI 2.0–8.0) (Fig. 8). The distribution of motor scores for both the DMSO and GM6001 treated dogs indicated that the majority of animals in these groups developed coordinated stepping movements with tail support and of those regaining movement many (6 of 12; 50%) walked without any support. Dogs that were treated with DMSO or GM6001 that regained pelvic limb movement typically (10 of 12; 83%) also recovered limb nociception. The extent of neurological recovery at 42 days post-injury was not significantly different in DMSO- and GM6001 (dissolved in DMSO)-treated groups. Such findings suggest that DMSO, rather than GM6001 contributed to enhanced recovery in these treatment groups.

Discussion

This study was designed as a large-scale clinical trial to evaluate MMP inhibition in a clinically relevant, naturally occurring canine SCI model. Using advanced technology to measure activity of MMP-2/MMP-9, we show that these proteases are elevated in serum of dogs across all levels of injury severity and that GM001, given as a single bolus subcutaneously, significantly reduced this activity. Despite the effectiveness of GM6001 in targeting early MMP activity, both GM6001, solubilized in DMSO, and DMSO

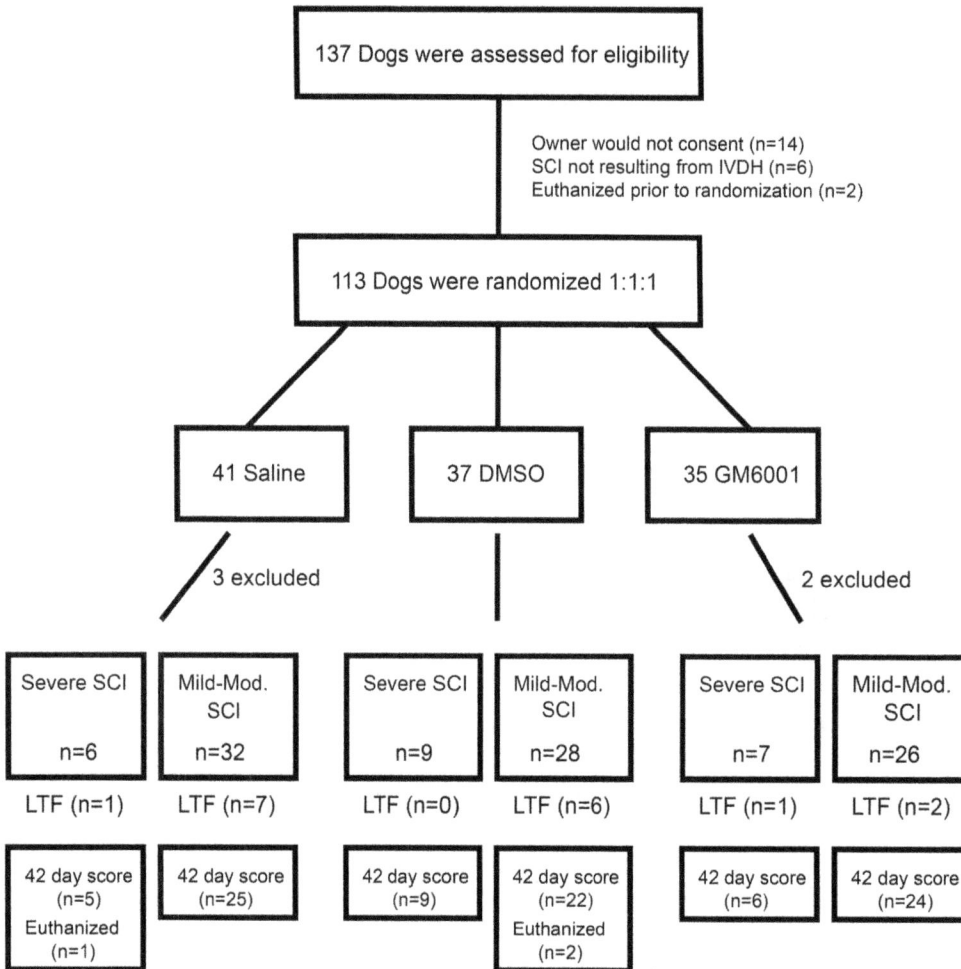

Figure 3. Consolidated Standards of Reporting Trials (CONSORT) Diagram. Flow diagram depicting progress through different phases of the clinical trial including enrollment, group allocation, and follow-up.

alone produced similar levels of neurological improvement in dogs with severe SCIs, relative to saline controls. At 42 days post-injury, these dogs showed robust stepping movements that were visible with tail support and many independently ambulated; saline-treated dogs either showed no movement or had minimal limb advancement without stepping. Together, these findings demonstrate that early blockade of MMPs did not improve long-term neurological recovery. Rather, DMSO alone was responsible for the beneficial outcomes in dogs with severe SCIs.

The clinical trial described here was designed to include dogs with both severe (paraplegia and absent nociception) and mild-to-moderate SCIs (non-ambulatory with intact nociception) for several reasons. First, there is an abnormal elevation of MMP-9 in serum [20], CSF [20,41] and spinal cords of dogs [42] with IVDH across a spectrum of injury severities. Second, while long-term recovery of ambulation is common (64 of 71 dogs in this trial walked independently) in the mild-to-moderate injury group, few animals normalize with reference to motor or postural scores [43].

Thus, there is an opportunity, even within animals that are likely to show marked recovery, to examine the effect of therapeutics. We chose to stratify our population based on SCI severity to examine the effect of treatment on neurologic recovery. This approach was necessary given the well-known difference in outcome between these populations (approximately 85–95% of mildly-to-moderately and 50–60% of severely injured dogs recover independent ambulation) and the potential for differential activation of secondary injury pathways based on SCI severity [30–33]. Stratification based on SCI severity is common and accepted in human clinical trials because of expected differences in recovery between injury groups and the potential impact of this difference on evaluation of effectiveness of therapies [44,45].

GM6001 is a broad-spectrum MMP inhibitor that has been shown to exert neuroprotection in rodent models of brain and SCIs, primarily via antagonism of MMP-9 associated with neutrophils [1]. Evidence supporting this position includes a temporal association between neutrophil trafficking and MMP-9

Table 1. Baseline characteristics did not differ significantly among treatment groups.

A. Continuous variables: Medians (range); P values from Kruskal-Wallis testing

Variable	Saline Controls	DMSO	Drug+DMSO	P value
	(N = 38)	*(N = 33)*	*(N = 33)*	
Age (years)	5 (2 to 13)	5 (3 to 13)	5 (2 to 14)	0.9833
Duration of signs prior to admission (hours)	24 (1 to 48)	18 (4 to 36)	12 (2 to 48)	0.2246
*MFS**	2 (0 to 3)	2 (0 to 3)	2 (0 to 3)	0.7409
TSCIS#	4 (0 to 10)	4 (0 to 11)	4 (0 to 10)	0.5907

B. Categorical variables: P values from chi-squared testing

Variable		DMSO	Drug+DMSO	P value
		(N = 38)	*(N = 37)*	*(N = 33)*	

Variable		DMSO *(N = 38)*	DMSO *(N = 37)*	Drug+DMSO *(N = 33)*	P value
Sex	Female	61% (23/38)	53% (19/36)	39% (13/33)	0.3039
	Male	39% (15/38)	47% (17/36)	61% (20/33)	
Neutered	No	16% (6/38)	22% (8/36)	18% (6/33)	0.9078
	Yes	84% (32/38)	78% (28/36)	82% (27/33)	
Breed	Dachshund	71% (27/35)	61% (22/36)	85% (28/33)	0.1560
	Other	29% (8/35)	39% (14/36)	15% (5/33)	
Chondrodystrophoid	Yes	89% (34/38)	86% (31/36)	88% (29/33)	0.9628
	Other	11% (4/38)	14% (5/36)	12% (4/33)	
Level of Spinal Cord Injury	T12-T13	34% (13/38)	36% (13/36)	24% (8/33)	0.6986
	T13-L1	29% (11/38)	25% (9/36)	33% (11/33)	0.8705
	L1-L2, L2-L3, or L3-L4	29% (11/38)	33% (12/36)	24% (8/33)	0.8390
T2-Weighted Hyperintensity (only available for 76 dogs)	Absent	62% (18/29)	76% (22/29)	50% (9/18)	0.3225
	Present	38% (11/29)	24% (7/29)	50% (9/18)	

Panel A summarizes continuous variables using medians (ranges) by group, with P values from Kruskal-Wallis tests; panel B describes categorical variables using proportions by group with P values from chi-squared testing.
* MFS = Modified Frankel Score; # TSCIS = Texas Spinal Cord Injury Score.

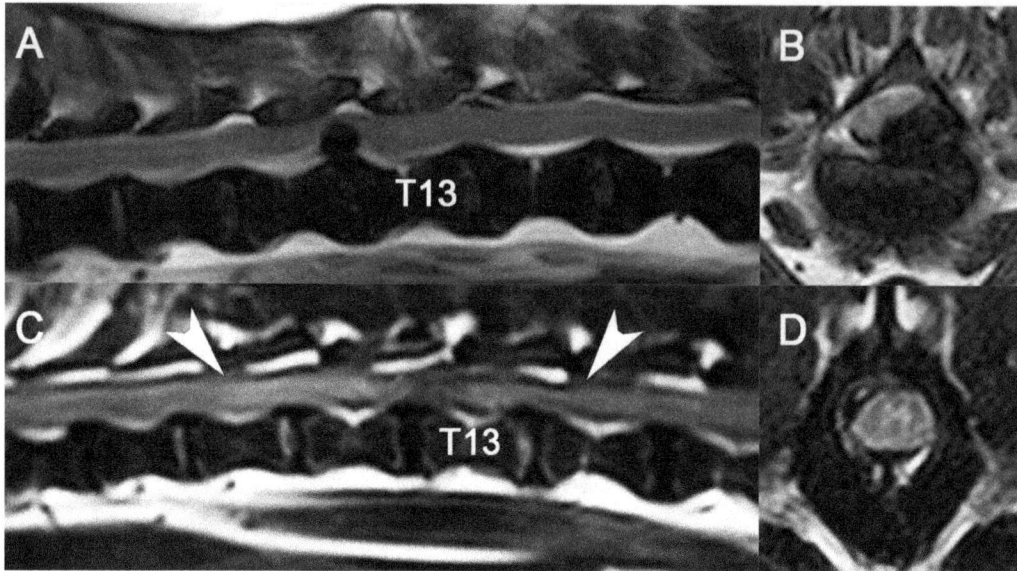

Figure 4. T2-weighted magnetic resonance images in dogs with spinal cord injuries from intervertebral disk herniation. In 1 dog (A, B) that was non-ambulatory with intact pelvic limb movement and sensation, there was focal ventrolateral spinal cord compression at the T12-T13 vertebral articulation without spinal cord signal change. A second dog (C, D) with paraplegia and absent pelvic limb deep nociception had compression at the T12-T13 vertebral articulation. There was extensive spinal cord T2-weighted hyperintensity (white arrows) visible on the sagittal image (C), suggestive of processes seen in contusion injuries such as edema, necrosis, hemorrhage, or cellular infiltrates. The transverse image (D, level of T13 vertebral body) indicated that T2-weighted hyperintensity was predominantly localized to the gray matter.

expression, reduced expression of MMP-9 in spinal cord injured mice that are neutrophil-depleted, and reduced neutrophil content within injured spinal cords of MMP-9 null mice [2,8,46]. In this

study, GM6001 was delivered SC using DMSO as a vehicle. While the high prevalence of injection site reactions and route of administration may have altered drug absorption in comparison to

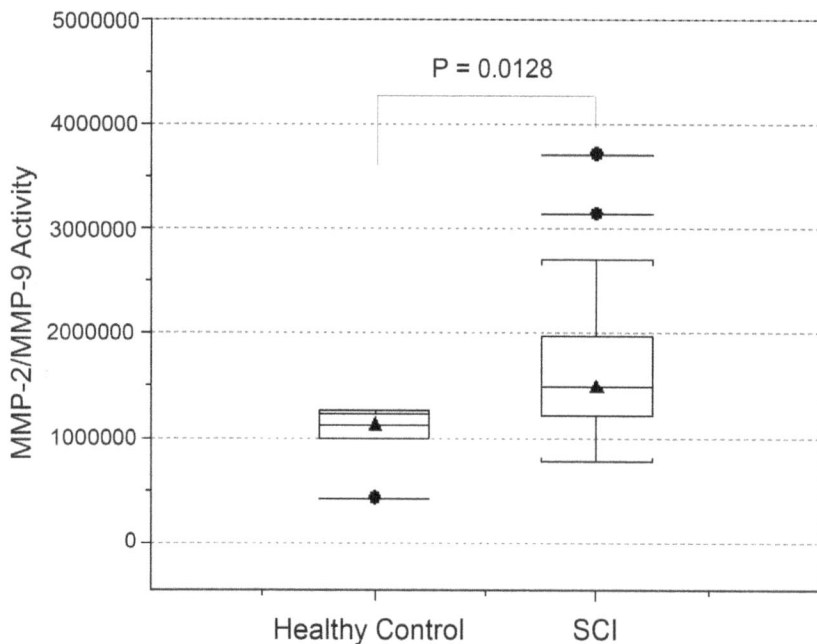

Figure 5. Serum MMP-2/MMP-9 activity in healthy and injured dogs. Box-and-whisker plots summarizing the distribution of MMP 2/9 activity for healthy control dogs (N = 5) and dogs with spinal cord injury (SCI; N = 42) that had serum collected. Values of serum MMP 2/9 activities were significantly (P = 0.0128) greater for dogs with SCI included in the trial than control dogs. The horizontal lines with triangles represent the median value; the horizontal lines at the bottom and top of the boxes represent the 25th and 75th percentiles of the data, respectively. The thin vertical lines extending up or down from the boxes to horizontal lines (so-called whiskers) extend to a multiple of 1.75× the distance of the upper and lower quartile, respectively. Horizontal lines with circles represent values outside the limits of the whiskers.

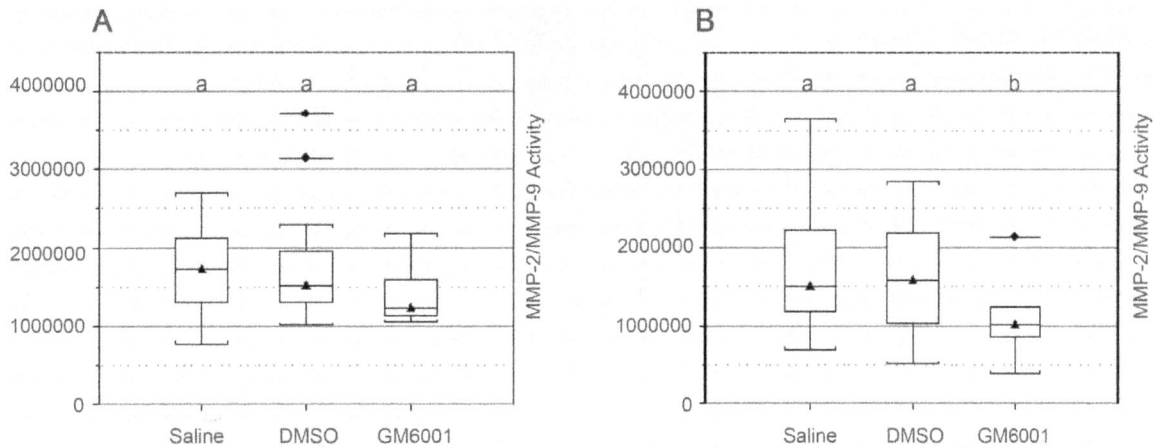

Figure 6. Serum MMP-2/MMP-9 activity pre- and post-drug delivery. Dogs were first randomized into 3 treatment groups, and serum was obtained prior to administration of saline, DMSO, or GM6001 (panel A). There were no differences in serum MMP-2/MMP-9 activity among treatment groups at the time of admission (panel A); however, at day 3, there was a significant (P = 0.0482) difference in serum activity between GM6001-treated dogs and the other treatment groups (panel B). See Figure 5 for a description of box-and-whisker plots. Groups marked with different letters differ significantly (P<0.05).

studies in other species, our data support favorable PK via SC administration of GM6001. Furthermore, relatively small plasma concentrations of GM6001 present 3 days post-delivery appear capable of modulating MMP-2/MMP-9 activity in study dogs.

Here we studied the effects of GM6001 on MMP-2/MMP-9 activity in serum. While there was no relationship between injury severity and level of MMP-2/9 activity in serum, spinal cord injured dogs showed an increase in these proteases relative to healthy controls. Moreover, the early elevation of serum MMP-2/MMP-9 activity was significantly reduced following treatment with

GM6001, a finding which serves to confirm the effectiveness of the drug in reducing proteolytic activity.

While MMP-2/MMP-9 activity was detected in the CSF of injured dogs, activity did not differ between healthy control dogs and those with SCI. The lack of a demonstrable difference in CSF MMP-2/MMP-9 between SCI and control groups may reflect the inability of this assay to distinguish between the 2 proteases. Based upon an earlier study using gelatin zymography [20], MMP-2 was found to be expressed in the CSF of normal dogs and remained unchanged after SCI. In contrast, MMP-9 was only detected in

Table 2. Values of serum MMP-2/MMP-9 activity were not significantly associated with various clinical variables.

Variable	Median (Range) of MMP-2/MMP-9 Activity in Serum		P value
Age	≤5 Years (N=28)	>5 Years (N=12)	
	1,519,998 (1,009,205–3,708,449)	1,315,180 (769,191–2,700,981	0.1458
Sex	Male (N=22)	Female (N=18)	
	1,504,968 (1,009,205–3,708,449)	1,455,587 (769,191–2,700,981)	0.2625
Neutered	Not neutered (N=9)	Neutered (N=31)	
	1,492,947 (1,009,205–2,266,638)	1,479,017 (769,191–3,708,449)	0.5881
Breed	Dachshund (N=28)	Other (N=12)	
	1,411,546 (769,191 - 3,144,395)	1,528,755 (941,766 - 3,708,449)	0.4932
Chondrodysplastic	Yes (N=38)	Other (N=2)	
	1,474,618 (769,191–3,708,449)	1,983,362 (1,975,379–1,991,345)	0.2564
Duration of clinical signs prior to admission	≤12 hours (N=12)	>12 hours (N=28)	
	1,453,961 (1,009,205 - 3,708,449)	1,485,982 (769,191–3,144,395)	0.9189
	≤24 hours (N=35)	>24 hours (N=5)	
	1,492,947 (941,766–3,708,449)	1,310,144 (769,191–2,306,259)	0.5243
T2-weighted hyperintensity	Absent (N=20)	Present (N=11)	
	1,507,977 (769,191–3,708,449)	1,523,790 (1,062,500–3,144,395)	0.6995
MFS at admission	≤2 (N=22)	>2 (N=18)	
	1,455,587 (1,009,205 - 2,292,539)	1,504,968 (769,191–3,708,449)	0.4924

Medians (and ranges) and P values derived from Wilcoxon-rank sum tests are reported for the categorical variables listed above. MMP=matrix metalloproteinase; MFS=Modified Frankel Score.

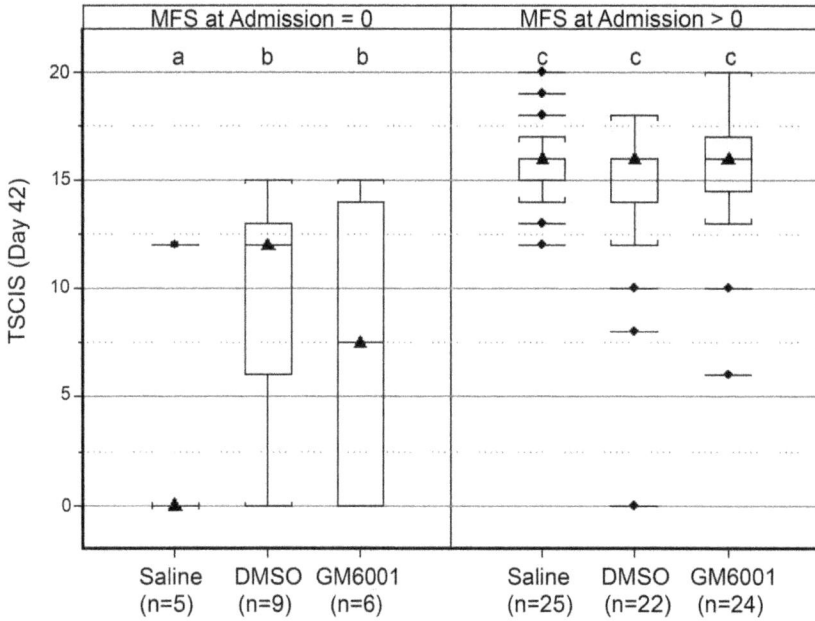

Figure 7. Evaluation of primary outcome in dogs with SCI. Box-and-whisker plots of TSCIS on day 42 by treatment group, stratified by MFS at admission (MFS = 0, left panel; or MFS >0, right panel). There were no significant differences in TSCIS among dogs with MFS score >0 (right panel), but TSCIS was significantly (P<0.05) greater for the GM6001 and the DMSO group than saline treated dogs with MFS = 0 (left panel). See Figure 5 for a description of box-and-whisker plots. Groups marked with different letters differ significantly (P<0.05).

spinal cord injured dogs [20,41]. Thus, in the current study, the absence of any differences between injured and control dogs may have been confounded by the constitutive activity of MMP-2 in CSF that may have masked any increase in MMP-9.

There are likely a number of possible explanations for why GM6001 failed to improve neurological recovery in spinal cord injured dogs. First, while GM6001 has been shown to improve neurological outcomes in various rodent models of brain and spinal cord injury [2,47,48], no studies to date have evaluated efficacy in dogs. Thus, there may be species differences in responsiveness to GM6001 and/or MMP-directed pathogenesis. Additionally, effects of GM6001 demonstrated in rodents may not

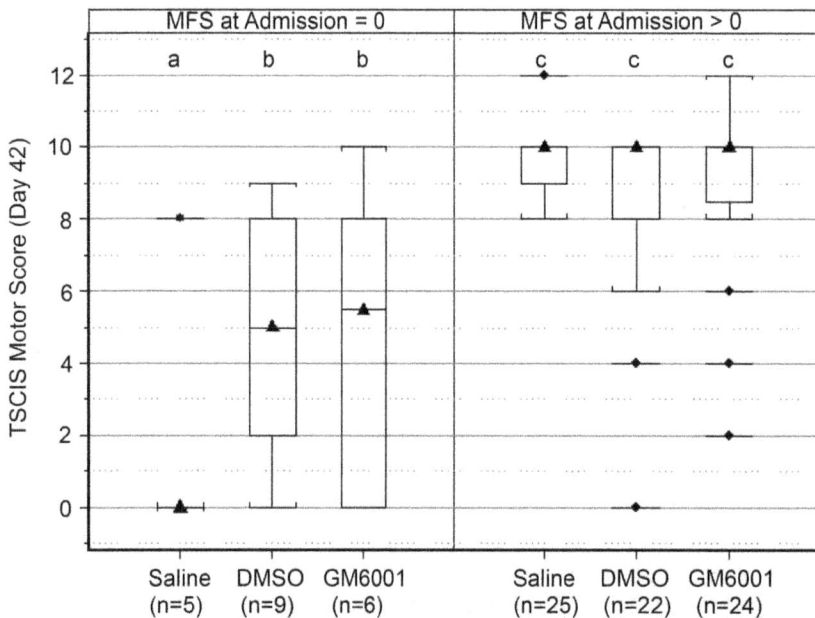

Figure 8. Evaluation of TSCIS motor score at day 42 following SCI. Box-and-whisker plots of TSCIS motor score on day 42 by treatment group, stratified by MFS at admission (MFS = 0, left panel; or MFS >0, right panel). There were no significant differences in motor score among dogs with MFS >0 (right panel), but motor score was significantly (P<0.05) greater for the GM6001 and the DMSO group than saline treated dogs with MFS = 0 (left panel). See Figure 5 for a description of box-and-whisker plots. Groups marked with different letters differ significantly (P<0.05).

be sufficiently robust to positively influence outcome under the clinical conditions of this study [49,50]. Second, the drug was active beyond the first several days post-injury and as such could have interfered with mechanisms underlying recovery in SCI. Pharmacokinetics in healthy dogs demonstrated that plasma concentration of GM6001, present at even the 96-hour time-point, approximated or exceeded that necessary to block MMP-9 *in vitro*. As some MMPs modulate the formation of a glial scar and axonal plasticity [4], their subacute/chronic blockade may result in adverse neurological outcomes. Third, the timing between SCI and administration of GM6001 may not have been optimal. The strong association between MMP-9 expression and neutrophils suggests that an optimal therapeutic window for GM6001 is defined by the early trafficking of neutrophils into the injured cord. Such a position is supported by evidence of pronounced neurological recovery when the drug was given beginning 3 hours post-injury in a murine model of SCI [2]. In dogs treated with GM6001, median delay between injury and enrollment was 12 hours, which may have exceeded the window of efficacy for GM6001. Finally, while the use of dogs with thoracic and lumbar spinal cord lesions could have influenced our ability to detect drug-related effects [51], the proportion of dogs with lumbar lesions was similar amongst treatment groups (Table 1). Additionally, the inclusion of lesion location (lumbar versus thoracic) in multivariable generalized linear modeling did not alter the significance or magnitude of observed treatment effects (data not shown).

We found that DMSO improved motor recovery in dogs with severe SCIs. This finding is perhaps not too surprising as DMSO, under defined dosing conditions, has the ability to function as a neuroprotectant [14] and in some cases when used as a vehicle, may be synergistic. In the setting of neurotrauma, neuroprotection is exemplified in a study by Di Giorgio et al [52] which compared the antioxidant curcumin, α-tocopherol, DMSO and saline in a model of traumatic brain injury. These authors reported similar levels of early neuroprotection across all agents relative to the saline control group. Beneficial effects of DMSO might also be indicated in studies where DMSO is used as a vehicle without any additional negative control group. For example, in a recent study the efficacy of an epidermal growth factor receptor inhibitor was assessed in a rodent model of SCI [53]. This inhibitor was compared against its vehicle, DMSO. Recovery of motor and bladder function was significantly greater in rats that received DMSO relative to the inhibitor. The authors concluded that the receptor inhibitor showed no efficacy relative to the "baseline" values as defined by DMSO. Based upon our study, an alternative explanation is that DMSO did not serve as the "baseline" but rather may have exerted a beneficial effect. Finally, DMSO, when co-administered with a candidate therapeutic, offers potential for synergism, by acting through separate and/or overlapping pathways. While we found no evidence of this in the current study, others have reported synergism in a model of brain ischemia where DMSO was either combined with fructose 1,6-disphosphate, an intermediate of anaerobic metabolism, or prostacyclin (PG_{I2}) which blocks aggregation of platelets and functions as a vasodilator [12,54].

The mechanisms underlying DMSO-mediated neuroprotection have been attributed to its ability to function as a free radical scavenger and suppress a variety of pathobiologic events including inflammation, calcium influx, and glutamate excitoxicity [14]. Such broad-based, temporally-defined targets may account for the extended window of efficacy (within 48 hours of injury) in spinal cord-injured dogs.

Dogs with severe SCIs and treated with either DMSO or GM6001 in DMSO showed a consistent (>80%), improvement in pelvic limb stepping. A critical question is whether this stepping was voluntary or mediated through the central pattern generator (i.e., spinal stepping). The vast majority of these dogs with motor recovery also regained pelvic limb nociception (10 of 12; 83%) and 50% walked independently (without tail support) when evaluated at 42 days post injury. These data would argue that pelvic limb movement was indeed voluntary in the majority of dogs with severe SCIs treated with either DMSO or GM6001.

In summary, while this study and others [12,13,52,54] underscore the potential utility of DMSO for the treatment of brain and SCI, there remain conflicting reports about the efficacy of DMSO. This is illustrated in recent studies reporting either no effects or reduced performance on behavioral tests after traumatic brain injury [55] and others suggesting improved learning ability in cerebellar mutant Lurcher mice [56]. As it is shrouded in controversy as a therapeutic yet commonly used as a vehicle, there is a need to rigorously evaluate DMSO from the standpoint of safety, dosing, and efficacy. Given that it is a common vehicle for drug delivery, there is opportunity to evaluate its synergistic properties. Such logic has been successfully applied to the treatment of human interstitial cystitis, where DMSO is given as part of multimodal regimen [57]. With FDA approval for the treatment of interstitial cystitis, there is potential for the repurposing of DMSO, capitalizing on its favorable properties as a solvent, in developing combinatorial therapies for SCI. The current study suggests that DMSO has an extended therapeutic window (up to 48 hours). As time to treatment for human SCI may be delayed for up to 1 to 3 days post-injury [58], a broader therapeutic window could potentially expand the population of spinal cord injured patients that would otherwise not qualify for treatments with more restricted windows of intervention.

Supporting Information

Figure S1 Rectal body temperature in healthy dogs delivered DMSO or GM6001. All dogs delivered GM6001 at 6–18 times the cumulative clinical trial dose (100–300 mg/kg six times) experienced body temperature elevations beyond normal. The elevation in body temperature qualitatively appeared greatest in dogs receiving higher doses of GM6001.

Figure S2 Drug delivery site diameters in healthy dogs receiving GM6001. Delivery site diameter appeared greatest one day after administration (panel A) and diminished by day 8 post-administration (panel B) in dogs receiving 6–18 times the cumulative clinical trial dose of GM6001.

Figure S3 Cerebrospinal fluid MMP-2/MMP-9 activity in healthy and spinal cord injured dogs. Although MMP-2/MMP-9 activity tended to be higher in dogs with spinal cord injuries (n = 40) than healthy controls (n = 5), the difference was not significant (P = 0.5011; Wilcoxon rank-sum test).

Figure S4 Texas Spinal Cord Injury Score (TSCIS) on day 3 following spinal cord injury. There were no significant differences in TSCIS based on treatment group for dogs with severe (MFS = 0) and mild-to-moderate (MFS >0) spinal cord injuries. Box-and-Whiskers with different letters differ significantly (P< 0.05).

Table S1 Frequency of adverse events and survival (died or euthanized) by treatment group. Injection site reactions were significantly associated with GM6001 delivery, but no other adverse events were significantly associated with treatments.

Table S2 Cerebrospinal MMP-2/MMP-9 activity in dogs with spinal cord injury. Cerebrospinal fluid MMP-2/MMP-9 activity in dogs with spinal cord injury was not significantly associated with signalment, duration of clinical signs, or MFS at the time of admission. Medians (and ranges) and P values derived from Wilcoxon-rank sum tests were reported for the categorical variables.

Acknowledgments

We thank Ms. Alisha Selix for coordinating canine trial enrollment and providing technical support for canine studies. We also thank Dr. George Lemieux for advice on the inhibitor. Finally, we would like to thank Matthew Tyndall for his assistance in developing the fluorescent electrophoretic assay to detect MMP-2/MMP-9 activity.

Author Contributions

Conceived and designed the experiments: JML NDC MH VRF GJL AAT AM ZW LJN. Performed the experiments: JML GJL SCK AM LJN. Analyzed the data: NDC VRF. Contributed reagents/materials/analysis tools: JML MH AM. Wrote the paper: JML NDC MH VRF GJL SCK AAT TMF ZW AM LJN.

References

1. Zhang H, Adwanikar H, Werb Z, Noble-Haeusslein LJ (2010) Matrix metalloproteinases and neurotrauma: evolving roles in injury and reparative processes. Neuroscientist 16: 156–170.
2. Noble LJ, Donovan F, Igarashi T, Goussev S, Werb Z (2002) Matrix metalloproteinases limit functional recovery after spinal cord injury by modulation of early vascular events. J Neurosci 22: 7526–7535.
3. Wells JE, Rice TK, Nuttall RK, Edwards DR, Zekki H, et al. (2003) An adverse role for matrix metalloproteinase 12 after spinal cord injury in mice. J Neurosci 23: 10107–10115.
4. Zhang H, Trivedi A, Lee JU, Lohela M, Lee SM, et al. (2011) Matrix metalloproteinase-9 and stromal cell-derived factor-1 act synergistically to support migration of blood-borne monocytes into the injured spinal cord. J Neurosci 31: 15894–15903.
5. Shigemori Y, Katayama Y, Mori T, Maeda T, Kawamata T (2006) Matrix metalloproteinase-9 is associated with blood-brain barrier opening and brain edema formation after cortical contusion in rats. Acta Neurochir Suppl 96: 130–133.
6. Lee JY, Kim HS, Choi HY, Oh TH, Yune TY (2012) Fluoxetine inhibits matrix metalloprotease activation and prevents disruption of blood-spinal cord barrier after spinal cord injury. Brain 135: 2375–2389.
7. Lee JY, Kim HS, Choi HY, Oh TH, Ju BG, et al. (2012) Valproic acid attenuates blood-spinal cord barrier disruption by inhibiting matrix metalloprotease-9 activity and improves functional recovery after spinal cord injury. Journal of neurochemistry 121: 818–829.
8. Stirling DP, Yong VW (2008) Dynamics of the inflammatory response after murine spinal cord injury revealed by flow cytometry. J Neurosci Res 86: 1944–1958.
9. Opdenakker G, Van den Steen PE, Dubois B, Nelissen I, Van Coillie E, et al. (2001) Gelatinase B functions as regulator and effector in leukocyte biology. J Leukoc Biol 69: 851–859.
10. Kobayashi H, Chattopadhyay S, Kato K, Dolkas J, Kikuchi S, et al. (2008) MMPs initiate Schwann cell-mediated MBP degradation and mechanical nociception after nerve damage. Mol Cell Neurosci 39: 619–627.
11. Sifringer M, Stefovska V, Zentner I, Hansen B, Stepulak A, et al. (2007) The role of matrix metalloproteinases in infant traumatic brain injury. Neurobiol Dis 25: 526–535.
12. De La Torre JC (1995) Treatment of head injury in mice, using a fructose 1,6-diphosphate and dimethyl sulfoxide combination. Neurosurgery 37: 273–279.
13. De La Torre JC, Johnson CM, Goode DJ, Mullan S (1975) Pharmacologic treatment and evaluation of permanent experimental spinal cord trauma. Neurology 25: 508–514.
14. Jacob SW, de la Torre JC (2009) Pharmacology of dimethyl sulfoxide in cardiac and CNS damage. Pharmacological reports : PR 61: 225–235.
15. Levine JM, Levine GJ, Porter BF, Topp K, Noble-Haeusslein LJ (2011) Naturally occurring disk herniation in dogs: an opportunity for pre-clinical spinal cord injury research. J Neurotrauma 28: 675–688.
16. Jeffery ND, Hamilton L, Granger N (2011) Designing clinical trials in canine spinal cord injury as a model to translate successful laboratory interventions into clinical practice. Vet Rec 168: 102–107.
17. Jeffery ND, Smith PM, Lakatos A, Ibanez C, Ito D, et al. (2006) Clinical canine spinal cord injury provides an opportunity to examine the issues in translating laboratory techniques into practical therapy. Spinal Cord 44: 1–10.
18. Griffiths IR (1972) Some aspects of the pathology and pathogenesis of the myelopathy caused by disc protrusions in dogs. J Neurol Neurosurg Psychiatry 35: 403–413.
19. Smith PM, Jeffery ND (2006) Histological and ultrastructural analysis of white matter damage after naturally-occurring spinal cord injury. Brain Pathol 16: 99–109.
20. Levine JM, Ruaux CG, Bergman RL, Coates JR, Steiner JM, et al. (2006) Matrix metalloproteinase-9 activity in the cerebrospinal fluid and serum of dogs with acute spinal cord trauma from intervertebral disk disease. Am J Vet Res 67: 283–287.
21. Riviere JE (1999) Study Design and Data Analysis. Comparative Pharmacokinetics: Principles, Techniques, and Applications. Ames, Iowa: Iowa State University Press. 239–258.
22. Lammertse D, Tuszynski MH, Steeves JD, Curt A, Fawcett JW, et al. (2007) Guidelines for the conduct of clinical trials for spinal cord injury as developed by the ICCP panel: clinical trial design. Spinal Cord 45: 232–242.
23. Moher D, Hopewell S, Schulz KF, Montori V, Gotzsche PC, et al. (2010) CONSORT 2010 explanation and elaboration: updated guidelines for reporting parallel group randomised trials. BMJ 340: c869.
24. Schulz KF, Altman DG, Moher D (2010) CONSORT 2010 statement: updated guidelines for reporting parallel group randomised trials. BMJ 340: c332.
25. Dobkin B, Barbeau H, Deforge D, Ditunno J, Elashoff R, et al. (2007) The evolution of walking-related outcomes over the first 12 weeks of rehabilitation for incomplete traumatic spinal cord injury: the multicenter randomized Spinal Cord Injury Locomotor Trial. Neurorehabil Neural Repair 21: 25–35.
26. Geisler FH, Dorsey FC, Coleman WP (1991) Recovery of motor function after spinal-cord injury–a randomized, placebo-controlled trial with GM-1 ganglioside. N Engl J Med 324: 1829–1838.
27. Blight AR, Toombs JP, Bauer MS, Widmer WR (1991) The effects of 4-aminopyridine on neurological deficits in chronic cases of traumatic spinal cord injury in dogs: a phase I clinical trial. J Neurotrauma 8: 103–119.
28. Laverty PH, Leskovar A, Breur GJ, Coates JR, Bergman RL, et al. (2004) A preliminary study of intravenous surfactants in paraplegic dogs: polymer therapy in canine clinical SCI. J Neurotrauma 21: 1767–1777.
29. Levine GJ, Levine JM, Budke CM, Kerwin SC, Au J, et al. (2009) Description and repeatability of a newly developed spinal cord injury scale for dogs. Prev Vet Med 89: 121–127.
30. Ferreira AJ, Correia JH, Jaggy A (2002) Thoracolumbar disc disease in 71 paraplegic dogs: influence of rate of onset and duration of clinical signs on treatment results. J Small Anim Pract 43: 158–163.
31. Ito D, Matsunaga S, Jeffery ND, Sasaki N, Nishimura R, et al. (2005) Prognostic value of magnetic resonance imaging in dogs with paraplegia caused by thoracolumbar intervertebral disk extrusion: 77 cases (2000–2003). J Am Vet Med Assoc 227: 1454–1460.
32. Olby N, Levine J, Harris T, Munana K, Skeen T, et al. (2003) Long-term functional outcome of dogs with severe injuries of the thoracolumbar spinal cord: 87 cases (1996–2001). J Am Vet Med Assoc 222: 762–769.
33. Ruddle TL, Allen DA, Schertel ER, Barnhart MD, Wilson ER, et al. (2006) Outcome and prognostic factors in non-ambulatory Hansen type I intervertebral disc extrusions: 308 cases. Vet Comp Orthop Traumatol 19: 29–34.
34. Basso DM, Beattie MS, Bresnahan JC (1995) A sensitive and reliable locomotor rating scale for open field testing in rats. J Neurotrauma 12: 1–21.
35. Levine JM, Fosgate GT, Rushing R, Nghiem PP, Platt SR, et al. (2009) Magnetic resonance imaging in dogs with neurologic impairment due to acute thoracic and lumbar intervertebral disk herniation. J Vet Intern Med 23: 1220–1226.
36. Miyanji F, Furlan JC, Aarabi B, Arnold PM, Fehlings MG (2007) Acute cervical traumatic spinal cord injury: MR imaging findings correlated with neurologic outcome - prospective study with 100 consecutive patients. Radiology 243: 820–827.
37. Lefkowitz RB, Schmid-Schonbein GW, Heller MJ (2010) Whole blood assay for elastase, chymotrypsin, matrix metalloproteinase-2, and matrix metalloproteinase-9 activity. Anal Chem 82: 8251–8258.
38. Lefkowitz RB, Schmid-Schonbein GW, Heller MJ (2010) Whole blood assay for trypsin activity using polyanionic focusing gel electrophoresis. Electrophoresis 31: 2442–2451.
39. Lefkowitz RB, Marciniak JY, Hu CM, Schmid-Schonbein GW, Heller MJ (2010) An electrophoretic method for the detection of chymotrypsin and trypsin activity directly in whole blood. Electrophoresis 31: 403–410.
40. Mahmood I (2010) Theoretical versus empirical allometry: Facts behind theories and application to pharmacokinetics. J Pharm Sci 99: 2927–2933.

41. Nagano S, Kim SH, Tokunaga S, Arai K, Fujiki M, et al. (2011) Matrix metalloprotease-9 activity in the cerebrospinal fluid and spinal injury severity in dogs with intervertebral disc herniation. Res Vet Sci 91: 482–485.

42. Bock P, Spitzbarth I, Haist V, Stein VM, Tipold A, et al. (2013) Spatio-temporal development of axonopathy in canine intervertebral disc disease as a translational large animal model for nonexperimental spinal cord injury. Brain Pathol 23: 82–99.

43. Olby N, Harris T, Burr J, Munana K, Sharp N, et al. (2004) Recovery of pelvic limb function in dogs following acute intervertebral disc herniations. J Neurotrauma 21: 49–59.

44. Lammertse DP (2013) Clinical trials in spinal cord injury: lessons learned on the path to translation. The 2011 International Spinal Cord Society Sir Ludwig Guttmann Lecture. Spinal Cord 51: 2–9.

45. Geisler FH, Coleman WP, Grieco G, Poonian D, Group SS (2001) Measurements and recovery patterns in a multicenter study of acute spinal cord injury. Spine 24S: S68–S86.

46. Zhang H, Chang M, Hansen CN, Basso DM, Noble-Haeusslein LJ (2011) Role of matrix metalloproteinases and therapeutic benefits of their inhibition in spinal cord injury. Neurotherapeutics 8: 206–220.

47. Wang J, Tsirka SE (2005) Neuroprotection by inhibition of matrix metalloproteinases in a mouse model of intracerebral haemorrhage. Brain 128: 1622–1633.

48. Gursoy-Ozdemir Y, Qiu J, Matsuoka N, Bolay H, Bermpohl D, et al. (2004) Cortical spreading depression activates and upregulates MMP-9. J Clin Invest 113: 1447–1455.

49. Kwon BK, Okon E, Hillyer J, Mann C, Baptiste D, et al. (2011) A systematic review of non-invasive pharmacologic neuroprotective treatments for acute spinal cord injury. J Neurotrauma 28: 1545–1588.

50. Kwon BK, Okon EB, Tsai E, Beattie MS, Bresnahan J, et al. (2010) A Grading System to Objectively Evaluate the Strength of Preclinical Data of Acute Neuroprotective Therapies for Clinical Translation in Spinal Cord Injury. J Neurotrauma 28: 1525–1543.

51. Magnuson DS, Lovett R, Coffee C, Gray R, Han Y, et al. (2005) Functional consequences of lumbar spinal cord contusion injuries in the adult rat. J Neurotrauma 22: 529–543.

52. Di Giorgio AM, Hou Y, Zhao X, Zhang B, Lyeth BG, et al. (2008) Dimethyl sulfoxide provides neuroprotection in a traumatic brain injury model. Restor Neurol Neurosci 26: 501–507.

53. Sharp K, Yee KM, Steward O (2012) A re-assessment of the effects of treatment with an epidermal growth factor receptor (EGFR) inhibitor on recovery of bladder and locomotor function following thoracic spinal cord injury in rats. Exp Neurol 233: 649–659.

54. de la Torre JC (1991) Synergic activity of combined prostacyclin: dimethyl sulfoxide in experimental brain ischemia. Can J Physiol Pharmacol 69: 191–198.

55. Budinich CS, Tucker LB, Lowe D, Rosenberger JG, McCabe JT (2013) Short and long-term motor and behavioral effects of diazoxide and dimethyl sulfoxide administration in the mouse after traumatic brain injury. Pharmacol Biochem Behav 108: 66–73.

56. Markvartova V, Cendelin J, Vozeh F (2013) Effect of dimethyl sulfoxide in cerebellar mutant Lurcher mice. Neurosci Lett 543: 142–145.

57. Stav K, Beberashvili I, Lindner A, Leibovici D (2012) Predictors of response to intravesical dimethyl-sulfoxide cocktail in patients with interstitial cystitis. Urology 80: 61–65.

58. Furlan JC, Tung K, Fehlings M (2013) Process Benchmarking Appraisal of Early Surgical Decompression of Spinal Cord following Traumatic Cervical Spinal Cord Injury: Opportunities to Enhance the Time to Definitive Treatment. J Neurotrauma 30: 487–491.

4

Temporal Profile of Endogenous Anatomical Repair and Functional Recovery following Spinal Cord Injury in Adult Zebrafish

Katarina Vajn[1]*, Denis Suler[1], Jeffery A. Plunkett[2], Martin Oudega[1,3,4]

1 Department of Physical Medicine and Rehabilitation, University of Pittsburgh School of Medicine, Pittsburgh, Pennsylvania, United States of America, 2 School of Science Technology and Engineering Management, St. Thomas University, Miami Gardens, Florida, United States of America, 3 Department of Bioengineering, University of Pittsburgh School of Medicine, Pittsburgh, Pennsylvania, United States of America, 4 Department of Neurobiology, University of Pittsburgh School of Medicine, Pittsburgh, Pennsylvania, United States of America

Abstract

Regenerated cerebrospinal axons are considered to be involved in the spontaneous recovery of swimming ability following a spinal cord injury in adult zebrafish. We employed behavioral analysis, neuronal tracing, and immunocytochemistry to determine the exact temporal relationship between swimming ability and regenerated cerebrospinal axon number in adult zebrafish with a complete spinal cord transection. Between two and eight weeks post-lesion, swimming gradually improved to 44% of sham-injured zebrafish. Neurons within the reticular formation, magnocellular octaval nucleus, and nucleus of the medial longitudinal fascicle grew their axon across and at least four millimeters beyond the lesion. The largest increases in swimming ability and number of regenerated cerebrospinal axons were observed between two and four weeks post-lesion. Regression analyses revealed a significant correlation between swimming ability and the number of regenerated axons. Our results indicate the involvement of cerebrospinal axons in swimming recovery after spinal cord injury in adult zebrafish.

Editor: Simone Di Giovanni, Hertie Institute for Clinical Brain Research, University of Tuebingen, Germany

Funding: Funding was provided by United States Department of Defense Grant W81XWH-11-0645 to JAP, U.S. Army Medical Research and Materiel Command/ Telemedicine and Advanced Technology Research Center (www.tatrc.org). The funders had no role in study design, data collection and analysis, decision to publish, or preparation of the manuscript.

Competing Interests: The authors have declared that no competing interests exist.

* Email: moudega@pitt.edu

Introduction

Adult zebrafish (*Danio rerio*) spontaneously recover coordinated swimming function after spinal cord injury [1–7]. This recovery is partial after a complete transection [1,3–6] and nearly full after a crush of the spinal cord [7], demonstrating the restorative potential of the central nervous system in adult zebrafish.

After an injury to the spinal cord in adult zebrafish, tissue forms to span the lesion site [5,7]. Ependymoradial glial cells have a central role in the formation and functioning of this tissue [5,7], which serves as a bridge for cerebrospinal axons that grow into the caudal spinal cord [2,4–9]. The reticular formation (RT), nucleus of the medial longitudinal fascicle (NMLF), and magnocellular octaval nucleus (MaON) are most regenerative with 30–50% of their neurons growing their axon across and beyond the lesion site [9].

We performed quantitative longitudinal analyses of spontaneous swimming restoration, tissue formation, and axonal regeneration in adult wild-type zebrafish after a complete spinal cord transection. Regression analysis was used to determine the relationship between swimming and regenerating cerebrospinal axons.

Materials and Methods

Animals

Adult zebrafish (*Danio rerio*; male or female wild-type AB* strain, 4–6 months old; <2.5 cm body length) were raised and kept on a 14 h light and 10 h dark cycle in 2.5-liter fish tanks in a double-barrier zebrafish facility with controlled air flow and room and water temperature (28.5°C). The experimental procedures were approved by the Institutional Animal Care and Use Committee at the University of Pittsburgh School of Medicine.

Spinal cord transection and maintenance

The zebrafish were anesthetized by immersion in 0.033% aminobenzoic acid ethylmethylester (Tricaine; Argent Laboratories, Redmond, WA) in phosphate-buffered saline (PBS; 0.1 M, pH 7.4) at 28.5°C for about 2 min. After removal of 2–3 scales at the left side at the mid-point between the brainstem-spinal cord junction and the rostral aspect of the dorsal fin, which corresponds with the eighth vertebra level (Fig. 1A), a 3 mm-long longitudinal incision was made and the muscles bluntly and gently retracted to provide access to the spinal column. With a sterilized surgical microknife (model 10055-12; Fine Science Tools, Foster City, CA) the spinal cord was completely transected between the eighth and ninth vertebra. Then, muscle tissue was cautiously maneuvered

A

spinal cord transection

8th vertebra

survival

B

open-field testing

1d

C

retrograde tracing

4mm

1wk

D

transcardial perfusion

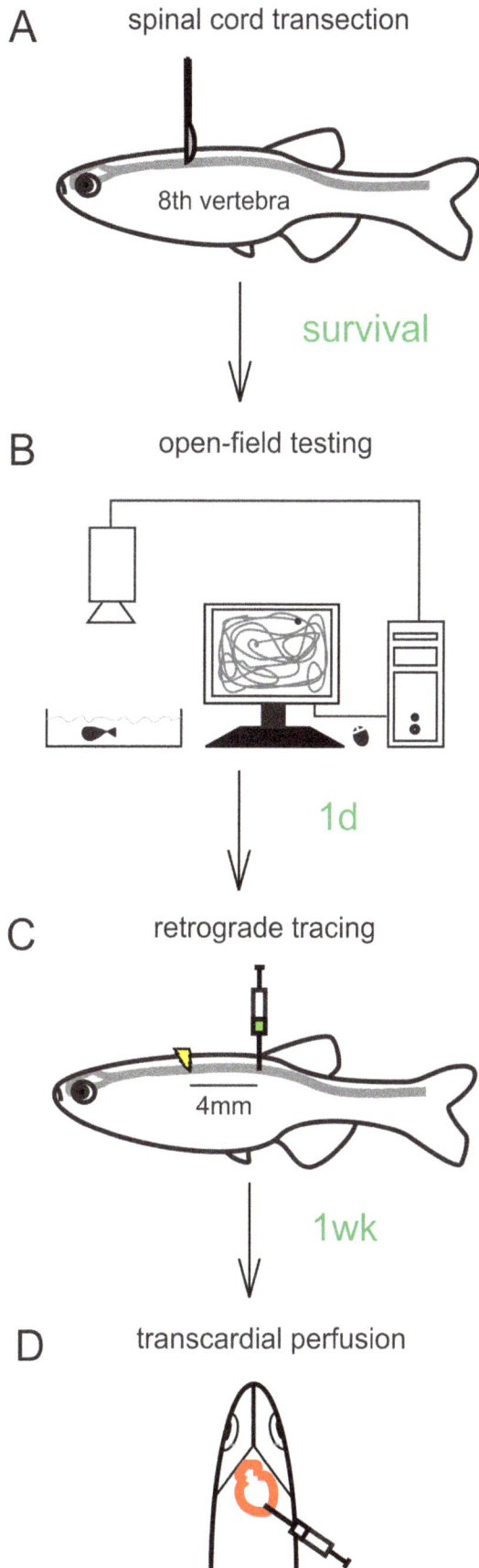

Figure 1. Schematic representation of the: (A) spinal cord transection, (B) open-field testing system, (C) retrograde tracing procedure, (D) transcardial perfusion. The spinal cord was cut between 8th and 9th vertebra. At different time points after transection ("survival"), average distance swam was measured for each fish using an open-field testing system. One day after swimming assessment Fluoroemerald was injected 4 mm caudally from the transection site. Unlesioned zebrafish were traced at the same level as lesioned zebrafish. A week after tracing, zebrafish were transcardially perfused and tissue collected for analysis. 1 d, 1 day; 1 wk, 1 week.

back in place and the wound closed with surgical glue (Histoacryl Blue; TissueSeal LLC, Ann Arbor, MI). The zebrafish were recovering in water at 28.5°C and, thereafter, kept individually in 2.5-liter fish tanks with Dura-Cross zebrafish breeding tank slotted inserts (Dynalon Labware, Rochester, NY) for the length of the experiment. The zebrafish were kept in the dark for the first 72 h without feeding and water change. Fungal infections were prevented with stabilized chlorine oxides (Maroxy; Sergeant's Pet Care Products, Inc., Omaha, NE; 66 µL/L). After transection each zebrafish was randomly assigned to a particular time point group ("survival", Fig. 1), the average swimming distance was assessed followed by retrograde tracing the next day and fixation one week later (Fig. 1).

Behavioral testing

Swimming ability was assessed using an open-field tracking system (Ethovision XT 9.0; Noldus Information Technology Inc., Leesburg, VA) at two, four, six and eight weeks post-lesion and in unlesioned zebrafish (Fig. 1B). The zebrafish were acclimated to the testing room for 1 h prior to the testing. During the assessments, zebrafish were kept in a $26 \times 15.5 \times 5$ cm tank with water (28.5°C) under constant lighting conditions. For each zebrafish at each of the time points, the swimming tracks were recorded and the average distance determined in two five-minute trials one hour apart.

Neuronal tracing

Zebrafish were anesthetized as described above and the spinal cord exposed 4 mm caudal to the transection. A capillary pulled from R-6 custom glass tubing (inner diameter: 0.2 mm; Drummond Scientific Company, Broomall, PA) was prefilled with 3% Fluoroemerald (FE, Life Technologies, Grand Island, NY) in MilliQ water, attached to a Pneumatic Picopump PV-820 (World Precision Instruments Inc., Sarasota, FL), and the tip gently inserted in the spinal cord 4 mm caudally from the transection site (Fig. 1C). Then, 15 nl fluoroemerald was injected at two (n = 20), four (n = 33), six (n = 34), and eight (n = 35) weeks post-transection and in controls without transection (n = 19). The zebrafish were recovered in water at 28.5°C and were kept in standard conditions with regular feeding schedule.

Histological procedures

One week after FE injection, the zebrafish were anesthetized as described above, perfused transcardially with PBS (0.1 M, pH 7.4) using a 1 ml insulin syringe (Fig. 1D). Then, the brain and spinal column were removed and post-fixed by immersion in 4% paraformaldehyde in PBS overnight. Next, the tissues were transferred to 30% sucrose in PBS for at least 24 h and then embedded (Richard Allen NEG50; Thermo Fisher Scientific, Waltham, MA). The brain (15 µm) and the spinal cord (10 µm) were sectioned using a cryostat (CM1950; Leica Microsystems

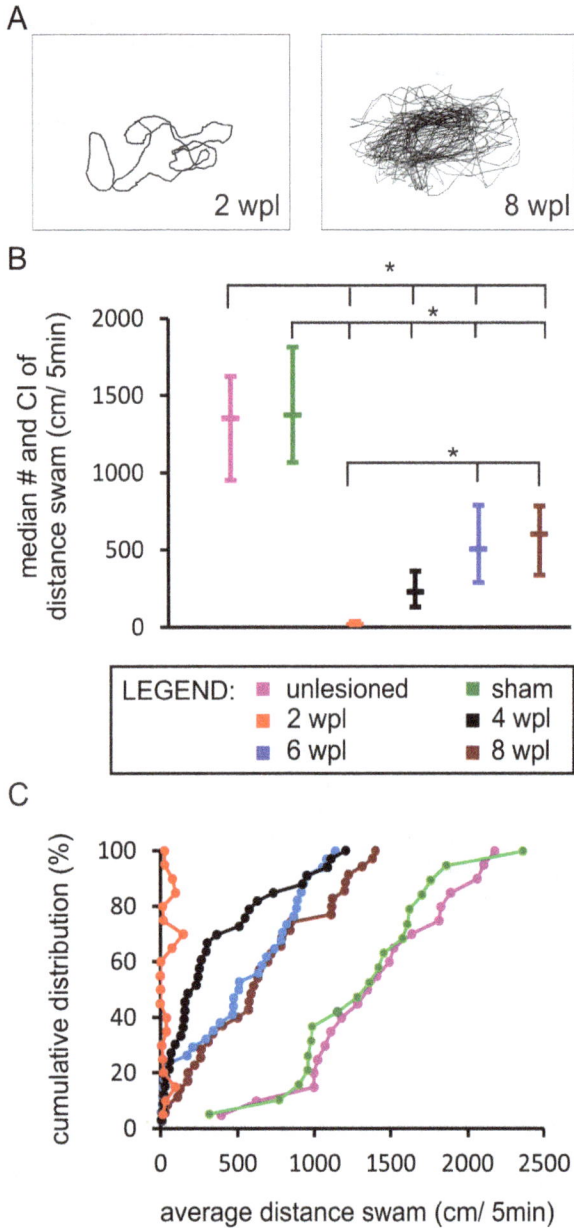

Figure 2. Swimming ability improves over a period of eight weeks after a complete spinal cord transection in adult zebrafish. (A) Examples of swimming path recorded in a five-min period at two- ("2 wpl") and eight ("8 wpl") weeks post-lesion. (B) Boxplot diagram demonstrating the median distance swam and confidence interval of the median during the five-min period. Asterisks indicate significant differences between groups (Kruskal-Wallis test, followed by Mann-Whitney U test with Bonferroni correction, p significant if ≤0.003). Two weeks post-lesion group is significantly different from all other groups. Normal (unlesioned) group is significantly different from all other groups. (C) A cumulative distribution plot illustrating the differences in the distribution of data between individual groups. (unlesioned (n = 19), sham-injured (n = 20), 2 wpl (n = 20), 4 wpl (n = 33), 6 wpl (n = 34), 8 wpl (n = 35).

Inc., Buffalo Grove, IL) and stored at –20°C until staining and/or examination.

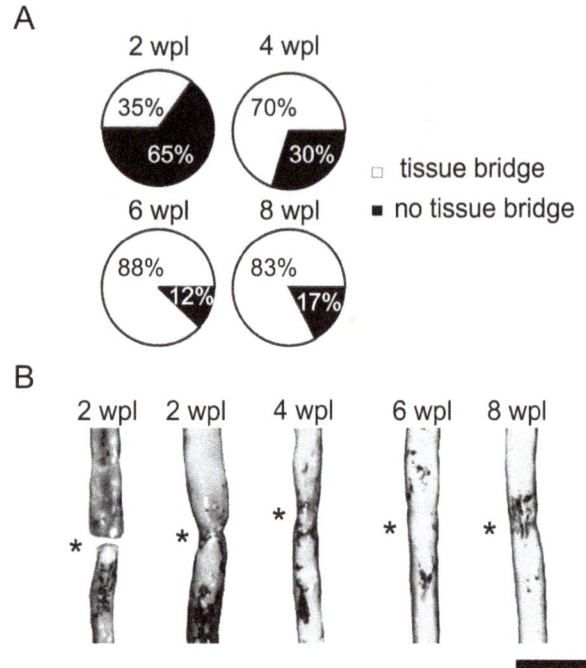

Figure 3. New tissue forms within the spinal cord transection site in adult zebrafish. (A) Percentage of zebrafish with (white) and without (black) a tissue bridge at the different time points post-lesion. (B) Photographs of dissected spinal cord showing the new tissue in the transection site (asterisks) and bridging the spinal cord stumps. Bar = 1 mm.

Immunohistochemistry

Spinal cord sections were incubated in 1% bovine serum albumin (Sigma-Aldrich, St. Louis, MO), 5% goat serum (Invitrogen, Carlsbad, CA) and 0.1% Triton X-100 (Sigma-Aldrich, St. Louis, MO) in PBS for 2 h. Next, the sections were incubated overnight with primary rabbit polyclonal antibodies against glial fibrillary acidic protein (GFAP, 1:200; DAKO North America Inc., Carpinteria, CA). After washing two times for 15 min in PBS primary antibody binding was detected with Alexa Fluor 546 Goat Anti-Rabbit IgG (H+L) (Life technologies, Grand Island, NY). The sections were then washed two times for 15 min, covered with glass slips in Fluorescence Mounting Medium (DAKO North America Inc., Carpinteria, CA), and stored at –20°C until examination.

Assessment of labeled neurons

A Zeiss Axioskop inverted microscope (Carl Zeiss Microscopy, LLC; Thornwood, NY) was used to identify FE-labeled neurons in the brain. All FE-labeled neurons were counted in brain including the NMLF, MaON, and RT. The RT included the superior reticular nucleus, intermediate reticular nucleus and the inferior reticular nucleus. CorelDraw 12 software (Corel Inc., Mountain View, CA) was used to assemble final figures, which were adjusted for contrast, intensity and brightness.

Statistical analysis

SPSS Statistics (IBM Software, Armonk, NY) was used for statistical analyses. Kolmogorov-Smirnov and Shapiro-Wilk's tests were used to determine whether the distribution of data was normal, and Levene's test was used to determine the homogeneity of variance. Upon determining the non-normality of distribution

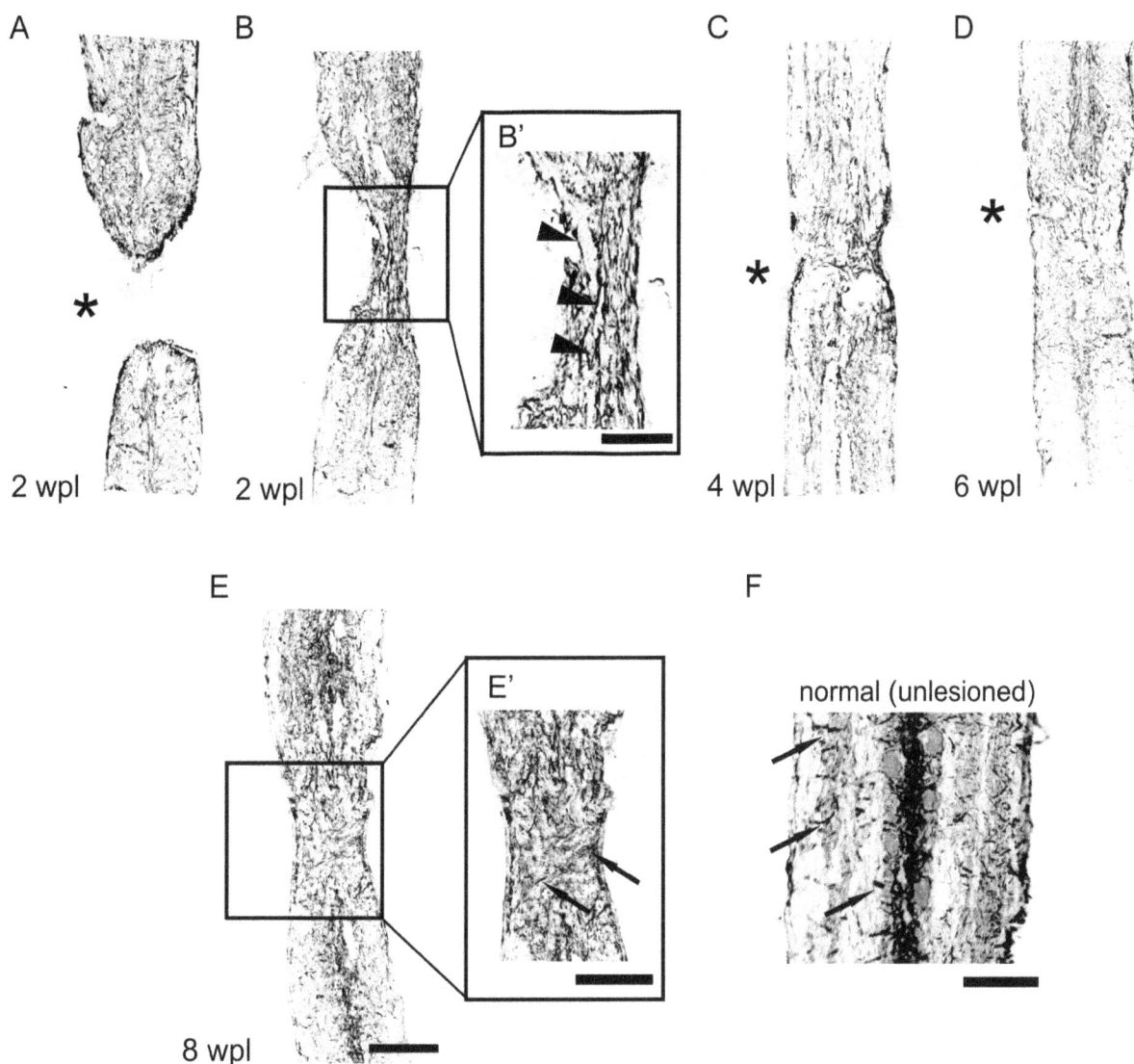

Figure 4. GFAP-positive cells form a tissue bridge at the spinal cord transection site. (A) Distribution and orientation of GFAP-positive cells and processes at two weeks post-lesion in zebrafish without the tissue bridge. Distribution and orientation of GFAP-positive cells and processes in zebrafish with the tissue bridge at two weeks post-lesion (B), four weeks post-lesion (C), six weeks post-lesion (D) and eight weeks post-lesion (E). (B') Enlarged view of the newly formed tissue from box in B. Arrowheads point at the longitudinally oriented GFAP-positive processes. (E') Enlarged view of the newly formed tissue from box in E. (F) Distribution of GFAP-positive cells and processes in normal (unlesioned) tissue. Arrows point at the radially oriented GFAP-positive processes. Transection site is denoted with asterisks. Bar = 100 μm in A–E and 50 μm in B', E', F.

and the non-homogeneity of variance, statistical significance was determined using the non-parametric Kruskal-Wallis test for multiple comparisons followed by Mann-Whitney-U tests for single comparisons with Bonferroni adjustment for the 10–15 comparisons that were conducted. Differences were considered significant with $p \leq 0.005$ (10 comparisons) or $p \leq 0.003$ (15 comparisons). Because the data was non-parametric, we used the median as a measure of central tendency with the variability given as a 95% confidence interval of the median. The cumulative frequency was calculated and plotted for the behavioral data to illustrate the non-normality/normality of distribution in individual groups. The neuron counts and average distance swam were ranked for each zebrafish in a group and Spearman's rho test was used to determine correlations between these two variables. Correlation was considered significant with $p < 0.05$.

Results

Swimming ability gradually increases after spinal cord transection

One day post-lesion the injured zebrafish mainly stayed still at the bottom of the tank and swam only for short periods of time using their pectoral fins (Movie S1). At 2 weeks post-lesion some fish exhibited smooth movements of the tail fin (Movie S2), but most still swam using their pectoral fins (Movie S3). Over the ensuing weeks, most of the injured fish demonstrated increasingly smooth coordinated movements of the tail fin (Movie S4) which resembled those of normal (unlesioned) fish (Movie S5).

With an open-field tracking system swimming was recorded and the distance measured (for the original data see Supporting Information S1). Examples of raw tracking data are provided in figure 2A. The median total swimming distance over a five min

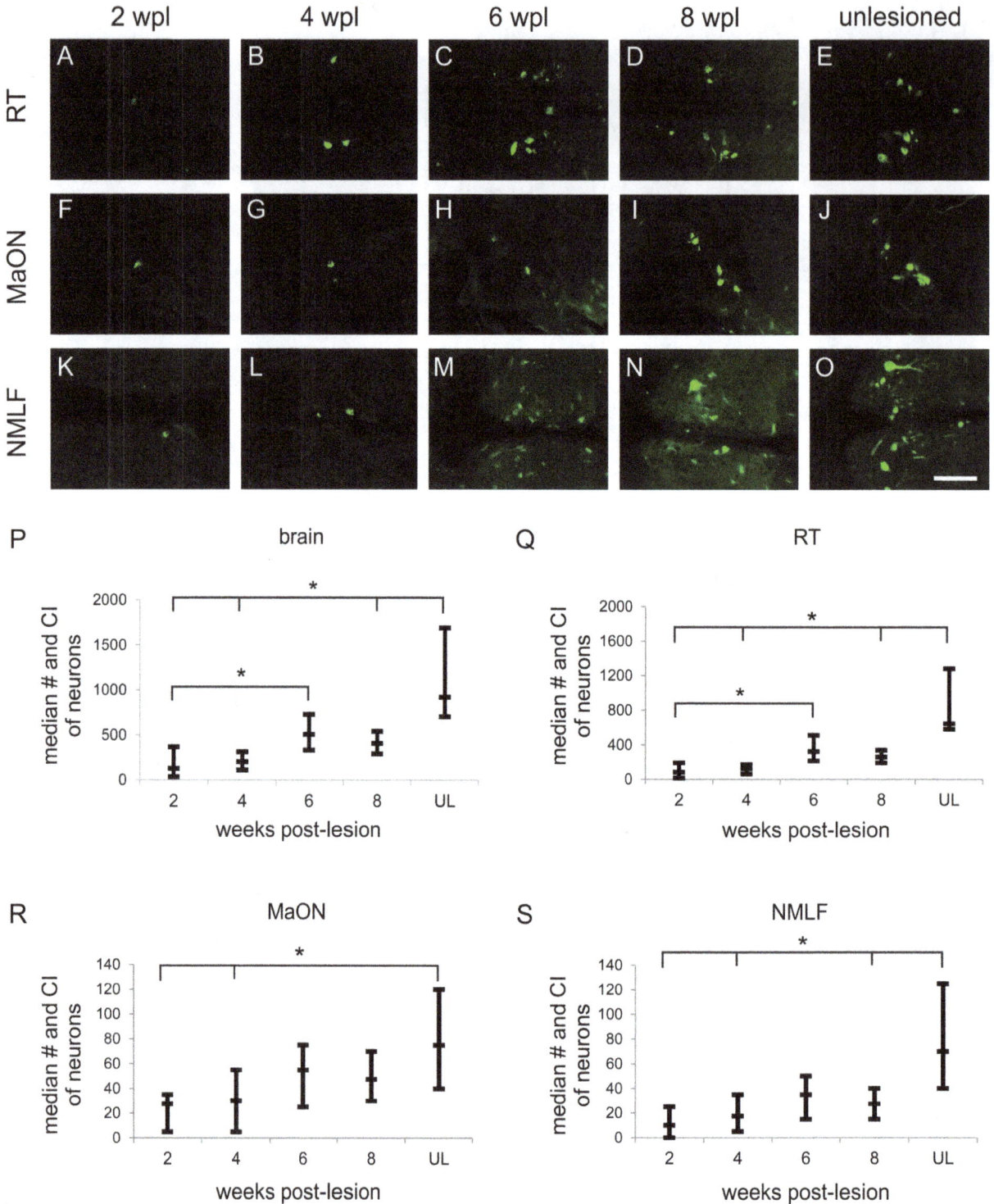

Figure 5. The number of cerebrospinal axons regenerated into the caudal spinal cord increases in time after the lesion. (A–E) Retrogradely labeled neurons in RT (A–E), MaON (F–J), and NMLF (K–O) at two (A, F, K, respectively), four (B, G, L, respectively), six (C, H, M, respectively), and eight (D, I, N, respectively) weeks post-lesion and in unlesioned zebrafish (E, J, O, respectively). Boxplot diagrams demonstrating the median number (and confidence interval of median) of FE-labeled neurons in zebrafish at two, four, six, and eight weeks post-lesion and in unlesioned zebrafish in the whole brain (P), RT (Q), MaON (R), and NMLF (S). Asterisks indicate significant differences between groups (Kruskal-Wallis test, followed by Mann-Whitney U test with Bonferroni correction, p significant if ≤ 0.005). The numbers of total FE-positive neurons and FE-positive neurons in RT are significantly different between two weeks post-lesion and six weeks post-lesion. The number of FE-positive neurons in normal (unlesioned) group is not significantly different from six weeks post-lesion in the whole brain and in each of the examined nuclei. 2 wpl (n = 20); 4 wpl (n = 21); 6 wpl (n = 20); 8 wpl (n = 20), unlesioned (n = 19). Bar = 100 μm in A–O.

Total n=142

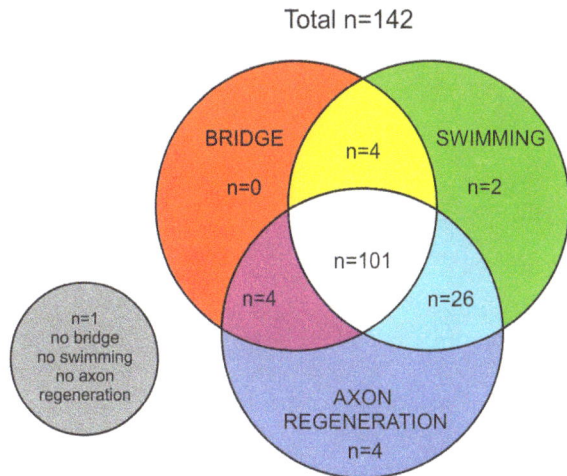

Figure 6. Venn diagram denoting the number of zebrafish belonging to each set. Zebrafish that had a nervous-like tissue bridge (set "BRIDGE"), zebrafish that swam ≥10 cm/5 min (set "SWIMMING"), and zebrafish that had ≥1 FE-positive neuron in brain (set "AXON REGENERATION").

period increased from 22 cm at two (95% CI [13.45, 38.84], n = 20), 229 cm at four (95% CI [131.23, 363.13], n = 33), 509 cm at six (95% CI [292.07, 792.60], n = 34), and 604 cm at eight (95% CI [338.69, 787.15], n = 35) weeks post-lesion (Fig. 2B). Compared with two weeks, swimming distance improved 10-fold at four, 23-fold at six, and 27-fold at eight weeks post-lesion. At each post-lesion time point, injured zebrafish swam less than uninjured zebrafish (median: 1355 cm; 95% CI [956.37, 1625.12], n = 19) (Fig. 2B) and sham-injured fish (median: 1376 cm; 95% CI [1069.26, 1817.34], n = 20) (Fig. 2B). A cumulative distribution plot (Fig. 2C) illustrates the distribution of data at six- and eight-weeks post-lesion approaching the distribution observed in the sham and unlesioned group. At eight weeks post-lesion, swimming ability had recovered to 44% of the sham-injured fish swimming ability. Our data show that swimming ability gradually recovers after a spinal cord transection with the largest relative improvement between two and four weeks post-lesion.

Generation of new tissue at the spinal cord transection site

After complete transection, the spinal cord stumps slightly retracted. In time, new tissue was generated in the lesion forming a bridge between the rostral and caudal spinal cord. The lesion was bridged by new tissue in 35% of the injured zebrafish at two weeks (Figs. 3A, 3B). An example of the spinal cord at two weeks post-lesion in which a tissue bridge is not yet present is provided in figure 4A. The advent of the tissue bridge correlated with the onset of swimming recovery. A tissue bridge was found in 70% of the zebrafish at four weeks, 88% at six weeks, and 83% at eight weeks post-lesion (Figs. 3A, 3B). At six weeks and later, the diameter of the tissue bridge was similar to the spinal cord at the comparable level in unlesioned zebrafish (Fig. 3B). GFAP-positive cells with longitudinally oriented processes appeared in the newly formed tissue during the second week post-lesion (Figs. 4B, 4B'). The GFAP pattern gradually developed into that seen in adult unlesioned zebrafish (Figs. 4C–F). The results show that new tissue gradually forms between the spinal cord stumps starting during the second week post-transection facilitating the onset of coordinated swimming recovery.

Axons regenerate beyond a complete spinal cord transection

To determine axonal regeneration across and beyond the newly formed tissue bridge, we used FE to retrogradely label neurons with an axon projecting into the caudal spinal cord. FE-labeled neurons were consistently found in the RT (Figs. 5A–D), MaON (Figs. 5F–I), and NMLF (Figs. 5K–N) at all times post-lesion. The presence of labeled neurons in the RT, MaON, and NMLF in unlesioned age-matched zebrafish is shown in figures 5E, J, and O, respectively. Lesioned fish also had FE-labeled neurons in the periventricular nucleus of posterior tuberculum, nucleus of the lateral lemniscus, anterior octaval nucleus, descending octaval nucleus, inferior raphe, and Mauthner neurons. The number of FE-labeled neurons in these nuclei was highly variable between zebrafish; we counted these together as 'other nuclei'. At eight weeks post-lesion, the mean total number of the FE-labeled neurons in these 'other nuclei' was 17% of that in the whole brain.

Quantification revealed that from two weeks post-lesion on, the number of FE-positive neurons gradually increased in the RT to a median of 263 (95% CI [190, 340], n = 20; Fig. 5Q), in the MaON to 48 (95% CI [30, 70], n = 20; Fig. 5R), and in the NMLF to 28 (95% CI [15, 40], n = 20; Fig. 5S) at eight weeks post-lesion. At this time point, the number of FE-labeled neurons in the whole brain had gradually increased to a median of 410 (95% CI [295, 540], n = 20; Fig. 5P). The total number of FE-labeled neurons was similar at six and eight weeks post-lesion. The total number of FE-labeled neurons at six weeks post-lesion was not significantly different than that in unlesioned (normal) adult zebrafish (Fig. 5P). At eight weeks, the number of labeled neurons compared with unlesioned zebrafish was 41% in the RT, 64% in the MaON, 40% in the NMLF, and 45% in the whole brain. The data show that cerebrospinal axons start regenerating across and beyond the newly formed tissue bridge in the second week post-lesion.

Axonal regeneration correlates with swimming capability

In order to test the hypothesis that swimming recovery is influenced by tissue bridge formation and cerebrospinal axon regeneration, we examined each of the analyzed zebrafish (n = 142) for presence of tissue bridge at dissection, average distance swam and the presence of FE-labeled neurons in the brain (Fig. 6). Since the transection has been performed at the 8th vertebra, the zebrafish have been able to use their pectoral fins and swim some distance right after the transection (Movie S1). Hence, for further analysis we defined all the zebrafish that swam ≤ 10 cm/5 min as 'not swimming' (n = 9). We found that most of the fish examined (n = 101) had a tissue bridge at dissection, swam ≥ 10 cm/5 min and had at least 1 FE-labeled neuron in the brain. About 23% of zebrafish (n = 32) swam some distance although they had either no tissue bridge (n = 28), no FE-labeled neurons in the brain (n = 6) or both (n = 2).

Next, after exclusion of the not swimming zebrafish we performed regression analyses to determine the exact relationship between the number of traced neurons and average swimming distance. Regression analyses revealed that, taking all zebrafish and all time points in account, the number of FE-labeled neurons correlated with swimming ability ($\rho^2 = .27$, p (one-tailed) <0.01; n = 132; Fig. 7A). A more detailed analysis showed that these two parameters correlated at four ($\rho^2 = .19$, p (one-tailed) <0.01; n = 32; Fig. 7C) and six ($\rho^2 = .27$, p (one-tailed) <0.01; n = 32; Fig. 7D) weeks post-lesion. A correlation between swimming and FE-labeled neurons was not found at two (Fig. 7B) and eight (Fig. 7E) weeks post-lesion or in unlesioned adult zebrafish (Fig. 7F). Investigating the individual nuclei, we found that

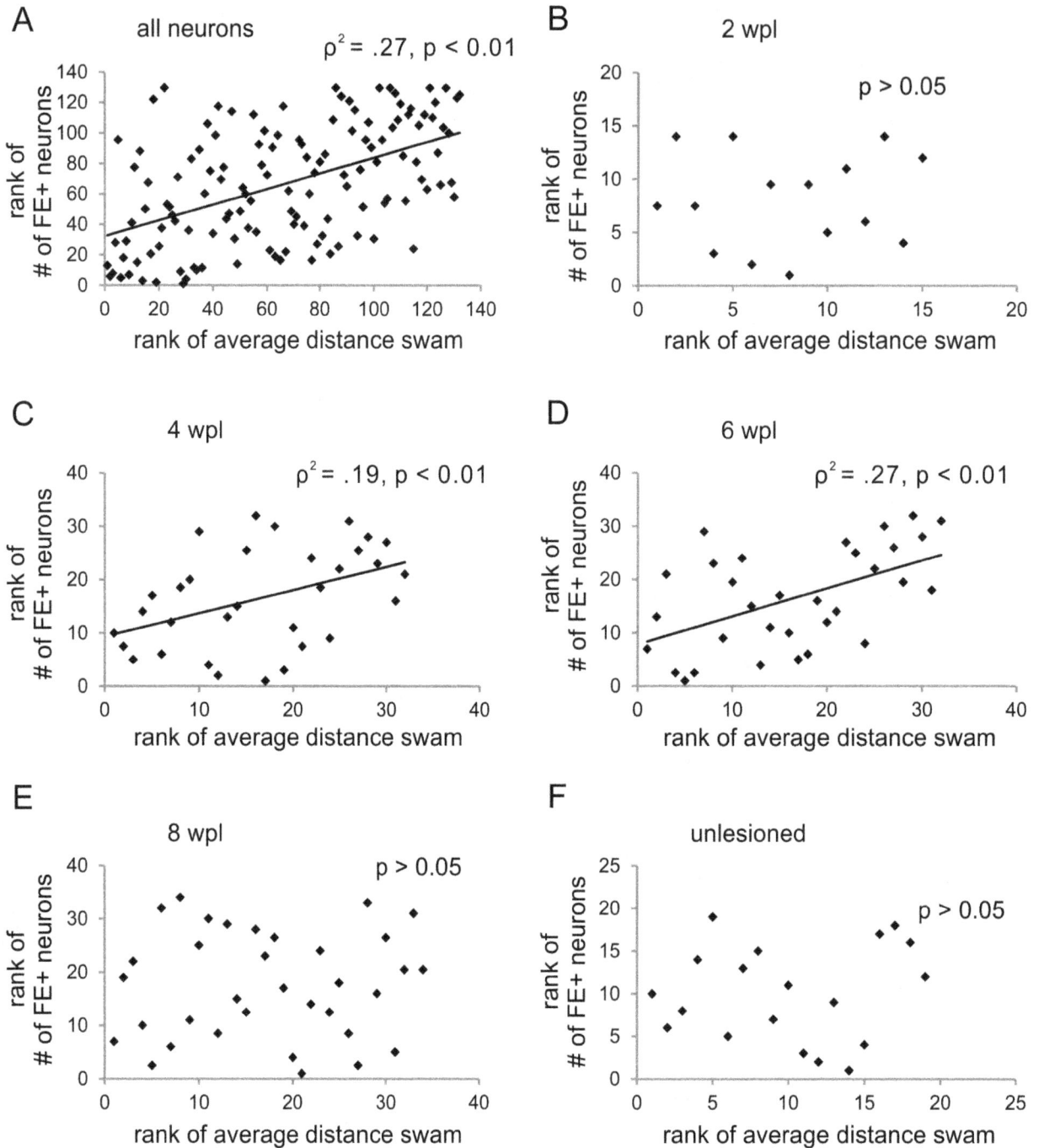

Figure 7. Cerebrospinal axon regeneration is correlated with swimming ability. (A) Rank of number of FE-positive neurons in the whole brain is correlated with the rank of average distance swam in all analyzed zebrafish (n = 132) and, specifically, at (C) four (n = 32) and (D) six (n = 32) weeks post-lesion. No correlation was observed at (B) two (n = 15) and (E) eight (n = 34) weeks post-lesion and in (F) normal (unlesioned) zebrafish (n = 19). Spearman's rho correlation, differences considered significant with p<0.05.

swimming ability correlated with the number of FE-positive neurons in the RT ($\rho^2 = .38$, p (one-tailed) <0.01, n = 92; Fig. 8A), MaON ($\rho^2 = .13$, p (one-tailed) <0.01, n = 92, Fig. 8B), and NMLF ($\rho^2 = .25$, p (one-tailed) <0.01, n = 92; Fig. 8C).

Discussion

Our data showed that adult zebrafish gradually regain their ability to generate coordinated swimming movements between two and eight weeks after a complete spinal cord transection. The largest relative improvement in swimming was found between the second and fourth week post-injury. Recovery was incomplete reaching a maximum of 44% of the swimming ability of sham-

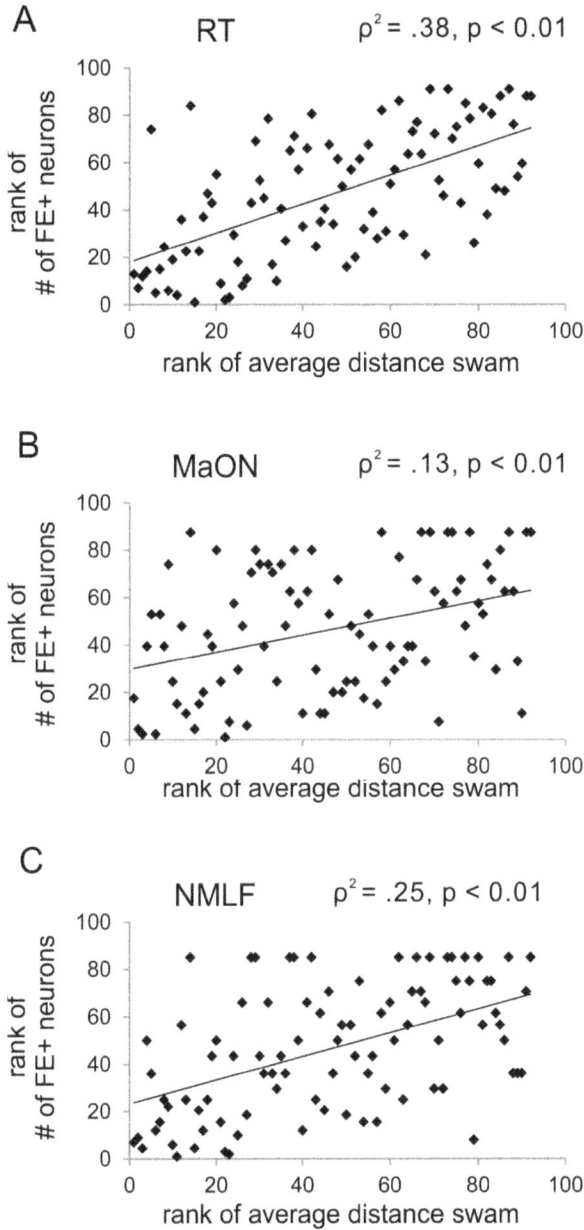

Figure 8. Axonal regeneration from specific brain nuclei is correlated with swimming ability. In all analyzed zebrafish, the rank of average distance swam is correlated with the rank of number of FE-positive neurons in the (A) RT, (B) MaON, and the (C) NMLF. Spearman's rho correlation, differences considered significant with p<0.05, n=92.

We demonstrated that cerebrospinal axons extend beyond the transection site starting from the second week post-injury. These axons derived mostly from existing brainstem neurons because a possible contribution of newly generated brainstem neurons is either small [9] or absent [6]. The largest relative growth was found between the second and fourth week post-injury. At six weeks, the total number of regenerated cerebrospinal axons reached its maximum at 55% of normal projection in unlesioned age-matched zebrafish. Among the examined nuclei, the RT contained the largest number of neurons projecting beyond the lesion and the MaON exhibited the largest relative regenerative capacity with 64% of its normal projection in unlesioned zebrafish.

This is the first quantitative study of the regenerative response of cerebrospinal axons during the first weeks after spinal cord injury in adult zebrafish. Our data is in agreement with the finding that neurons in the RT, MaON, and NMLF are most regenerative in adult zebrafish after spinal cord injury [9]. The percentage of regenerating neurons at six weeks post-lesion is largely similar between our and this previous study [9]. However, the total number of retrogradely-labeled (regenerating) neurons is higher in the present study, which could be due to the use of different retrograde tracers; Fluoroemerald in the present study and biocytin in the previous study [9]. An alternative explanation may be that in time regenerated axons are pruned from the caudal spinal cord which would explain lower overall number of back-filled neurons with tracer injections at later time points. Indeed, our finding of lower numbers of labeled neurons in the whole brain and in the examined nuclei, at 8 weeks as compared to 6 weeks, supports such a pruning mechanism.

Our data showed that, with time, newly formed tissue bridged the spinal cord stumps in an increasing number of zebrafish, indicating variability in the ability to generate new tissue. From six weeks on, this bridge had a similar diameter and appeared essentially similar as the unlesioned spinal cord at the same spinal cord segment. We found that in the new tissue, an early mostly longitudinal pattern of GFAP-positive processes developed gradually into a more typical radial pattern, which is congruent with previously published data [5]. The consecutive longitudinal and radial pattern of GFAP-positive processes reflected the initial presence of elongated bipolar glial cells bridging the spinal cord stumps and the final presence of radial glia, a hallmark of normal unlesioned spinal cord tissue, which was apparent around week six post-lesion when a central canal had been reconstructed [5]. Interestingly, we found the tissue bridge permissive to axon growth starting around two weeks post-lesion, which was before its architecture had finalized in that typical for unlesioned nervous tissue. In fact, the longitudinal GFAP-positive processes facilitated axon regeneration across the bridge [5]. It is also possible that radially oriented GFAP-processes impeded axon regeneration, which could explain the relative lower regenerative responses at later post-lesion time points. Altogether, it is likely that the development of the new tissue into mature-appearing nervous tissue at least in part determined the magnitude of the axon growth process and thus of the overall swimming recovery. Cellular or molecular manipulation of this maturation process may therefore be used as a tool to influence the overall repair and recovery after spinal cord injury.

The onset of coordinated swimming was noticed around two weeks post-lesion which correlates with the time when new tissue was found spanning the lesion and when the first cerebrospinal axons were found in the caudal spinal cord. The temporal profiles of swimming recovery and axon regeneration were largely similar with a progressive increase that starts to plateau after six weeks post-lesion. For both swimming and axon regeneration around

injured age-matched zebrafish at eight weeks post-injury. These data on the recovery of swimming after a complete spinal cord transection were largely in agreement with previous studies [1,4]. The average post-lesion swimming distance in our study was shorter than that reported at comparable time-points which may account for the lower maximum recovery of 44% vs. 57% [1] or 78% [4]. The lack of an adaptation period prior to measuring swimming distance in our study may explain these overall shorter distances [4]. Also, the use of a shorter time interval between trials [1] may have contributed to the observed difference in swimming distances.

50% of the maximum was reached at four weeks post-lesion. This means that in most fish at this time point, at least half of the axons were still actively regenerating.

Taking all post-lesion time points into account, regression analysis confirmed the presence of a significant correlation between swimming distance and cerebrospinal axon number. When specific post-lesion time points were analyzed, the correlation between swimming and cerebrospinal axon number was present at four and six weeks, but not at two and eight weeks post-lesion. The lack of a relationship at two weeks post-lesion may reflect the relatively small number of axons that regenerated beyond the lesion at this early time point. Also, at two weeks, 65% of all zebrafish had not yet formed a complete tissue bridge between the spinal cord stumps. The lack of a relationship between swimming and axon number at eight weeks post-lesion could have been due to a pruning effect that was apparent at this time point.

Dopaminergic and serotonergic axons from neurons in diencephalic and raphe nuclei, respectively, have been implicated in swimming ability in adult zebrafish [2]. However, these nuclei project only a few axons to spinal cord and rarely regenerate axons as evidenced by Beckers et al. [9] and confirmed by our own data. Additionally, these types of neurons regenerate their axon over relatively short distances beyond the transection site [2]. In contrast, the significant correlation between the number of regenerated axons originating from RT, MaON and NMLF and the average swimming distance suggests that these nuclei are the most likely candidates in the descending control of locomotion. These nuclei have a large number of neurons projecting to mid-thoracic level of spinal cord and have been shown to consistently regenerate about half of that projection to at least 4 mm beyond the lesion by six weeks post-lesion.

Supporting the idea that RT, MaON and NMLF are the principal nuclei involved in the descending control of zebrafish swimming is a recent study by Kyriakatos et al. [10] Using a model of fictive locomotion, they investigated the origin of descending inputs to central pattern generators of the spinal cord in the adult unlesioned zebrafish. While the stimulated nuclei were not anatomically identified, the position of the electrodes in their paper indicates that they most likely stimulated reticular nuclei and/or the medial longitudinal fasciculus. Additionally, it was also recently shown that reticulospinal glutamatergic V2a neurons are involved in the excitation of spinal locomotor circuits during larval zebrafish swimming [11].

The key finding of this study is that the axons of RT, MaON and NMLF actively regenerate between the second and fourth week post-lesion. A comprehensive gene expression data on populations of regenerating vs. non-regenerating neurons, collected during this period, may provide us with key molecules involved in the axonal regeneration. The information on molecules involved in the successful axonal regeneration can further be used to create transgenic zebrafish with labeled regenerating axons to aid future functional and connectomics studies.

Supporting Information

Movie S1   Zebrafish swimming at one day post-lesion.

Movie S2   Zebrafish swimming at two weeks post-lesion (with smooth movements of the tail fin).

Movie S3   Zebrafish swimming at two weeks post-lesion (without smooth movements of the tail fin).

Movie S4   Zebrafish swimming at four weeks post-lesion.

Movie S5   Unlesioned zebrafish swimming.

Supporting Information S1   Original data.

Acknowledgments

We thank Tabitha Novosat for help with behavioral analysis, tissue processing, and general zebrafish maintenance.

Author Contributions

Conceived and designed the experiments: KV MO DS JAP. Performed the experiments: KV DS. Analyzed the data: KV MO. Contributed reagents/materials/analysis tools: JAP. Contributed to the writing of the manuscript: KV MO JAP.

References

1. Becker CG, Lieberoth BC, Morellini F, Feldner J, Becker T, et al. (2004) L1.1 is involved in spinal cord regeneration in adult zebrafish. The Journal of neuroscience: the official journal of the Society for Neuroscience 24: 7837–7842.
2. Kuscha V, Barreiro-Iglesias A, Becker CG, Becker T (2012) Plasticity of tyrosine hydroxylase and serotonergic systems in the regenerating spinal cord of adult zebrafish. The Journal of comparative neurology 520: 933–951.
3. van Raamsdonk W, Maslam S, de Jong DH, Smit-Onel MJ, Velzing E (1998) Long term effects of spinal cord transection in zebrafish: swimming performances, and metabolic properties of the neuromuscular system. Acta histochemica 100: 117–131.
4. Fang P, Lin JF, Pan HC, Shen YQ, Schachner M (2012) A surgery protocol for adult zebrafish spinal cord injury. J Genet Genomics 39: 481–487.
5. Goldshmit Y, Sztal TE, Jusuf PR, Hall TE, Nguyen-Chi M, et al. (2012) Fgf-dependent glial cell bridges facilitate spinal cord regeneration in zebrafish. The Journal of neuroscience: the official journal of the Society for Neuroscience 32: 7477–7492.
6. Ogai K, Hisano S, Mawatari K, Sugitani K, Koriyama Y, et al. (2012) Upregulation of anti-apoptotic factors in upper motor neurons after spinal cord injury in adult zebrafish. Neurochem Int 61: 1202–1211.
7. Hui SP, Dutta A, Ghosh S (2010) Cellular response after crush injury in adult zebrafish spinal cord. Dev Dyn 239: 2962–2979.
8. Becker T, Wullimann MF, Becker CG, Bernhardt RR, Schachner M (1997) Axonal regrowth after spinal cord transection in adult zebrafish. The Journal of comparative neurology 377: 577–595.
9. Becker T, Becker CG (2001) Regenerating descending axons preferentially reroute to the gray matter in the presence of a general macrophage/microglial reaction caudal to a spinal transection in adult zebrafish. The Journal of comparative neurology 433: 131–147.
10. Kyriakatos A, Mahmood R, Ausborn J, Porres CP, Buschges A, et al. (2011) Initiation of locomotion in adult zebrafish. The Journal of neuroscience: the official journal of the Society for Neuroscience 31: 8422–8431.
11. Kimura Y, Satou C, Fujioka S, Shoji W, Umeda K, et al. (2013) Hindbrain V2a neurons in the excitation of spinal locomotor circuits during zebrafish swimming. Curr Biol 23: 843–849.

5

The Effects of Controlled Release of Neurotrophin-3 from PCLA Scaffolds on the Survival and Neuronal Differentiation of Transplanted Neural Stem Cells in a Rat Spinal Cord Injury Model

Shuo Tang[1⑤]**, Xiang Liao**[2⑤]**, Bo Shi**[3]**, Yanzhen Qu**[4]**, Zeyu Huang**[1]**, Qiang Lin**[5]*****, Xiaodong Guo**[4]*****, Fuxing Pei**[1]*****

1 Department of Orthopaedics, West China Hospital, Sichuan University, Chengdu, China, 2 Department of Pain Medicine, Shenzhen Nanshan Hospital, Shenzhen, China, 3 Department of Orthopaedics, Mianyang Center Hospital, Mianyang, China, 4 Department of Orthopaedics, Union Hospital, Tongji Medical College, Huazhong University of Science and Technology, Wuhan, China, 5 Department of Orthopaedics, Guangdong hospital of traditional Chinese medicine, Guangzhou, China

Abstract

Neural stem cells (NSCs) have emerged as a potential source for cell replacement therapy following spinal cord injury (SCI). However, poor survival and low neuronal differentiation remain major obstacles to the use of NSCs. Biomaterials with neurotrophic factors are promising strategies for promoting the proliferation and differentiation of NSCs. Silk fibroin (SF) matrices were demonstrated to successfully deliver growth factors and preserve their potency. In this study, by incorporating NT-3 into a SF coating, we successfully developed NT-3-immobilized scaffolds (membranes and conduits). Sustained release of bioactive NT-3 from the conduits for up to 8 weeks was achieved. Cell viability was confirmed using live/dead staining after 14 days in culture. The efficacy of the immobilized NT-3 was confirmed by assessing NSC neuronal differentiation in vitro. NSC neuronal differentiation was 55.2±4.1% on the NT-3-immobilized membranes, which was significantly higher than that on the NT-3 free membrane. Furthermore, 8 weeks after the NSCs were seeded into conduits and implanted in rats with a transected SCI, the conduit+NT-3+NSCs group achieved higher NSC survival (75.8±15.1%) and neuronal differentiation (21.5±5.2%) compared with the conduit+NSCs group. The animals that received the conduit+NT-3+NSCs treatment also showed improved functional outcomes, as well as increased axonal regeneration. These results indicate the feasibility of fabricating NT-3-immobilized scaffolds using the adsorption of NT-3/SF coating method, as well as the potential of these scaffolds to induce SCI repair by promoting survival and neuronal differentiation of transplanted NSCs.

Editor: Wenhui Hu, Temple University School of Medicine, United States of America

Funding: This work was financially supported by the National Natural Science Foundation of China (NSFC, No. 81401787, 81371939 and 81000812), the International Science & Technology Cooperation Program of China (2013DFG32690), as well as the Science & Technology Bureau of Chengdu City-West China Hospital Joint Foundation (ZH13034). The funders had no role in study design, data collection and analysis, decision to publish, or preparation of the manuscript.

Competing Interests: The authors have declared that no competing interests exist.

* Email: qiang_linm@163.com (QL); xiaodongguo@hust.edu.cn (XDG); peifuxing@vip.163.com (FXP)

⑤ These authors contributed equally to this work.

Introduction

Trauma-induced spinal cord injuries (SCI) resulting in significant motor impairment or paralysis remain a critical public health concern with approximately 100,000 new cases each year [1]. SCI interrupts connections between the brain and the spinal cord, which transmit motor control and somatic sensory signals. Victims of SCI often suffer from severe neurological disabilities. However, effective treatment is currently limited because of the complexity of the pathophysiology of the injured spinal cord. SCI triggers a series of events, including systemic and local inflammatory responses, subsequent death of neuronal and glial cells, and formation of cavities and glial scars in the injury site [2].

Cell transplantation therapy provides a potential source of cells to repopulate the damaged spinal cord and aid in functional recovery by replacing damaged circuits, increasing plasticity, and promoting cell survival and regeneration of host axons [3]. Neural stem cells (NSCs) have the potential to proliferate, migrate, and differentiate into the three major cell types of the central nerve system, oligodendrocytes, astrocytes, and neurons, to replace lost cells or rescue dysfunctional cells [4,5]. However, poor cell survival and uncontrolled differentiation of transplanted NSCs are the current limitations of this approach [6]. Transplanted NSCs have a much greater tendency to astrocytically differentiate, and they rarely undergo neuronal differentiation. Neurons that have differentiated from transplanted NSCs can extend axons into the host spinal cord in both rostral and caudal directions over remarkably long distances, and connections with the host axons are then formed. The host axons can also regenerate into the sites of transplanted NSCs and promote host-to-graft connectivity [7]. The differentiation into oligodendrocytes can promote remyelination of regenerated axons [8]. However, the differentiation of transplanted NSCs into astrocytes may be problematic because reactive gliosis is believed to be an inhibitor of regeneration [9].

Therefore, increasing the rate of survival and differentiation of NSCs into neuronal cells is important.

Neurotrophins (NTs), such as nerve growth factor (NGF), brain-derived neurophic factor, and neurotrophin-3 (NT-3), are important in neuronal survival and differentiation [10,11]. Among these factors, NT-3 facilitates the differentiation of NSCs into neurons and supports the survival and maturation of neurons [12]. Combining NSC transplantation with NT-3 is considered a potentially useful approach for the treatment of SCI [13]. NSC transplantation and soluble NT therapies are limited by the poor survival of injected cells and the short half-life of injected NTs. The external pump/catheter system is used as a controlled release system for delivering drugs into the intrathecal space through a catheter. However, this method is prone to infection and has not been approved for long-term delivery in SCI patients in the USA [14]. To address these issues, tissue-engineered scaffolds have been developed for the treatment of SCI. Biodegradable scaffolds and NSC transplantation each have unique advantages as therapeutic strategies for SCI. Biodegradable scaffolds have many advantages as a delivery system, not only for sustained NT-3 delivery but also for the delivery of NSCs to the injured spinal cord [15]. Furthermore, scaffolds can also bridge the lesion with a 3D permissive environment, which can fill the tissue gap and concomitantly support axonal regeneration [16].

Thus, the incorporation of NT-3 within a biodegradable scaffold offers an opportunity to promote the survival and differentiation of NSCs. Most of the current approaches in incorporating growth factors in biomaterials include physically entrapping soluble growth factors into the scaffolds or covalently immobilizing growth factors onto synthetic polymer scaffolds [17]. By immobilizing growth factors within scaffolds, the growth factors are protected against cellular inactivation and digestion [18]. As a result, the immobilized growth factors can overcome the diffusional limitations of soluble factors, thereby allowing sustained activity. However, most of the covalent immobilization methods require the use of organic solvents or cross-linking agents, which may limit the biological activity of the growth factors. Furthermore, by using these methods, the immobilization of growth factors is not a simple task [19].

Silk fibroin (SF), a natural protein, has been recently found to be biocompatible, slowly biodegradable, and endowed with excellent mechanical properties and processability [20]. SF matrices can successfully deliver growth factors while preserving their potency [21]. Interestingly, SF in aqueous solution can precipitate due to β-sheet formation. SF adsorbs onto various substrates spontaneously and forms a layer, which eventually forms a robust and stable coating through mild all-aqueous processes [22]. Growth factors can be incorporated into the SF matrix during these processes. With the degradation of SF, growth factors can be released. In our previous study, Poly(ε-caprolactone)-block-poly(l-lactic acid-co-ε-caprolactone) (PCLA) scaffolds with precise hierarchical pore architectures were fabricated using injection molding combined with thermally induced phase separation [23]. In the present study, the PCLA scaffolds (membranes and conduits) were fabricated first, and then NT-3 was immobilized within the scaffolds by coating the scaffold with a solution of SF and NT-3. NSCs were cultured in vitro, and their differentiation into neural cells was measured after seeding on the NT-3-immobilized membranes. A rat spinal cord transection model was utilized to evaluate the efficacy of the NT-3 immobilized conduit with the adhered NSCs in vivo.

Materials and Methods

Ethics Statement

All experimental protocols were approved by the Ethics Committee in Sichuan University (protocol # 2013-C-206). The animals were maintained on a standard laboratory diet in plastic cages at ambient temperature, and allowed free mobilization in compliance with the requirements of the International Council on Laboratory Animal Science.

Scaffold fabrication and NT-3 immobilization

PCLA: [PCL27-b-P(LLA405- co-CL14) (PCLA); Mn = 8.8×10^4, PDI = 1.22, T = 171.2°C, and ΔH = 39.3 J/g. PCLA was first dissolved in dioxane with a concentration of 60 mg/ml at 50°C, and the mold was chilled to the preset temperature of −40°C. The hot PCLA/dioxane solution was quickly injected into the cold mold using a syringe, as previously described [24]. The temperature of the system was maintained at −40°C for 2 h to induce the solid-liquid phase separation of the polymer solution. Then, the temperature of the cold trap was adjusted to −20°C, and the solvents were sublimated through a two-day lyophilizing process. Finally, the mold was removed, and the 2D scaffolds (membranes) and the 3D scaffolds (conduits) for in vitro and in vivo studies, respectively, were obtained. The prepared conduit had an inner diameter of 3.0 mm, a wall thickness of 0.5 mm and a length of 2.0 mm.

The SF aqueous solution was prepared as previously described [22]. Briefly, cocoons from *Bombyx mori* were boiled in ultra-purified water (UPW) containing 0.02 M Na_2CO_3, thoroughly rinsed with distilled water to extract the glue-like sericin proteins and wax, and then dissolved in 9 M LiBr at 55°C to obtain a 3% (w/v) aqueous SF solution. NT-3 (PeproTech, Rocky Hill, NJ, USA) was embedded by adding 20 µg of NT-3 to 1 ml of SF solution. The NT-3/SF solution was subsequently sterilized using a 0.22 µm filter (Millipore, Tullagreen, Ireland). The scaffolds were immersed in the NT-3/SF solution for 2 h at room temperature. Then, the scaffolds were freeze-dried overnight and subsequently treated with 90% (v/v) methanol in UPW for 15 min to induce formation of SF crystalline β-sheet structure. The scaffolds were stored in a desiccator and rinsed with sterile PBS three times before use.

Determination of kinetics of NT-3 release from NT-3 immobilized PCLA scaffold

Five conduits were separately immersed in 500 µl PBS (10 mM, pH 7.4) and kept in a gently shaking incubator (20 rpm) at 37°C for various time periods up to 8 weeks. The release of NT-3 was examined on day 1, with further measurements after 2, 3, 4, 5, 6, and 7 days. After that, continuous measurements were performed for 8 weeks at 1 week intervals. At each time interval, the supernatant was removed completely and replaced with fresh buffer. The amounts of NT-3 in the collected supernatants were measured using enzyme-linked immunosorbent assay (ELISA; Becton Dickinson, Franklin Lakes, NJ, USA) in accordance with the manufacturer's instructions. The absorbance was measured at 450 nm using a plate reader (Model 680; Bio-RAD, Hercules, CA, USA). The NT-3 concentration was determined by comparing the reading to the standard curve. The amounts of NT-3 in each conduit were calculated based on the cumulative amounts of bioactive NT-3 released in PBS and normalized by the mass of the conduit.

Isolation and culture of rat brain-derived NSCs

Primary NSCs were isolated from E14 Sprague-Dawley (SD) rats, expressing green fluorescent protein (GFP) for the in vivo study and non-GFP for the in vitro study. The transgenic SD rats expressing GFP were purchased from Cyagen Biotechnology Company Ltd. (Guangzhou, China). Whole hippocampi were dissected and dissociated in Hanks' balanced salt solution (HBSS). After centrifugation at 1000 rpm for 5 min, the supernatant containing cell debris was removed. The pelleted cells were resuspended in growth medium, which contained Neurobasal media (Gibco-Invitrogen, Carlsbad, CA, USA), B27 neural supplement (Gibco-Invitrogen), 2 mM L-glutamine (Sigma-Aldrich, St Louis, MO, USA), 1% penicillin-streptomycin (Sigma-Aldrich), 20 ng/ml epidermal growth factor (Gibco-Invitrogen), and 20 ng/ml bFGF (Gibco-Invitrogen). The cells were then plated onto 75 ml culture flasks, with fresh medium every 3 days. The cultured cells typically grew as suspending neurospheres and were passaged once a week. The expression of nestin, a marker of NSCs, was assessed by immunocytochemistry.

PCLA membrane studies

PCLA membrane were placed in 24-well plates and sterilized with 70% ethanol for 5 min, followed by washing three times with PBS solution prior to use. NSCs were spun down at 1500 rpm for 5 min, and the resultant pellet was re-suspended and dissociated in fresh growth media. The cell solution was then added so that each well contained 10 000 cells, and the final volume of media in the wells was 500 μl. After 24 h, the media was removed and replaced with differentiation media – Neurobasal media containing B27 supplement, L-glutamine, penicillin-streptomycin, and 1% fetal bovine serum (FBS). Half-volume media changes were performed every 48 h thereafter.

The viability of cells on the membranes was determined using a live/dead assay (Molecular Probes, Eugene, OR), in accordance with the manufacturer's protocol. Briefly, after 14 days of culture, the PCLA membranes were rinsed with 0.1 M PBS (pH 7.4) three times, followed by staining in 2 ml 0.1 M PBS containing 2 mM of calcein-AM and 4 mM ethidium homodimer (EthD-III) for 30 min at 37°C. The cells were washed again with PBS and then imaged using an Olympus fluorescent microscope. Live cells stained with calcein-AM showed a green color, and dead cells stained with EthD-III showed a red color. Cell viability was calculated by counting the percentage of calcein-AM-positive cells over the total number of cells from five randomly chosen fields of view per sample.

Differentiation was determined using immunocytochemistry staining following the standard protocol. The following primary antibodies were used for immunohistochemical analysis: rabbit anti-2',3'-cyclic nucleotide 3'-phosphodiesterase (CNPase, 1:100, Cell Signaling Technology, Beverly, MA), mouse anti-glial fibrillary acidic protein (GFAP; 1:500, Sigma, St. Louis, MO) for astrocytes, and rabbit anti-microtubule-associated protein 2 (MAP2; 1:500, Sigma, St. Louis, MO) for neurons. Briefly, the samples were fixed in 4% paraformaldehyde for 20 min at 4°C and then permeabilized with 0.3% Triton X-100 for 5 min. Non-specific binding was blocked with 10% goat serum and 1% bovine serum albumin (BSA) for 1 h at room temperature. The samples were subsequently incubated with the primary antibodies overnight at 4°C. After washing with PBS, the samples were incubated at room temperature for 2 h with secondary fluorescent antibodies: Alexa Fluor 488-conjugated goat anti-rabbit IgG or Alexa Fluor 594-conjugated goat anti-mouse IgG (1:500, Invitrogen, Carlsbad, CA, USA). The nuclei were stained with 4',6-diamidino-2-phenylindole (DAPI; Sigma-Aldrich, St Louis, MO, USA). The samples were viewed under an Olympus fluorescent microscope. Cell differentiation was calculated by counting the percentage of MAP2-, GFAP- and CNPase-positive cells from five randomly chosen fields of view per sample using ImageJ software (National Institutes of Health, Bethesda, MD).

Seeding of NSCs into PCLA conduits

Sterile conduits were incubated in complete media overnight, prior to cell seeding. Before seeding the NSCs into the conduits, the NSCs were digested into single cell suspension. The media inside the tubes were then replaced with 80 μl of cell suspension, which contained GFP-positive cells (passage 4) at a cell density of 4×10^6 cells per 80 μl. For the in vivo study, the conduits containing the neurosphere suspension were rotated manually every 15 min for 1 hour to achieve uniform cell seeding. These conduits were then transferred to new wells, which contained growth media, and incubated for 24 h prior to implantation into the transected spinal cords. Scanning electron microscopy (SEM, JSM-5800LV) (JEOL, Tokyo, Japan) was used to observe the cell morphology after 24 h of culture. The cell density inside the channels was not uniform and covered mainly the lower half of the channels due to gravity.

Animal surgery and post-operative care

All of the animal experiments were approved and performed according to the regulations of the Animal Ethical Committee of our university. Adult male rats (220–250 g, purchased from the Experimental Animals Center of Sichun University) were divided randomly into three groups. 1, conduit+NT-3+NSCs group (n = 8): the transected spinal cord was bridged by an NT-3 immobilized conduit with NSCs; 2, conduit+NSCs group (n = 7): the transected spinal cord was bridged by a conduit with NSCs; 3, conduit+NT-3 group (n = 7): the transected spinal cord was bridged by an NT-3 immobilized conduit without NSCs. Each rat was anesthetized with an intraperitoneal injection of sodium pentobarbital (50 mg/kg) before the operation. We performed all of the surgical procedures under a microscope and under sterile conditions. The backs of rats were shaved and aseptically prepared. After checking of the lowest lumbar level, a laminectomy was performed to expose the T8-10 spinal segments. The posterior aspect of the spinal cord was exposed and the dura was cut vertically using microforceps and microscissors. An angled microscissor was used to transect the spinal cord competely and the stumps were retracted, creating a 2.0-mm gap in the spinal cord of T9. To prevent unexpected reflex movements and bleeding, we applied two drops of 1% lidocaine with epinephrine onto the spinal cord. The conduit was grafted into the lesion site in a manner such that the cut ends of both spinal stumps were apposed to the NSCs-containing conduit. The exposed spinal cord with the implanted conduit was covered with muscles and fascia. The skin was repositioned and closed with sutures.

After surgery, the rats were injected with 5.0 ml saline subcutaneously and allowed to recuperate. Buprenorphine (0.03 mg/kg) was administered subcutaneously for 3 days to minimize pain. Enroflaxacin (2.5 mg/kg) was administered subcutaneously for 7 days for prophylactic treatment against postoperative infections. Bladders were manually expressed thrice daily for the duration of the experiment. Functional recovery was assessed weekly during the 8 week survival period using the Basso, Beattie, Bresnahan (BBB) open field locomotor scale [25]. BBB scoring was conducted by two observers blinded to the experimental groups. All of the animals were evaluated weekly for 8 weeks.

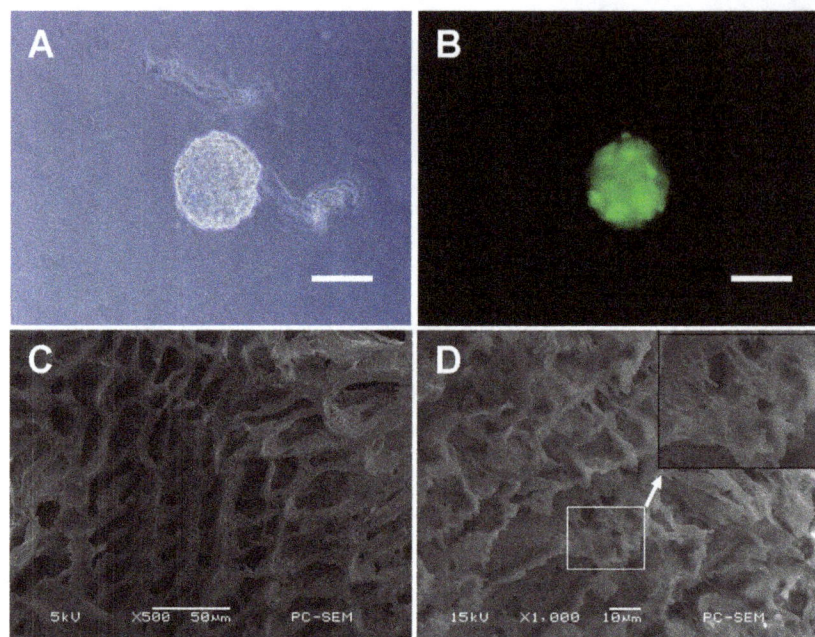

Figure 1. Neurosphere and PCLA scaffold. (A) A neurosphere visualized under a light microscope. (B) GFP-positive neurosphere visualized under a fluorescent microscope. (C) SEM images of the inner wall of the PCLA conduit without NSCs. (D) NSCs adhered to the inner wall of the PCLA conduit. The black box show representative cells from the white box at higher magnification to enhance visualization of cellular morphology under SEM. Scale bars = 100 μm in A–B, 50 μm in C, and 10 μm in D.

Tissue preparation and cell counts of GFP-positive cells

The animals were sacrificed via transcardial perfusion with 4% paraformaldehyde in 0.1 M PBS at 8 weeks after implantation. The spinal cords were carefully removed, postfixed in 4% paraformaldehyde for 5 h, and then transferred to 0.1 M PBS containing 30% sucrose at 4°C overnight. Afterwards, they were frozen and embedded in an optimal cutting temperature (OCT) compound (Sakura, Tokyo, Japan), and then cut into 15 μm sections on a freezing microtome for cell count and histological analysis.

To quantify cell survival, every tenth equidistant frozen section of the spinal cord was selected from each animal and counterstained with the nuclear dye DAPI. The samples were examined using a Zeiss LSM 710 laser scanning confocal microscope (LSCM; Zeiss, Oberkochen, Germany). A minimum of five random fields containing the GFP-positive transplanted NSCs were photographed over multiple tissue sections of each animal. Cell survival was calculated by manually counting GFP-positive cells associated with DAPI stained nuclei across the sample.

Histological analysis

In addition to the antibodies previously described, mouse anti-neurofilament 200 (NF200; 1:500, Sigma, St. Louis, MO) for axons was also used. The secondary antibodies were Alexa Fluor 594-conjugated goat anti-mouse or goat anti-rabbit IgG antibodies (1:500, Invitrogen, Carlsbad, CA, USA). The sections were washed with PBS and permeabilized with 0.3% Triton X-100 for 5 min. Non-specific binding was blocked using 10% goat serum and 1% BSA for 1 h at room temperature. After washing with PBS, the sections were incubated in primary antibody overnight at 4°C. Afterwards, sections were washed with 0.1 M PBS, and corresponding secondary antibodies was added for 1 h at 25°C. After another series of washes, the nuclei were stained with DAPI. Finally, the immunostained samples were mounted

onto glass slides with mounting medium and viewed under the LSCM. In all the immunohistochemistry procedures, appropriate negative controls were used without the primary antibodies.

For histological analysis, every tenth equidistant frozen section of the spinal cord was selected from each animal. A minimum of five random fields containing the GFP-positive transplanted NSCs were photographed per sample. Phenotypic analysis of transplanted NSCs was calculated based on identification of GFP-positive cells associated with a DAPI stained nucleus and the immunohistological marker of interest. The number of NF200-positive axons in the conduits was also counted.

Statistical analysis

Analysis of variance (ANOVA) was used to test for the statistical significance, and the results were accepted when two-tailed $P < 0.05$. Tukey's post-test was performed to compare individual pairs of means if ANOVA $P < 0.05$. The results are presented as mean ± standard deviation.

Results

Isolation and culture of NSCs

NSCs were isolated from the whole hippocampi of E14 SD rats. The NSCs aggregated as free-floating neurospheres (Fig. 1A), as observed under a phase contrast microscope after 5 days of culture. The formation of neurospheres is considered the gold standard for the identification of NSCs. Then, the NSCs were assessed using nestin, a marker for neural precursors. The immunocytochemistry results indicated that the neurospheres showed positive immunoreactivity to nestin, a known protein marker of NSCs (Fig. 1B). These data indicated that NSCs maintained their undifferentiated status in the defined medium. The NSCs grafted into the NT-3-immobilized PCLA conduits were shown in Fig. 1C and D.

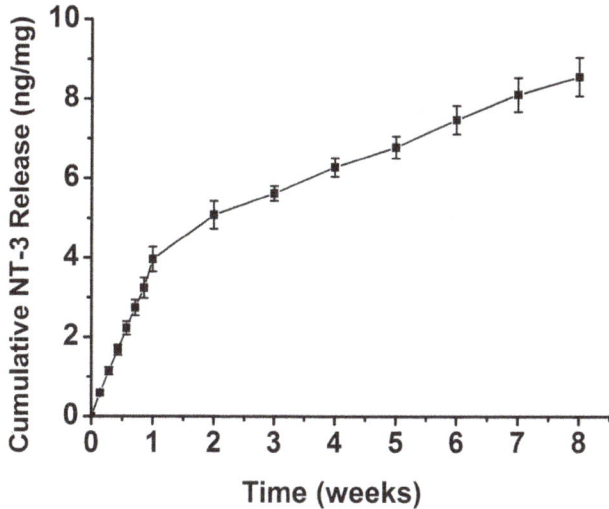

Figure 2. Cumulative release profile of bioactive NT-3 from NT-3-immobilized PCLA-SF conduits in vitro. n = 3.

Determination of kinetics of NT-3 release from NT-3 immobilized scaffolds

NT-3 was released from NT-3-immobilized conduits in vitro for at least 8 weeks (Fig. 2). The release profile was composed of two parts, an initial burst in the first week followed by a sustained release. After an initial burst release in the first week, the NT-3-immobilized conduits released NT-3 at a stable and constant rate in the following seven weeks. The cumulative amount of released NT-3 was 8.56 ng/mg.

Viability and differentiation of NSCs on NT-3-immobilized PCLA membranes

To determine the viability of the NSCs on the membranes, the seeded cells were cultured for 14 days, and then stained with calcein-AM and EthD-III. The cell viability on PCLA-SF-NT-3, PCLA-SF, and PCLA membranes were determined to be 94.52±3.37%, 87.12±2.63%, and 86.86±3.61%, respectively (Fig. 3A–D). The percentage of live cells was highest on PCLA-SF-NT-3 membranes. No significant difference in viability was found between the PCLA-SF and PCLA membranes.

To evaluate the differentiation of seeded NSCs on the NT-3-immobilized PCLA membranes, we stained the cells with MAP-2, GFAP, and CNPase (Fig. 4A–I). At day 14, the percentages of MAP-2-positive cells on PCLA, PCLA-SF, and PCLA-SF-NT-3 membranes were determined to be 18.6±2.2%, 25.3±3.2%, 55.2±4.1%, respectively. The percentages of GFAP-positive cells and CNPase-positive cells were the lowest in the PCLA-SF-NT-3 group, compared with the PCLA and PCLA-SF groups (Fig. 4J).

Long-term survival and differentiation of NSCs after SCI

The surgical procedures are shown in Fig. 5A and B. During the experiment, no rats exhibited wound complications. At explantation, no inflammatory signs or adverse tissue reactions were observed. General observation of both ends of the lesion site revealed reparative tissue completely filling the gap between the transected cord stumps 8 weeks after implantation (Fig. 5C).

At 8 weeks after implantation, NSC survival was observed in the conduit+NT-3+NSCs and conduit+NSCs groups. Fluorescent microscopy of frozen sections showed GFP-positive transplanted NSCs in the bridge tissue (Fig. 5D, E). The overall survival of the transplanted NSCs was quantified for each group. The conduit+NT-3+NSCs group exhibited an average GFP-positive cell density of 75.8±15.1%, whereas the conduit+NSCs group exhibited only

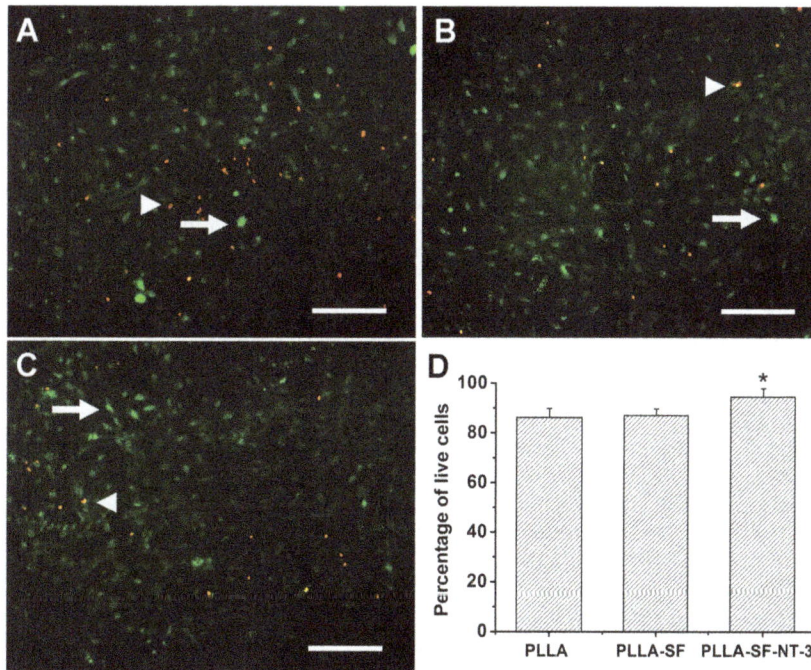

Figure 3. Fluorescent staining for cell viability of NSCs grown on PCLA (A), PCLA-SF (B), and PCLA-SF-NT-3 (C) membranes for 14 days. Living cells (white arrows) were in green and dead cells (white arrowheads) were in red. (D) The percentage of live cells. Scale bars = 100 µm; *P<0.05; n = 4.

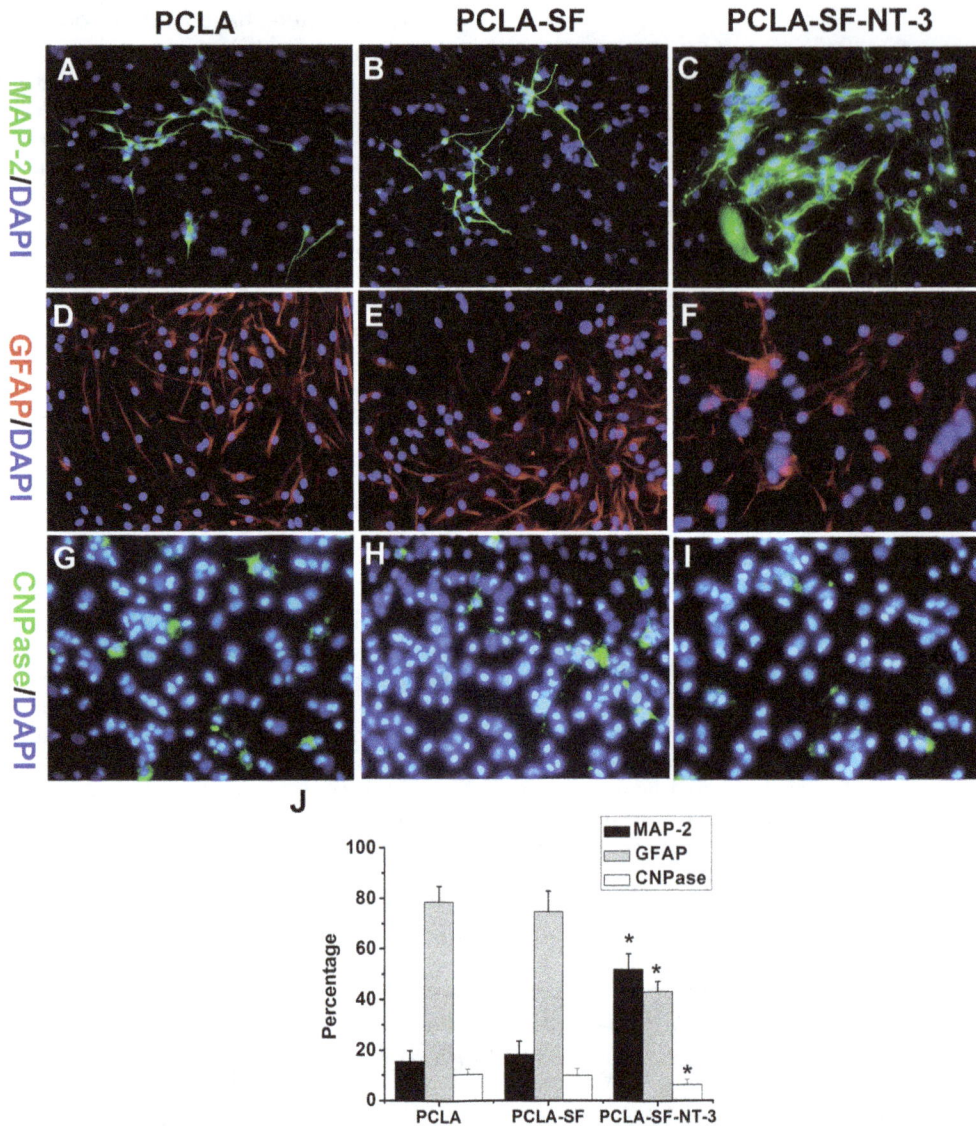

Figure 4. Differentiation of NSCs in vitro. (A–I) Cells cultured on PCLA (A, D, G), PCLA-SF (B, E, H), and PCLA-SF-NT-3 (C, F, I) membrane were immunostained with MAP-2 for neurons (A–C), GFPA for astrocytes (D–F), CNPase for oligodendrocytes (G–I). The nuclei were stained with DAPI. (J) Quantitative analysis of the NSC differentiation in vitro. Scale bars = 25 μm, *$P<0.05$; n = 4.

32.3±10.2% GFP positive cell density (Fig. 5F). The conduit+NT-3+NSCs group showed significantly improved long-term survival of NSCs compared with the conduit+NSCs group.

NSC differentiation after 8 weeks was examined. Immunofluorescent images showed that GFP-positive cells co-localized with MAP-2 positive mature neurons, GFAP-positive astrocytes, or CNPase-positive oligodendrocytes of the conduit+NT-3+NSCs and conduit+NSCs groups (Fig. 6A–F). The results are summarized in Fig. 6G. MAP-2 staining for neurons showed that 21.5±5.2% neuronal differentiation of NSCs in the conduit+NT-3+NSCs group, which was higher than that in the conduit+NSCs group. In contrast, the percentages of GFAP-positive cells and CNPase-positive cells in the conduit+NT-3+NSCs group were lower, compared with the conduit+NSCs group.

Axon regeneration

Axon regeneration across the bridge was identified by NF200 staining at 8 weeks after implantation. Fluorescent microscopy showed that the regenerating axons were visible in the conduit+NT-3+NSCs group, whereas few regenerating axons were found in the conduit+NSCs group (Fig. 7A and B). The number of NF-200 positive axons in the NSCs contained conduit was determined to be 75.3±7.2 in the conduit+NT-3+NSCs group, and 48.3±6.2 in the conduit+NSCs group. The difference in the number of NF200-positive axons between the two groups was statistically significant (Fig. 7C).

Locomotor function recovery

Animals were monitored weekly for hindlimb function using the BBB open field locomotor scale. BBB scores were 0 when the spinal cord was completely transected. A time-dependent increase

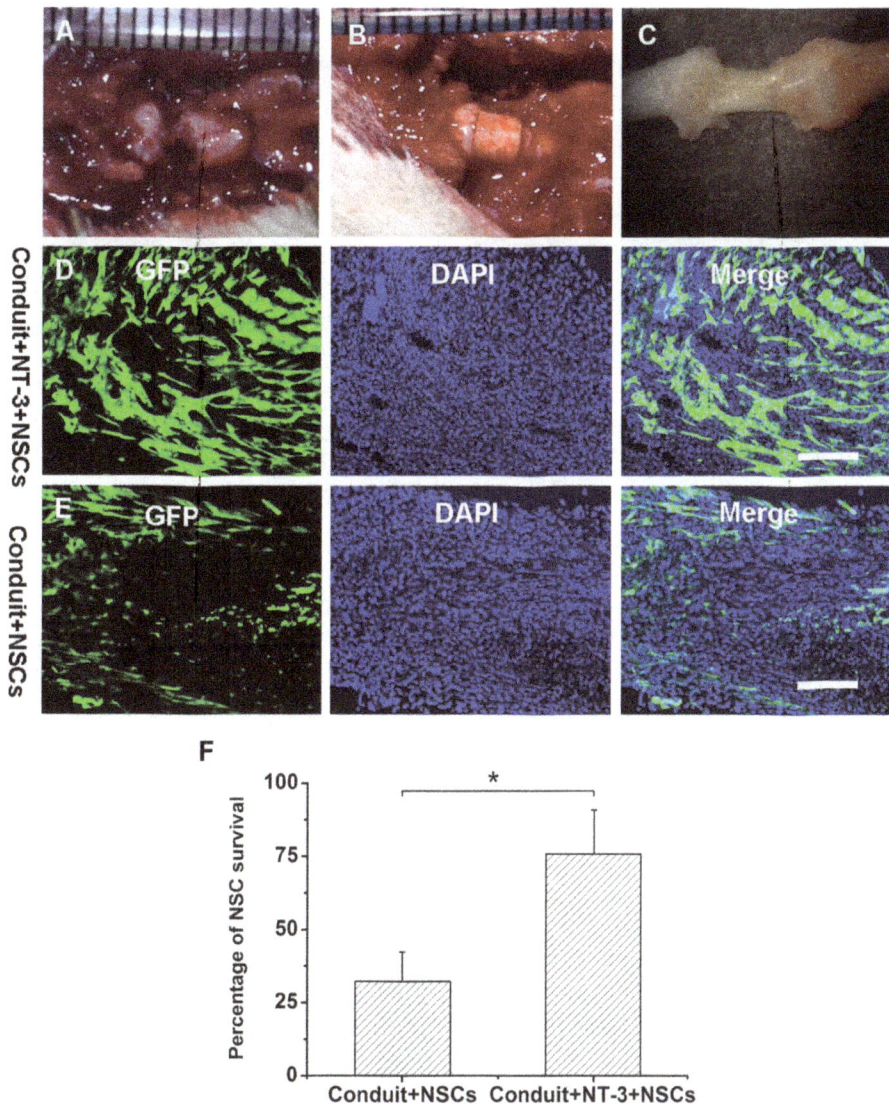

Figure 5. Conduit implantation after spinal cord transection facilitates tissue bridging and NSC survival. (A–B) Surgical procedure for implantation of conduits into completely transected rat spinal cords. (C) Gross appearance of spinal cords 8 weeks after implantation of the conduits. (D–E) Confocal fluorescent images of NSC survival in the conduit+NT-3+NSCs (D) and conduit+NSCs (E) groups 8 weeks after implantation. (F) Percentage of NSC survival for each group. Scale bar = 100 µm; *$P<0.05$; n=7.

in the BBB scores was displayed in the conduit+NT-3+NSCs, conduit+ NSCs, and conduit+NT-3 groups.

No significant difference was observed among the three groups until 3 weeks. However, at 4 weeks and thereafter, the conduit+ NT-3+NSCs group displayed significant behavioral improvement compared with the other two groups (Fig. 8).

Discussion

NSCs-based transplantation therapy is currently considered a potentially useful approach for SCI treatment [26]. A major challenge in NSCs-based transplantation therapy is to increase the rate of survival and neuronal differentiation of grafted NSCs. NT-3 is one of the best candidates in stimulating the survival and differentiation of NSCs. However, NT-3 has a short half-life and easily diffuses through tissue and cerebrospinal fluid. Moreover, maintaining a sufficient concentration of NT-3 at the injury site to

elicit an effect is difficult [27]. In the present study, we utilized SF β-sheet formation to immobilize NT-3 within the PCLA scaffolds, in which the bioactivity of NT-3 can be maintained, and its release can be controlled for 8 weeks. We then investigated the effects of NT-3-immobilized scaffolds on the survival and neuronal differentiation of NSCs in vitro and in a rat spinal cord transection model. The results showed that the NT-3-immobilized scaffolds enhanced the survival and neuronal differentiation of NSCs in vitro and 8 weeks after implantation in rats. Functional recovery and regeneration of NF200-positive axons were also promoted.

Maintaining the integrity and activity of NT-3 is critical for effective NT-3 delivery. In this study, NT-3 ELISA kits were used to quantify the release of growth factors from the conduits. The release profiles showed that the release of bioactive NT-3 was sustained over 8 weeks. The sustained release is due to the proteolytic degradation of SF coating [28]. The rate of NT-3 release was highest in the first 7 d, and NT-3 release continued at a

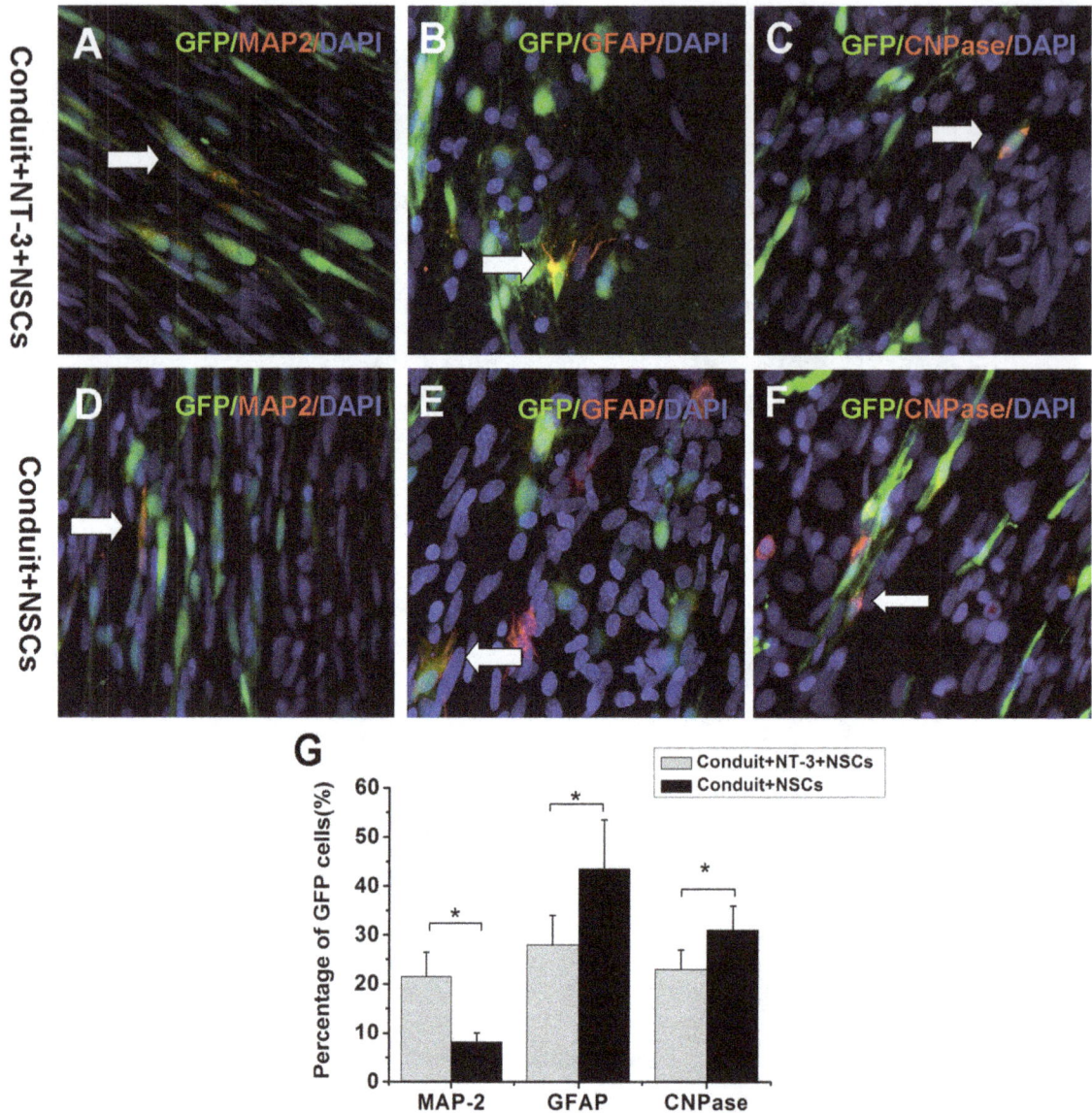

Figure 6. Differentiation profiles of NSCs in vivo. (A–F) Tissue samples were immunostained with MAP-2 for neurons (A, D), GFAP for astrocytes (B, E), and CNPase for oligodendrocytes (C, F) from the conduit+NT-3+NSCs (A–C) and conduit+NSCs groups (D–F). White arrows indicate the representative differentiated cells. (G) Quantification of NSC differentiation profile for each group. Scale bar = 20 μm. *$P<0.05$; n = 7.

slower rate for up to 8 wks. This can be ascribed to the inactive of released NT-3 in PBS during the testing interval, and ELISA can only detect the intact NT-3. In the present study, a daily testing interval was initially set, and then the testing interval was changed to weekly.

Currently, the development of biomaterials for neural tissue regeneration and stem cell implantation is a prominent research focus in regenerative medicine. SF has been shown to have excellent biocompatibility both in vitro and in vivo, good mechanical properties, and a slow biodegradation rate [20]. The crystal structure of SF is composed of hydrophilic domains (silk I) and hydrophobic domains (silk II). Hydrophobic blocks make up the crystalline regions of SF due to their ability to form intermolecular β-sheets. Methanol treatement dehydrates and destabilizes the unstable silk I state of SF, leading to a switch to the silk II (predominant) conformation, which is more stable and characterized by an increase in β-sheet content [29]. Therefore, by

treating the adsorbed SF/NT-3 molecules on the surface of the scaffolds with methanol, the NT-3 molecules are entrapped in the SF coating. In the present study, SF coating was used as NT-3 reservoir, which played an important role in stabilizing the bioactivity of NT-3. No obvious cytotoxicity of the biomaterials could be observed for the NSCs, due to the biocompatibility of the scaffold and the sustained release of NT-3. In our previous work, we also immobilized NGF within nanofibrous nerve conduits in a concentration gradient pattern by SF coating to guide the dorsal root ganglia (DRG) neurite outgrowth [23]. In sum, the NT-3-immobilized PCLA-SF scaffold is a promising NT-3 delivery system, which increases NSC survival.

SCI results in loss of both sensory and motor neuron function, even neuronal damage and death, as well as axonal demyelination. Despite the presence of endogenous NSC populations within the adult spinal cord, the extent of neuronal differentiation from these endogenous precursor cells, even after infusion of exogenous

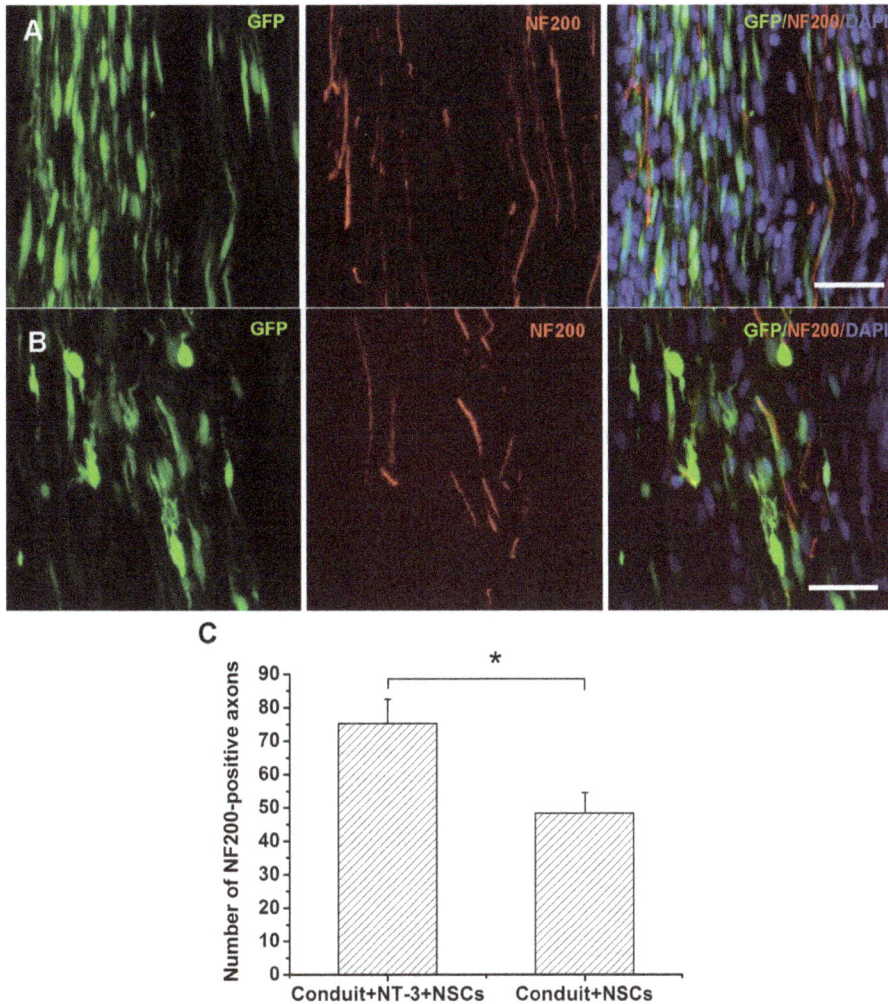

Figure 7. Axonal regeneration. NF200-positive axons were observed in the conduit+NT-3+NSCs (A) and conduit+NSCs (B) groups 8 weeks after implantation. (C) Histograms showing the number of NF200-positive axons for each group. Scale bar = 20 μm, *$P<0.05$; n = 7.

growth factors, is not sufficient to stimulate neuroplasticity, and rescue neuronal loss after SCI [30]. Thus, restoration of the neuron population by cell transplantation therapy is an attractive strategy in constructing a neural network after SCI. In the present study, enhanced survival and differentiation of transplanted NSCs in vitro and in vivo was achieved using the NT-3 delivery system. Each conduit was seeded with NSCs prior to implantation, and cell survival was assayed 8 weeks after implantation. The conduit+NT-3+NSCs group had a higher density of GFP-positive cells, compared with the conduit+NSCs group. Hence, the NT-3-immobilized scaffolds enhanced the survival of the NSCs not only in vitro but also in vivo.

On the NT-3-immobilized membranes, NSCs differentiated into neurons with a significantly high percentage in vitro. However, when the NT-3-immobilized scaffolds were implanted into the injured spinal cord, this differentiation percentage decreased in vivo, yet was still significantly higher than the control group. Despite this lower cell survival in vivo, the NT-3 group still had the highest effect in terms of NF200-positive axon regeneration and functional recovery. Therefore, although this differentiation percentage was lower in vivo than in vitro, the NT-3 delivery system is still meaningful.

Complete spinal cord transection is the most severe injury model and results in loss of hindlimb movement immediately after injury. In the present study, the conduit+NT-3+NSCs group showed a statistically significant improvement in hindlimb function, resulting in some movement of hindlimb joints. Immunohistochemistry showed that the NF200-positive axons were densest across the tissue bridge. Axon regeneration has been demonstrated in several SCI models [31,32]. We believe that this finding is important because these axons may provide a structural basis for re-establishment of a neuronal network for physiological signal transduction across the injury site. Lu et al. seeded NSCs derived from human fetal spinal cord in growth-factor-containing fibrin to derive neurons [7]. The graft-derived neurons were found to extend large numbers of axons into the host spinal cord in both rostral and caudal directions. These axons in the host spinal cord formed dense bouton-like terminals around the host dendrites and cell bodies. Synapse formation was identified by immunohistochemistry and electron microscopy, which supported the observed enhanced functional recovery [33]. In our study, the enhanced functional recovery in the conduit+NT-3+NSCs group can be ascribed to the relatively high amount of NF200-positive axons.

Remarkable progress in guiding neuronal differentiation has been achieved by priming NSCs to neuron-restricted progenitor

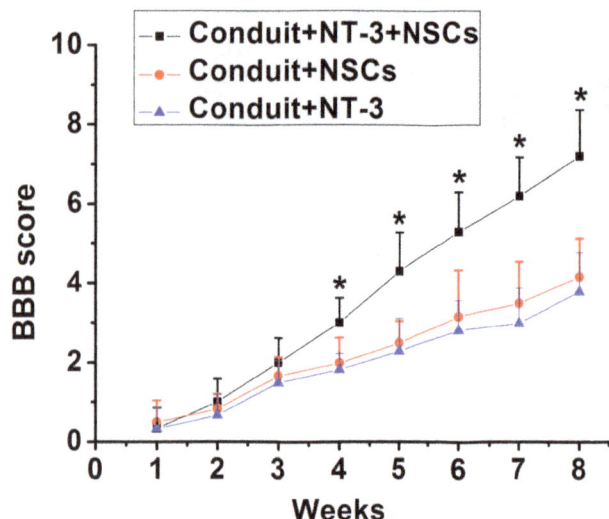

Figure 8. BBB locomotor scores were evaluated weekly for 8 weeks after SCI. At 4 weeks and thereafter, the conduit+NT-3+NSCs group displayed significant behavioral improvement compared with the other two groups. *$P<0.05$; $n=6$.

cells in vitro and addition of growth factors, including NTs, sonic hedgehog protein, and retinoid acid [34,35]. NTs, particularly NT-3, are considered to be the most promising strategy for future clinical application. NT-3 could not only facilitate the survival and proliferation of NSCs, but also induce the differentiation of NSCs into neurons. NT-3 acts via its corresponding receptor tyrosine kinases (TrkA, TrkB, and TrkC). NT-3 preferentially binds to TrkC, and then activates the Akt/MAP kinase signal pathway, which is involved in neurotransmitter regulation and neural peptide synthesis [36]. In several investigations, genetically modified NSCs were utilized to overexpress NT-3 to affect the survival and differentiation of surrounding cells. However, gene transduction is limited by various problems, including concerns about the safety and efficiency of gene transfection and the

potential adverse effects of exogenous gene expression [37]. In contrast, PCLA-SF has several advantages for NT-3 delivery. First, SF adsorption and β-sheet formation is a simple method to immobilize growth factors. Multiple growth factors can also be immobilized simultaneously with SF coating, which synergistically improve functional recovery. Furthermore, drugs that eliminate the inhibitory environment or enhance the regenerative ability of axons could also be included. Second, the present NT-3 delivery system is safe. Both PCLA and SF are recommended scaffold materials because of their unique features, such as biocompatibility and biodegradability, for tissue engineering for the repair and regeneration of injured tissues [38,39].

Conclusions

By incorporating NT-3 into SF coating, we successfully developed an NT-3-immobilized PCLA scaffold as a delivery system. Seeding NSCs within these NT-3-immobilized PCLA scaffolds not only enhanced the survival of grafted cells but also promoted neuronal differentiation both in vitro and in a rat SCI model. At 8 weeks after implantation, the conduit+NT-3+NSCs group showed significant improvement in axon regeneration and functional recovery. Our results suggest that PCLA conduits immobilized with NT-3 have the potential for SCI repair by promoting survival and neuronal differentiation of transplanted NSCs. In addition, SF adsorption and coating are simple methods for immobilizing bioactive molecules. In the future, drugs that eliminate the inhibitory environment and enhance regeneration can be immobilized within the scaffolds for a synergistic effect.

Acknowledgments

The authors appreciate Jixiang Zhu (Department of Biomedical Engineering, Guangzhou Medical University, China) for his kind help in material fabrication.

Author Contributions

Conceived and designed the experiments: XG. Performed the experiments: ST XL ZH. Analyzed the data: BX YQ. Contributed reagents/materials/analysis tools: QL. Wrote the paper: FP.

References

1. Adams M, Cavanagh JF (2004) International Campaign for Cures of Spinal Cord Injury Paralysis (ICCP): another step forward for spinal cord injury research. Spinal Cord 42: 273–280.
2. Fleming JC, Norenberg MD, Ramsay DA, Dekaban GA, Marcillo AE, et al. (2006) The cellular inflammatory response in human spinal cords after injury. Brain 129: 3249–3269.
3. Johnson PJ, Tatara A, McCreedy DA, Shiu A, Sakiyama-Elbert SE (2010) Tissue-engineered fibrin scaffolds containing neural progenitors enhance functional recovery in a subacute model of SCI. Soft Matter 6: 5127–5137.
4. Kim H, Zahir T, Tator CH, Shoichet MS (2011) Effects of dibutyryl cyclic-AMP on survival and neuronal differentiation of neural stem/progenitor cells transplanted into spinal cord injured rats. PLoS One 6: e21744.
5. Yang Z, Duan H, Mo L, Qiao H, Li X (2010) The effect of the dosage of NT-3/chitosan carriers on the proliferation and differentiation of neural stem cells. Biomaterials 31: 4846–4854.
6. Abematsu M, Tsujimura K, Yamano M, Saito M, Kohno K, et al. (2010) Neurons derived from transplanted neural stem cells restore disrupted neuronal circuitry in a mouse model of spinal cord injury. J Clin Invest 120: 3255–3266.
7. Lu P, Wang Y, Graham L, McHale K, Gao M, et al. (2012) Long-distance growth and connectivity of neural stem cells after severe spinal cord injury. Cell 150: 1264–1273.
8. Guo X, Zahir T, Mothe A, Shoichet MS, Morshead CM, et al. (2012) The effect of growth factors and soluble Nogo-66 receptor protein on transplanted neural stem/progenitor survival and axonal regeneration after complete transection of rat spinal cord. Cell Transplant 21: 1177–1197.
9. Johnson PJ, Tatara A, Shiu A, Sakiyama-Elbert SE (2010) Controlled release of neurotrophin-3 and platelet-derived growth factor from fibrin scaffolds containing neural progenitor cells enhances survival and differentiation into neurons in a subacute model of SCI. Cell Transplant 19: 89–101.
10. Weishaupt N, Blesch A, Fouad K (2012) BDNF: the career of a multifaceted neurotrophin in spinal cord injury. Exp Neurol 238: 254–264.
11. Chao MV (2003) Neurotrophins and their receptors: a convergence point for many signalling pathways. Nat Rev Neurosci 4: 299–309.
12. Yang Z, Duan H, Mo L, Qiao H, Li X (2010) The effect of the dosage of NT-3/chitosan carriers on the proliferation and differentiation of neural stem cells. Biomaterials 31: 4846–4854.
13. Wang JM, Zeng YS, Wu JL, Li Y, Teng YD (2011) Cograft of neural stem cells and schwann cells overexpressing TrkC and neurotrophin-3 respectively after rat spinal cord transection. Biomaterials 32: 7454–7468.
14. Wang Y, Lapitsky Y, Kang CE, Shoichet MS (2009) Accelerated release of a sparingly soluble drug from an injectable hyaluronan-methylcellulose hydrogel. J Control Release 140: 218–223.
15. Krych AJ, Rooney GE, Chen B, Schermerhorn TC, Ameenuddin S, et al. (2009) Relationship between scaffold channel diameter and number of regenerating axons in the transected rat spinal cord. Acta Biomater 5: 2551–2559.
16. Straley KS, Foo CW, Heilshorn SC (2010) Biomaterial design strategies for the treatment of spinal cord injuries. J Neurotrauma 27: 1–19.
17. Tang S, Zhao J, Xu S, Li J, Teng Y, et al. (2012) Bone induction through controlled release of novel BMP-2-related peptide from PTMC(11)-F127-PTMC(11) hydrogels. Biomed Mater 7.
18. Chiu LL, Weisel RD, Li RK, Radisic M (2011) Defining conditions for covalent immobilization of angiogenic growth factors onto scaffolds for tissue engineering. J Tissue Eng Regen Med 5: 69–84.
19. Meade KE, White KJ, Pickford CE, Holley RJ, Marson A, et al. (2013) Immobilization of heparan sulfate on electrospun meshes to support embryonic stem cell culture and differentiation. J Biol Chem 288: 5530–5538.
20. Wenk E, Merkle HP, Meinel L (2011) Silk fibroin as a vehicle for drug delivery applications. J Control Release 150: 128–141.

21. Shchepelina O, Drachuk I, Gupta MK, Lin J, Tsukruk VV (2011) Silk-on-silk layer-by-layer microcapsules. Adv Mater 23: 4655–4660.
22. Uebersax L, Mattotti M, Papaloizos M, Merkle HP, Gander B, et al. (2007) Silk fibroin matrices for the controlled release of nerve growth factor (NGF). Biomaterials 28: 4449–4460.
23. Tang S, Zhu J, Xu Y, Xiang AP, Jiang MH, et al. (2013) The effects of gradients of nerve growth factor immobilized PCLA scaffolds on neurite outgrowth in vitro and peripheral nerve regeneration in rats. Biomaterials 34: 7086–7096.
24. He L, Zhang Y, Zeng C, Ngiam M, Liao S, et al. (2009) Manufacture of PLGA multiple-channel conduits with precise hierarchical pore architectures and in vitro/vivo evaluation for spinal cord injury. Tissue Eng Part C Methods 15: 243–255.
25. Basso DM, Beattie MS, Bresnahan JC (1995) A sensitive and reliable locomotor rating scale for open field testing in rats. J Neurotrauma 12: 1–21.
26. Yang Z, Duan H, Mo L, Qiao H, Li X (2010) The effect of the dosage of NT-3/ chitosan carriers on the proliferation and differentiation of neural stem cells. Biomaterials 31: 4846–4854.
27. Willerth SM, Rader A, Sakiyama-Elbert SE (2008) The effect of controlled growth factor delivery on embryonic stem cell differentiation inside fibrin scaffolds. Stem Cell Res 1: 205–218.
28. Lu Q, Wang X, Hu X, Cebe P, Omenetto F, et al. (2010) Stabilization and release of enzymes from silk films. Macromol Biosci 10: 359–368.
29. Taddei P, Monti P (2005) Vibrational infrared conformational studies of model peptides representing the semicrystalline domains of Bombyx mori silk fibroin. Biopolymers 78: 249–258.
30. Obermair FJ, Schroter A, Thallmair M (2008) Endogenous neural progenitor cells as therapeutic target after spinal cord injury. Physiology (Bethesda) 23: 296–304.
31. Steward O, Sharp K, Selvan G, Hadden A, Hofstadter M, et al. (2006) A re-assessment of the consequences of delayed transplantation of olfactory lamina propria following complete spinal cord transection in rats. Exp Neurol 198: 483–499.
32. Kim D, Adipudi V, Shibayama M, Giszter S, Tessler A, et al. (1999) Direct agonists for serotonin receptors enhance locomotor function in rats that received neural transplants after neonatal spinal transection. J Neurosci 19: 6213–6224.
33. Abematsu M, Tsujimura K, Yamano M, Saito M, Kohno K, et al. (2010) Neurons derived from transplanted neural stem cells restore disrupted neuronal circuitry in a mouse model of spinal cord injury. J Clin Invest 120: 3255–3266.
34. Lowry N, Goderie SK, Lederman P, Charniga C, Gooch MR, et al. (2012) The effect of long-term release of Shh from implanted biodegradable microspheres on recovery from spinal cord injury in mice. Biomaterials 33: 2892–2901.
35. Santos T, Ferreira R, Maia J, Agasse F, Xapelli S, et al. (2012) Polymeric nanoparticles to control the differentiation of neural stem cells in the subventricular zone of the brain. ACS Nano 6: 10463–10474.
36. Lim MS, Nam SH, Kim SJ, Kang SY, Lee YS, et al. (2007) Signaling pathways of the early differentiation of neural stem cells by neurotrophin-3. Biochem Biophys Res Commun 357: 903–909.
37. Lu HX, Hao ZM, Jiao Q, Xie WL, Zhang JF, et al. (2011) Neurotrophin-3 gene transduction of mouse neural stem cells promotes proliferation and neuronal differentiation in organotypic hippocampal slice cultures. Med Sci Monit 17: R305–R311.
38. Sandker MJ, Petit A, Redout EM, Siebelt M, Muller B, et al. (2013) In situ forming acyl-capped PCLA-PEG-PCLA triblock copolymer based hydrogels. Biomaterials 34: 8002–8011.
39. Wang X, Hu X, Daley A, Rabotyagova O, Cebe P, et al. (2007) Nanolayer biomaterial coatings of silk fibroin for controlled release. J Control Release 121: 190–199.

6

Genome Wide Expression Profiling during Spinal Cord Regeneration Identifies Comprehensive Cellular Responses in Zebrafish

Subhra Prakash Hui[1¤a], **Dhriti Sengupta**[1], **Serene Gek Ping Lee**[2], **Triparna Sen**[3¤b], **Sudip Kundu**[1], **Sinnakaruppan Mathavan**[2], **Sukla Ghosh**[1]*

1 Department of Biophysics, Molecular Biology and Bioinformatics, University of Calcutta, Kolkata, India, 2 Genome Institute of Singapore, Singapore, Singapore, 3 Chittaranjan National Cancer Research Institute, Kolkata, India

Abstract

Background: Among the vertebrates, teleost and urodele amphibians are capable of regenerating their central nervous system. We have used zebrafish as a model to study spinal cord injury and regeneration. Relatively little is known about the molecular mechanisms underlying spinal cord regeneration and information based on high density oligonucleotide microarray was not available. We have used a high density microarray to profile the temporal transcriptome dynamics during the entire phenomenon.

Results: A total of 3842 genes expressed differentially with significant fold changes during spinal cord regeneration. Cluster analysis revealed event specific dynamic expression of genes related to inflammation, cell death, cell migration, cell proliferation, neurogenesis, neural patterning and axonal regrowth. Spatio-temporal analysis of *stat3* expression suggested its possible function in controlling inflammation and cell proliferation. Genes involved in neurogenesis and their dorso-ventral patterning (*sox2* and *dbx2*) are differentially expressed. Injury induced cell proliferation is controlled by many cell cycle regulators and some are commonly expressed in regenerating fin, heart and retina. Expression pattern of certain pathway genes are identified for the first time during regeneration of spinal cord. Several genes involved in PNS regeneration in mammals like *stat3*, *socs3*, *atf3*, *mmp9* and *sox11* are upregulated in zebrafish SCI thus creating PNS like environment after injury.

Conclusion: Our study provides a comprehensive genetic blue print of diverse cellular response(s) during regeneration of zebrafish spinal cord. The data highlights the importance of different event specific gene expression that could be better understood and manipulated further to induce successful regeneration in mammals.

Editor: Ryan Thummel, Wayne State University School of Medicine, United States of America

Funding: This work was supported by Department of Science and Technology, Department of Biotechnology (BT/PR13953/AAQ/03/523/2010), Ministry of Science and Technology (INT/CP-STIO/2006-2007/39/2006), Govt. of India to SG and DIC (Establishment…BT/BI/04/001/93), and the Department of Biophysics, Molecular Biology and Bioinformatics at the University of Calcutta. Generous funding was extended by the Genome Institute of Singapore for zebrafish array work. The funders had no role in study design, data collection and analysis, decision to publish, or preparation of the manuscript.

Competing Interests: The data in this study represents microarray data, which the authors may seek a patent for (few target genes) in the future.

* E-mail: suklagh2010@gmail.com

¤a Current address: Victor Chang Cardiac Research Institute, Darlinghurst, New South Wales, Australia
¤b Current address: Indian Institute of Chemical Biology, Kolkata, India

Introduction

Among the vertebrate, urodele amphibians and teleost fish have ability to regenerate their spinal cord after injury. In mammals following spinal cord injury (SCI) there are overwhelming inflammatory responses which trigger several other secondary tissue damage, neuronal and glial loss, progressive cavitation and glial scarring. These processes lead to functional decline and paralysis. Zebrafish is a powerful vertebrate model organism to elucidate gene function during regeneration, since they have extraordinary ability to regenerate their fins [1,2], heart muscle [3] and central nervous system (CNS) [4–9] after injury. Adult zebrafish, in contrast to mammals, can re-grow axons readily after

SCI and re-establish appropriate connections to recover significant functions [4,6,10]. In order to understand the mechanisms of inducing CNS regeneration in mammals, studies involving regeneration competent model organism is a prerequisite.

Regeneration of spinal cord has been studied by various groups using expression analysis of candidate genes or by generating transgenic zebrafish [11,12]. However, parallel analysis of gene expression during different phases of regenerative events in spinal cord using high-density dedicated zebrafish arrays has not been attempted. In Medaka, another teleost fish, a small scale cDNA microarray screen during fin regeneration was reported using 2,900 expressed sequence tags (ESTs), which shared no homology to known genes [13]. Attempts have been made to employ

Affymetrix arrays containing 14,900 transcripts representing 10,000 genes to study regeneration of fin, heart and retina in zebrafish [5,14,15]. High density arrays have been used to profile the transcriptome dynamics during embryogenesis [16] but such high-density microarray for genome-wide gene expression analysis has not previously been attempted for studying regeneration in adult zebrafish. For the present study, we have used a custom designed high-density oligonucleotide microarray for zebrafish (Agilent platform; 44000 probes) and determined the expression dynamics during the process of spinal cord regeneration at five different time points. We have tried to focus on the analysis of gene expression during different cellular events spanning all stages of regeneration. Previously we have characterized cellular events that include infiltration of blood cells, inflammation, cell death, proliferative response, neurogenesis and axonal regrowth during spinal cord regeneration in zebrafish [6]. Our present analysis, for the first time, reports a comprehensive genome wide expression analysis of regenerating zebrafish spinal cord after giving crush injury and we focused on event specific expression analysis during regeneration. We report here the genes that are differentially expressed in 5 different time points of regeneration and their involvement in the cellular events that modulate the process.

Results and Discussion

Previously we have studied time course analysis of spinal cord regeneration after giving crush injury [6] which revealed that immediately after injury there is infiltration of various blood cells until 5 day post injury (dpi). Among them macrophage played a pivotal role in devouring and clearing apoptotic cells as well as myelin debris. Apoptotic cell death has been recognized very early within 6 hrs of injury and peaked around 24 hrs; subsequently it declined. Infiltration and cell death is followed by ependymal sealing and other regenerative response like migration and accumulation of cells near the injury epicenter. Injury induced proliferation is a key event after SCI in zebrafish [6,12]. Proliferative response after injury is quite robust and initiated at 3 dpi cord, peaked at 7 dpi cord and later decreases gradually at 10 and 15 dpi cord. Ependymal cells are highly proliferative in nature and contribute to successful neurogenesis, which may include radial glia. Axonal regrowth can be seen in 15 dpi cord and remyelination is aided by the presence of Schwann cells. Both neurogenesis and axonogenesis is leading to successful regeneration in this species. We have studied the basic cellular events to uncover the molecular basis of some of the events characterized during spinal cord regeneration.

Analysis of differentially expressed genes during spinal cord regeneration in zebrafish

To identify the underlying molecular events following crush injury, we have focused on gene expression profile during different stages of zebrafish spinal cord regeneration. The whole data represents gene expression in uninjured spinal cord (control) and injured spinal cord at five different time points of regeneration (Day 1, Day 3, Day 7, Day 10 and Day 15).

Following SAM and GeneSpring analysis of the microarray data, a total 3842 (fold change ≥ 2, FDR < 0.05) differentially expressing unique genes were identified. From this unique set of annotated genes 304, 727, 1093, 551 and 263 genes are up-regulated at 1 dpi, 3 dpi, 7 dpi, 10 dpi and 15 dpi cords, respectively. On the other hand 93, 65, 1342, 666 and 226 genes are down-regulated at the above mentioned time points respectively (Fig. 1A, Table S1). Maximum numbers of genes are differentially expressed at 7 dpi cord (Fig. 1A). It is also evident

that in early phases (Day 1 and Day 3) of regeneration, higher numbers of genes are up-regulated whereas in the later time point (Day 7 and Day 10) more genes are down-regulated. The differentially expressing genes at various points of regeneration are very dynamic in nature. Among the 3842 differentially expressed genes, as many as 2073 genes are up-regulated at certain stages of regeneration and down-regulated at other stages; whereas 864 and 905 genes are exclusively up-regulated and down-regulated, respectively.

The differentially expressed genes are clustered by using k-mean clustering algorithm (using the Cluster3.0). We have optimized 'k' = 7 (the selection of k was done using an R package for cluster validation named clValid) and number of iterations = 5000 for the genes expressed across the 5 time points of regeneration. Distinctly, 7 clusters are generated and are viewed using TreeView (Fig. 1B). The average value of each cluster is also displayed in the same figure. Cluster I and Cluster VII include genes that are maximally up-regulated in 3 dpi compared to other time points and consist of 1314 and 531 genes, respectively. The genes in cluster VII showed higher level of up or down regulation than Cluster I in all the time points. The genes in Cluster IV are unique (425 genes); these genes respond significantly immediately after injury (Day 1) and are subsequently down-regulated in all time points. The genes that are upregulated at 7 dpi are clustered in 4 groups viz. Cluster II, Cluster III, Cluster V and Cluster VI, containing 699, 586, 225 and 52 genes, respectively. Though these four clusters showed similar basic pattern of expression displaying maximum expression at 7 dpi compared to other stages of regeneration, the degree of average expression levels varied in these clusters (eg. Cluster VI from −5.9 to 2.0).

Analysis of biological functional groups and enriched pathways

Cluster wise analysis of different functional groups. We intended to perform functional enrichment analysis on the clusters to study the functional groups that are largely activated during the process of regeneration. We have used Ingenuity Pathway Analysis (IPA) to identify functional groups. We provided both up and down-regulated genes of each cluster as input and selected 12 significantly enriched groups that are related to regeneration. All these groups are highly enriched in the clusters. Some of the enriched functions that we identified are 'cell death', 'cellular growth and proliferation', 'cellular development', 'cell cycle', 'DNA replication and repair', 'nervous system development' etc (Fig. 2A; Figure S1 and Table S2).

Functional group analysis in five different time points after injury. The set of differentially expressed genes, both up and down-regulated, are also grouped on the basis of their highest expression at a particular time point during regeneration. For instance, when a differentially expressing gene shows highest expression at 3 dpi, it is assigned to the 3 dpi group. Similarly, the whole data is divided into 5 groups (1, 3, 7, 10 and 15 dpi groups) and each group is subjected to IPA analysis. We observed that same set of functional groups are significantly enriched in these day-wise groups (Fig. 2A; Figure S2 and Table S2). To analyze the data in more detail and relate information to the different phases of regeneration, we have analyzed the functional enrichments during the stages of regeneration (Fig. 2A). It is evident that different functional groups are enriched in different time points suggesting their involvement with particular event(s) in regeneration. Early time points like 1 and 3 dpi showed enrichment of similar functional groups like 'cell death', 'cell growth and proliferation' and 'cellular development'. Whereas in 7 dpi, which is the proliferative phase of regeneration, other functional groups

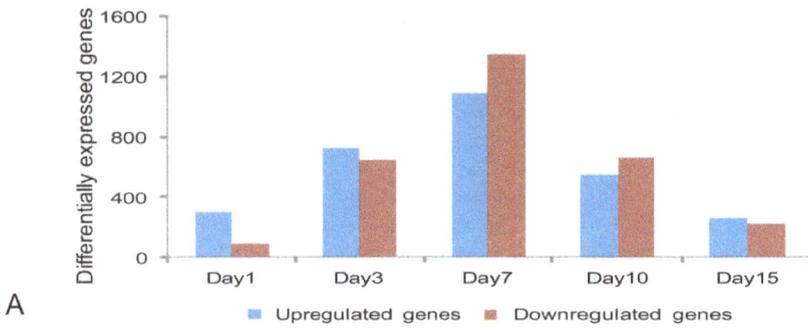

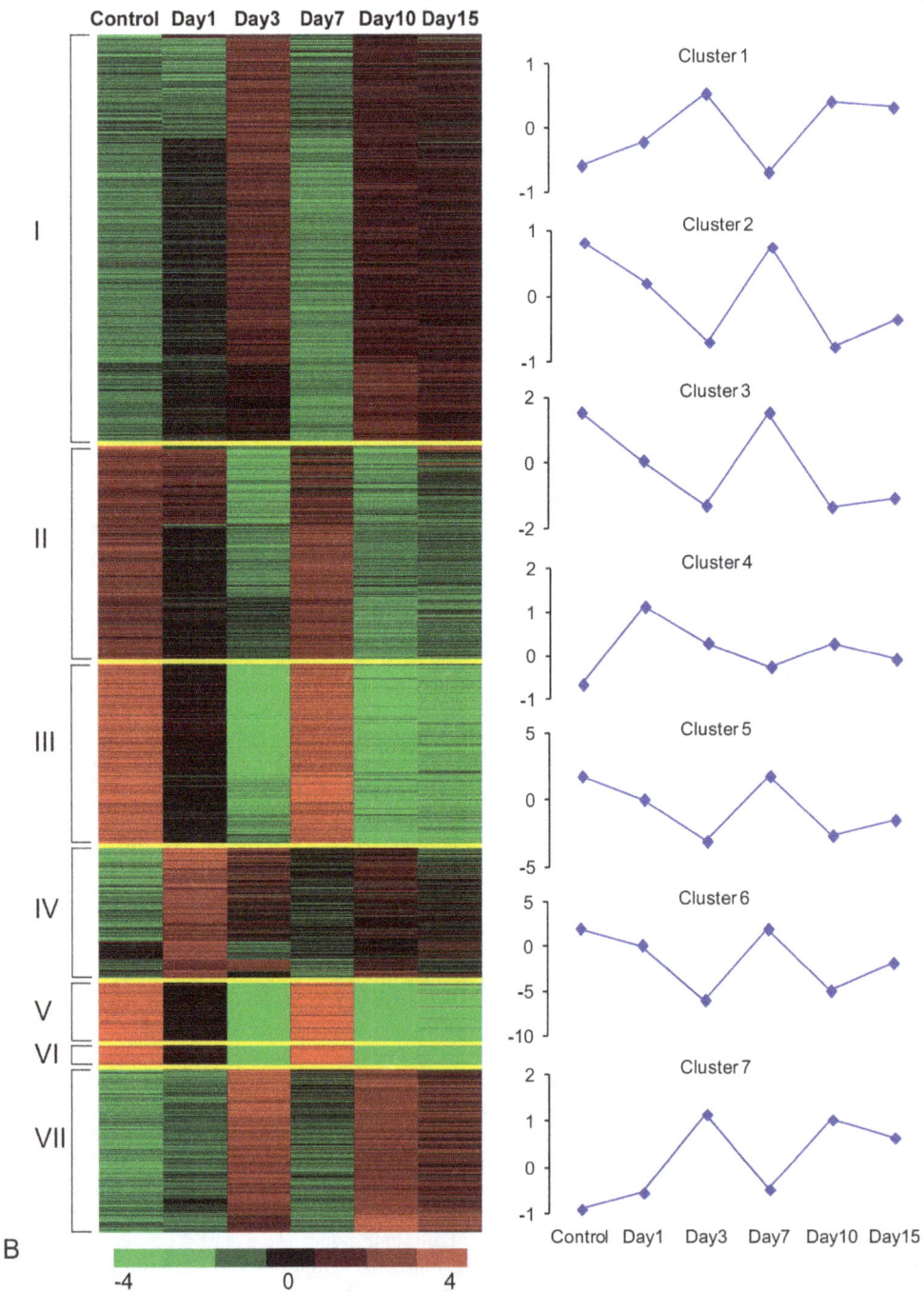

Figure 1. K-means Clustering Analysis of Differentially Expressed Genes before and after SCI in zebrafish. A) Distribution of differentially expressed genes both up-regulated and down-regulated after SCI at different time points. B) A set of 3,842 genes are identified as differentially expressed in at least one time point and are clustered into seven groups using the k-means algorithm. In the figure, horizontal lines indicate the expression pattern of each gene and the vertical columns indicate the time points after injury. The color chart indicates mean fold change of gene expression in each time points. Red and green colors represent increased and decreased expression respectively. Control = uninjured cord, Day 1 = 1 dpi cord, Day 3 = 3 dpi cord, Day 7 = 7 dpi cord, Day 10 = 10 dpi cord and Day 15 = 15 dpi cord. The clusters are separated by fine yellow lines. The average expression value of each cluster is plotted and shown in the line graph.

like 'cell cycle', 'cell growth and proliferation', 'DNA replication and repair' are significantly enriched. Similarly, in late regenerative phase that is related to tissue repatterning, enriched functional groups are 'nervous system development and function', 'tissue development' and 'organ development'.

IPA analysis also allowed us to identify enrichment of genes in canonical pathways during the process of regeneration. Some of the important canonical pathways that are enriched at different time points of regeneration are Wnt, axonal guidance, interleukin, purine-pyrimidine biosynthesis, G-protein coupled receptor signaling, human embryonic stem cell pluripotency signaling and several other signaling pathways (Fig. 2B; Figure S3 and Table S3). Interleukin (IL) signaling molecules are highly enriched in very early and late stages of regeneration and involved all different signaling pathways like Il-8, Il-6, Il-22, Il-10 and Il-k. Molecules related to axonal guidance signaling are highly enriched in 3 dpi, 10 dpi and 15 dpi cord, where highest enrichment is observed in 3 dpi cord. Embryonic stem cell pluripotency is enriched at several time points 3 dpi, 7 dpi and 10 dpi cord. We find a high predominance of molecules related to purine and pyrimidine metabolism in 7 dpi, when cell proliferation is at its highest peak. Similarly, cAMP mediated signaling is enriched in late time points, in 10 dpi and 15 dpi cord where axonal regeneration is initiated and maintained. Interestingly we observed that many signaling pathways are enriched in the initial time points (Day 1 and Day 3) and also in late time points (Day 10 and Day 15). Another salient observation is enrichment of few but very interesting pathways like 'One Carbon Pool by Folate' and 'N-Glycan Biosynthesis' at 7 dpi cord (Figure S3).

Events involved in different phases of regeneration: Analysis of event specific genes

Regeneration of spinal cord involves highly coordinated cellular and molecular events. There are different phases like early regeneration phase, proliferative and growth phase and late regeneration phase. We have tried to identify genes involved in these different phases. The fold change and q-value for genes are provided in supporting information files.

Early regeneration phase involves events like inflammation, macrophage infiltration, cell death, cell migration and dedifferentiation. These events are initiated immediately after injury (0 hr- 1day) and continue at least until Day 3. Immediately after injury there is infiltration of blood cells (predominantly macrophages) and a brief inflammatory response and cell death. The expression of different genes would reflect these specific events after injury.

Control of inflammatory response. Inflammatory response is known to be controlled by members of cytokine, chemokine signaling pathways in mammalian SCI and other diseased state [17–19]. Here we found 27 differentially expressed genes (Fig. 3A, Table S4), among them, 21 genes were expressed their maximum level at 1 dpi or 3 dpi cord. Some of the differentially expressed important cytokines and chemokines are *ccl1, ccrl1a, cmklr1, crfb2, crfb8, cxcl12b, cxcr3.2, socs3a, socs3b, il1b, il4r, il22, irf10, irf11, irf8* and *irf9*. Molecules like *il4r, ifnα, tgfβ* are upregulated both in mammalian CNS [20] and in zebrafish spinal

cord after injury as studied by us, but their temporal pattern and level of expression varies. For example, *tgfβ1* in mammalian brain after hypoxic injury shows 0.54 fold changes in 8 hr compared to 4 fold changes in 1 dpi zebrafish cord. On the contrary, *il10*, which is a neuroprotective interleukin, is downregulated in mammalian SCI [21] but upregulated in 1 dpi zebrafish cord (*il10* data not shown due to low fold change 1.36). The *tgfβ1* and *il10* play critical role in suppressing immune response [22,23]. We observed that *socs3, stat3* and *tgfβ1* are highly upregulated in 1 dpi zebrafish cord that is in early phase of regeneration (Fig. 3 and 4, Table S4).

The array data of *stat3* and *tgfβ1* molecules have been further validated by qRT-PCR, immunohistochemistry and ELISA analysis (Fig. 3 and 4). Both *stat3* and *tgfβ1* show highest upregulation in 1 dpi cord and array hybridization data is confirmed by qRT-PCR, immunohistochemistry and ELISA analysis. STAT3 expression can be localized in injured cord, predominantly in the grey matter both in ependymal cells and in neuronal cells. It is important to mention that expression was observed exclusively at the injury site of 1 dpi and 3 dpi cord (Fig. 3D, E, I, M) and absent in the normal part of same cord. Colocalization study of STAT3 with GFAP (Fig. 3E–H, Q–T) and HuC/D (Fig. 3I–L, U–X) in 3 dpi cord suggests expression both in radial glia and in neurons, although we found that a higher number of STAT3 positive cells are HuC/D positive newly formed neurons [6] (Fig. 3K, X, Y; Table S5). We have also analyzed STAT3 colocalization with BrdU in 3 dpi cord, which is the beginning of proliferation stage and found that many STAT3+ cells are BrdU+ proliferating cells (Fig. 3M–P). There is also a population of STAT3 positive cells which are not colocalized with HuC/D and GFAP and they are probably inflammatory cells present in the injury epicenter of both 1 and 3 dpi cord. Our expression analysis of *tgfβ1* expression showed highest level of expression in 1 dpi cord and it was present in both grey and white matter of adjacent part of the epicenter (Fig. 4A–G). TGFβ, a multi-potent cytokine, plays critical role in suppressing the immune response after CNS injury in mammals [23–26]. Furthermore, it also plays a role in epithelial-mesenchymal transition (EMT) after SCI, expressed in M2 type macrophages [27] and may induce initiation of cell proliferation during tail regeneration in *Xenopus* [28].

Other analysis in mammalian CNS injury refers to importance of complement factors and MHC class I and II molecules expression [20,29]. We observed upregulation of two complement factors *c1qc* and *c1a13b* early after injury (Table S4). Between these two factors prominent role of *c1qc* in activation of phagocytosis of macrophage/microglia in mammalian CNS is well known [30] which may suggest a similar role in zebrafish SCI where we observe increased phagocytosis by macrophage in 3 dpi cord [6]. Unlike mammalian CNS injury, where both MHC class I and II molecules are upregulated, we only found upregulation of MHC class I molecules like *mhc1uba, mhc1aa* and *mhc1ze* in early time points in zebrafish cord regeneration (Table S4).

Pro- and anti-inflammatory macrophages. Our previous study highlighted importance of macrophage during early phase of regeneration in zebrafish spinal cord. In mammalian SCI presence of both pro- and anti- inflammatory macrophages are related to

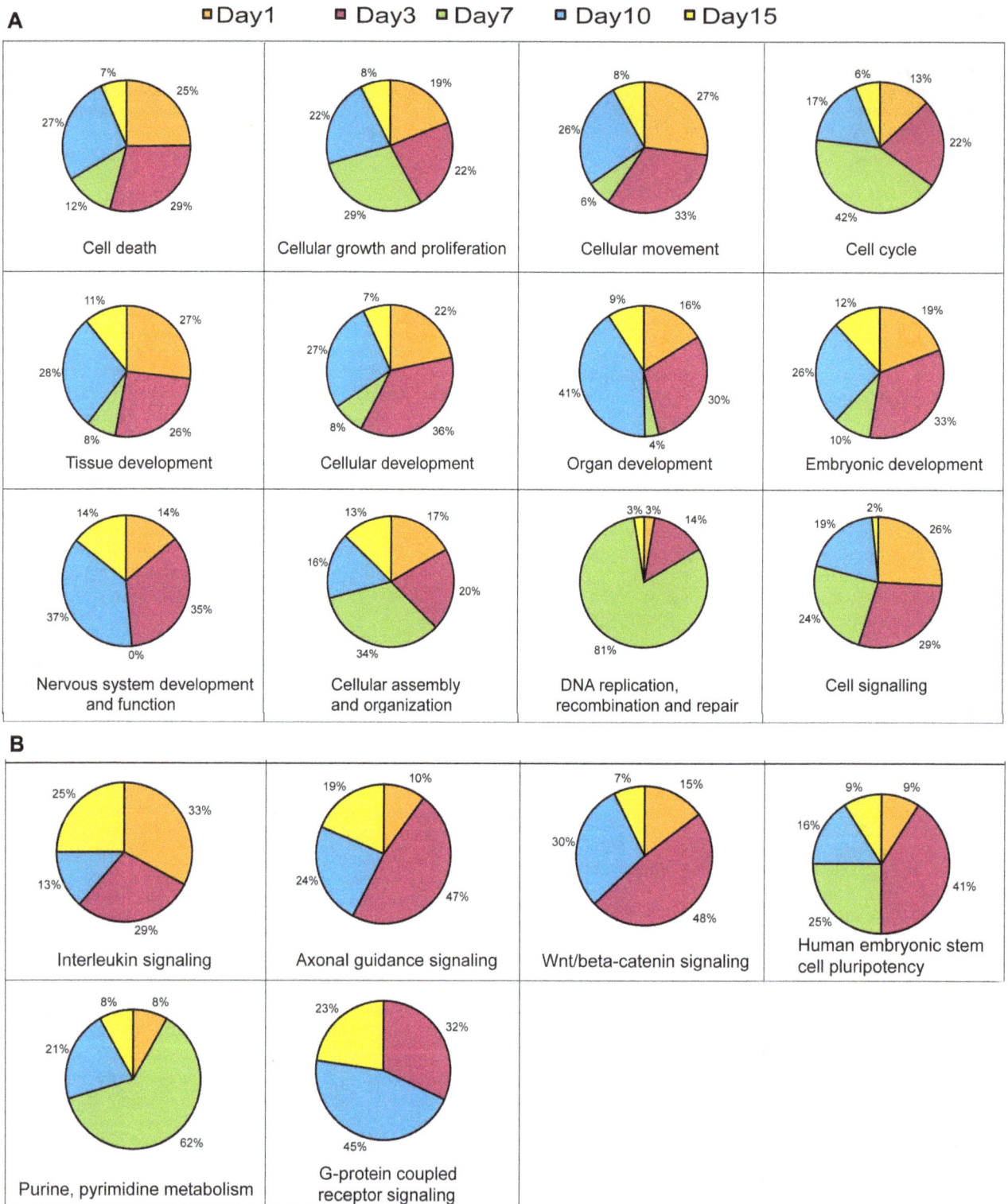

Figure 2. IPA analysis of biological functional groups and enriched pathways. A) Pie charts showing the percentage of genes that are differentially expressed (both up and down regulated) at different time points for the various enriched functional groups in IPA analysis. B) Pie charts showing the percentage of genes that are differentially expressed (both up and down regulated) for the various enriched signaling pathways in IPA analysis at different time points after SCI.

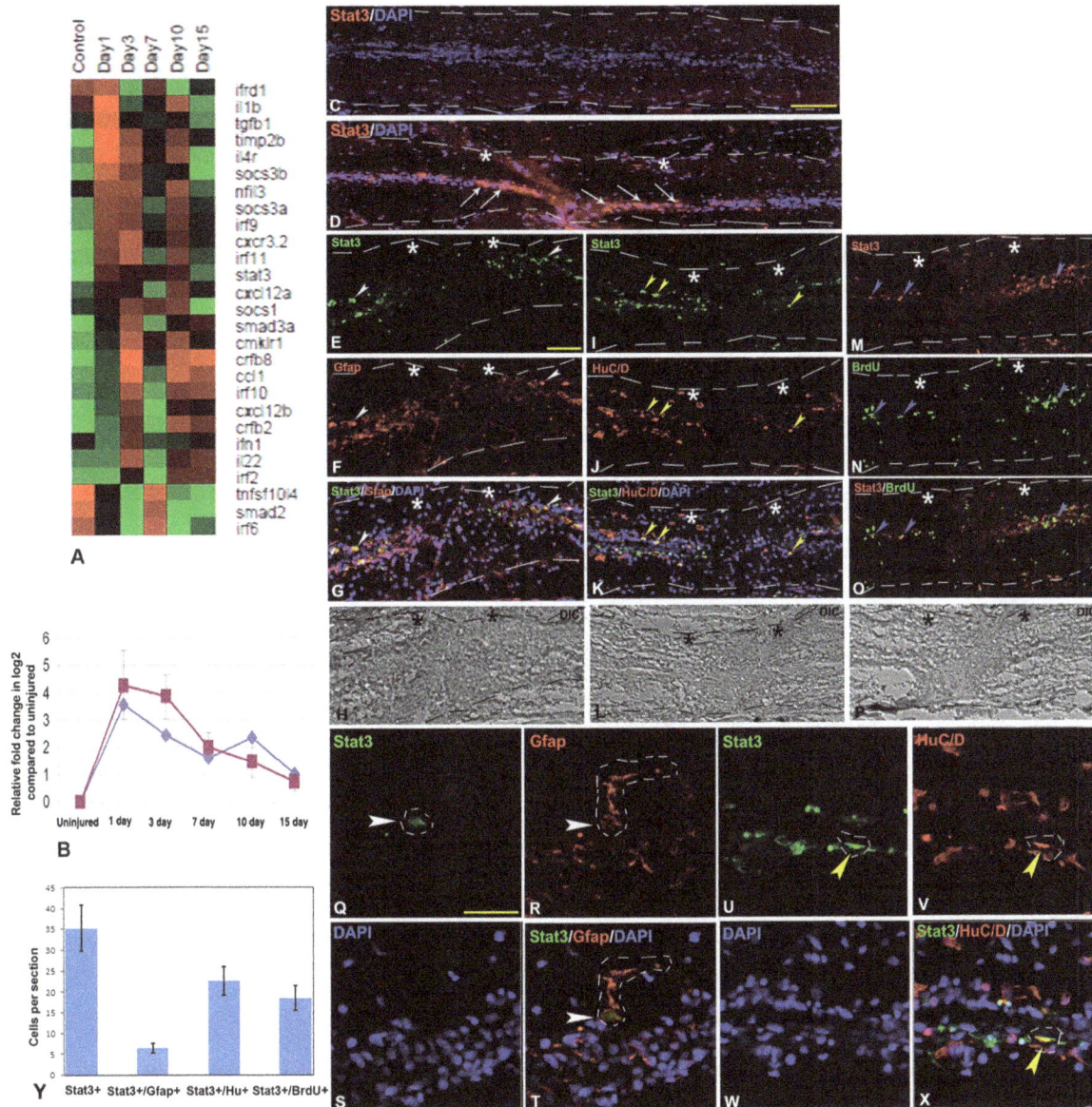

Figure 3. Differentially expressed genes related to inflammatory response and validation of *stat3* expression in uninjured and injured zebrafish spinal cord. A) Dendrogram representing genes related to regulation of inflammation. Each horizontal line indicates the expression pattern of each gene and the vertical columns indicate the uninjured control and time points after SCI. The color chart indicates mean fold change of gene expression in each time points. Red and green colors represent increased and decreased expression respectively. B) Quantitative RT-PCR of *stat3* expression showing fold change (red graph) and pattern of expression at different time points after injury. The temporal expression pattern of qRT-PCR (red graph) was compared with results of microarray analysis (blue graph). Error bars represent SEM, n = 3, p<0.01. C) A longitudinal section of uninjured cord stained with STAT3 and DAPI. D) A longitudinal section of 1 dpi cord showing many STAT3 positive cells (white arrows) close to the injury epicenter (double white stars) counter stained with DAPI. E–H) A longitudinal section of 3 dpi cord double stained with STAT3 and radial glial marker- GFAP, showing individual panels of STAT3 (E), GFAP (F), merge with DAPI (G) and DIC (Differential interference contrast) (H). A few STAT3$^+$ cells are colocalized with GFAP$^+$ cells (white arrowheads) close to injury epicenter. I–L) A longitudinal section of 3 dpi cord showing colocalization of STAT3 and newly formed neuronal marker, HuC/D with individual panels of STAT3 (I), HuC/D (J), merge with DAPI (K) and DIC (L). Some of the STAT3$^+$ cells are colocalized with HuC/D$^+$ cells (yellow arrowheads) close to the injury epicenter. M–P) A longitudinal section of 3 dpi cord colocalized with STAT3 and proliferating cell marker, BrdU shows individual panels of STAT3 (M), BrdU (N), merge (O) and DIC (P). Proliferating BrdU$^+$ cells are also colocalized with STAT3$^+$ cells (blue arrowheads) close to the injury epicenter. White dashed line in panel C to P mark the boundary of spinal cord tissue. Q–T) A representative higher magnification of 3 dpi cord section shows individual panels like STAT3 (Q), GFAP (R), DAPI (S) and merge (T). A STAT3$^+$ cell (white arrowhead; the boundary of the cell nucleus is marked by white dashed line) is colocalized with GFAP$^+$ radial glia (white arrowhead; the boundary of the cytoplasm of radial glia is marked by white dashed line). U–X) A representative higher magnification of 3 dpi cord section shows individual panels like STAT3 (U), HuC/D (V), DAPI (W) and merge (X). A STAT3$^+$ cell (yellow arrowhead; the boundary of the cell nucleus is marked by white dashed line) is colocalized with HuC/D$^+$ newly formed neuron close to ependyma (yellow arrowhead; the boundary of the cell nucleus is marked by white dashed line). Y) Quantitative analysis of STAT3$^+$, STAT3$^+$/GFAP$^+$, STAT3$^+$/HuC/D$^+$ and STAT3$^+$/BrdU$^+$ cells in 3 dpi cord in longitudinal sections. The value represented as Mean±SEM of individual longitudinal section, n = 5 cord, p<0.01.Scale bar = 200 μm (C–D); 50 μm (E–P), 20 μm (Q–X).

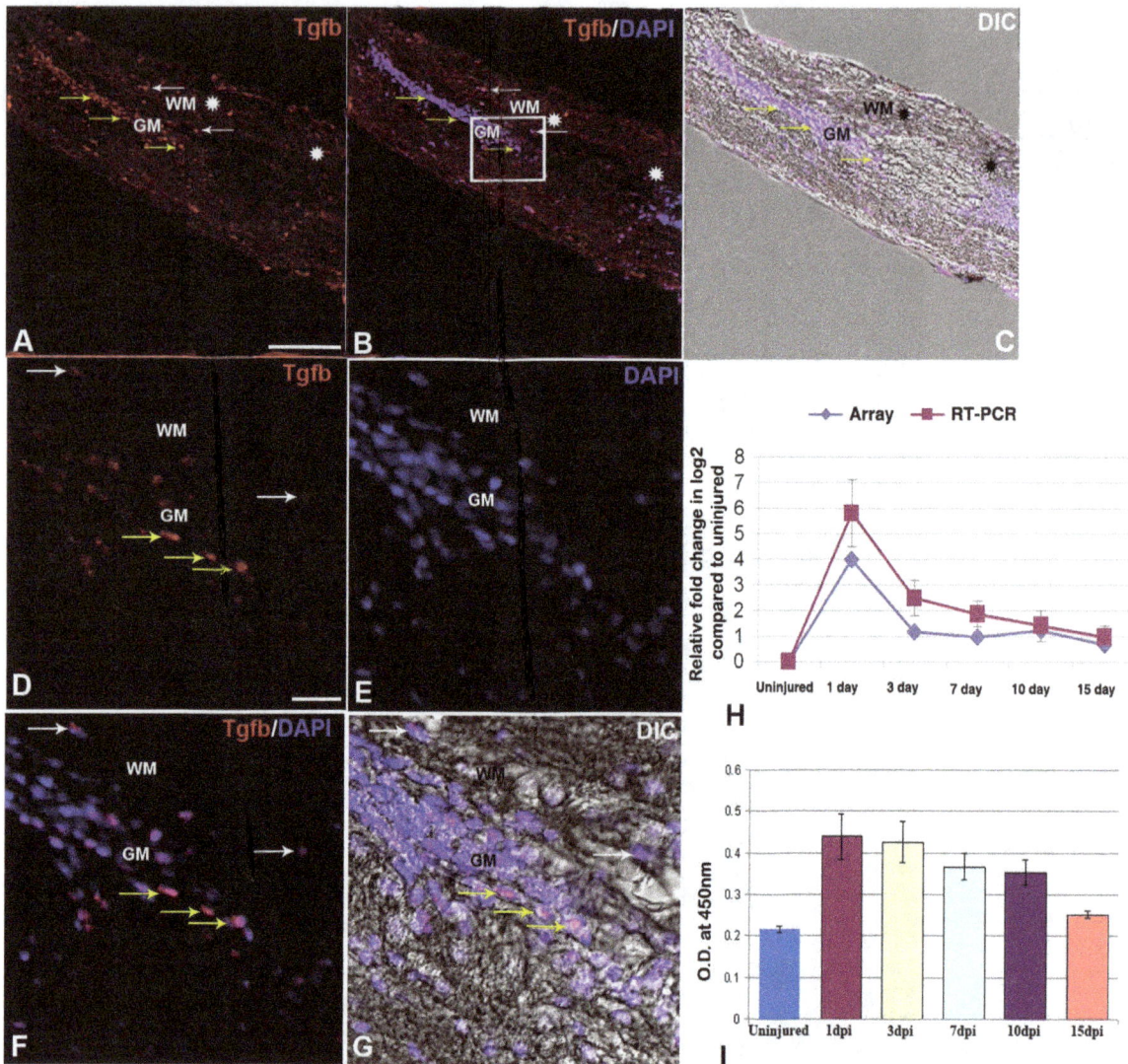

Figure 4. TGFβ expression in uninjured and injured zebrafish spinal cord. A) A longitudinal section of 1 dpi cord showing TGFβ positive cells in both grey matter (GM, yellow arrows) and white matter (WM, white arrows) of the cord at injury epicenter (double white star) and adjacent part. B) Same section merged with DAPI. C) Same section merged with DIC. D–G) Higher magnification of the boxed area of the section in B showing many TGFβ positive cells in both grey matter (GM, yellow arrows) and white matter (WM, white arrows) regions of the cord represented in individual panels of TGFβ (D), DAPI (E), merge of both (F) and merge with DIC (G). H) Quantitative RT-PCR of *tgbβ1* expression showing fold change (red graph) and pattern of expression at different time points after injury. The temporal expression pattern of qRT-PCR (red graph) was compared with results of microarray analysis (blue graph). Error bars represent SEM, n = 3, p<0.05. I) Quantification of TGFβ expression in uninjured and injured cord at different time points by ELISA. Error bars represent SEM, n = 5, p<0.01. Scale bar = 50 μm (A–C); 10 μm (D–G).

neuroprotective and neurodegenerative response [27]. In this context, it is worth mentioning that M1 macrophages are pro-inflammatory as characterized by pro-inflammatory cytokine release [31] and M2 macrophages as characterized by presence of scavenger receptors, IL-1 receptor antagonist [32] resulting in decreased production of pro-inflammatory cytokines like *il-1β* and upregulation of anti-inflammatory cytokines like *il-4* and *il-13* [27,33]. We observed presence of a higher number of M2 type macrophage related genes (anti-inflammatory) compared to M1 type (pro-inflammatory) (Table S6). M2 type macrophage related genes include *scarb1, scarb2, il4r, tgfβ1, vegfa, tgif1, arg2* and many of them are upregulated in 1 dpi and 3 dpi cord.. Only two of the genes related to M1 type macrophage (*caspa* and *nos2*) are expressed. Suppression of *nos2* limit self-damage of phagocytic

macrophages [34]. Similarly, we also found *nos2* expression as a consequence of inflammatory response.

Activated macrophage are known to play a role in wound healing, allergic reaction and proliferation and arginase activity controls the role of activated macrophages after injury [35–37]. Inflammatory response is complex as we observe both pro- and anti-inflammatory types of molecules, although a bias towards anti-inflammatory response was observed as we see strong upregulation of many M2 type macrophage related molecules. Macrophage may also enhance axonal growth by secreting several molecules like cytokines and neurotrophic factors and allowing Schwann cell migration as it happens in peripheral nervous system (PNS) [38]. Macrophage along with Schwann cell helps in clearing myelin and axonal debris as reported by others and us [6,39–41]. Macrophage may also induce MMP-9, which is playing important role in debris clearance and preventing collagen scar formation [42,43]. Our present data highlight the importance of macrophage as a key player in controlling inflammation, debris clearance and creation of permissive environment for axonal regrowth during regeneration.

Cell death.   In mammalian SCI cell death contributes to huge neuronal and glial loss and involves distinct necrotic and apoptotic pathways. Apoptotic cell death is common to both mammalian and zebrafish SCI but in a different spatio-temporal pattern [6,44]. We have identified many cell death related genes, their regulators and anti-apoptotic genes with differential expression during regeneration (Table S7). Two members, *tnfα* induced protein and *fasl*, which are upregulated in different time points and may have dual role in controlling apoptotic and necrotic pathway. Apoptotic cell death in mammalian CNS injury is regulated by Caspase and Calpain family of genes [45,46] and we observed upregulation of *caspa, caspb, casp7, capn9* in 1 dpi and 3 dpi zebrafish cord. Upregulation of 12 apoptotic genes in early time points like 1 dpi and 3 dpi are probably induced as a consequence of injury, as these genes are absent in control, and are significantly downregulated in 7 dpi cord. Among these 12 genes, *capn9* and *traf4a* are upregulated in 10 dpi and 15 dpi cord. Significance of expression of these molecules in late time points during regeneration is not well understood although these are implicated in zebrafish CNS development [47]. Mammalian anti-apoptotic protein Bcl-X$_L$ is known to control cell death and cell survival [48]. We also observed that many anti-apoptotic genes like *bcl2l13, mcm5, bag3, tnfaip6* and *igf1ra* [49–52] are upregulated in different time points after injury.

Cell migration and epithelial-mesenchymal transition.   Cell migration is one of the key phenomena in early regeneration time points as we showed that accumulation of cells in the injury epicenter occur as early as Day 3 and continues at least until Day 7 post injury [6]. Molecules like fibronectin, integrin, laminin, cadherin, matrix metalloproteinase(s) (MMPs) and collagen are known to be involved in cell adhesion, cell migration in developing and regenerating organs [5,14,15,53–57]. Our data showed that most of the genes related to cell migration are up-regulated either in 1 dpi (*fn1b, mmp13, mmp9*) or in 3 dpi (*itgav, vim, itgb4, itgb3a, cdh2, cdh23, lamb4, lamb1, cxcl12b*) cord (Table S8). Many genes are also upregulated in different regenerating organs probably indicate their common role in tissue remodeling [15,54–56]. Epithelial-mesenchymal transition (EMT) or interaction during regeneration is well known [54,58,59]. A similar EMT is probably operating during early phases of regenerating zebrafish spinal cord although it has not been characterized yet. We see expression of 8 EMT related genes which are upregulated in zebrafish cord after SCI (Table S8). A separate group of six genes represents Adam and Integrins of which *adam8a* and *adam9* show their upregulation in early time point (Table S8). Genes like *cdh2, cdh23, lamb4, lamb1, cxcl12b* are highly upregulated in 3 dpi cord. Further upregulation of these genes at 10 dpi or at 15 dpi cord, may suggest their role in different types of cell migration. In this context, it is important to refer that both neuronal migration and Schwann cell migration [60,61] is known to occur at later time points after injury.

Epithelial-mesnchymal (EM) interaction is a phenomenon during dedifferentiation phase. We see expression of some of the genes related to dedifferentiation process (like *msx-c, msx-e* and *vim*) in 3 dpi zebrafish cord (Table S9).

Proliferative response after injury in spinal cord.   Injury induced proliferation has been documented previously and proliferation is necessary to replace the lost neural cells. The proliferative response is controlled by many genes, which have been categorized as genes related to cell cycle and other regulators, involved in proliferation (Fig. 5; Table S10). As many as 48 genes

associated with cell cycle are differentially regulated. Interestingly almost all genes expressed in uninjured control are also represented in 7 dpi cord, but are not expressed in other injury time points. Exception among these patterns is *hsp90a.1* and *hsp90a.2*, which are upregulated in uninjured cord and 1 dpi but down regulated in other injury time points (Fig. 5A). A high number of genes are Cyclins and Cdc/Cdks (Fig. 5A; Table S10). Based on cell counts of colocalized BrdU/H3P along with DAPI indicate that in uninjured cord there are a low number of cells in S-phase (2%) and M-phase (1%) compared to Go-G1 phase (97%). Number of cells in both S-phase and M-phase, increases after injury, although percentage of cells entering into S-phase are higher in both 3 dpi and 7 dpi cord (8% and 12% respectively) when compared to percentage of cells in M-phase (2% and 5% respectively) (Figure S4). Our present data on array analysis corroborated with the cell count data and showed that genes involved in G1-S phase transition are selectively upregulated either in 3 dpi (*ccnd1, ccni* and *myca*) and 7 dpi (*cdk2, cdk7, ccne* and *ccnh*) cord and all 3 genes associated with S-phase (*ccna2, pcna, uhrf1*) are upregulated only in 7 dpi cord when highest number of proliferating cells are in S-phase. Both the uninjured and injured cord showed expression of *cdk2, ccnh, ccne* and *ccna2*, but fold change varies, expression level is higher in injured than uninjured cord. Among 12 genes involved in G2-M transition, 10 genes (*ccnb1, ccnb2, cdc20, klf11a, mcm6, mcm2, mad2l1, ttk, plk1, kifc1*) which are M-phase related are expressed in both uninjured control and higher in 7 dpi cord. Expression of four genes have been further validated by qRT-PCR which confirms upregulation of *ccnd1* within 1 dpi to 3 dpi cord and *ccne, cdk2* and *ccnb1* in 7 dpi cord (Fig. 5C–F). Cell cycle regulators like *myca* and *ccnd1* both are down regulated in uninjured cord but upregulated early after injury and *myca* is known to upregulate its downstream molecules *ccnd1* and *cdk2* [62]. Cell cycle regulators like *cdc20* have a role in degradation of *ccnb1* during mitosis [63]; both *cdc20* and *ccnb1* are expressed in uninjured cord and highly upregulated in 7 dpi cord and subsequent downregulation of *ccnb1* in 10–15 dpi cord probably refers to reduction of cell proliferation and down regulation of mitosis markers at late stage of regeneration [6]. Cell cycle regulators also include members of *Mcm* families, members of *Hsp* families, *plk1, ttk, klf11a, ppp1r3b* and *ppp1r7* (approximately 19 genes) are upregulated both in uninjured control and 7 dpi cord and many of them are M-phase regulators.

As mentioned earlier that proliferative response are being controlled by cell cycle regulators along with a second category of genes, which include cell proliferation related genes (Fig. 5B; Table S10). 30 genes are further separated into four different subgroups based on their temporal expression pattern and known function. There are 11 genes, which are known to be negative regulators of cell cycle progression, mostly upregulated in 1 dpi and 3 dpi cords. Among them *anxa1a, cebpd* and *cebpb* are all upregulated in 1 dpi cord and may play a role in arresting of G1-S transition [64,65]. Another important functional group of genes involved in positive regulation of cell cycle progression includes 12 genes. *Atf-3* is one of the highly upregulated genes in 1 dpi and 3 dpi cord compared to uninjured cord. A similar elevated expression of *atf-3* was demonstrated after injury in optic nerve [66], in dorsal root ganglia (DRG) and in motor neurons [67].

Differentially expressed genes involved in neurogenesis and neuronal differentiation.   Many genes related to neurogenesis are differentially regulated during the process of regeneration. Previously we showed that generation of new neurons is related to cell proliferation and Hu$^+$/Brdu$^+$ cells are continuously present in 3 dpi, 7 dpi and 10 dpi cord. Some of these cells become NeuroD positive and have undergone full neuronal

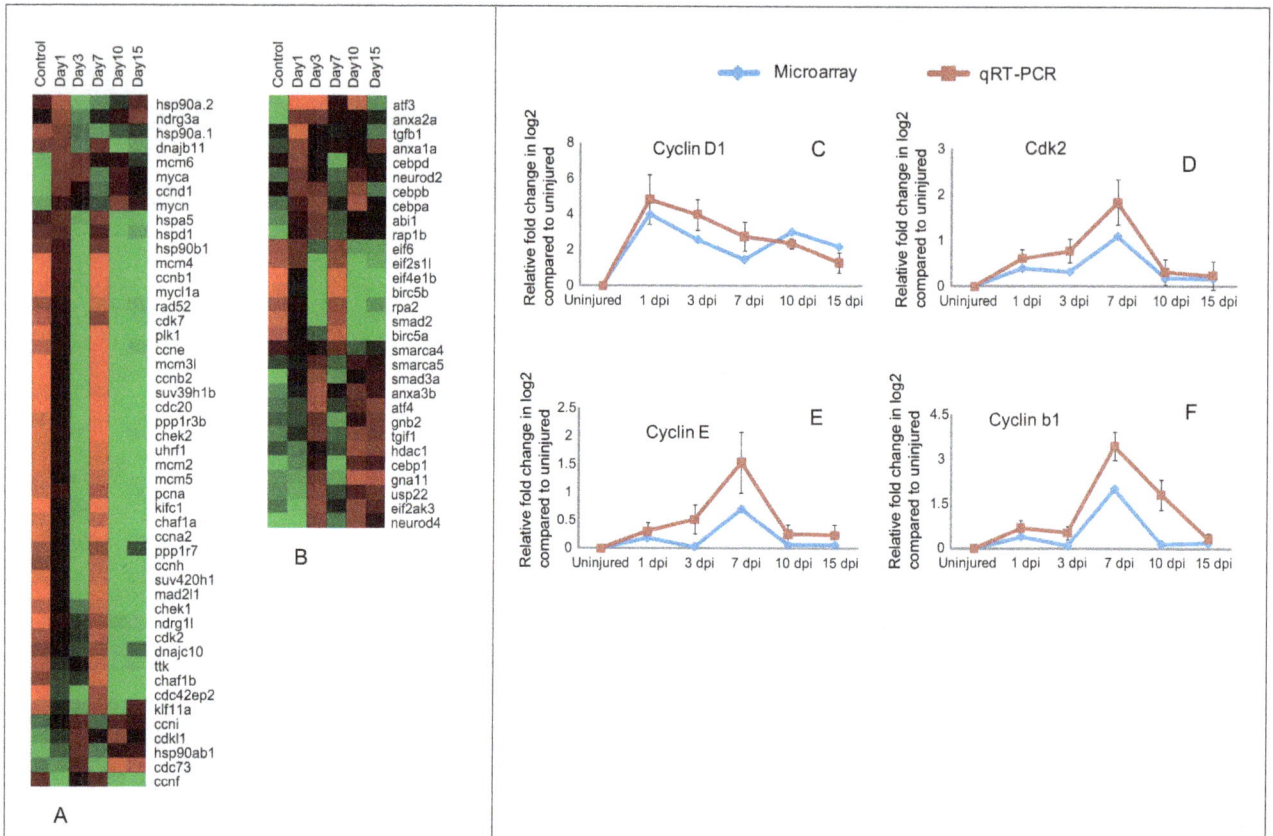

Figure 5. Differentially expressed genes related to cell proliferation in zebrafish spinal cord after injury and validation of cell cycle regulators. A) Dendrogram representing a group of cell cycle regulators directly involved with different cell cycle phases. B) Same representing group of genes indirectly control cell proliferation which include both negative and positive regulators. Each horizontal line indicates the expression pattern of each gene and the vertical columns indicate the uninjured control and time points after SCI. The color chart indicates mean fold change of gene expression in each time points. Red and green colors represent increased and decreased expression respectively. C–F) Quantitative RT-PCR analysis of *ccnd1* (C), *cdk2* (D), *ccne* (E) and *ccnb1* (F) showing fold change and pattern of expression at different time points after injury. The temporal expression pattern of qRT-PCR (red graph) was compared with results of microarray analysis (blue graph). Error bars represent SEM, n = 3, p<0.05.

differentiation [6]. Molecular analysis showed at least 54 genes are differentially expressed (Fig. 6Q; Table S11) and among them 41 genes are transcription factors (Figure S5). All the 54 genes are categorized in different groups based on their temporal pattern of expression. Group-I includes *her2*, *dab2*, *pou5f1*, *emx3*, *bmi*, *paxip*, *sox19b* and *sox21a* that are expressed in uninjured control and are upregulated in 7 dpi cord, when we also observe a very high level of proliferation, which contributes significantly to neurogenesis [6]. Among these genes, expressions of *her2* and *dab2* have been reported during retinal neurogenesis and in proliferating neuro-epithelium of developing CNS [68,69]. Group-II consists of large number of genes (36 genes) that are upregulated in 3 dpi, 10 dpi and 15 dpi cord and down regulated in uninjured control and 7 dpi cord. These are injury induced since these are not expressed in uninjured control. Genes like *notch1a*, *jagg1a*, *deltab* and *deltad* are all upregulated in 3 dpi and 10 dpi cord whereas proneural genes like *neurog1*, *neurod2*, *neurod4* and *olig2* are all upregulated in 10 dpi cord. Many of the genes in this group are members of Notch signaling pathway. Similar to developing CNS the above mentioned genes may promote differentiation of progenitors selectively to different neural fate and maintenance of reserve pools. Group-III consists of 10 genes *neurod2*, *nrarpa*, *hes5*, *nkx3.2*, *ascl1a*, *numb1*, *hesx*, *shhb*, *bdnf* and *gadd45a* all of these are highly upregulated in 1 dpi but downregulated in uninjured cord.

Many members of Sox gene family are differentially controlled during neurogenesis. There are two distinct pattern of expression within Sox family members. *Sox19b* and *sox21a* are upregulated both in uninjured cord and in 7 dpi cord. Others Sox family members (*sox2*, *sox4a*, *sox9a*, *sox9b*, *sox10*, *sox11a*, *sox14*, *sox21b* and *sox32*) are injury induced since they are upregulated in 3 dpi, 10 dpi and 15 dpi cord but down regulated in uninjured and 7 dpi cord. The highest expression values are different for different *sox* genes suggesting multiple functions during regeneration. Sox2, one of the key transcription factors is expressed in the neuroepithelium of the developing mammalian CNS and adult zebrafish brain. Its function in neural stem cell (NSC) maintenance, proliferation and specifying their identity [70–73] is well known. Our real-time PCR analysis showed that there is upregulation of *sox2* after injury at Day 3 compared to uninjured cord (Fig. 6P). The immunohisto-chemical analysis showed that in uninjured cord SOX2 positive cells are present both in ventricular region and in subependymal region of grey matter (Fig. 6A–C). A higher number of SOX2 positive cells have been found in the grey matter of 3 dpi cord (Fig. 6D–H) compared to uninjured cord. These cells are situated mostly in ependyma and few are in subependyma. A subpopula-tion of SOX2 positive cells are radial glia since they co-localize with GFAP with appropriate morphology (Fig. 6G–H; Table S12). When we co-localize SOX2 positive cells with a neuronal marker

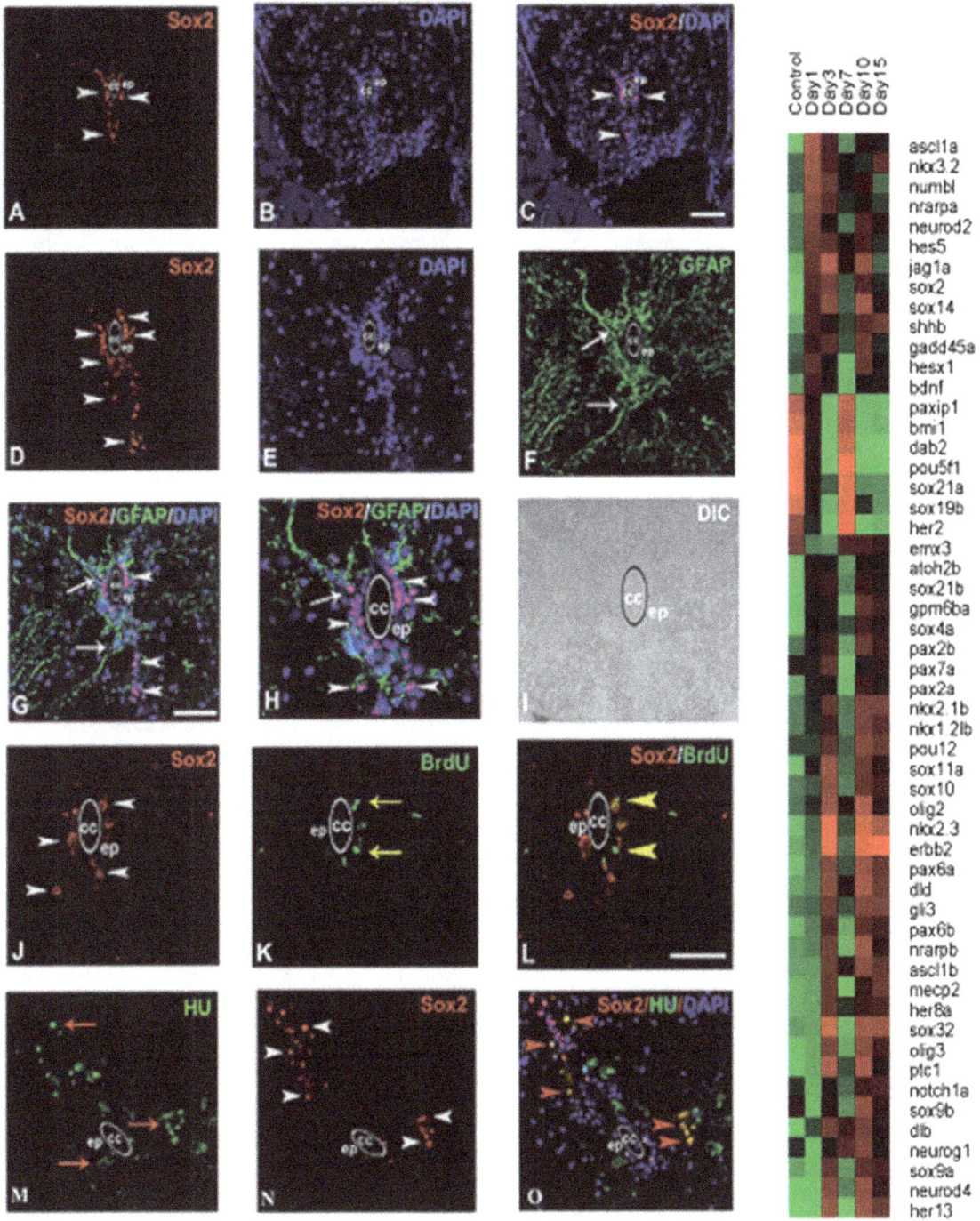

SOX2

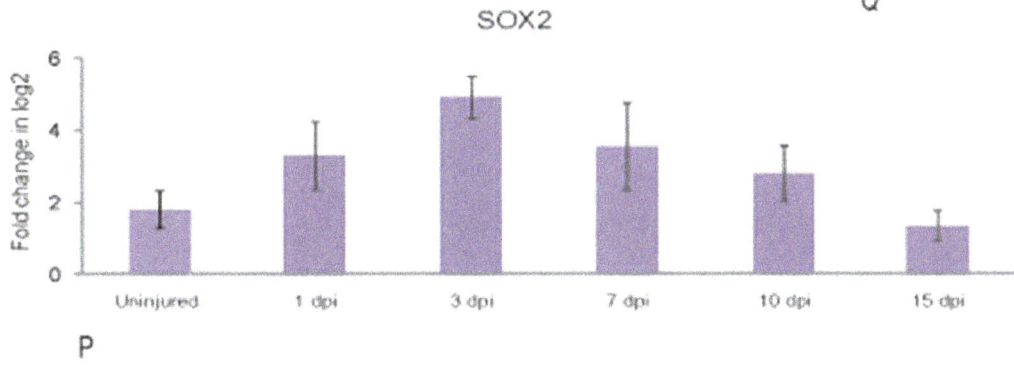

Figure 6. Differentially expressed genes involved in neurogenesis and neuronal differentiation after injury in zebrafish spinal cord and validation of Sox2 expression by immunohistochemistry and qRT-PCR analysis. A–C) A cross section of uninjured cord showing SOX2 positive cells (white arrowhead) in ependyma (ep) around the central canal (cc), counter stained with DAPI (B) and merge (C). D) A cross section of 3 dpi cord showing higher number of SOX2 positive cells compared to uninjured (A) in grey matter (white arrowhead) mostly in ependyma (ep) around the central canal (cc). E–F) Same 3 dpi cord section counter stained with DAPI (E) and stained with radial glial marker GFAP (F). G) Same 3 dpi cord section showing both SOX2 positive cells (arrowheads) and their colocalization with GFAP (arrow). H) Same section (G) in higher magnification showing colocalized SOX2 and GFAP positive cells (arrow) around the central canal (cc), I) DIC of same section in H. J–L) 3 dpi cord section showing SOX2 positive cells (J, arrowheads) and BrdU positive cells (K, yellow arrow) in the grey matter and many of them are SOX2$^+$/BrdU$^+$ (L, yellow arrowheads) in ependyma (ep) around the central canal (cc). M–O) A 3 dpi cord section showing many HuC/D positive neuronal cells (M, red arrow) and SOX2 positive cells (N, white arrowheads) in the grey matter. Same section showing colocalization of SOX2 and HuC/D (O, red arrowheads). P) qRT-PCR of *sox2* in uninjured cord and in injured cord at different time points. Error bars represent SEM, n = 3, p<0.05. Q) Dendrogram showing differentially expressed genes involved in neurogenesis and neuronal differentiation after injury. Each horizontal line indicates the expression pattern of each gene and the vertical columns indicate the uninjured control and time points after SCI. The color chart indicates mean fold change of gene expression in each time points. Red and green colors represent increased and decreased expression respectively. Scale bar = 50 μm (A–G and M–O), 20 μm (H–L).

(HuC/D), we found that many newly formed HuC/D$^+$ neuronal cells (as they are morphologically smaller than specified mature neuron) in the grey matter are SOX2 positive (Fig. 6M–O; Table S12). The colocalization of SOX2 with BrdU identified many cells present in both ventricular and subventricular region (Fig. 6J–L; Table S12) thus confirming presence of proliferating neural progenitors in regenerating cord.

Differentially expressed genes involved in repatterning
Regeneration is a complex process of rebuilding diverse tissue that involves patterning process and the mechanism substantially represents recapitulation of developmental pattern formation. The repatterning event has been studied in amphibian limb and spinal cord [74–77]. We have identified 84 pattern-forming genes that are differentially regulated (Fig. 7; Figure S6 and Table S13). Based on the temporal expression pattern we have separated 84 genes in 4 different groups. Highest numbers of genes (63 genes) are upregulated in 3 dpi, 10 dpi and 15 dpi cord that are downregulated in uninjured cord. Another category of genes (8) is upregulated in 1 dpi cord and gradually downregulated in later time points. All these genes are also down regulated in uninjured cord. The third and fourth groups, which include eight and five genes respectively, are upregulated in 7 dpi and 10/15 dpi cord. Genes belonging to these two groups are also upregulated in uninjured control unlike the first two categories (Figure S6 and Table S13).

Based on the studies on different species, combinatorial expression of different genes involved in dorso-ventral patterning of spinal cord have been identified [78–81]. Most importantly gradient of Shh induces five distinct classes of ventral neurons namely V_3, V_{MN}, V_2, V_1, V_0 from neural progenitors [78,80] and ventral cell types are determined by expression of different transcription factors. A gradient of SHH-N establishes a dorso-ventral domain by modulating expression of transcription factors of class-I and class-II proteins. SHH gradient is ventrally high and dorsally low, it represses class-I proteins creating an opposite gradient of *pax6, pax7, dbx1, dbx2, irx*. Similarly same SHH gradient activates class-II proteins namely nkx6.1 and nkx2.2 [79,80]. Our present array analysis data indicates that upregulation of *shh* during regeneration probably creating gradient similar to development. Most of the genes involved in specification of different neuronal subtypes in ventral cord (Fig. 7G; Figure S6 and Table S13). For example *dbx2, irx3* and *pax6*, all involved in V_0 and V_1 neuronal patterning, are upregulated in regenerating cord similar to developing zebrafish spinal cord [82]. Similarly, *olig2, pax6, hlxb9* and *isl2*, involved in motor neuron progenitor domain, are also upregulated in regenerating cord. The neuronal populations identified in the dorsal domain is specified by expression of Mash, Math, Neurogenin and LIM homeobox proteins in developing vertebrate cord [81]. In regenerating cord

we also observed upregulation of *neurog1, lim1* and *lim3b* (Fig. 7). We have validated three genes *dbx2, pax6a* and *shhb* by ELISA (Fig. 7E–F), qRT-PCR (Fig. 7B–D) and in situ hybridization analysis (Fig. 7H–K). Our qRT-PCR analysis revealed highest upregulation of all three genes in 10 dpi cord and significantly down regulated in control (Fig. 7B–D) and it suggests involvement of these genes in late events like repatterning of spinal cord. ELISA results of PAX6 and SHH confirms the expression pattern observed in array hybridization and qRT-PCR. *Dbx2* is another transcription factor involved in patterning of ventral spinal cord and specification of V_0 and V_1 domain interneurons during development [81]. Our array analysis and qRT-PCR data showed up-regulation of *dbx2* in 10 dpi and 15 dpi cord (fold change 8 and 6 respectively) and down regulation in other injured time points and uninjured control (Fig. 7D). In situ hybridization data reveals presence of few *dbx2* positive cells in the grey matter of uninjured cord and whereas 3 dpi cord showed complete absence of *dbx2* positive cells. The numbers of *dbx2* positive cells have increased significantly in 10 dpi cord compared to uninjured cord (Fig. 7H and J). *Dbx2* positive cells can be localized in the grey matter more ventrally, suggesting its possible role in respecifying ventral neuron during regeneration.

We have identified 52 genes, which are thought to be related to A–P patterning during CNS development in different species [83–85]. These genes are again differentially regulated at different time points after SCI. Based on the temporal expression pattern we observed three different groups. Majority of the genes (38 genes) showed upregulation in 3 dpi, 10 dpi and 15 dpi cord (21 genes are showing highest expression in 10 dpi and 15 dpi) but downregulated in uninjured control. Another set of genes showed upregulation both in uninjured control and 7 dpi cord but down regulated in other time points (Fig. 7A; Figure S6 and Table S13). A high number of genes (approximately 24) implicated in conferring A–P polarity of CNS belongs to four *hox* clusters. In regenerating zebrafish cord we observed six genes, viz. *hoxb7a, hoxb8a, hoxc8a, hoxd10a, hoxa11b, hoxd11a* which are all upregulated in 3 dpi, 10 dpi and 15 dpi cord. Upregulation of above mentioned *hox* genes in injured cord at later time points might suggest that they are probably involved in respecification of caudal spinal cord during regeneration. Furthermore, other patterning genes like *cdx1a* and *gdf11* are also upregulated in regenerating 3 dpi cord which are known to be involved in caudal spinal cord patterning during development [86,87]. Thus, different *hox* genes with overlapping rostro-caudal domain of expression in the developing cord establish different region along the A–P axis [88,89]. We inflicted injury at approximately 15th–16th vertebrae level of adult spinal cord that is more caudal and any repatterning during regeneration would require respecification of spinal cord by combinatorial expression of relevant *hox* codes. More experimental

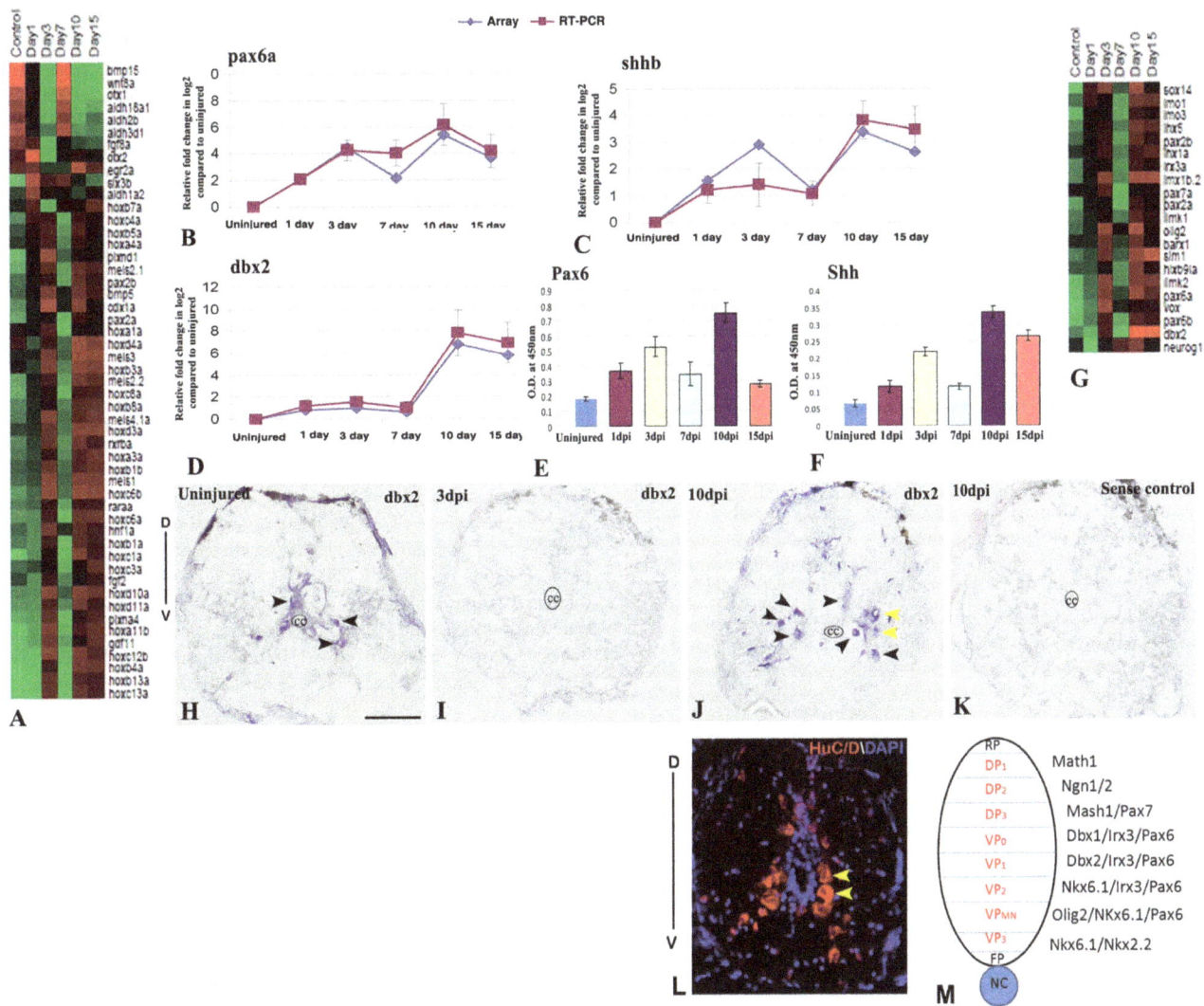

Figure 7. Differential expression of pattern forming genes during zebrafish spinal cord regeneration and validations of *pax6a*, *shhb* and *dbx2*. A) Represents known genes related to anterio-posterior patterning in CNS that are differentially expressed at different time points after SCI. The color chart indicates mean fold change of gene expression in each time points. Red and green colors represent increased and decreased expression respectively. B–D) Quantitative RT-PCR analysis of *pax6a*, *shhb* and *dbx2* respectively showing fold change and differential pattern of expression in various time points after injury and compared with the temporal expression patterns of microarray data. Error bars represent SEM, n = 3, p<0.01. E–F) Quantitative analysis of PAX6 and SHH expression by ELISA in uninjured and injured cord at different time points. Error bars represent SEM, n = 5, p<0.001. G) Represents known genes related to dorso-ventral patterning in CNS that are differentially expressed at different time points after SCI. The color chart indicates mean fold change of gene expression in each time points. Red and green colors represent increased and decreased expression respectively. H–K) In situ hybridization of *dbx2* in uninjured (H), 3 dpi (I) and 10 dpi (J) cord section shows presence of *dbx2* transcripts in few neurons (black arrowheads) in uninjured cord but complete absence of *dbx2* transcripts in 3 dpi cord and reappearance of *dbx2* transcripts in many neurons in 10 dpi cord (black arrowheads). Significantly, higher numbers of *dbx2* positive cells are present in the ventral side of the 10 dpi cord compared to uninjured cord. Yellow arrows indicate neurons of ventral progenitor domain. Section in K represents sense control of *dbx2* in a 10 dpi cord. The mark 'cc' denotes central canal of the cord. 'D' and 'V' indicates dorsal and ventral side of the cord respectively. L) Representative transverse section of 10 dpi cord stained with HuC/D and DAPI showing the distribution of regenerated neurons in the dorso-ventral axis of the cord. Yellow arrows indicate neurons of ventral progenitor domain. M) A schematic diagram of various progenitor domains in dorso-ventral axis of spinal cord on the basis of spatial distribution and gene expression, adapted from Wilson and Maden [81]. 'D' and 'V' indicates dorsal and ventral side of the cord respectively. RP = Roof plate, FP = Floor plate, NC = Notochord, DP = Dorsal progenitor, VP = Ventral progenitor. Scale bar = 50 μm.

validations involving different *hox* genes family members need to be done to corroborate our expression analysis.

Differentially expressed genes involved in axonal regrowth and guidance. Time course analysis of regeneration demonstrated axonal regrowth and substantial functional recovery after SCI in zebrafish [4,6,10]. We can see reconnected axons at 15 dpi cord although molecular events related to initiation of axonal regrowth may start early [6]. In the present study, we have

identified many genes involved in axonogenesis and axonal guidance. There are at least 80 genes involved in axonal regrowth and guidance that also include many transcription factors (Figure S7 and Table S14). Based on temporal expression patterns, we have found 3 different groups. Group-I consists of 11 genes and they are upregulated both in uninjured control and 7 dpi cord. Group-II consists of 13 genes and they are particularly downregulated in control but upregulated in 1 dpi cord and gradually downregulated in later injury time points. In Group-III, highest number (56) of genes showed upregulation in 3 dpi, 10 dpi and 15 dpi cord but downregulated in uninjured control. It is important to note that IPA analysis also showed high enrichment of axonal guidance signaling genes in all three above mentioned time points (Fig. 2; Figure S2 and Table S3). Similar to developing nervous system there is also a complex mechanism of axonal pathfinding during axonal regrowth that include different axonal guidance molecules with attractive, repulsive and adhesive properties [90]. For example molecules like *robo1*, *robo2*, *slit1b*, *slit3*, *sema3ab* and *sema3h* all are with repellent properties and are all upregulated in 3 dpi, 10/15 dpi cord. Axonal attractant molecules like *netrin1a*, *netrin1b*, *plexina4*, are also upregulated in 3 dpi and 10 dpi cord. Cell adhesion molecules like *ncam* show slightly different expression pattern, as they are upregulated in 3 dpi and 10/15 dpi cord. Ephrins and receptor tyrosine kinases are known to be involved in organization of axons in different topographic planes during development of CNS [91,92]. *Efnb1* and *efnb3* are upregulated in 3 dpi and 10 dpi cord whereas *rtk6* are upregulated in 1 dpi and 3 dpi cord but all remained downregulated in uninjured control. In developing zebrafish, motor guidance and target recognition molecules include CAMs [85], *semaphorins* [93,94], *netrins* [93], robo, *slit* [95], ephrin and *rtk* [91]. Another gene *atf-3* is also highly upregulated in 1 dpi, 3 dpi and 10 dpi cord and may be involved in axonal regrowth as indicated in various reports [66,96]. Induction of *atf-3* in both PNS injury and optic nerve injury is implicated in creation of permissive environment for axonal regeneration. Interestingly in zebrafish SCI, there is also creation of PNS like environment in CNS. As many as six genes (like *atf3*, *fgf2*, *mmp-9*, *stat3*, *socs3* and *sox11*), which are related to PNS regeneration, are upregulated after injury. Similar to the previous studies on axonal regeneration in zebrafish CNS [5,97] *contactin1b* and *gefiltin* are also upregulated in either 10/15 day after injury. All these molecules are upregulated in regenerating cord during axonogenesis suggesting similar mechanism of axonal growth and guidance are probably being employed in directing axonal regrowth. In adult, functional analysis of identified genes during axonogenesis would provide some clue to understand regrowth of axonal tracts in regenerating cord.

Expression of genes in signaling pathways during spinal cord regeneration

We have analyzed expression profiles of different members of Wnt, BMP/TGF beta and JAK-STAT pathway and validated expression of few genes from the respective pathways (Fig. 3, 4, 8; Figure S8 and Table S15). Other signaling pathways such as Hedgehog, Notch and FGF also appear to play critical role in regeneration (Figure S8 and Table S15).

Wnt signaling. Many members of Wnt signaling pathway are differentially regulated at different time points suggesting their diverse role in cellular events of regeneration (Fig. 8H; Figure S8 and Table S15). Several Wnt members like *wnt4a*, *wnt4b*, *wnt7a*, *wnt8a*, *wnt9a*, *wnt11* and *β-catenin* are upregulated at different time points after injury. Other members of Wnt signaling pathway represent Frizzled like (*fzd2*, *fzd3i* and *celsr2*; zebrafish homolog of mouse *flamingo*) which are mostly upregulated in 3 dpi and 10 dpi cord. Both *wnt4a* and *wnt9a* are upregulated in 3 dpi and either in 10 and or 15 dpi cord and downregulated in other time points of regeneration. On the other hand, *wnt8a* showed upregulation in control and 7 dpi cord and down regulated in other time points. Regulators of Wnt signaling genes like *dixdc1*, *gsk3b*, *tcf7l1* and *tcf7l2* are all differentially upregulated in 3 dpi, 10 dpi and 15 dpi cord and down regulated in 7 dpi cord. There are different

inducible targets of different Wnt, β-catenin or Frizzled, which include *myca*, *mycn*, *myc11a*, *jun*, *ccnd1*, retinoic acid receptors and many members of *sox* family genes. Role of different Wnts like *wnt3a*, *wnt5a*, *wnt5b*, *wnt7a*, *wnt8a*, *wnt10a* are well documented in different regenerating tissues [56,98–101]. In regenerating fin, over expression of *wnt8a* caused activation of *β-catenin* and which leads to increased proliferative response and accelerated regeneration [100]. We have validated array expression data of *wnt8a* and *β-catenin* by qRT-PCR and in situ hybridization experiments (Fig. 8). The qRT-PCR analysis shows both *wnt8a* and *β-catenin* are upregulated in 7 dpi cord, where we see highest rate of proliferation (Fig. 8A–B). In situ hybridization analysis with *wnt8a* transcript showed high expression in 7 dpi cord and absent in uninjured and 3 dpi cord. Many cells with *wnt8a* mRNA transcript are present around the central canal and are ependymal cells (Fig. 8F) which are thought to be precursors [12]. These data confirm our previous observation where we have showed the presence of proliferating BrdU$^+$ precursors in ependyma [6]. Few *wnt8a* expressing cells are also present in white matter of 7 dpi cord (Fig. 8F and F.1). The spatio-temporal distribution of *wnt8a* transcript in regenerating cord suggests that it is upregulated predominantly in ependymal cells, which actively proliferates following injury. Another member of Wnt family *wnt7a* is upregulated in wound epidermis, cartilage, spinal cord and muscle in regenerating tail in urodele [102]. Both *wnt7a* and *wnt4b* are highly upregulated in regenerating cord in early time points and validated by qRT-PCR (Fig. 8C–D. Apart from the positive regulators there are many negative regulators in Wnt signaling pathway like *dixdc1*, *gsk3*, *sfrp1*, *sfrp1b* and *sfrp5* suggesting both presence of pro and negative Wnt signaling during spinal cord regeneration.

BMP/TGF beta signaling. Members of BMP/TGF beta signaling pathways are differentially up or down regulated during the different events of regeneration (Figure S8A and Table S15). This list contains both TGFβ signaling genes and their target genes. We observe different group of genes based on temporal expression pattern. Among members of TGFβ signaling family, temporal expression pattern of *tgfβ1* gene is distinctly different being upregulated immediately after injury (1 dpi cord) and down regulated in subsequent time periods. This gene is associated with inflammatory process early during regeneration phase as discussed previously in section 3A. Members of BMPs and growth and differentiation factor 11 (Gdf11) are known to control neurogenesis in olfactory neuroepithelia and help in maintenance of progenitor population by replacing dying neurons [103,104]. We have also found *bmp5* and *gdf11* both are upregulated in 3 dpi and 10 dpi cord and these genes are known to play key role in this pathway.

JAK-STAT signaling. Three members of JAK-STAT pathway like stat1b, stat5.2 and stat3 are upregulated during regeneration of zebrafish spinal cord (Figure S8B and Table S15). Stat5.2 and stat1b are both upregulated at 3 dpi and 10 dpi cord and down regulated in uninjured control and other injury time points. Stat3 showed different temporal expression pattern than others and uprgulated in 1 dpi and 3 dpi cord. Similarly, stat3 interacting genes like rtk6 and target genes like socs3a and socs3b, mapk2l and ptpn6 all are upregulated in 1 dpi and 3 dpi cords. Stat3 expression has been validated and described previously (Fig. 3), which is an important regulator of inflammation and may promote cell survival and proliferation. The temporal expression of stat3 and its downstream targets like socs3a and socs3b are similar and may indicate the immunomodulatory role of socs3 by regulating JAK-STAT signaling as suggested earlier [105].

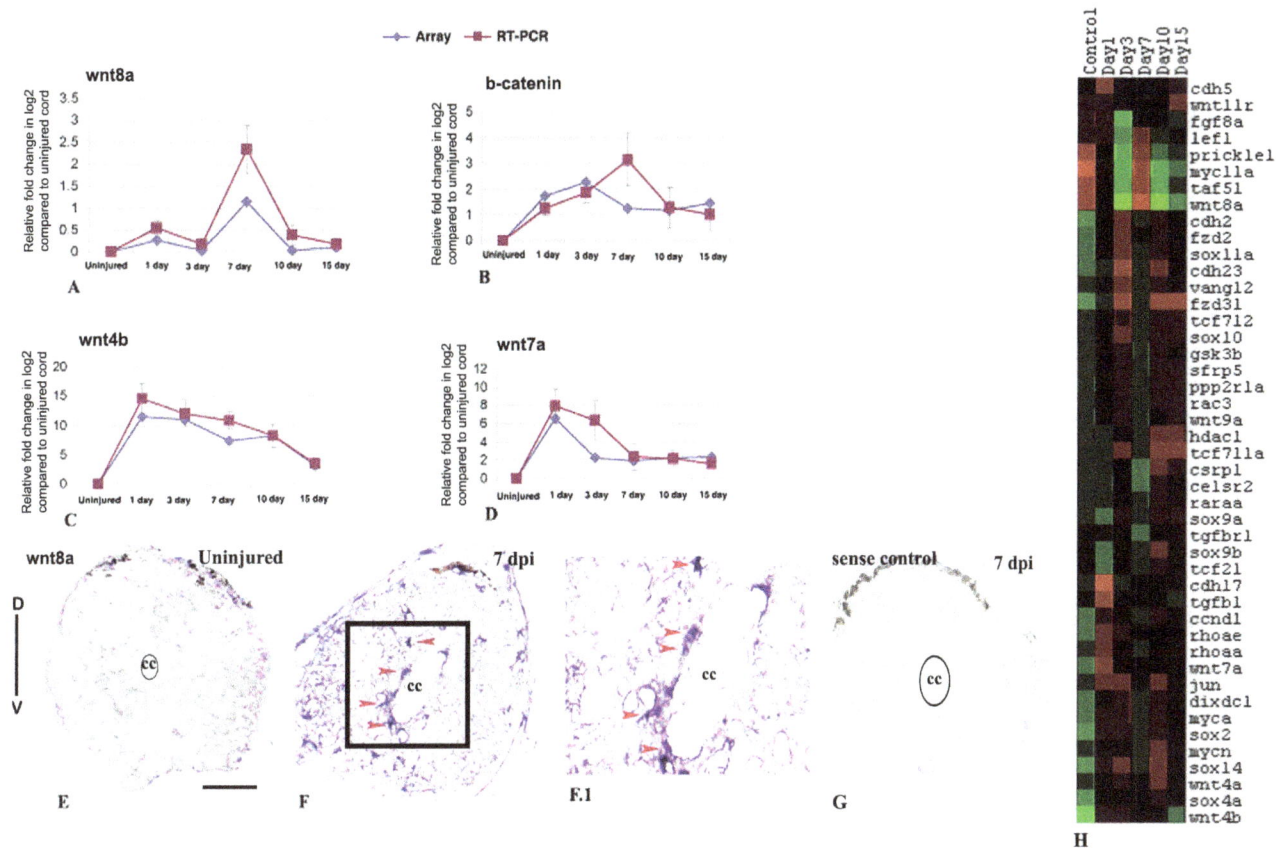

Figure 8. Differentially expressed genes involved in Wnt signaling pathway in zebrafish spinal cord after injury and validation of *wnt8a, wnt4b, wnt7a* and *b- catenin*: A–D) Quantitative RT-PCR analysis of *wnt8a*, *b-catenin*, *wnt4b* and *wnt7a* respectively showing fold change (red graph) and temporal expression pattern after injury. Pattern of expression was compared with microarray data (blue graph). Error bars represent SEM, n = 3, p<0.01. E–F) In situ hybridization with *wnt8a* anti-sense probe showed absence and presence of mRNA transcripts in uninjured and 7 dpi cord respectively. F.1) Higher magnification of the boxed area in section F shows *wnt8a* expression in ependymal cells (red arrowheads). G) In situ hybridization of 7 dpi section with *wnt8a*sense probe as control. 'D' and 'V' indicates dorsal and ventral side of the cord respectively. The mark 'cc' denotes central canal of the cord. H) Represents temporal expression pattern of genes after SCI related to Wnt signaling pathway. The color chart indicates mean fold change of gene expression in each time points. Red and green colors represent increased and decreased expression respectively. Scale bar = 50 µm.

Identification of conserved genes differentially expressed during spinal cord, retina, fin and heart regeneration in zebrafish

To identify the conserved genes involved in regeneration, we compared the gene identified in regenerating spinal cord with the set of genes identified in other regenerating tissues like heart, fin and retina. Among the 3842 genes that are differentially expressed during spinal cord regeneration, 156, 297 and 835 genes are commonly expressed during heart, fin and retinal regeneration respectively (Fig. 9A; Table S16). Both spinal cord and retina regeneration involve related common process like proliferation and neurogenesis and they shared maximum number of common genes during the regeneration. It is evident from the figure 9A that these tissues share a significant number of genes among themselves whether they are compared in twos or threes. When we consider all the four tissues at a time, we find they share 29 common genes (Fig. 9B). However there are also 2952, 2362, 427 and 511 genes that are specific to regenerating spinal cord, retina, fin and heart respectively (Fig. 9A).

There are five known genes *plk1* (polo-kinase 1), *ttk1/mps1* (monopolar spindle 1, a kinase required for mitotic check point regulation), *cdc20, ccna2* and *atf-3* commonly expressed in different regenerating organs like fin, heart, retina and spinal cord (Fig. 9B; Table S16). Among these genes, expression of *mps1* has been reported to be present in fin blastema [3], regenerating heart [15] and retina [5] during proliferation phase. We report low and high expression of mps1 in uninjured and 7 dpi cord respectively. Similarly, M-phase regulators like *plk1, cdc20,* and *ccna2* are also upregulated in 7 dpi cord. These data suggest that there is a common mechanism regulating cell proliferation in all these regenerating organs and all the three M-phase regulators are tightly controlled during proliferation. *Atf3* is another common gene which is highly upregulated in regenerating cord compared to normal uninjured cord.

Hdac1 is yet another common cell cycle regulator known to repress expression of *ccnd1* and *ccne2* [106] and expressed in regenerating CNS like retina [107] and in developing CNS [108]. Temporal expression pattern of *hdac1* shows two different upregulated peaks in 3 dpi and 10/15 dpi cord and may be related to gradual repression of *ccnd1* from 3 dpi to 15 dpi cord. Furthermore, second peak of *hdac1* expression in 10 dpi and 15 dpi cords is suggestive of its role in differentiation of neurons and glia as observed in zebrafish retina [106,107].

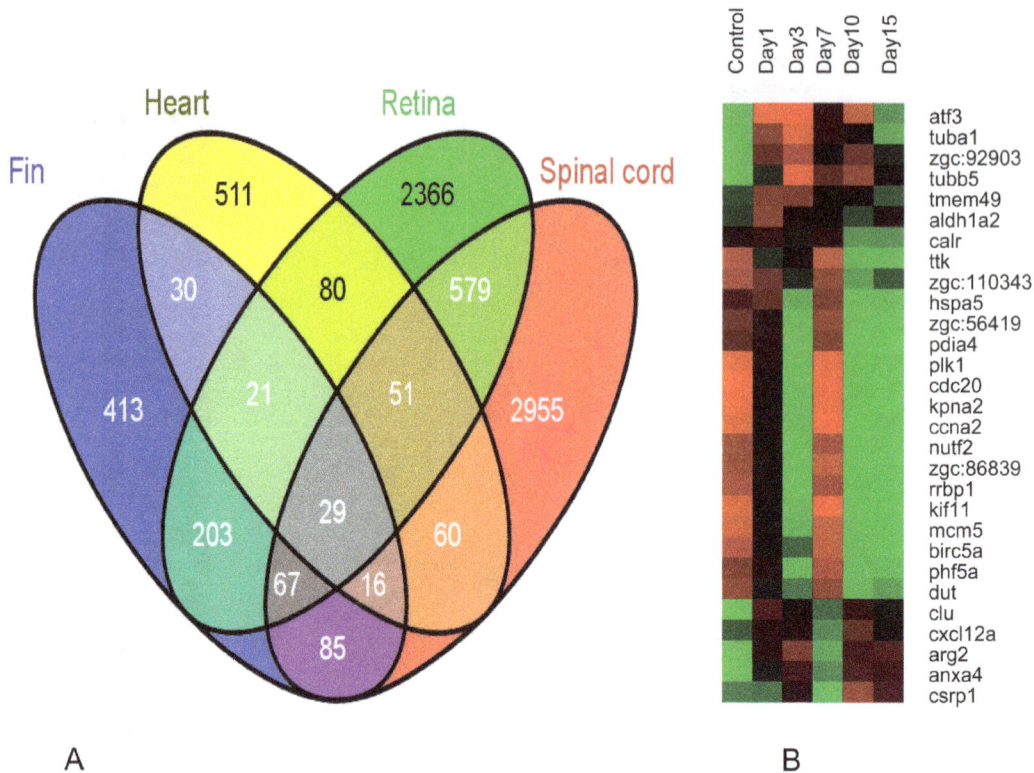

Figure 9. Common genes differentially expressed in spinal cord, fin, retina and heart during regeneration in zebrafish. A) Vein diagram illustrates number of genes that are expressed (uniquely as well as shared) during regeneration of the four different tissues like fin, heart, retina and spinal cord. B) Differential expression pattern of the 29 common genes in uninjured and injured zebrafish spinal cord with different time points. The color chart indicates mean fold change of gene expression in each time points. Red and green color represents increased and decreased expression respectively.

Many genes involved with one-carbon folate metabolism, N-glycan biosynthesis and ion transport were differentially expressed during spinal cord regeneration

Based on the IPA analysis we have identified and clustered at least 44 genes which are involved in ion transport and are also differentially expressed during regeneration (Figure S9 and Table S17). This particular group includes genes of sodium, potassium and calcium channel proteins; glutamate, glycine and purinergic receptors and other associated ion transport proteins.

The IPA analysis also identified two novel signaling pathways like one-carbon folate metabolism and N-glycan biosynthesis from the array data and the genes involved in these signaling pathways have been identified (Figure S9 andTable S17). All the five genes (*tyms, dhfr, shmt1, atic* and *amt*) involved with one-carbon folate metabolism are upregulated in uninjured zebrafish cord and 7 dpi cord. Following transection injury to the rat spinal cord, increased expression of folate receptor 1 (FOLR1) promotes methylation of spinal cord DNA [109,110]. Two genes, *tyms* and *dhfr* are also involved in de novo purine-pyrimidine biosynthesis. Temporal expression pattern of these 5 genes further corroborates with our finding in IPA analysis that enrichment of purine-pyrimidine metabolism pathway genes are highest (63%) at 7 dpi cord.

Among the genes related to N-glycan biosynthesis pathway, four genes are upregulated in both uninjured and 7 dpi cord. Only *b4galt1* is upregulated in 3 dpi and 10/15 dpi cord and remained downregulated in uninjured control and other injured time points.

All the five genes (*b4galt1, st6gal1, alg3, alg1* and *mgat3*) in this group are enzymes related to glycosylation of proteins.

Identification and validation of some unannotated genes involved in spinal cord regeneration

We have identified 91 genes that are totally uncharacterized and unannotated from the list of differentially expressed genes. Although these genes have unique Unigene ID their functions are not properly annotated; few of them have unannotated/validated human homolog. As of now, it appears that these are fish specific genes that are involved in regeneration process. Identification of human homolog for these fish specific genes will give new target genes, which may be crucial in regeneration process. Among the 91 uncharacterized genes, we selected 9 genes that show a high fold change and are distributed among the 7 clusters represented in figure 1 (Fig. 10; Table S18). Expression pattern of these genes are represented in treeview (Fig. 10A) and are validated by qRT-PCR (Fig. 10B). We have BLAST searched the proteins of these nine genes to find their putative homologues in human and assigned functions to them based on these homologues. The expression patterns and the human homologous functions of the genes are described below. Among these nine genes, four are upregulated both in uninjured and 7 dpi cord which are zgc:66483 (zinc finger protein 389), si:dkeyp-50f7.2 (ZPA domain containing protein), zgc:162945 (Putative nuclease Harbi1) and zgc:110788 (Vesicle transport protein Sft2B). zgc:110179 (Ras signaling related protein) is upregulated in 7 dpi and 15 dpi cord. zgc:111821 (Spp1 protein or Osteopontin) and zgc:112054 (cAMP responsive

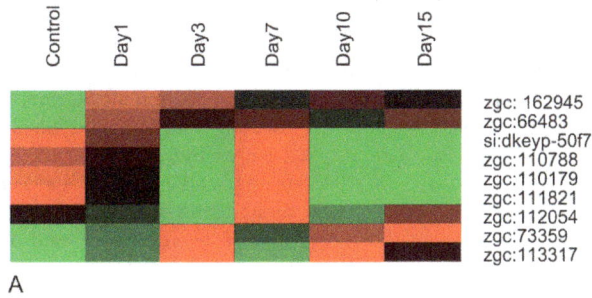

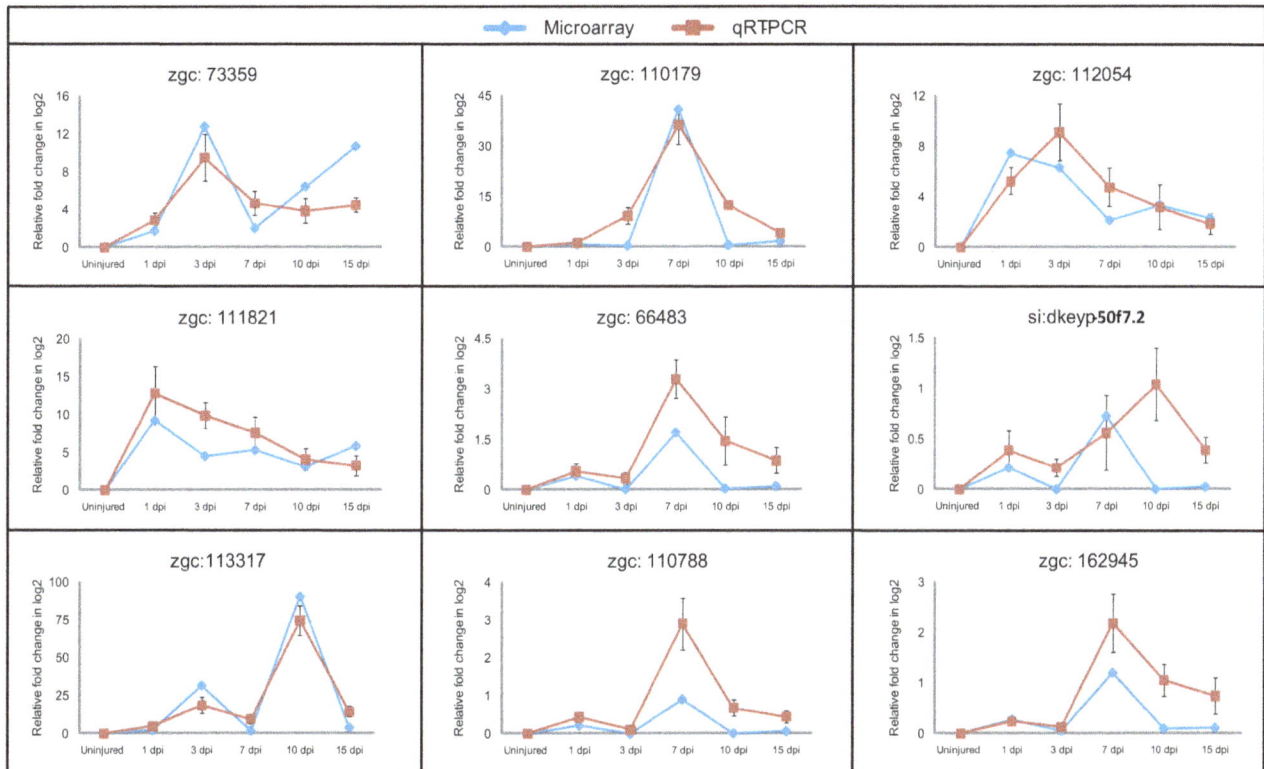

B

Figure 10. Validation of unannotated genes differentially expressed in array hybridization during regeneration of zebrafish spinal cord. A) Cluster of nine differentially expressed unannotated genes. Each horizontal line indicates the expression pattern of each gene and the vertical columns indicate the uninjured control and time points after SCI. The color chart indicates mean fold change of gene expression in each time points. Red and green colors represent increased and decreased expression respectively. B) Comparative gene expression analysis by microarray (Blue) and qRT-PCR (Red) of nine unannotated genes at different injury time points. Error bars represent SEM, n = 3, p<0.05.

element) are upregulated in 1 dpi and 3 dpi cord. Other two genes are upregulated in 3 dpi and 10/15 dpi cord which are zgc:73359 (Retinal rod rhodopsin sensitive cGMP) and zgc:113317 (Amine sulfotransferase) (Fig. 10).

We have used zebrafish as a regeneration competent model and combined the transcriptome profiling to uncover the molecular mechanisms underlying spinal cord regeneration. Our analysis is based on different cellular events occurring during regeneration and thus allowed us to specify molecular basis of different cellular events that are different from one another. A schematic diagram represents the different cellular events and upregulation of some important genes expression (Fig. 11). The diagram also highlights the similarity and dissimilarity of the events between zebrafish and mammalian SCI thus providing more insight on how to approach for possible future therapeutic strategy. In summary, some of the key events analyzed are inflammatory response, cell proliferation

& neurogenesis and axonal growth and inhibition. Early inflammatory response was induced after injury both in zebrafish and in mammals, although nature of cells involved in inducing inflammatory response varies. Some of the genes (*tgfb1*, *stat3* and *casp3*) are conserved in responding to injury between the two species. In mammalian SCI, astrogliosis and microglial activation is key to regeneration failure. In fish CNS, microglial activation is rapid but transient and proved to be beneficiary [9]. One of the expression markers of glia, GFAP is downregulated after SCI [6] whereas GFAP upregulation has been observed in mammalian SCI [111]. Proliferative response is high following injury in zebrafish cord. Expression of different cell cycle regulators and transcription factors points towards their contribution in neurogenesis. In comparison, proliferative response in mammals predominantly targets astrocytes and inflammatory cells [112]. Failure of axonal regeneration in mammal is controlled by absence of permissive niche, apoptosis, demyelination followed by accumulation of myelin debris and Wallerian degeneration [113,114]. We observed limited apoptosis, rapid debri clearance, and absence of Nogo (Our unpublished observation) and generation of permissive niche. Expression of appropriate genes responsible for axonal regrowth has also been documented in zebrafish cord.

Conclusions

The present study has identified 3,842 differentially expressed genes during spinal cord regeneration in zebrafish by using high-density oligonucleotide based microarray. Events specific cluster analysis further identified many important genes involved in controlling different processes in regeneration like inflammation, cell death, cell migration, cell proliferation and neurogenesis followed by axonogenesis and repatterning of the regenerating spinal cord tissue. Comprehensive event specific analysis during spinal cord regeneration is a key to define therapeutic strategy to be adapted in higher vertebrates. Possibility of using a combinatorial approach may include targeting of genes a) to control secondary degenerative response after injury, b) to induce controlled cell proliferation, c) to induce selective neurogenesis and axonogenesis and d) for creation of permissive niche. All the cellular events mentioned here are to be taken care of simultaneously in order to deliver appropriate therapy after SCI in mammals. There are also lessons to be learnt about the evolutionarily common genetic program operating in different organs and information on tissue specific gene expression that could be used selectively for regeneration of specific organs.

Materials and Methods

Zebrafish husbandry and surgical procedure to inflict spinal cord injury

Zebrafish were obtained (~3–4 cm) either from local pet shop or bred in our animal house facility. Fish were kept in separate groups of 10 in the aquatic system maintained at 28°C on a 14 hr

light/10 hr dark cycle. Fish were anaesthetized for 5 minutes in 0.02% tricaine (MS222; Sigma, USA) before giving SCI. A longitudinal lesion was made at the side of the fish to expose vertebral column at the level of dorsal fin, which corresponds to 15/16th vertebrae. The spinal cord has been injured by crushing dorso-ventrally for 1 sec with a number 5 Dumont forceps at the same level (Figure S10). Later the wound were sealed by placing a suture. Both spinal cord injured and sham operated fish were allowed to regenerate and the progress of regeneration was observed after 1, 3, 7, 10 and 15 days of injury. During the process of regeneration, operated fish were incubated in normal aquarium at 28°C . This study was carried out in accordance with the recommendation in the guidelines provided by CPCSEA (Committee for the Purpose of Control and Supervision of Experiments on Animals, Ministry of Environments and Forests, Government of India). The protocol (Part B), which includes all the details of surgical processes inflicted and anesthesia requirement for injuring and sacrificing animals, was approved by the Institutional Animal Ethics committee, Department of Biophysics, Molecular Biology and Bioinformatics, University of Calcutta under the registration number with CPCSEA (CPCSEA/ORG/CH/Reg No. 925/295).

Tissue collection and RNA extraction for microarray analysis

Control fishes and spinal cord injured fishes were anesthetized deeply for 5 minutes in 0.1% tricaine (MS222; Sigma, USA) and approximately 1 mm length of spinal cord both rostrally and caudally from injury epicenter were dissected out from 50–60 fishes in each batch and pooled for RNA extraction. RNA was extracted from the control and regenerating spinal cords of the experimental fishes using Trizol (Invitrogen,15596018) and quality of RNA was checked on Agilent 2100 Bioanalyzer (Agilent RNA 6000 Nano Assay). RNA was prepared from a minimum of 3 biological replicates. For each biological replicate, spinal cord

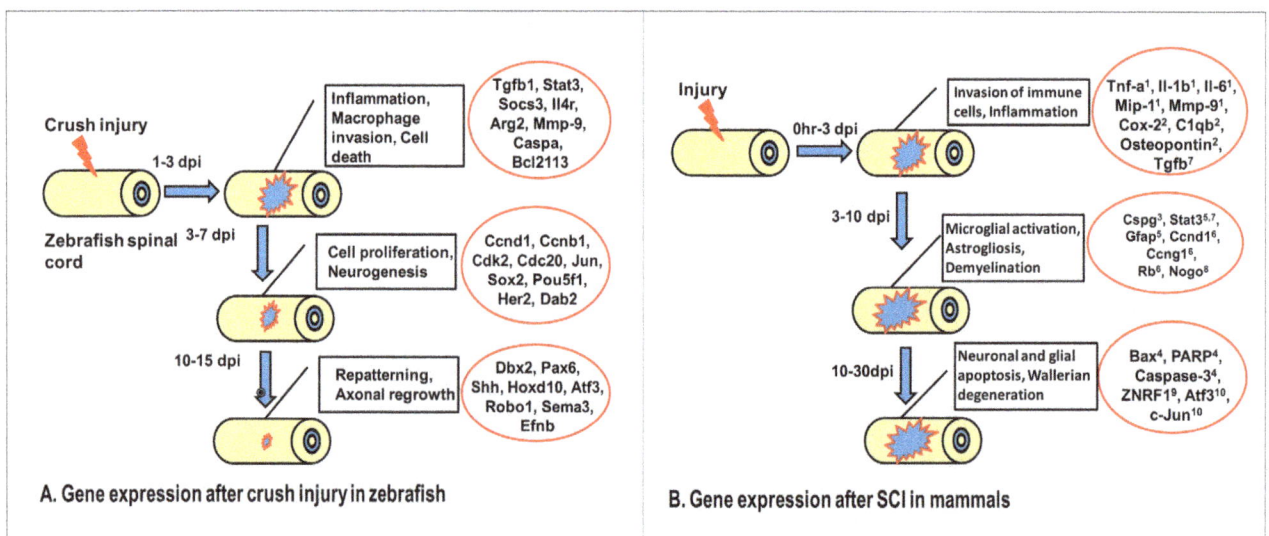

Figure 11. Comparative analysis of cellular events and upregulation of genes following SCI in zebrafish and mammals. A) Schematic representation of different events and underlying expression of some important genes during zebrafish spinal cord regeneration. B) Schematic representation of different events and corresponding upregulation of genes in mammalian spinal cord after inflicting different modes of injury. The expressions of gene(s) are compiled based on previous evidences, which are known to regulate different cellular events. (1. [120]; 2. [121]; 3. [122]; 4. [123]; 5. [111]; 6. [112]; 7. [124]; 8. [125]; 9. [126]; 10. [127].).

from about, 50–60 fishes were pooled in the control and in the regenerating samples.

Oligonucleotide probe design and microarray design

Microarray was performed using Agilent platform. Zebrafish microarray was custom designed for gene-expression, containing ~44,000 probes (60 mer long; including positive and negative controls designed by Agilent and beta-actin controls). All procedures were carried out using standard recommended protocols from Agilent. The microarrays were performed following Agilent's One-Color Microarray-Based Gene Expression Analysis (Quick Amp Labeling) protocol (Version 5.7, March 2008) and RNA Spike-In-One Color. We used about 400 ng total RNA as the starting material for amplification and labelling. After cDNA and cRNA synthesis, the Cy3 labeled cRNA samples were column purified, and checked for yield and those passed the QC (1.65 μg and specific activity >9.0 pmol Cy3 per μg cRNA) were used for hybridization to the arrays. Arrays were hybridized at 65°C for 17 hours in a slow rotating hybridization chamber. The slides were washed as described in Agilent's protocol and scanned on Agilent's DNA Microarray Scanner. The scanned images were analyzed using Agilent Feature Extraction Software (v10.5.1.1). Feature extracted data were analyzed using the tools in Gene-Spring. Full microarray data were deposited in GenBank, GEO accession number is GSE39295 and it is available in following link http://www.ncbi.nlm.nih.gov/geo/query/acc.cgi?acc = GSE39295.

Statistical analysis and selection of differentially expressed genes

Statistically significant gene expressions were identified using Significance Analysis of Microarrays (SAM 3.05) for each successive time point [115]. Stringent values of fold-change and other thresholds are taken into account while identifying differentially expressing genes. The threshold values we selected are stringent, where the fold change is always greater than or equal to 2 and the q-value is always less than 0.8. The predicted false discovery rate (FDR) never exceeded 0.05%. FDR indicates the expected proportion of false positives among the declared significant results. A final set of differentially expressed genes was then obtained after removing all the repetitions. A PERL script is used to filter out the annotated differentially expressed genes from the un-annotated genes.

Annotation of genes

Annotations of genes were done using the "Unigene & Gene Ontology Annotation Tool" available at GIS site (link: http://123.136.65.67/). We have mapped the Unigene IDs against this database and retrieved the zebrafish UniGene description (UniGene build 119), Entrez Gene ID, Official Gene symbol, GO term and Human homologues information (Unigene ID and Descriptions).

Identification of gene expression pattern

The expression values of the technical replicates of each gene was then averaged and then used for further analyses. Next, we have identified the peaks for each gene (i.e. time point where the expression value of the gene is highest in the array). Genes with similar functions may show similar expression pattern, at least similar time of highest activity. Therefore, we have grouped the genes with similar peak expression time point, performed the cluster analysis using Gene Cluster 3.0 [116], viewed using the software Java TreeView [117], and then carried out the functional enrichment analysis for each cluster using the GO annotation.

Functional event wise clustering of differentially expressed genes by IPA analysis

The differentially expressed genes were subjected to Ingenuity Pathways Analysis (IPA) to identify the enrichment of genes in specific functional groups and pathways (IPA, Version 4, Ingenuity Systems, http://www.ingenuity.com). IPA can accept zebrafish as well as Human UniGene IDs as input for data analysis. We used IPA to find functional and pathway enrichment in the gene sets that are differentially up and down regulated at different time points of regeneration. The clusters resulting after k-means clustering were also analyzed using IPA.

Microarray validation by using quantitative real-Time RT-PCR (qRT-PCR)

The total RNA was extracted from both normal and injured spinal cord by RNaqeous-4PCR kit (Ambion, USA) and cDNA was synthesized using 2 steps RT-PCR (Retroscript, Ambion, USA) with equal amounts of total RNA and by using specific oligo dT primers. Real-Time quantitative RT-PCR using relative quantitation by the comparative C_T method was used to determine mRNA expression. 3 μl of cDNA was subjected to Real-Time quantitative RT-PCR using the Real Time PCR (ABI-7500, USA) with SYBR Green as a fluorescent reporter using the qPCR master-mix plus for SYBR Assay I Low ROX (Eurogentec, USA). The specific gene primers (zebrafish *sox2, stat3, tgfβ1, dbx2, wnt8a, cdk2, ccnb1, ccne, ccnd1, pax6a, shhb, wnt4b, wnt7a* and *β-catenin*) and the internal control gene *β-actin* (beta-actin) were amplified in separate reaction tubes. The details of all known gene primers used are tabulated in Table S19. From the microarray dataset, the genes that do not have UniGene annotation (unannotated genes) were also validated by qRT-PCR. The details of specific gene primers for each gene and the internal control gene *β-actin* (beta-actin) are listed in Table S20. Threshold cycle number (C_T), of triplicate reactions, was determined using the ABI-7500 software and the mean C_T of triplicate reactions was determined. The levels of specific gene expression was normalized to beta-actin levels using the formula $2^{-ΔΔC_T}$, where $ΔΔC_T$ = $ΔC_T$ (sample)−$ΔC_T$ (calibrator) and $ΔCT$ is the C_T of the housekeeping gene (beta-actin) subtracted from the C_T of the target genes. The calibrator used in our experiments is the uninjured spinal cord tissue and the samples are injured spinal cord tissue of same time points as used in microarray. The $ΔC_T$ values are being inversely proportional to the mRNA expression of the samples. No primer -dimers were obtained for either the target genes or beta-actin as assessed by melt curve analysis. The specificity of the products was also confirmed by melt curve analysis. The PCR cycles in all cases were started with Taq activation at 94°C for 5 mins and followed by final extension of 72°C for 7 mins. All experimental data are expressed as Mean±''' SEM. The data obtained were compared using unpaired two-sided Student's *t*-test, Significance was set at $P<0.05$. Data were analyzed using Excel software.

Immunohistochemistry

Spinal cord tissues were dissected out and fixed in 4% paraformaldehyde (Sigma, USA) for 8 hr or overnight at 4°C. Both injured and uninjured spinal cord tissues were embedded either in paraffin or in a mixture of PEG and hexadecanol (9:1, Sigma) or in O.C.T compound (Leica, Germany) and sectioned at 5–7 micron. Immunostaining was performed as described previously [6] by using the following primary antibodies shown to specifically recognize fish, amphibian and human proteins: anti-HuC/D (1:50, Molecular Probes, USA), anti- TGFβ (1:100, Santa

Cruz Biotech, USA), anti- STAT3 (1:100, Santa Cruz, USA), anti-GFAP (1:400, DAKO), anti- SOX2 (1:200, Abcam, USA), anti-BrdU (1:200, Sigma, USA), anti- Phospho-histone H3 (H3P, 1:400, Cell Signaling Technology, USA). Tissue sections were briefly rehydrated in phosphate buffered saline (PBS) and given several washes in PBS with 0.1% Tween-20 or Triton X-100 (PBST). The sections were first incubated with blocking solution for 1 hr (5% goat/rabbit/donkey serum, 1% BSA in PBS) and then with primary antibody for either 1 hr at room temperature or overnight at 4°C. Antigen retrieval was done wherever appropriate by keeping the slides in 85°C water bath for 15 min either in sodium-citrate buffer (pH 6.0) or Tris buffer (pH 8.0) before incubation with the primary antibody. The following secondary antibodies were used: Rhodamine-conjugated goat anti-rabbit antibody (1:100, Santa Cruz, USA), rhodamine-conjugated donkey anti-goat antibody (1:100, Santa Cruz, USA), rhodamine-conjugated goat anti-mouse IgG antibody (1:100, Jackson ImmunoResearch Laboratories, USA), FITC-conjugated goat anti-mouse (1:50, Santa Cruz, USA) and FITC-conjugated goat anti-rabbit IgG antibody (1:100, Jackson ImmunoResearch Laboratories, USA). Nuclei were counter-stained either with bisbenzimide H 33258 fluorochrome (Hoechst nuclear stain) or with DAPI (1:1000, Sigma, USA). We injected 50 μl volume of BrdU (Bromo-deoxy- Uridine, Sigma-Aldrich, USA) at the concentration 2.5 mg/ml to the adult fish intra-peritoneally, 24 hr before the collection of tissues at different injury time points. Spinal cord tissue equivalent of approximately 1 mm length was collected from both injured and uninjured animals. Tissue samples from injured cord was collected in such a way that epicenter of the lesion is going approximately through middle of the cord and included normal part on the both sides of the injury. BrdU immunohistochemistry on uninjured and injured spinal cord was done according to Hui et al. [6]. Paraformaldehyde fixed paraffin sections were washed in PBST twice for 10 min, followed by incubation in 2N HCl (pH 2.0) for 30 min at 37°C. Sections were washed in PBS and blocked with 5% normal goat serum in 0.5% PBST for 1 hr at room temperature. The mouse monoclonal anti-BrdU primary antibody (1:300, Sigma, USA) was applied for 2 hr at room temperature or overnight at 4°C. This was followed by washes in PBS and incubated with secondary anti-mouse FITC/TRITC conjugated antibody for 2 hr at room temperature. After washing in PBS, the sections were mounted with Aqua Vectashield (Vector labs, USA) and kept in the dark. During H3P and BrdU colocalization study, the quantification of cells was done from all optical images by using a Zeiss LSM 510 Meta (inverted) confocal microscope. We have used approx. 4 mm length of tissues both from uninjured (n = 4) and injured cords (n = 4), sectioned the whole cord and all the sections were stained with both H3P along with BrdU and counter-stained with DAPI. All quantification data are expressed as Mean±SEM. using Excel software. The data obtained were compared using unpaired two-sided Student's t-test, Significance was set at P<0.05.

Enzyme linked immunosorbant assay (ELISA)

Analysis of TGFβ, PAX6 and SHH by using ELISA assay was done according to Dutta et al. [118]. Tissue extract of spinal cord were added to wells (65 μg protein/well) of the ELISA plate and incubated overnight at 4°C. After non-specific sites were blocked with blocking buffer (1% BSA in PBS), the wells were incubated with primary antibodies like anti- TGFβ (1:100, Santa Cruz Biotech, USA), anti- PAX6 (1:30, Developmental Studies Hybridoma Bank, USA), anti- SHH (1:50, Developmental Studies Hybridoma Bank, USA) for 1 hr at 37°C, and washed thrice in washing buffer (0.5% BSA, 0.5% NP-40 in PBS). The HRP coupled anti- goat, anti- mouse, anti-rabbit antibodies (1:1000 dilution) were used for incubating the plates at 37°C for 1 hr, then washed several times in washing buffer and substrate tetramethyl benzedine (TMB) was added in dark. The reaction was stopped by adding 1M H_2SO_4. The optical density was measured at 450 nm by using an ELISA reader (Bio Rad, USA). Data are expressed as Mean±SEM using Excel software. The data obtained were compared using unpaired two-sided Student's t-test, Significance was set at P<0.05.

In situ hybridization on zebrafish tissue section

To obtain riboprobes for in situ hybridization pCRIITOPO vector (Invitrogen) containing wnt8a and dbx2 cDNA clones were obtained from Genome Institute of Singapore, zebrafish genome resources. Both sense and antisense RNAprobes were generated using a digoxigenin (DIG) RNA labeling kit (Roche Diagnostics, Laval, Que'bec, Canada) following the manufacturer's instructions. The probes were used to detect dbx2 and wnt8a mRNA in zebrafish tissue section. For tissue sections, both uninjured and injured cord were excised and quickly fixed in precooled 4% paraformaldehyde prepared with DEPC-PBS in RNAse free condition, cryo protected with 20% sucrose in PBS and frozen with OCT compound and subsequently stored at −80°C. Cryostat sections (10 μm) were cut and fixed to poly-L-lysine-coated slides and allowed to dry. In situ hybridizations were performed following the protocol of Braissant and Wahli [119], with the addition of a 5 minutes digestion with proteinase- K (5 μg/ml) diluted in 50 mM Tris HCl (pH 8, 5 mM EDTA) step before prehybridization. Briefly, after fixation in 4% paraformaldehyde, tissue sections were washed and prehybridized for 2 h at 58°C in 5 × saline sodium citrate (SSC)/formamide (1:1) containing 40 μg/ml salmon sperm DNA, 50 μg/ml yeast tRNA, 4 mM EDTA, 2.5% dextran sulfate). The sections were then incubated overnight at 58°C in SSC/formamide containing 1 μg/ml DIG-labeled dbx2 sense or antisense RNA probe and at 60°C in SSC/formamide containing 1 μg/ml DIG-labeled wnt8a sense or antisense RNA probe. After hybridization, sections were washed in 2× SSC at room temperature (RT) and then 2× and 0.1× SSC at 65°C. After Blocking with in situ blocking reagent (Roche Diagnostics, Laval, Que'bec, Canada) at 37°C for 2 hrs, sections were washed again in 0.1× SSC and incubated with an anti-DIG antibody (Roche; 1:5000 dilution) for overnight in 4°C. Color was developed using 5-bromo-4-chloro-3-indoyl-phosphate/4-nitro blue tetrazolium chloride (NBT-BCIP, SIGMA) for 2 to 12 hrs at room temperature (RT). Photographs were taken under light microscope using an Olympus microscope (model; BX 51) and a Leica Microsystem microscope with build camera (DFC 290).

Supporting Information

Figure S1 Pie charts showing the percentage of functionally enriched genes that are differentially expressed in the seven clusters.

Figure S2 Pie charts show the percentage of functionally enriched genes that are differentially expressed at different time points after SCI in zebrafish.

Figure S3 Pie charts showing the percentage of canonical pathway enriched genes that are differentially expressed at different time points after SCI in zebrafish.

Figure S4   Quantification of cells present in different cell cycle phases in uninjured and injured cord based on BrdU, H3P and DAPI colocalization study. A) In uninjured cord only 2% and 1% of cells are in S-phase and M-phase respectively. B) In 3 dpi cord the percentage of S-phase cells have been increased significantly to 8% than uninjured cord and only 2% cells are in M-phase. C) In 7 dpi cord 12% of total populations are in S-phase and 5% of total populations are in M-phase.

Figure S5   Dendrogram represents differential expression pattern of transcription factors involved in neurogenesis and neuronal specification during regeneration of zebrafish spinal cord. Each horizontal line indicates the expression pattern of each gene and the vertical columns indicate the uninjured control and time points after SCI. The color chart indicates mean fold change of gene expression in each time points. Red and green color represents increased and decreased expression respectively.

Figure S6   Differentially expressed genes related to pattern formation are represented in two dendograms in regenerating zebrafish spinal cord. Each horizontal line indicates the expression pattern of each gene and the vertical columns indicate the uninjured control and time points after SCI. The color chart indicates mean fold change of gene expression in each time points. Red and green colors represent increased and decreased expression respectively.

Figure S7   Differentially expressed genes related to axonogenesis and axonal guidance is represented in two different dendrograms (A and A1) in regenerating zebrafish spinal cord. Dendrogram (B) represents differential expression pattern of transcription factors involved in axonogenesis and axonal guidance. Each horizontal line indicates the expression pattern of each gene and the vertical columns indicate the uninjured control and time points after SCI. The color chart indicates mean fold change of gene expression in each time points. Red and green colors represent increased and decreased expression respectively.

Figure S8   Differentially expressed genes involved in different signaling pathways in zebrafish spinal cord after injury. A–E) Dendrograms representing genes related to BMP/TGFβ signaling, JAK/STAT signaling, Shh signaling, Notch signaling and FGF signaling respectively. Each horizontal line indicates the expression pattern of each gene and the vertical columns indicate the uninjured control and time points after SCI. The color chart indicates mean fold change of gene expression in each time points. Red and green colors represent increased and decreased expression respectively.

Figure S9   Differential expression pattern of genes involved in Ion channel transport, One carbon folate metabolism and N-glycan biosynthesis pathway during regeneration of zebrafish spinal cord.

Figure S10   A) Adult zebrafish showing the dorsal fin level where a wound has been made. B) Inside wound showing uninjured spinal cord, spinal cord after giving control crush injury. C) Skeletal preparation of adult zebrafish stained with Alcian Blue and Alizarine Red, where vertebrae at dorsal fin level are clearly visible. D) Skeletal preparation of adult zebrafish after crush injury in spinal cord at dorsal fin level showing the injured vertebra.

Table S1   List of genes differentially expressed during zebrafish spinal cord regeneration.

Table S2   Table representing number of genes, p-value at different time point related to different enriches functional group in figure 2A.

Table S3   Table represents number of genes, p-value at different time point related to different enriched signaling pathways in figure 2B.

Table S4   List of differentially expressed genes related to inflammation regulation, MHC molecules and complement factors after SCI in zebrafish.

Table S5   Table represents quantification of STAT-3 positive cells along with different markers.

Table S6   List of differentially expressed genes related to M1 and M2 type macrophages after SCI in zebrafish.

Table S7   List of differentially expressed genes related to cell death and anti-apoptosis after SCI in zebrafish.

Table S8   List of differentially expressed genes related to cell migration after SCI in zebrafish.

Table S9   List of differentially expressed genes related to cellular dedifferentiation process after SCI in zebrafish.

Table S10   List of differentially expressed genes related to cell cycle and cell proliferation regulation after SCI in zebrafish.

Table S11   List of differentially expressed genes related to neurogenesis and neuronal differentiation after SCI in zebrafish.

Table S12   Table represents quantification of SOX2 positive cells along with different markers.

Table S13   List of differentially expressed genes related to anterior-posterior and dorso-ventral pattern formation after SCI in zebrafish.

Table S14   List of differentially expressed genes related to axonogenesis and axonal guidance after SCI in zebrafish.

Table S15   List of differentially expressed genes related to different signaling pathways after SCI in zebrafish.

Table S16 List of differentially expressed genes commonly expressed in fin, retina, heart and spinal cord regeneration in zebrafish.

Table S17 List of differentially expressed genes related to N-glycan biosynthesis, one carbon folate metabolism and ion channel transport after SCI in zebrafish.

Table S18 List of differentially expressed unannotated genes after SCI in zebrafish.

Table S19 List of primers, Tm, primer annealing time and product length of annotated genes used for qRT-PCR.

Table S20 List of primers, Tm, primer annealing time and product length of unannotated genes used for qRT-PCR.

Author Contributions

Conceived and designed the experiments: SG SM. Performed the experiments: SPH TS SGPL. Analyzed the data: DS SK. Contributed reagents/materials/analysis tools: SG SM. Wrote the paper: SG .

References

1. Akimenko MA, Mari-Beffa M, Becerra J, Geraudie J (2003) Old questions, new tools, and some answers to the mystery of fin regeneration. Dev Dyn 226: 190–201.
2. Padhi BK, Joly L, Tellis P, Smith A, Nanjappa P, et al. (2004) Screen for genes differentially expressed during regeneration of the zebrafish caudal fin. Dev Dyn 231: 527–541.
3. Poss KD, Wilson LG, Keating MT (2002) Heart regeneration in zebrafish. Science 298: 2188–2190.
4. Becker T, Wullimann MF, Becker CG, Bernhardt RR, Schachner M (1997) Axonal regrowth after spinal cord transection in adult zebrafish. J Comp Neurol 377: 577–595.
5. Cameron DA, Gentile KL, Middleton FA, Yurco P (2005) Gene expression profiles of intact and regenerating zebrafish retina. Mol Vis 11: 775–791.
6. Hui SP, Dutta A, Ghosh S (2010) Cellular response after crush injury in adult zebrafish spinal cord. Dev Dyn 239: 2962–2979.
7. Kizil C, Kaslin J, Kroehne V, Brand M (2012) Adult neurogenesis and brain regeneration in zebrafish. Dev Neurobiol 72: 429–461.
8. Marz M, Schmidt R, Rastegar S, Strahle U (2011) Regenerative response following stab injury in the adult zebrafish telencephalon. Dev Dyn 240: 2221–2231.
9. Baumgart EV, Barbosa JS, Bally-Cuif L, Gotz M, Ninkovic J (2012) Stab wound injury of the zebrafish telencephalon: a model for comparative analysis of reactive gliosis. Glia 60: 343–357.
10. Bernhardt RR (1999) Cellular and molecular bases of axonal regeneration in the fish central nervous system. Exp Neurol 157: 223–240.
11. Goldman D, Hankin M, Li Z, Dai X, Ding J (2001) Transgenic zebrafish for studying nervous system development and regeneration. Transgenic Res 10: 21–33.
12. Reimer MM, Sorensen I, Kuscha V, Frank RE, Liu C, et al. (2008) Motor neuron regeneration in adult zebrafish. J Neurosci 28: 8510–8516.
13. Nishidate M, Nakatani Y, Kudo A, Kawakami A (2007) Identification of novel markers expressed during fin regeneration by microarray analysis in medaka fish. Dev Dyn 236: 2685–2693.
14. Schebesta M, Lien CL, Engel FB, Keating MT (2006) Transcriptional profiling of caudal fin regeneration in zebrafish. ScientificWorldJournal 6 Suppl 1: 38–54.
15. Lien CL, Schebesta M, Makino S, Weber GJ, Keating MT (2006) Gene expression analysis of zebrafish heart regeneration. PLoS Biol 4: e260.
16. Mathavan S, Lee SG, Mak A, Miller LD, Murthy KR, et al. (2005) Transcriptome analysis of zebrafish embryogenesis using microarrays. PLoS Genet 1: 260–276.
17. Ghirnikar RS, Lee YL, Eng LF (1998) Inflammation in traumatic brain injury: role of cytokines and chemokines. Neurochem Res 23: 329–340.
18. Coussens LM, Werb Z (2002) Inflammation and cancer. Nature 420: 860–867.
19. Profyris C, Cheema SS, Zang D, Azari MF, Boyle K, et al. (2004) Degenerative and regenerative mechanisms governing spinal cord injury. Neurobiol Dis 15: 415–436.
20. Hedtjarn M, Mallard C, Hagberg H (2004) Inflammatory gene profiling in the developing mouse brain after hypoxia-ischemia. J Cereb Blood Flow Metab 24: 1333–1351.
21. Brewer KL, Bethea JR, Yezierski RP (1999) Neuroprotective effects of interleukin-10 following excitotoxic spinal cord injury. Exp Neurol 159: 484–493.
22. Moore KW, de Waal Malefyt R, Coffman RL, O'Garra A (2001) Interleukin-10 and the interleukin-10 receptor. Annu Rev Immunol 19: 683–765.
23. Li MO, Wan YY, Sanjabi S, Robertson AK, Flavell RA (2006) Transforming growth factor-beta regulation of immune responses. Annu Rev Immunol 24: 99–146.
24. Mattson MP, Barger SW, Furukawa K, Bruce AJ, Wyss-Coray T, et al. (1997) Cellular signaling roles of TGF beta, TNF alpha and beta APP in brain injury responses and Alzheimer's disease. Brain Res Brain Res Rev 23: 47–61.
25. Yoshimura A, Wakabayashi Y, Mori T (2010) Cellular and molecular basis for the regulation of inflammation by TGF-beta. J Biochem 147: 781–792.
26. Willis BC, Borok Z (2007) TGF-beta-induced EMT: mechanisms and implications for fibrotic lung disease. Am J Physiol Lung Cell Mol Physiol 293: L525–534.
27. Kigerl KA, Gensel JC, Ankeny DP, Alexander JK, Donnelly DJ, et al. (2009) Identification of two distinct macrophage subsets with divergent effects causing either neurotoxicity or regeneration in the injured mouse spinal cord. J Neurosci 29: 13435–13444.
28. Ho DM, Whitman M (2008) TGF-beta signaling is required for multiple processes during Xenopus tail regeneration. Dev Biol 315: 203–216.
29. Popovich PG, Wei P, Stokes BT (1997) Cellular inflammatory response after spinal cord injury in Sprague-Dawley and Lewis rats. J Comp Neurol 377: 443–464.
30. Fraser DA, Pisalyaput K, Tenner AJ (2010) C1q enhances microglial clearance of apoptotic neurons and neuronal blebs, and modulates subsequent inflammatory cytokine production. J Neurochem 112:733–743.
31. Ding AH, Nathan CF, Stuehr DJ (1988) Release of reactive nitrogen intermediates and reactive oxygen intermediates from mouse peritoneal macrophages. Comparison of activating cytokines and evidence for independent production. J Immunol 141: 2407–2412.
32. Deonarine K, Panelli MC, Stashower ME, Jin P, Smith K, et al. (2007) Gene expression profiling of cutaneous wound healing. J Transl Med 5: 11.
33. Sica A, Schioppa T, Mantovani A, Allavena P (2006) Tumour-associated macrophages are a distinct M2 polarised population promoting tumour progression: potential targets of anti-cancer therapy. Eur J Cancer 42 : 717–727.
34. Colton CA (2009) Heterogeneity of microglial activation in the innate immune response in the brain. J Neuroimmune Pharmacol 4: 399–418.
35. Mills CD, Kincaid K, Alt JM, Heilman MJ, Hill AM (2000) M-1/M-2 macrophages and the Th1/Th2 paradigm. J Immunol 164: 6166–6173.
36. Mori M, Gotoh T (2000) Regulation of nitric oxide production by arginine metabolic enzymes. Biochem Biophys Res Commun 275: 715–719.
37. Mantovani A, Sica A, Sozzani S, Allavena P, Vecchi A, et al. (2004) The chemokine system in diverse forms of macrophage activation and polarization. Trends Immunol 25: 677–686.
38. Luk HW, Noble LJ, Werb Z (2003) Macrophages contribute to the maintenance of stable regenerating neurites following peripheral nerve injury. J Neurosci Res 73: 644–658.
39. Stoll G, Griffin JW, Li CY, Trapp BD (1989) Wallerian degeneration in the peripheral nervous system: participation of both Schwann cells and macrophages in myelin degradation. J Neurocytol 18: 671–683.
40. Lu X, Richardson PM (1993) Responses of macrophages in rat dorsal root ganglia following peripheral nerve injury. J Neurocytol 22: 334–341.
41. Hu P, McLachlan EM (2003) Distinct functional types of macrophage in dorsal root ganglia and spinal nerves proximal to sciatic and spinal nerve transections in the rat. Exp Neurol 184: 590–605.
42. Ling C, Zou T, Hsiao Y, Tao X, Chen ZL, et al. (2006) Disruption of tissue plasminogen activator gene reduces macrophage migration. Biochem Biophys Res Commun 349: 906–912.
43. Zou T, Ling C, Xiao Y, Tao X, Ma D, et al. (2006) Exogenous tissue plasminogen activator enhances peripheral nerve regeneration and functional recovery after injury in mice. J Neuropathol Exp Neurol 65: 78–86.
44. McEwen ML, Springer JE (2005) A mapping study of caspase-3 activation following acute spinal cord contusion in rats. J Histochem Cytochem 53: 809–819.
45. Yakovlev AG, Knoblach SM, Fan L, Fox GB, Goodnight R, et al. (1997) Activation of CPP32-like caspases contributes to neuronal apoptosis and neurological dysfunction after traumatic brain injury. J Neurosci 17: 7415–7424.
46. Springer JE, Azbill RD, Knapp PE (1999) Activation of the caspase-3 apoptotic cascade in traumatic spinal cord injury. Nat Med 5: 943–946.
47. Kedinger V, Alpy F, Tomasetto C, Thisse C, Thisse B, et al. (2005) Spatial and temporal distribution of the traf4 genes during zebrafish development. Gene Expr Patterns 5: 545–552.

48. Motoyama N, Wang F, Roth KA, Sawa H, Nakayama K, et al. (1995) Massive cell death of immature hematopoietic cells and neurons in Bcl-x-deficient mice. Science 267: 1506–1510.

49. Liao Q, Ozawa F, Friess H, Zimmermann A, Takayama S, et al. (2001) The anti-apoptotic protein BAG-3 is overexpressed in pancreatic cancer and induced by heat stress in pancreatic cancer cell lines. FEBS Lett 503: 151–157.

50. Song HD, Sun XJ, Deng M, Zhang GW, Zhou Y, et al. (2004) Hematopoietic gene expression profile in zebrafish kidney marrow. Proc Natl Acad Sci U S A 101: 16240–16245.

51. Ryu S, Holzschuh J, Erhardt S, Ettl AK, Driever W (2005) Depletion of minichromosome maintenance protein 5 in the zebrafish retina causes cell-cycle defect and apoptosis. Proc Natl Acad Sci U S A 102: 18467–18472.

52. Schlueter PJ, Peng G, Westerfield M, Duan C (2007) Insulin-like growth factor signaling regulates zebrafish embryonic growth and development by promoting cell survival and cell cycle progression. Cell Death Differ 14: 1095–1105.

53. Sheppard AM, Brunstrom JE, Thornton TN, Gerfen RW, Broekelmann TJ, et al. (1995) Neuronal production of fibronectin in the cerebral cortex during migration and layer formation is unique to specific cortical domains. Dev Biol 172: 504–518.

54. Chernoff EA, Stocum DL, Nye HL, Cameron JA (2003) Urodele spinal cord regeneration and related processes. Dev Dyn 226: 295–307.

55. Bai S, Thummel R, Godwin AR, Nagase H, Itoh Y, et al. (2005) Matrix metalloproteinase expression and function during fin regeneration in zebrafish: analysis of MT1-MMP, MMP2 and TIMP2. Matrix Biol 24: 247–260.

56. Monaghan JR, Walker JA, Page RB, Putta S, Beachy CK, et al. (2007) Early gene expression during natural spinal cord regeneration in the salamander *Ambystoma mexicanum*. J Neurochem 101: 27–40.

57. Smith A, Zhang J, Guay D, Quint E, Johnson A, et al. (2008) Gene expression analysis on sections of zebrafish regenerating fins reveals limitations in the whole-mount in situ hybridization method. Dev Dyn 237: 417–425.

58. Brockes JP (1997) Amphibian limb regeneration: rebuilding a complex structure. Science 276: 81–87.

59. Poss KD, Keating MT, Nechiporuk A (2003) Tales of regeneration in zebrafish. Dev Dyn 226: 202–210.

60. Nona SN, Thomlinson AM, Bartlett CA, Scholes J (2000) Schwann cells in the regenerating fish optic nerve: evidence that CNS axons, not the glia, determine when myelin formation begins. J Neurocytol 29: 285–300.

61. Tysseling VM, Mithal D, Sahni V, Birch D, Jung H, et al. (2011) SDF1 in the dorsal corticospinal tract promotes CXCR4+ cell migration after spinal cord injury. J Neuroinflammation 8: 16.

62. Daksis JI, Lu RY, Facchini LM, Marhin WW, Penn LJ (1994) Myc induces cyclin D1 expression in the absence of de novo protein synthesis and links mitogen-stimulated signal transduction to the cell cycle. Oncogene 9: 3635–3645.

63. Yudkovsky Y, Shteinberg M, Listovsky T, Brandeis M, Hershko A (2000) Phosphorylation of Cdc20/fizzy negatively regulates the mammalian cyclosome/APC in the mitotic checkpoint. Biochem Biophys Res Commun 271: 299–304.

64. Harris TE, Albrecht JH, Nakanishi M, Darlington GJ (2001) CCAAT/enhancer-binding protein-alpha cooperates with p21 to inhibit cyclin-dependent kinase-2 activity and induces growth arrest independent of DNA binding. J Biol Chem 276: 29200–29209.

65. Alldridge LC, Bryant CE (2003) Annexin 1 regulates cell proliferation by disruption of cell morphology and inhibition of cyclin D1 expression through sustained activation of the ERK1/2 MAPK signal. Exp Cell Res 290: 93–107.

66. Saul KE, Koke JR, Garcia DM (2010) Activating transcription factor 3 (ATF3) expression in the neural retina and optic nerve of zebrafish during optic nerve regeneration. Comp Biochem Physiol A Mol Integr Physiol 155: 172–182.

67. Tsujino H, Kondo E, Fukuoka T, Dai Y, Tokunaga A, et al. (2000) Activating transcription factor 3 (ATF3) induction by axotomy in sensory and motorneurons: A novel neuronal marker of nerve injury. Mol Cell Neurosci 15: 170–182.

68. Raymond PA, Barthel LK, Bernardos RL, Perkowski JJ (2006) Molecular characterization of retinal stem cells and their niches in adult zebrafish. BMC Dev Biol 6: 36.

69. Cheung KK, Mok SC, Rezaie P, Chan WY (2008) Dynamic expression of Dab2 in the mouse embryonic central nervous system. BMC Dev Biol 8: 76.

70. Avilion AA, Nicolis SK, Pevny LH, Perez L, Vivian N, et al. (2003) Multipotent cell lineages in early mouse development depend on SOX2 function. Genes Dev 17: 126–140.

71. Graham V, Khudyakov J, Ellis P, Pevny L (2003) SOX2 functions to maintain neural progenitor identity. Neuron 39: 749–765.

72. Ferri AL, Cavallaro M, Braida D, Di Cristofano A, Canta A, et al. (2004) Sox2 deficiency causes neurodegeneration and impaired neurogenesis in the adult mouse brain. Development 131: 3805–3819.

73. Adolf B, Chapouton P, Lam CS, Topp S, Tannhauser B, et al. (2006) Conserved and acquired features of adult neurogenesis in the zebrafish telencephalon. Dev Biol 295: 278–293.

74. Muneoka K, Bryant SV (1982) Evidence that patterning mechanisms in developing and regenerating limbs are the same. Nature 298: 369–371.

75. Stocum DL (1996) A conceptual framework for analyzing axial patterning in regenerating urodele limbs. Int J Dev Biol 40: 773–783.

76. Schnapp E, Kragl M, Rubin L, Tanaka EM (2005) Hedgehog signaling controls dorsoventral patterning, blastema cell proliferation and cartilage induction during axolotl tail regeneration. Development 132: 3243–3253.

77. Tanaka EM, Ferretti P (2009) Considering the evolution of regeneration in the central nervous system. Nat Rev Neurosci 10: 713–723.

78. Jessell TM (2000) Neuronal specification in the spinal cord: inductive signals and transcriptional codes. Nat Rev Genet 1: 20–29.

79. Briscoe J, Pierani A, Jessell TM, Ericson J (2000) A homeodomain protein code specifies progenitor cell identity and neuronal fate in the ventral neural tube. Cell 101: 435–445.

80. Poh A, Karunaratne A, Kolle G, Huang N, Smith E, et al. (2002) Patterning of the vertebrate ventral spinal cord. Int J Dev Biol 46: 597–608.

81. Wilson L, Maden M (2005) The mechanisms of dorsoventral patterning in the vertebrate neural tube. Dev Biol 282: 1–13.

82. Guner B, Karlstrom RO (2007) Cloning of zebrafish nkx6.2 and a comprehensive analysis of the conserved transcriptional response to Hedgehog/Gli signaling in the zebrafish neural tube. Gene Expr Patterns 7: 596–605.

83. Lufkin T (1996) Transcriptional control of Hox genes in the vertebrate nervous system. Curr Opin Genet Dev 6: 575–580.

84. Prince VE, Joly L, Ekker M, Ho RK (1998) Zebrafish hox genes: genomic organization and modified colinear expression patterns in the trunk. Development 125: 407–420.

85. Koshida S, Shinya M, Mizuno T, Kuroiwa A, Takeda H (1998) Initial anteroposterior pattern of the zebrafish central nervous system is determined by differential competence of the epiblast. Development 125: 1957–1966.

86. van den Akker E, Forlani S, Chawengsaksophak K, de Graaff W, Beck F, et al. (2002) Cdx1 and Cdx2 have overlapping functions in anteroposterior patterning and posterior axis elongation. Development 129: 2181–2193.

87. Liu JP (2006) The function of growth/differentiation factor 11 (Gdf11) in rostrocaudal patterning of the developing spinal cord. Development 133: 2865–2874.

88. Carpenter EM (2002) Hox genes and spinal cord development. Dev Neurosci 24: 24–34.

89. Dasen JS, Liu JP, Jessell TM (2003) Motor neuron columnar fate imposed by sequential phases of Hox-c activity. Nature 425: 926–933.

90. Tessier-Lavigne M, Goodman CS (1996) The molecular biology of axon guidance. Science 274: 1123–1133.

91. Xu Q, Alldus G, Macdonald R, Wilkinson DG, Holder N (1996) Function of the Eph-related kinase rtk1 in patterning of the zebrafish forebrain. Nature 381: 319–322.

92. Flanagan JG (2006) Neural map specification by gradients. Curr Opin Neurobiol 16: 59–66.

93. Winberg ML, Mitchell KJ, Goodman CS (1998) Genetic analysis of the mechanisms controlling target selection: complementary and combinatorial functions of netrins, semaphorins, and IgCAMs. Cell 93: 581–591.

94. Roos M, Schachner M, Bernhardt RR (1999) Zebrafish semaphorin Z1b inhibits growing motor axons in vivo. Mech Dev 87: 103–117.

95. Devine CA, Key B (2008) Robo-Slit interactions regulate longitudinal axon pathfinding in the embryonic vertebrate brain. Dev Biol 313: 371–383.

96. Seijffers R, Mills CD, Woolf CJ (2007) ATF3 increases the intrinsic growth state of DRG neurons to enhance peripheral nerve regeneration. J Neurosci 27: 7911–7920.

97. Schweitzer J, Gimnopoulos D, Lieberoth BC, Pogoda HM, Feldner J, et al. (2007) Contactin1a expression is associated with oligodendrocyte differentiation and axonal regeneration in the central nervous system of zebrafish. Mol Cell Neurosci 35: 194–207.

98. Poss KD, Shen J, Keating MT (2000) Induction of lef1 during zebrafish fin regeneration. Dev Dyn 219: 282–286.

99. Kawakami Y, Rodriguez Esteban C, Raya M, Kawakami H, Marti M, et al. (2006) Wnt/beta-catenin signaling regulates vertebrate limb regeneration. Genes Dev 20: 3232–3237.

100. Stoick-Cooper CL, Moon RT, Weidinger G (2007) Advances in signaling in vertebrate regeneration as a prelude to regenerative medicine. Genes Dev 21: 1292–1315.

101. Ghosh S, Roy S, Seguin C, Bryant SV, Gardiner DM (2008) Analysis of the expression and function of Wnt-5a and Wnt-5b in developing and regenerating axolotl (Ambystoma mexicanum) limbs. Dev Growth Differ 50: 289–297.

102. Caubit X, Nicolas S, Le Parco Y (1997) Possible roles for Wnt genes in growth and axial patterning during regeneration of the tail in urodele amphibians. Dev Dyn 210: 1–10.

103. Shou J, Rim PC, Calof AL (1999) BMPs inhibit neurogenesis by a mechanism involving degradation of a transcription factor. Nat Neurosci 2: 339–345.

104. Wu HH, Ivkovic S, Murray RC, Jaramillo S, Lyons KM, et al. (2003) Autoregulation of neurogenesis by GDF11. Neuron 37: 197–207.

105. Jarnicki A, Putoczki T, Ernst M (2010) Stat3: linking inflammation to epithelial cancer - more than a "gut" feeling? Cell Div 5: 14.

106. Stadler JA, Shkumatava A, Norton WH, Rau MJ, Geisler R, et al. (2005) Histone deacetylase 1 is required for cell cycle exit and differentiation in the zebrafish retina. Dev Dyn 233: 883–889.

107. Yamaguchi M, Tonou-Fujimori N, Komori A, Maeda R, Nojima Y, et al. (2005) Histone deacetylase 1 regulates retinal neurogenesis in zebrafish by suppressing Wnt and Notch signaling pathways. Development 132: 3027–3043.

108. Harrison MR, Georgiou AS, Spaink HP, Cunliffe VT (2011) The epigenetic regulator Histone Deacetylase 1 promotes transcription of a core neurogenic programme in zebrafish embryos. BMC Genomics 12: 24.

109. Iskandar BJ, Rizk E, Meier B, Hariharan N, Bottiglieri T, et al. (2010) Folate regulation of axonal regeneration in the rodent central nervous system through DNA methylation. J Clin Invest 120: 1603–1616.

110. Kronenberg G, Endres M (2010) Neuronal injury: folate to the rescue? J Clin Invest 120: 1383–1386.

111. Herrmann JE, Imura T, Song B, Qi J, Ao Y, et al. (2008) STAT3 is a critical regulator of astrogliosis and scar formation after spinal cord injury. J Neurosci 28: 7231–7243.

112. Byrnes KR, Stoica BA, Fricke S, Di Giovanni S, Faden AI (2007) Cell cycle activation contributes to post-mitotic cell death and secondary damage after spinal cord injury. Brain 130: 2977–2992.

113. Horner PJ, Gage FH (2000) Regenerating the damaged central nervous system. Nature 407: 963–970.

114. Thuret S, Moon LD, Gage FH (2006) Therapeutic interventions after spinal cord injury. Nat Rev Neurosci 7: 628–643.

115. Tusher VG, Tibshirani R, Chu G (2001) Significance analysis of microarrays applied to the ionizing radiation response. Proc Natl Acad Sci U S A 98: 5116–5121.

116. Eisen MB, Spellman PT, Brown PO, Botstein D (1998) Cluster analysis and display of genome-wide expression patterns. Proc Natl Acad Sci U S A 95: 14863–14868.

117. Saldanha AJ (2004) Java Treeview–extensible visualization of microarray data. Bioinformatics 20: 3246–3248.

118. Dutta A, Sen T, Banerji A, Das S, Chatterjee A (2009) Studies on Multifunctional Effect of All-Trans Retinoic Acid (ATRA) on Matrix Metalloproteinase-2 (MMP-2) and Its Regulatory Molecules in Human Breast Cancer Cells (MCF-7). J Oncol 2009: 627840.

119. Braissant O, Wahli W (1998) Differential expression of peroxisome proliferator-activated receptor-alpha, -beta, and -gamma during rat embryonic development. Endocrinology 139: 2748–2754.

120. Hausmann ON (2003) Post-traumatic inflammation following spinal cord injury. Spinal Cord 41: 369–378.

121. Byrnes KR, Washington PM, Knoblach SM, Hoffman E, Faden AI (2011) Delayed inflammatory mRNA and protein expression after spinal cord injury. J Neuroinflammation 8: 130.

122. Carmichael ST, Archibeque I, Luke L, Nolan T, Momiy J, et al. (2005) Growth-associated gene expression after stroke: evidence for a growth-promoting region in peri-infarct cortex. Exp Neurol 193: 291–311.

123. Ahn YH, Lee G, Kang SK (2006) Molecular insights of the injured lesions of rat spinal cords: Inflammation, apoptosis, and cell survival. Biochem Biophys Res Commun 348: 560–570.

124. Aimone JB, Leasure JL, Perreau VM, Thallmair M (2004) Spatial and temporal gene expression profiling of the contused rat spinal cord. Exp Neurol 189: 204–221.

125. Mladinic M, Lefevre C, Del Bel E, Nicholls J, Digby M (2010) Developmental changes of gene expression after spinal cord injury in neonatal opossums. Brain Res 1363: 20–39.

126. Wakatsuki S, Saitoh F, Araki T (2011) ZNRF1 promotes Wallerian degeneration by degrading AKT to induce GSK3B-dependent CRMP2 phosphorylation. Nat Cell Biol 13: 1415–1423.

127. Hunt D, Hossain-Ibrahim K, Mason MR, Coffin RS, Lieberman AR, et al. (2004) ATF3 upregulation in glia during Wallerian degeneration: differential expression in peripheral nerves and CNS white matter. BMC Neurosci 5: 9.

7

Modified Cytoplasmic Ca^{2+} Sequestration Contributes to Spinal Cord Injury-Induced Augmentation of Nerve-Evoked Contractions in the Rat Tail Artery

Hussain Al Dera[1,2], Brid P. Callaghan[1], James A. Brock[1]*

1 Department of Anatomy and Neuroscience, University of Melbourne, Victoria, Australia, **2** Basic Medical Sciences, College of Medicine, King Saud bin Abdulaziz University for Health Sciences, Riyadh, Saudi Arabia

Abstract

In rat tail artery (RTA), spinal cord injury (SCI) increases nerve-evoked contractions and the contribution of L-type Ca^{2+} channels to these responses. In RTAs from unoperated rats, these channels play a minor role in contractions and Bay K8644 (L-type channel agonist) mimics the effects of SCI. Here we investigated the mechanisms underlying the facilitatory actions of SCI and Bay K8644 on nerve-evoked contractions of RTAs and the hypothesis that Ca^{2+} entering via L-type Ca^{2+} channels is rapidly sequestered by the sarcoplasmic reticulum (SR) limiting its role in contraction. *In situ* electrochemical detection of noradrenaline was used to assess if Bay K8644 increased noradrenaline release. Perforated patch recordings were used to assess if SCI changed the Ca^{2+} current recorded in RTA myocytes. Wire myography was used to assess if SCI modified the effects of Bay K8644 and of interrupting SR Ca^{2+} uptake on nerve-evoked contractions. Bay K8644 did not change noradrenaline-induced oxidation currents. Neither the size nor gating of Ca^{2+} currents differed between myocytes from sham-operated (control) and SCI rats. Bay K8644 increased nerve-evoked contractions in RTAs from both control and SCI rats, but the magnitude of this effect was reduced by SCI. By contrast, depleting SR Ca^{2+} stores with ryanodine or cyclopiazonic acid selectively increased nerve-evoked contractions in control RTAs. Cyclopiazonic acid also selectively increased the blockade of these responses by nifedipine (L-type channel blocker) in control RTAs, whereas ryanodine increased the blockade produced by nifedipine in both groups of RTAs. These findings suggest that Ca^{2+} entering via L-type channels is normally rapidly sequestered limiting its access to the contractile mechanism. Furthermore, the findings suggest SCI reduces the role of this mechanism.

Editor: Nicole Beard, University of Canberra, Australia

Funding: This work was supported by grants from the National Health and Medical Research Council of Australia (Grant ID GNT1024485) and the Transport Accident Commission (Victoria). H. Al Dera was supported by a postgraduate award from King Saud Bin Abdulaziz University for Health Sciences, College of Medicine (Riyadh, Saudi Arabia). The funders had no role in study design, data collection and analysis, decision to publish, or preparation of the manuscript.

Competing Interests: The authors have declared that no competing interests exist.

* Email: j.brock@unimelb.edu.au

Introduction

In spinal cord injured (SCI) patients with high thoracic or cervical lesions, spinal reflex-evoked vasoconstriction elicited by distension of visceral organs, or by some other unheeded afferent input from caudal to the lesion, is exaggerated leading to large increases in blood pressure (autonomic dysreflexia (AD); [1]). AD is normally attributed to excessive sympathetic nerve activity resulting from plasticity of connections within the damaged spinal cord [2]. However, in SCI subjects with AD, bladder compression or electrical stimulation of abdominal skin elicits only brief bursts of cutaneous vasoconstrictor nerve activity [3]. These bursts produced prolonged reductions in skin blood flow compared to those in able-bodied subjects [3], suggesting that the vasculature becomes hyperresponsive to sympathetic activity. Accordingly, in SCI rats that also display AD, neurovascular transmission is markedly increased in arteries isolated from both cutaneous and splanchnic vascular beds [4,5,6].

We have demonstrated that SCI markedly increases nerve-evoked constriction of rat tail artery and that this change is

associated with an increase in sensitivity of these responses to inhibition by the L-type Ca^{2+} channel blocker nifedipine [6,7]. Furthermore, in tail arteries from uninjured rats, we demonstrated that Ca^{2+} entry via L-type Ca^{2+} channels normally plays a relatively minor role in nerve-evoked contractions and that the enhancement of nerve-evoked contractions produced by the L-type Ca^{2+} channel agonist Bay K8644 mimics that produced by SCI [7]. Together these findings suggest that SCI augments nerve-evoked contractions by increasing the contribution of Ca^{2+} influx via L-type Ca^{2+} channels to contraction, but the mechanisms underlying this enhancement have not been determined.

Investigations of noradrenaline (NA) release from sympathetic nerve terminals in a range of tissues, including the rat tail artery, indicate that it is dependent primarily on Ca^{2+} entering through N-type Ca^{2+} channels and does not normally involve Ca^{2+} influx through L-type Ca^{2+} channels [8]. However, electrophysiological studies have demonstrated that postganglionic sympathetic neurons express functional L-type Ca^{2+} channels [9,10] and stimulation of these channels with Bay K8644 can increase action potential-evoked NA release in rabbit ear artery [11]. Therefore an increase in neurotransmitter release could contribute to the augmentation of nerve-evoked contractions produced by Bay K8644.

The question remains why L-type Ca^{2+} channels, whose activity is increased by Bay K8644, normally play a relatively minor role in nerve-evoked contractions of the tail artery. Previous studies in tail artery have suggested that Ca^{2+} entering through L-type Ca^{2+} channels is rapidly sequestered by the sarcoplasmic reticulum (SR), limiting its access to the contractile machinery [12]. Therefore Bay K8644 by augmenting Ca^{2+} influx may overcome this Ca^{2+} buffering role of the SR, increasing access of Ca^{2+} entering via L-type Ca^{2+} channels to the contractile mechanism.

In the present study we investigated the mechanisms by which SCI and Bay K8644 increase nerve-evoked contractions and the possibility that reducing Ca^{2+} sequestration by the SR increases the contribution of L-type Ca^{2+} channels to these responses. The findings demonstrate that SCI does not change the size or gating of Ca^{2+} channel currents recorded in tail artery myocytes. In addition, the findings demonstrate that depleting the SR Ca^{2+} store with ryanodine or interrupting Ca^{2+} uptake into the SR with the SR Ca^{2+}-ATPase (SERCA) inhibitor cyclopiazoinc acid selectively increases nerve-evoked contractions in tail arteries from sham-operated rats and also increases the sensitivity of these responses to nifedipine.

Methods

All experimental procedures were approved by the University of Melbourne Animal Experimentation Ethics Committee and they conformed to the Australian Code of Practice for the Care and Use of Animals for Scientific Purposes.

Spinal cord transection

The spinal cord was transected in 17 female Sprague Dawley rats (~8 weeks of age; supplied by Biomedical Sciences Animal Facility, University of Melbourne) that were anaesthetized with isoflurane (2–3% in oxygen). A full description of the surgery is described in Al Dera et al [7] and is briefly outlined here. A laminectomy was performed to remove the dorsal aspect of the T10 vertebrum and the spinal cord transected at the T11 spinal level. This lesion severs all bulbospinal connections to the preganglionic neurons that control the tail artery, which are located in the T13-L2 spinal segments [13,14]. The laminectomy site was closed and postoperatively animals received sterile saline (2 mL) and analgesic (0.06 mg kg^{-1} buprenorphine; Reckitt Benckiser, Sydney, Australia) by subcutaneous injection. Additional injections of saline and analgesic were administered daily for the first 3 post-operative days. Bladders were manually expressed 3 times daily until the animals regained the ability to empty their own bladders. In 17 age-matched sham-operated female rats, the laminectomy was performed to expose the spinal cord and post-operative treatments were similar except for bladder management. SCI and sham-operated rats were maintained for six weeks post surgery.

Tissue collection

Rats were deeply anaesthetized with the volatile anesthetic isoflurane and killed by decapitation. The tail artery was dissected from 20–40 mm distal to the base of the tail. After isolation, arteries were maintained in physiological saline with the following composition (in mmol/L): Na^+, 150.6; K^+, 4.7; Ca^{2+}, 2; Mg^{2+}, 1.2; Cl^-, 144.1; $H_2PO_4^-$, 1.3; HCO_3^-, 16.3; glucose, 7.8. This solution was gassed with 95% O_2 - 5% CO_2 and warmed to 36–37°C.

Mechanical responses

Segments of artery (~1.5 mm long) were mounted isometrically between stainless steel wires (50 μm diameter) in two 4-chamber myographs (Multi Myograph 610 M, Danish Myo Technology, Denmark) as previously described [7]. As there was some variation in the lengths of the artery segments studied, contractions were measured as increases in wall tension (force/2×vessel length; [see 15]). After equilibration for 30–45 mins, contractions to phenylephrine (3 μM) were used to test the vascular smooth muscle function of arteries from sham-operated and SCI rats. We have previously demonstrated that SCI does not change the EC_{50} or maximum contraction of tail arteries to phenylephrine [6,7]. In addition, carbachol (1 μM) induced vasorelaxation of phenylephrine constricted vessels was used to assess the vasorelaxatory action of activating the endothelium.

Electrically evoked contractions

The perivascular nerves were electrically stimulated with trains of 100 pulses (20 V, 0.2 ms pulse width) at 1 Hz applied through platinum plate electrodes mounted either side of the tissue. In preliminary experiments, it was confirmed that these stimulus parameters were supramaximal for activating the perivascular sympathetic axons and that contractions produced by electrical stimulation were fully blocked by tetrodotoxin (0.5 μM), confirming they are mediated by action potential-evoked neurotransmitter release. In all experiments assessing the effects of drugs on nerve-evoked contractions, the effects of each added drug was assessed 25 mins after its addition.

Electrochemical recording

The release of endogenous NA was monitored using continuous amperometry in tail arteries from unoperated rats as described previously [8,16]. Briefly, artery segments ~10 mm in length were pinned to the Sylgard (Dow-Corning) covered base of a 2 ml recording chamber that was perfused continuously at 3–5 ml min^{-1} with physiological saline. The proximal end of the artery was drawn into a suction stimulating electrode and the perivascular nerves were electrically activated (20 V, 0.2 ms pulse width). Recordings were made at a site 1–2 mm distal to the mouth of the suction electrode with a carbon fibre electrode (7 μm diameter) that was mounted so that the first 100–200 μm from the tip of the fibre was in contact with the adventitial surface of the artery. The electrode was connected to an AMU130 Nanoamperometer (Radiometer-Analytical SA, Villeurbanne Cedex, France) and a potential difference of +0.3 V was applied between the recording electrode and an Ag/AgCl pellet placed in the recording chamber medium. The current required to maintain this voltage was monitored.

In these experiments, the physiological saline contained the α_1-adrenoceptor antagonist, prazosin (0.1 μM), to inhibit contractions due to released NA and the neuronal NA transporter inhibitor, desmethylimipramine (0.1 μM), to inhibit neuronal reuptake of released NA. During the experiments, the arteries were stimulated at 1 min intervals with 10 pulses at 10 Hz and Bay K8644 (0.1 μM) or cyclopiazonic acid (CPZ; 1 μM) was added to the superfusing solution following the 10th train of stimuli and left in contact with the artery for a further 20 trains. At the end of the experiments, the Ca^{2+} channel blocker, Cd^{2+} (0.1 mM), was added to verify that the signals recorded were due to Ca^{2+}-dependent release of NA [see 8]. As a positive control, S_2/S_1 ratios were also determined in tissues treated with the α_2-adrenoceptor antagonist, idazoxan (0.1 μM), which increases NA release in the rat tail artery by interrupting α_2-adenoceptor-mediated autoinhibition [see 16].

Isolation of rat tail artery myocytes

After dissection, tail arteries were cut open lengthwise and divided into small segments (~2 mm in length) in Hanks buffer (Ca^{2+} free; Sigma-Aldrich, Castle Hill, NSW, Australia). The segments were incubated in dispersion solution (Hanks buffer (Ca^{2+} free) containing 0.7 mg ml^{-1} collagenase Type IA (Sigma-Aldrich), 0.5 mg ml^{-1} protease Type XIV (Sigma-Aldrich) and 2 mg ml^{-1} bovine serum albumin (Sigma-Aldrich)) for 10–14 min at 37°C in a 5% CO_2 incubator. The tissue was then rinsed 4 times using Hanks buffer containing 2 mg ml^{-1} BSA. Smooth muscle cells (SMCs) were dispersed by gentle trituration of the segments with a wide-tipped fire-polished Pasteur pipette. The cell suspension was stored in Hanks buffer containing bovine serum albumin (2 mg ml^{-1}) and Ca^{2+} (0.1 mM) at 4°C and used within 8 h.

Electrophysiology

Ba^{2+} currents (I_{Ba}) in myocytes were measured using the perforated patch configuration. The bath solution used to record I_{Ba} was composed of (in mmol/L) NaCl 130, KCl 5.4, $BaCl_2$ 10, glucose 10, EGTA 0.1 and HEPES 10 (pH adjusted to 7.4 with NaOH). The pipette solution for perforated patch recording contained (in mmol/L) $CsMeSO_4$ 120, tetraethylammonium Cl 20, EGTA 1, and HEPES 20 (pH adjusted to 7.2 with CsOH). Nystatin (10 mg/mL) was dissolved in dimethylsulfoxide (DMSO), sonicated, and diluted to give a final concentration of 150 μg/mL in the pipette solution. Inward currents were measured at room temperature using an Axopatch-1D patch-clamp amplifier, digitized with a 16-bit analog to digital converter (Model DIGIDATA 1322, Axon Instruments), and controlled by pClamp8 (Axon Instruments).

Data analysis

The output from the myograph and amperometer was recorded and analyzed using a PowerLab data acquisition system and the program Chart (ADInstruments, Bella Vista, NSW, Australia). Because the contractions to 100 pulses at 1 Hz have both an initial phasic and a later tonic component, the amplitude of these responses was measured at both the 10th and 100th pulse. As electrical stimulation produced an artefact (revealed in Cd^{2+}) that lasted up to 500 ms following the last stimulus in the train, the amplitude of the NA-induced oxidation currents were measured 1 s following the last stimulus. The mean amplitudes of the three responses immediately before (S_1) and 17–20 mins following the addition of Bay K8644 or CPZ (S_2) were determined. The S_2/S_1 ratios in Bay K8644 or CPZ treated tissues were compared with those determined at the same points in control experiments with no drug added.

To construct I–V relationships, cells were voltage-clamped at −80 mV and then stepped from −80 mV to +60 mV in 10 mV increments evoked 20 seconds apart. Activation relationships for the Ca^{2+} channels were determined by calculating the peak conductance at each test potential by using the equation $I_{Ba} = g_{Ba} \times (V - E_{rev})$, where g_{Ba}, V, and E_{rev} are peak conductance, test potential, and reversal potential, respectively. A double-pulse protocol was used to measure inactivation of Ca^{2+} channel current as a function of membrane potential. Conditioning steps from −80 to 30 mV (in 10 mV intervals) were applied for 3.5 s. After a 25 ms step to −80 mV, the membrane potential was stepped to 0 mV for 250 ms. Resulting currents were normalized to the maximum current obtained after a conditioning potential of −80 mV (I/I_{max}) and plotted as a function of the conditioning potential. The data were fitted by the Boltzmann equation using GraphPad Prism (GraphPad Software, Inc. CA, USA).

All statistical comparisons were made using SPSS 22 (IBM corporation, NY, USA. For experiments investigating the effects of drugs in control or SCI arteries comparisons were made with Student's paired t-tests. When multiple effects were assessed in a single experiment, the data was first subjected to repeated measures ANOVA and the P values for pairwise comparisons were adjusted using the false discovery rate procedure [17]. Comparison between the measures in control and SCI arteries were made with either Student's unpaired tests or Mann Whitney U-tests if the variation differed significantly between groups of data (assessed by Levine's test). Data are presented as mean and standard error (SE) or as median and interquartile range (IQR) when the Mann Whitney U-test was used. P values <0.05 were considered to indicate significant differences. Unless otherwise indicated in the text, P values were obtained using unpaired t-tests. In all cases, n indicates the number of animals studied.

Drugs

Bay K8644, nifedipine, phenylephrine HCl, prazosin, desmethylimipramine, carbachol, cyclopiazonic acid and nystatin were supplied by Sigma Aldrich (Castle Hill, NSW, Australia). Ryanodine was supplied by Tocris Bioscience (Bristol, UK). Drugs were prepared as stock solutions in water (phenylephrine, desmethylimipramine, carbachol), ethanol (nifedipine, Bay K8644) or DMSO (ryanodine, cyclopiazonic acid, prazosin). In all experiments, the highest concentration of ethanol or DMSO applied was 0.1% (w v^{-1}).

Results

Basal conditions for the experiments investigating nerve-evoked contractions

Mechanical responses were recorded in artery segments from twelve sham-operated rats (control arteries) and twelve SCI rats (SCI arteries). The estimated lumen diameter of the artery segments after the normalization procedure (calculated from the measured lumen circumference) was significantly smaller for the SCI arteries (control: 831±29 μm; SCI: 737±20 μm; $P<0.01$). As a consequence the basal wall tension was larger for control arteries (4.3±0.2 mN mm^{-1}) than it was for SCI arteries (3.7±0.2 mN mm^{-1}; $P<0.01$). These effects of SCI are similar to those previously reported [6,7]. The increase in wall tension produced by 3 μM phenylephrine did not differ between control and SCI arteries (control: 8.4±0.6 mN mm^{-1}; SCI: 7.7±0.7 mN mm^{-1}; $P=0.29$). Furthermore, when contracted with phenylephrine (3 μM), the % relaxation produced when the endothelium was stimulated with carbachol (1 μM) did not differ between control (47±7%) and SCI arteries (58±5%; $P=0.1$).

Bay K8644 produces a smaller facilitation of nerve-evoked contractions in SCI arteries

Using tail arteries from unoperated rat we have previously reported that the L-type Ca^{2+} channel agonist Bay K8644 mimics the effects of SCI on nerve-evoked contractions. Here we investigated the facilitatory effects of Bay K8644 (0.1 μM) on contractions evoked by 100 pulses at 1 Hz in control ($n=6$) and SCI ($n=6$) arteries. As previously reported [6,7], contractions of SCI arteries evoked by 100 pulses at 1 Hz were markedly larger than those of control arteries (**Fig. 1A, B;** $P<0.01$). In both groups of vessels, Bay K8644 increased the amplitude of contractions to this stimulus (**Fig. 1A, B**). However, the percentage increase in contraction amplitude measured at the 100th pulse was much larger in control arteries (median 403%, IQR 194–609%) than SCI arteries (median 124%, IQR 117–138%, Mann

Whitney U-test $P<0.05$). We have previously reported that the facilitatory effect of Bay K8644 on nerve-evoked contractions is completely blocked by nifedipine [7], confirming that it is mediated by an increase L-type Ca^{2+} channel activity. The finding that the facilitatory effect of Bay K8644 was much greater in control than SCI arteries may indicate that Ca^{2+} channel activity is elevated prior to adding this agent in SCI arteries.

Bay K8466 does not increase NA release

In situ amperometry was used to assess the possibility that Bay K8644 (0.1 µM) augments nerve-evoked contraction by increasing NA release from the sympathetic nerve terminals. These experiments used tail artery segments from unoperated rats that were stimulated with trains of 10 pulses at 10 Hz. The stimulation artifacts during the periods of stimulation prevented NA-induced oxidation currents evoked by individual stimuli being discerned, but summation of these signals produced a slowly decaying oxidation current following the last stimulus in the train (**Fig. 2A**). In comparison with time-matched controls ($n = 6$), Bay K8644 ($n = 6$) did not change NA release (assessed by S_2/S_1 ratios, see methods) whereas blockade of prejunctional α_2-adrenoceptors with idazoxan (0.1 µM, $n = 6$) significantly increased the NA release (**Fig. 2B**). The stimulus-evoked oxidation currents were abolished by the Ca^{2+} channel blocker Cd^{2+} (0.1 mM, **Fig. 2A**). These finding demonstrate that Bay K8644 does not increase NA release.

The depolarization-evoked inward Ba^{2+} current did not differ between SMCs from SCI and control rats

Perforated patch recordings were used to determine if the depolarization-evoked Ba^{2+} currents carried by Ca^{2+} channels differed between SMCs isolated from control and SCI arteries.

When tail artery SMCs are depolarized from -80 mV, it has been reported that ~60% of the Ca^{2+} channel current carried by Ba^{2+} is sensitive to nifedipine (i.e. is due to activation of L-type Ca^{2+} channels; [18]). Inward currents had similar amplitudes in SMCs isolated from both groups of arteries (**Fig. 3A–C**) and the peak Ba^{2+} currents elicited at +10 mV did not differ significantly (control: -3.07 ± 0.2 pA/pF, 8 cells, $n = 5$; SCI: -3.44 ± 0.5 pA/pF, 9 cells, $n = 5$; $P = 0.62$). Membrane capacitance also was similar (control: 38.94 ± 2.3 pF; SCI: 36.6 ± 1.72 pF; $P = 0.60$). Voltage pulse protocols were used to obtain the activation and inactivation curves for control and SCI SMCs (**Fig. 3D**). These analyses provided similar values for the half-maximal ($V_{1/2}$) current activation (control: -1.7 ± 1.6 mV; SCI: -0.8 ± 2.3 mV; $P = 0.70$) and inactivation (control: -22.6 ± 1.5 mV; SCI: -29.27 ± 2.4 mV; $P = 0.73$) in control and SCI SMCs. In addition, in both groups of SMCs, application of Bay K8644 (1 µM) approximately doubled the amplitude of Ba^{2+} currents measured at 10 mV (**Fig. 3E, F**), consistent with their primarily being mediated by L-type Ca^{2+} channels. These findings indicate that SCI does not detectably change Ca^{2+} channel density in SMCs or modify the gating of these channels.

Interrupting Ca^{2+} sequestration by the sarcoplasmic reticulum selectively increased the size of nerve-evoked contractions in control arteries

The possibility that a reduction in Ca^{2+} sequestration by the SR contributes to the augmentation nerve-evoked contractions in SCI arteries was investigated by assessing the effects of depleting the ryanodine-sensitive Ca^{2+} store (with 10 µM ryanodine) and by inhibiting Ca^{2+} uptake into the SR with the SERCA inhibitor CPZ (1 µM). In these experiments, the tissues were stimulated

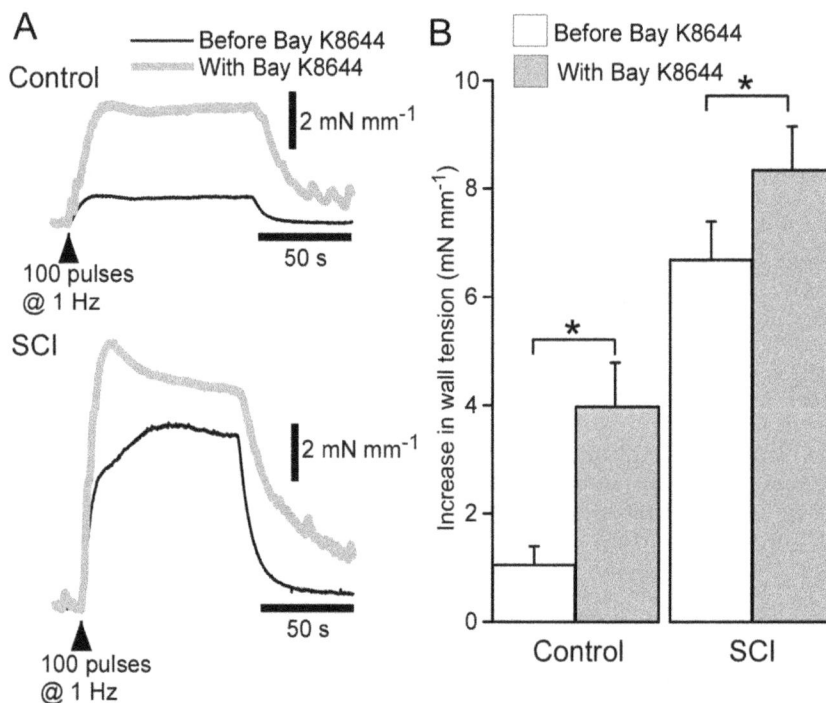

Figure 1. The facilitation of nerve-evoked contraction produced by Bay K8644 (0.1 µM) was greater in arteries from sham-operated rats (control arteries) than in arteries from spinal cord injured rats (SCI arteries). (A) Averaged traces showing contractions to 100 pulses at 1 Hz in control (*upper traces*) and SCI arteries (*lower traces*) before (*black line*) and during (*grey line*) application of Bay K8644 (0.1 µM). (B) Increases in wall tension measured at the 100th pulse during the trains stimuli in control ($n = 6$) and SCI ($n = 6$) arteries before (*white bars*) and during (*grey bars*) application of Bay K8644. Data are presented as means and SEs and statistical comparisons were made with paired *t*-tests. *$P<0.05$.

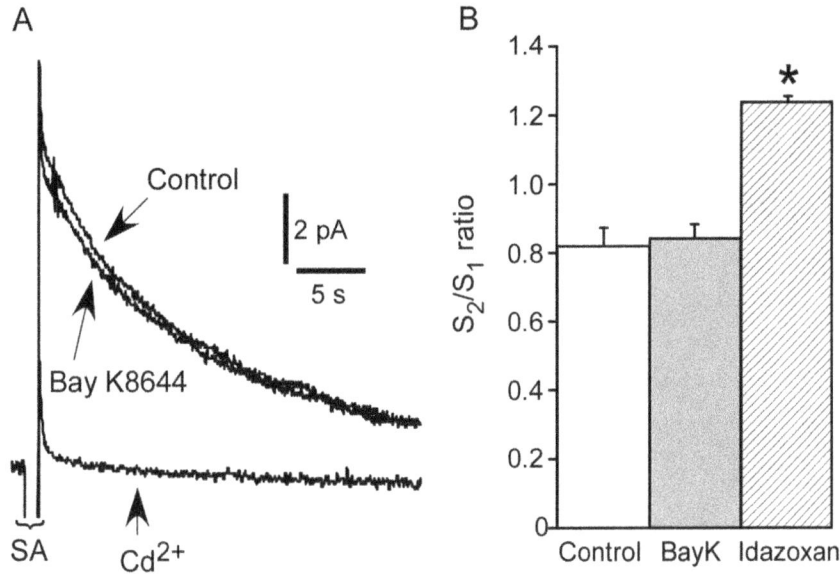

Figure 2. Bay K8644 did not change noradrenaline (NA)-induced oxidation currents evoked by nerve stimulation. (A) Overlaid averaged traces showing NA-induced oxidation currents that followed the stimulus artifacts (SA) before and during application of Bay K8644 (0.1 μM). In addition, **(A)** shows an averaged trace recorded during the subsequent addition of Cd^{2+} (0.1 mM) to block neurotransmitter release. **(B)** Mean stimulus period 2 to stimulus period 1 (S_2/S_1) ratios in tissues with Bay K8644 (BayK) added between the stimulus periods ($n = 6$; *grey bar*) and time-matched control tissues ($n = 6$; *white bar*). This graph also shows that S_2/S_1 ratios increased significantly in tissues treated with the $α_2$-adrenoceptor antagonist idazoxan (Idaz) between the stimulus periods (0.1 μM, $n = 6$; *hatched bar*). The data are presented as means and SE and statistical comparisons with control were made with unpaired t-tests. *$P < 0.05$.

with trains of 100 pulses at 1 Hz. In control arteries, both ryanodine ($n = 6$) and CPZ ($n = 6$) did not change the size of contractions measured at the 10th pulse during the trains of stimuli (**Fig. 4B, E**), but increased those measured at the 100th pulse (**Fig. 4A, C, D, F**). This effect of ryanodine and CPZ was not observed in SCI arteries ($n = 6$), where neither agent changed the size of nerve-evoked contractions (**Fig. 4 A, C, D, F**). Importantly, in the presence of either ryanodine or CPZ, the size of the contractions measured at the 100th pulse did not differ significantly between control and SCI arteries (**Fig. 4C, F**; Ryanodine $P = 0.31$, CPZ $P = 0.45$). Because both ryanodine and CPZ selectively increased the size of nerve-evoked contractions in control arteries, these findings suggest that reduced Ca^{2+} sequestration by the SR contributes to the augmentation nerve-evoked contractions in SCI arteries.

A possible alternative explanation for the increase in nerve-evoked contraction produced by ryanodine and CPZ is if they act at a prejunctional site to increase neurotransmitter release. Previously it has been reported that 10 μM ryanodine does not change NA release in the rat tail artery [19]. However, 5 μM CPZ has been reported to produce a small (~20%) increase in NA release in this artery [20]. To test whether 1 μM CPZ increases NA release in arteries from unoperated rats we used *in situ* amperometry. In comparison with S_2/S_1 ratios for NA-induced oxidation currents in time-dependent controls (0.84 ± 0.04, $n = 6$), those in tissues that were treated with CPZ did not differ significantly (0.90 ± 0.03, $n = 6$, $P = 0.27$). Therefore a prejunctional site of action for ryanodine and CPZ can be excluded in the present study.

Both ryanodine and CPZ increased the blockade of nerve-evoked contractions produced by nifedipine

To test the hypothesis that Ca^{2+} sequestration by the SR limits the contribution of Ca^{2+} entering via L-type Ca^{2+} channels to

nerve-evoked contraction, the effects of nifedipine (1 μM) were investigated in absence and in the presence of either ryanodine (10 μM) or CPZ (1 μM). In the absence of these agents, the % blockade of contractions produced by nifedipine at 10th pulse during trains of stimuli at 1 Hz was similar in control and SCI arteries (**Fig. 5D**; $P = 0.48$). By contrast, at the 100th pulse, the % blockade produced by nifedipine was greater in SCI arteries than in control arteries (**Fig. 5E**; $P < 0.05$). The absolute size of the nifedipine-sensitive component of contraction at the 100th pulse was also larger in SCI arteries (**Fig. 1A, Table 1**). The nifedipine-resistant contractions of SCI arteries measured at the 10th pulse were still larger than control, whereas those measured at 100th pulse had a tendency to be larger but this difference was not statistically significant (**Fig. 5A, Table 1**).

In ryanodine-pretreated control ($n = 6$) and SCI ($n = 6$) arteries, the % blockade of nerve-evoked contractions produced by nifedipine was increased at both the 10th and 100th pulse (**Fig. 5 D, E**). At the 10th pulse in the presence of ryanodine, the absolute size of the nifedipine-sensitive component of contraction was larger in SCI arteries than in control arteries (**Fig. 5B, Table 1**). By contrast, at the 100th pulse, the absolute size of the nifedipine-sensitive component in the presence of ryanodine did not differ between control and SCI arteries (**Fig. 5B, Table 1**). The nifedipine-resistant component of contraction did not differ between the ryanodine-treated control and SCI arteries at either the 10th and 100th pulse (**Fig. 5B, Table 1**).

CPZ did not significantly change the % blockade of contractions produced by nifedipine at the 10th pulse in both control ($n = 6$) and SCI arteries ($n = 6$; **Fig. 5D**). At the 100th pulse, CPZ selectively increased the % blockade of contractions by nifedipine in control arteries (**Fig. 5E**). At this time point the absolute size of the nifedipine-sensitive and nifedipine-resistant components of contraction did not differ between control and SCI arteries (**Fig. 5C, Table 1**). Together these findings indicate that disruption of Ca^{2+}

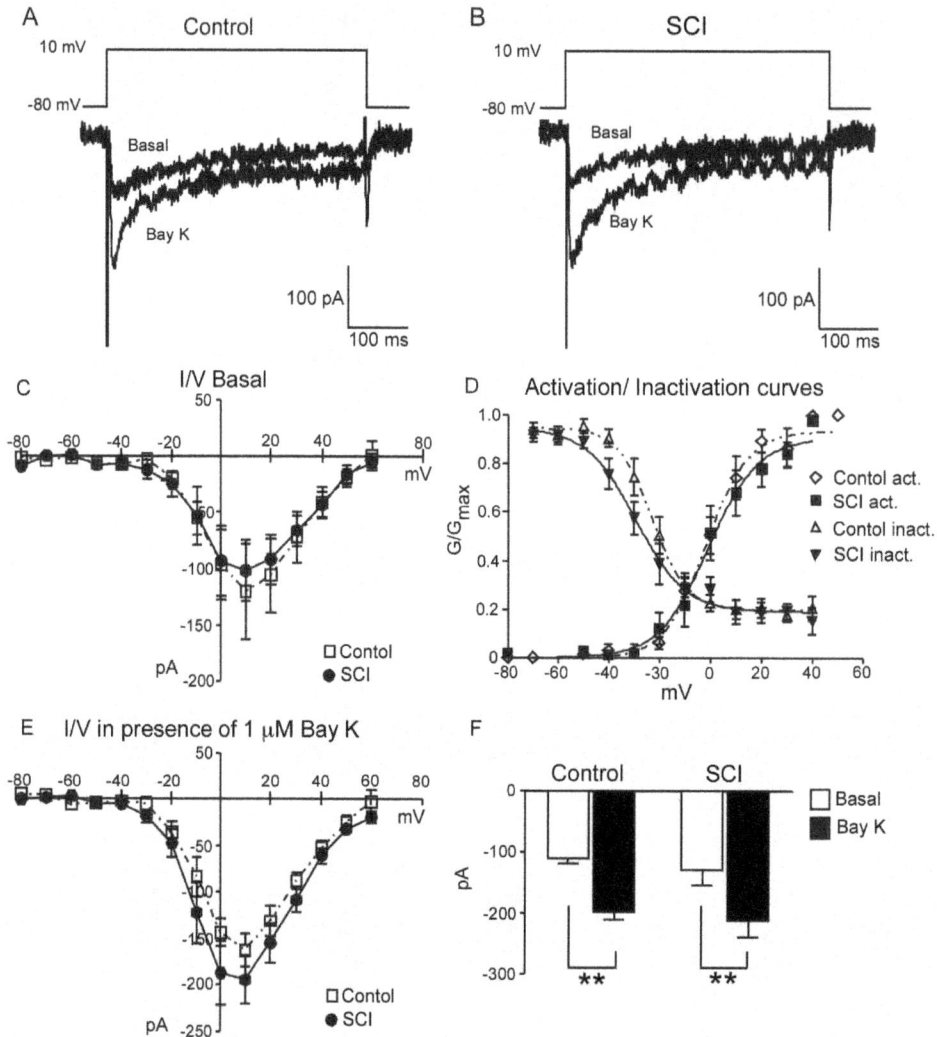

Figure 3. Calcium channel currents recorded from tail artery vascular smooth muscle cells (SMCs) are not changed by spinal cord injury (SCI). (A, B) Ba^{2+} currents elicited by a 250 ms depolarizing step to +10 mV from a holding potential of −80 mV in a representative SMC from a sham-operated (control) rat (**A**) and a SCI rat (**B**) before (basal) and during application of Bay K8644 (1 μM). (**C**) Leak-subtracted current-voltage relations in control and SCI SMCs under basal conditions (control: 8 cells, $n = 5$; SCI: 9 cells, $n = 5$). (**D**) Normalized conductance-voltage relations for currents from control and SCI SMCs. The activation and inactivation curves in each case are the least squares-fit to the Boltzmann equation. (**E**) Current-voltage relations in control and SCI SMCs in the presence of Bay K8644 (1 μM) (control: 8 cells, n = 5; SCI: 9 cells, n = 5). (**F**) Mean increase in current amplitude produced stepping from −80 mV to +10 mV in the absence and in the presence of Bay K8644 (control: 10 cells, n = 5; SCI: 9 cells, n = 5). The data are presented as means and SE and statistical comparisons were made with paired t-tests. **$P<0.01$.

buffering by the SR increases the contribution of Ca^{2+} influx via L-type Ca^{2+} channels to nerve-evoked contractions.

Discussion

The primary finding of this study is that the increased sensitivity of nerve-evoked contractions of tail arteries from SCI rats to nifedipine is not explained by an increase in functional membrane expression of L-type Ca^{2+} channels in SMCs. Furthermore, the greater augmentation of nerve-evoked contractions produced by Bay K8644 in control arteries does not appear to be explained by a greater stimulatory effect of this agent on L-type Ca^{2+} channel activity. Instead, the selective augmentation of nerve-evoked contractions produced by ryanodine and CPZ in control arteries, together with their greater sensitivity to nifedipine in the presence of these agents, suggests that Ca^{2+} entering via L-type Ca^{2+} channels is normally rapidly sequestered into the SR limiting its

access to the contractile mechanism. As neither ryanodine nor CPZ increased nerve-evoked contractions of SCI arteries, we assume that Ca^{2+} entering via L-type Ca^{2+} channels is less susceptible to sequestration by the SR in these vessels and more freely accesses the contractile mechanism.

Bay K8644 did not change the amplitude of nerve-evoked NA-induced oxidation currents, which provide a real time measure of NA release [8]. This finding accords with previous reports that Bay K8644 does not change NA release from sympathetic nerve terminals in other rat tissues [21,22]. As nerve-evoked contractions of both control and SCI arteries are mediated almost entirely by NA [6,7], the facilitatory action of Bay K8644 on these responses cannot be attributed to increased neurotransmitter release from the sympathetic nerve terminals.

The size of the whole cell Ba^{2+} current carried by voltage-activated Ca^{2+} channels did not differ between SMCs from control

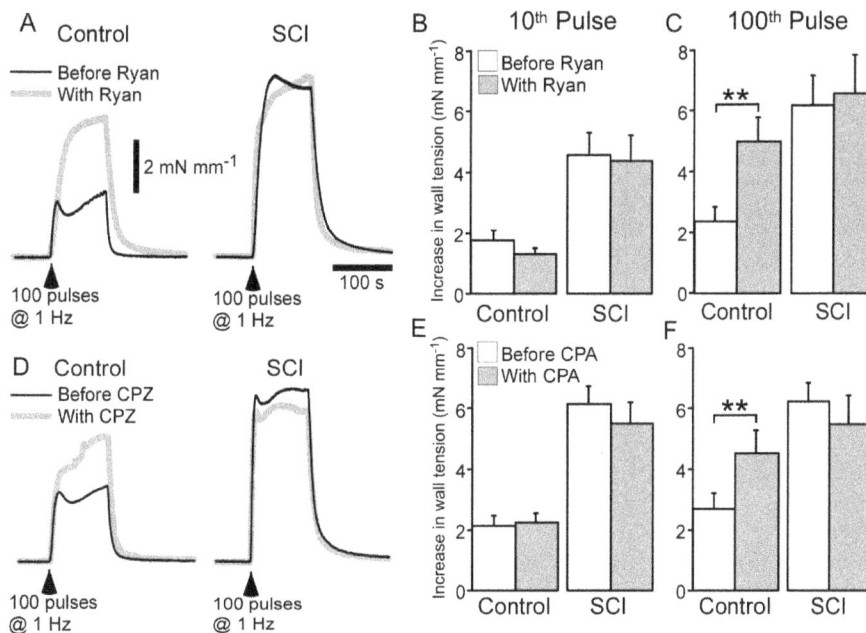

Figure 4. Both ryanodine (Ryan; 10 μM) and cyclopiazonic acid (CPZ; 1 μM) increased the amplitude of nerve-evoked contractions in arteries from sham-operated rats (control arteries) but not in those from spinal cord injured rats (SCI arteries). (A, D) Averaged traces showing contractions to 100 pulses at 1 Hz in control (*left traces*) and SCI arteries (*right traces*) before (*black line*) and during (*grey line*) application of ryanodine (**A**) or CPZ (**D**). (**B, C, E, F**) Increases in wall tension measured at the 10th (**B, E**) and 100th pulse (**C, F**) during the trains of stimuli in control (n = 6) and SCI (n = 6) arteries before (*white bars*) and during (*grey bars*) application of ryanodine (**B, C**) or CPZ (**E, F**). Data are presented as means and SEs and statistical comparisons were made with paired *t*-tests. **$P < 0.01$.

and SCI tail arteries. There was also no difference in the voltage for half-maximal activation and inactivation of the Ba^{2+} current between the two groups of SMCs. When depolarized from -80 mV most of the Ba^{2+} current in tail artery SMCs is carried by L-type Ca^{2+} channels but there is also a component that is carried by T-type Ca^{2+} channels [18,23]. Bay K8644 selectively enhances the L-type Ca^{2+} channel current in rat tail artery [23,24]. In both control and SCI SMCs, the increase in Ba^{2+} current produced by BayK8644 was similar, consistent with there being a similar contribution of L-type Ca^{2+} channel activation to the increase in Ca^{2+} conductance. Together these findings indicate that increased L-type Ca^{2+} channel expression in SMCs is unlikely to explain the greater contribution of these ion channels to neural activation of SCI tail arteries. The findings also indicate that the greater augmentation of nerve-evoked contractions produced by Bay K8644 in control arteries, compared to SCI arteries, is not explained by greater stimulation of L-type Ca^{2+} channel activity in these vessels.

In control arteries, but not SCI arteries, both ryanodine and CPZ increased the size of nerve-evoked contractions measured at the end of the trains of 100 pulses at 1 Hz. As Bay K8644 increased the size of contractions in SCI arteries, the failure of ryanodine and CPA to increase these responses cannot be attributed to the muscle already being maximally activated. At the 100th pulse, both ryanodine and CPZ also produced a greater increase the % blockade of nerve-evoked contractions by nifedipine in control arteries. As a consequence, while in the absence of these agents the absolute size of the nifedipine-sensitive component of contraction at the 100th pulse was much larger in SCI arteries than in control arteries, in their presence it did not differ between these groups of vessels. These findings indicate that impairing the ability of the SR to accumulate and/or release Ca^{2+} increases the contribution of L-type Ca^{2+} channels to nerve-

evoked contractions. Furthermore, as ryanodine and CPZ more markedly increased the contribution of L-type Ca^{2+} channels to neural activation of control arteries, this suggests that in these vessels Ca^{2+} entering via L-type Ca^{2+} channels is more susceptible to regulation by the SR than in SCI arteries.

It has previously been demonstrated that ryanodine does not change NA release in the tail artery [19] or other sympathetically innervated tissues in the rat [25,26]. While it has been reported that CPZ increases NA-release in the tail artery [20], in the present study this effect was not observed. A likely explanation is that Tsai et al. [20] used 5 μM CPZ whereas 1 μM CPZ was used in the present study. Therefore the augmentation of nerve-evoked contractions produced by ryanodine and CPZ cannot be attributed to an increase in neurotransmitter release.

Ryanodine at 10 μM depletes Ca^{2+} from the SR by locking the ryanodine receptor channels open [27]. This action of ryanodine inhibits the contribution of Ca^{2+}-induced Ca^{2+} release to activation of vascular muscle. In addition, the leak of Ca^{2+} from the SR induced by ryanodine prevents it from storing any Ca^{2+} accumulated by SERCA [27]. While both ryanodine and CPZ did not change the amplitude of contractions measured at the 10th pulse, ryanodine selectively and similarly increased the % blockade of contraction produced by nifedipine in both control and SCI arteries. Furthermore in the presence of ryanodine, the small nifedipine-resistant contractions measured at the 10th pulse did not differ between the groups of arteries. This selective action of ryanodine at the 10th pulse suggests that Ca^{2+}-induced Ca^{2+} release contributes to the early phase of contraction in the rail artery. A similar suggestion has been made in rat mesenteric arteries where the early phasic contraction to long trains of nerve stimuli was inhibited by ryanodine but this agent did not affect the later tonic phase of contraction [25].

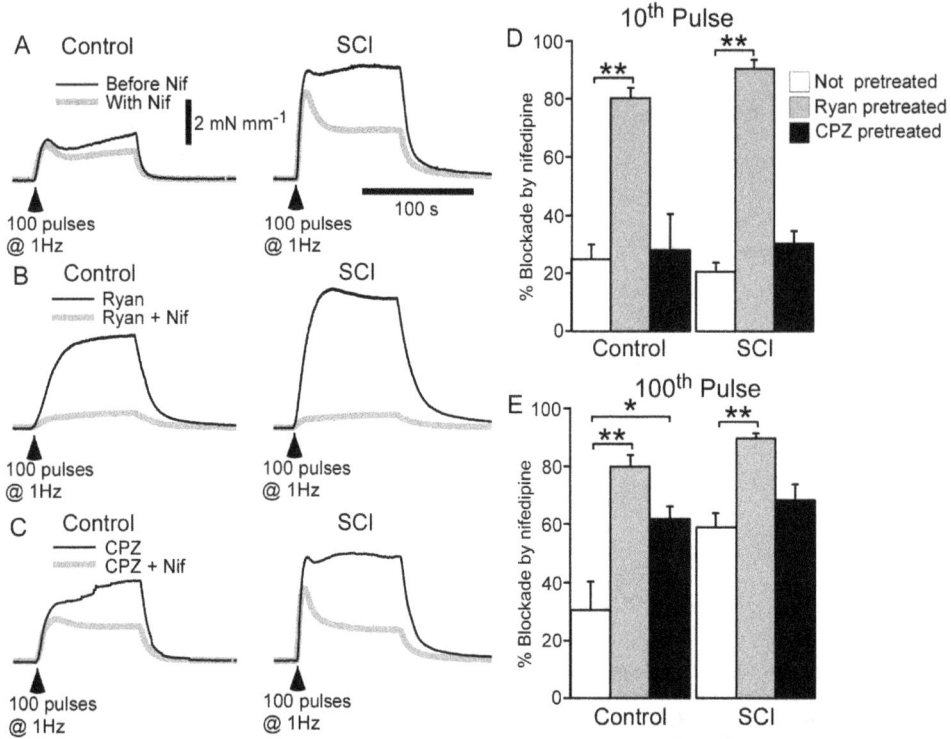

Figure 5. Both ryanodine (Ryan; 10 μM) and cyclopiazonic acid (CPZ; 1 μM) increased the blockade of nerve-evoked contractions produced by nifedipine (Nif; 1 μM) in arteries from sham-operated rats (control arteries). By contrast, only ryanodine increased the blockade of nerve-evoked contractions produced by nifedipine in arteries from spinal cord injured rats (SCI arteries). (A–C) Averaged overlaid traces showing contractions to 100 pulses at 1 Hz in control (*left traces*) and SCI arteries (*right traces*) in absence (A; *black line*) or in the presence of ryanodine (B; *black line*) or CPZ (C; *black line*) and following addition of nifedipine (*grey lines*). (D, E) The % blockade of contractions produced by nifedipine at the 10th (D) and 100th pulse (E) during the trains of stimuli in control (n = 6) and SCI (n = 6) arteries in the absence (*white bars*) or in the presence of ryanodine (*grey bars*) or CPZ (*black bars*). Data are presented as means and SEs and statistical comparisons were made with unpaired *t*-tests. *P<0.05, **P<0.01.

Table 1. The nifedipine-sensitive and nifedipine-resistant components of contractions evoked by 100 pulses at 1 Hz in control and SCI arteries with no pretreatment or pretreated with ryanodine (Ryan; 10 μM) or cyclopiazonic acid (CPZ; 1 μM).

		10th Pulse		100th Pulse	
		Nifedipine-sensitive contraction	Nifedipine-resistant contraction	Nifedipine-sensitive contraction	Nifedipine-resistant contraction
		mN mm⁻¹	mN mm⁻¹	mN mm⁻¹	mN mm⁻¹
Not pretreated	Control (n = 6)	0.44 ± 0.09	1.23 (1.02–1.68)	0.79 ± 0.35	1.34 (1.10–1.73)
	SCI (n = 6)	1.10 ± 0.18	4.59 (3.64–4.97)	3.14 ± 0.46	2.25 (1.59–2.74)
	P value	<0.01*	<0.01*	<0.01*	0.17
Ryan pretreated	Control (n = 6)	1.13 (0.73–1.39)	0.21 ± 0.04	3.65 ± 0.58	0.67 ± 0.11
	SCI (n = 6)	3.86 (2.54–5.90)	0.33 ± 0.09	5.56 ± 1.12	0.58 ± 0.15
	P value	<0.05*	0.24	0.16	0.63
CPZ pretreated	Control (n = 6)	0.56 ± 0.28	1.69 ± 0.36	2.27 ± 0.47	1.67 ± 0.30
	SCI (n = 6)	1.55 ± 0.27	3.65 ± 0.53	3.55 ± 0.67	1.53 ± 0.39
	P value	<0.05*	<0.05*	0.15	0.79

Data are presented as mean ± SE or median and interquartile range (in parentheses) and comparisons between control and SCI values were made with Student's unpaired *t*-tests or Mann Whitney U-tests respectively (* indicates significant P values).

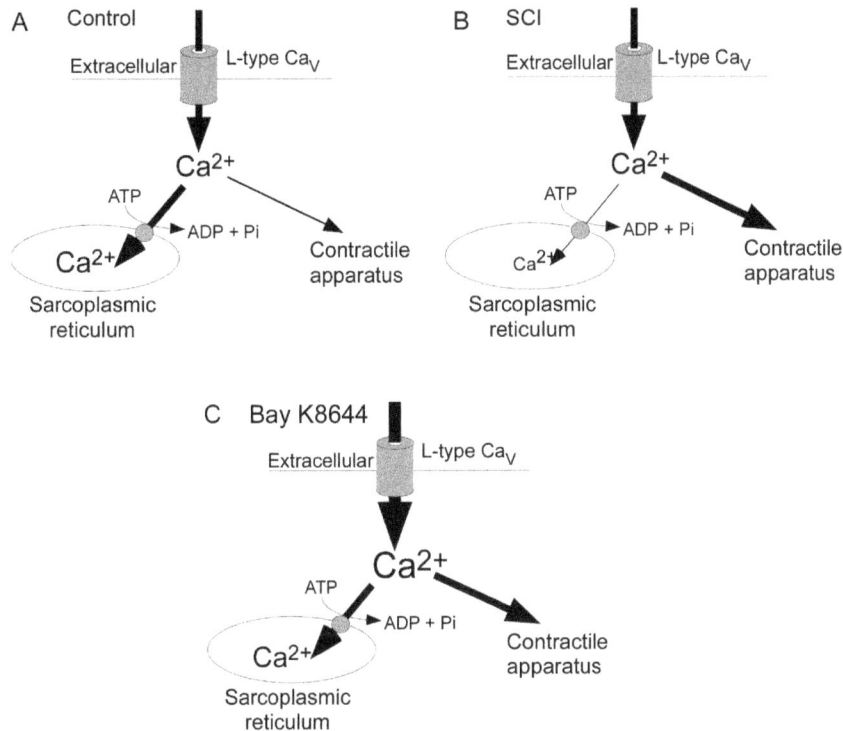

Figure 6. Schematic representations of the mechanisms regulating the contribution of Ca^{2+} influx via L-type Ca^{2+} channels to nerve-evoked contractions. (A) In control arteries, much of the Ca^{2+} entering the cell via L-type Ca^{2+} channels is rapidly sequestered into the sarcoplasmic reticulum (SR) limiting its access the contractile mechanism. (B) In SCI arteries, less of the Ca^{2+} entering through L-type Ca^{2+} channels is sequestered into the SR increasing its access to the contractile mechanism. (C) Bay K8644 increases Ca^{2+} entry via L-type Ca^{2+} channels overcoming the Ca^{2+} buffering capacity of the SR.

Previously it has been reported that both ryanodine and CPZ increase the contribution of Ca^{2+} influx via L-type Ca^{2+} channels to activation of tail artery smooth muscle [12]. To explain this finding Nomura and Asano [12] suggested that Ca^{2+} entering the cell via L-type Ca^{2+} channels is rapidly sequestered into the SR limiting its access to the contractile machinery (see also [28]). As CPZ did not change nerve-evoked contractions of SCI arteries or their sensitivity to nifedipine, it is possible that the activity of SERCA in these vessels is lower than in control arteries. This change would explain the greater sensitivity of SCI arteries to nifedipine. An increase in the contribution of L-type Ca^{2+} channels to contraction following depletion of the intracellular Ca^{2+} stores has also been demonstrated in rat mesenteric veins [29]. In SMCs from rat mesenteric veins, intracellular Ca^{2+} chelation with BAPTA increased L-type Ca^{2+} channel activity recorded in cell attached patches. Therefore Thakali et al. [29] concluded that Ca^{2+} released from the intracellular stores normally inactivates L-type Ca^{2+} channels. This process of inactivation is mediated via the Ca^{2+} sensor protein calmodulin, which binds to the intracellular C terminus of the Cav1.2 α_1-subunit to cause a conformational change that enables channel inactivation [30,31]. Perhaps the increase in the nifedipine-sensitive contraction produced by ryanodine at the 10th pulse in both control and SCI arteries indicates that Ca^{2+} released from a ryanodine-sensitive store normally inhibits L-type Ca^{2+} channel activity at this time point.

The effects of SCI on sympathetic nerve-mediated activation of the tail artery are similar to those produced when the postganglionic sympathetic neurons supplying this vessel are decentralized by lesioning their preganglionic inputs [32]. Therefore the changes in neurovascular function produced by SCI are almost certainly caused by the decrease in ongoing sympathetic nerve activity that is known to occur caudal to a spinal cord lesion [33]. The effects of decentralization on regulation of intracellular Ca^{2+} in vascular muscle cells are unknown. In rat vas deferens, the increase in smooth muscle reactivity produced by denervation is associated with a reduction in both SERCA Ca^{2+} uptake activity and protein expression of SERCA2 [34]. Down-regulation of SERCA has also been reported in denervated skeletal muscle [35]. In rat vas deferens homogenates, denervation also reduced the density of ryanodine binding sites but not their affinity [34]. As the effects of decentralization and denervation on smooth muscle reactivity are similar in the rat tail artery [36], it is possible that they are mediated, at least in part, by a down-regulation of SR proteins involved in intracellular Ca^{2+} homeostasis.

In conclusion, the increase in both nerve-evoked contraction amplitude and sensitivity to nifedipine produced by disrupting cytoplasmic Ca^{2+} buffering by the SR in control arteries suggests that Ca^{2+} entering via L-type Ca^{2+} channels is normally rapidly sequestered, reducing its access to the contractile mechanism (**Fig. 6A**). As nerve-evoked contractions of SCI arteries were larger and more sensitive to nifedipine, and disruption of Ca^{2+} buffering did not increase the size of these responses, it appears that sequestration of Ca^{2+} entering via L-type Ca^{2+} channels is lower in these vessels (**Fig. 6B**). If this interpretation is correct, the more marked facilitatory effect Bay K8644 on nerve-evoked contraction in control arteries is readily explained by the increase in Ca^{2+} influx overcoming the Ca^{2+} buffering role of the SR (**Fig. 6C**). In vascular muscle, there is also evidence that Ca^{2+} released from intracellular stores inhibits the activity of L-type

Ca^{2+} channels and that this is prevented by impairing ability of the SR to accumulate and release Ca^{2+} [29]. Therefore this mechanism could provide an alternative explanation for the effects of ryanodine and CPZ observed in the present study.

Acknowledgments

We thank Nicole Kerr for her technical assistance.

Author Contributions

Conceived and designed the experiments: HAD BPC JAB. Performed the experiments: HAD BPC JAB. Analyzed the data: HAD BPC JAB. Contributed to the writing of the manuscript: HAD BPC JAB.

References

1. Mathias CJ, Frankel HL (1999) Autonomic disturbances in spinal cord lesions. In: Mathias CJ, Banister R, editors. Autonomic Failure. Oxford: Oxford University Press. 494–519.

2. Weaver LC, Marsh DR, Gris D, Brown A, Dekaban GA (2006) Autonomic dysreflexia after spinal cord injury: central mechanisms and strategies for prevention. Prog Brain Res 152: 245–263.

3. Wallin BG, Stjernberg L (1984) Sympathetic activity in man after spinal cord injury. Outflow to skin below the lesion. Brain 107: 183–198.

4. Brock JA, Yeoh M, McLachlan EM (2006) Enhanced neurally evoked responses and inhibition of norepinephrine reuptake in rat mesenteric arteries after spinal transection. Am J Physiol Heart Circ Physiol 290: H398–405.

5. Rummery NM, Tripovic D, Mclachlan EM, Brock JA (2010) Sympathetic vasoconstriction is potentiated in arteries caudal but not rostral to a spinal cord transection in rats. J Neurotrauma 27: 2077–2089.

6. Yeoh M, McLachlan EM, Brock JA (2004) Tail arteries from chronically spinalized rats have potentiated responses to nerve stimulation in vitro. J Physiol 556: 545–555.

7. Al Dera H, Habgood MD, Furness JB, Brock JA (2012) A prominent contribution of L-type Ca^{2+} channels to cutaneous neurovascular transmission that is revealed after spinal cord injury augments vasoconstriction. Am J Physiol Heart Circ Physiol 302: H752–H762.

8. Brock JA, Cunnane TC (1999) Effects of Ca^{2+} concentration and Ca^{2+} channel blockers on noradrenaline release and purinergic neuroeffector transmission in rat tail artery. Br J Pharmacol 126: 11–18.

9. Davies PJ, Ireland DR, McLachlan EM (1996) Sources of Ca^{2+} for different Ca^{2+}-activated K^+ conductances in neurones of the rat superior cervical ganglion. J Physiol 495: 353–366.

10. Martinez-Pinna J, Lamas JA, Gallego R (2002) Calcium current components in intact and dissociated adult mouse sympathetic neurons. Brain Res 951: 227–236.

11. Pan M, Scriabine A, Steinsland OS (1988) Effects of BAY K 8644 on the responses of rabbit ear artery to electrical stimulation. J Cardiovasc Pharmacol 11: 127–133.

12. Nomura Y, Asano M (2000) Ca^{2+} buffering function of sarcoplasmic reticulum in rat tail arteries: comparison in normotensive and spontaneously hypertensive rats. Jpn J Pharmacol 83: 335–343.

13. Rathner JA, McAllen RM (1998) The lumbar preganglionic sympathetic supply to rat tail and hindpaw. J Auton Nerv Syst 69: 127–131.

14. Smith JE, Gilbey MP (1998) Segmental origin of sympathetic preganglionic neurones regulating the tail circulation in the rat. J Auton Nerv Syst 68: 109–114.

15. Mulvany MJ, Halpern W (1977) Contractile properties of small arterial resistance vessels in spontaneously hypertensive and normotensive rats. Circ Res 41: 19–26.

16. Brock JA, Tan JH (2004) Selective modulation of noradrenaline release by alpha 2-adrenoceptor blockade in the rat-tail artery in vitro. Br J Pharmacol 142: 267–274.

17. Curran-Everett D (2000) Multiple comparisons: philosophies and illustrations. Am J Physiol Regul Integr Comp Physiol 279: R1–8.

18. Wilkinson MF, Earle ML, Triggle CR, Barnes S (1996) Interleukin-1β, tumor necrosis factor-α, and LPS enhance calcium channel current in isolated vascular smooth muscle cells of rat tail artery. FASEB J 10: 785–791.

19. Bao JX, Gonon F, Stjarne L (1993) Frequency- and train length-dependent variation in the roles of postjunctional α_1- and α_2-adrenoceptors for the field stimulation-induced neurogenic contraction of rat tail artery. Naunyn Schmiedebergs Arch Pharmacol 347: 601–616.

20. Tsai H, Pottorf WJ, Buchholz JN, Duckles SP (1998) Adrenergic nerve smooth endoplasmic reticulum calcium buffering declines with age. Neurobiol Aging 19: 89–96.

21. Somogyi GT, Zernova GV, Tanowitz M, de Groat WC (1997) Role of L- and N-type Ca^{2+} channels in muscarinic receptor-mediated facilitation of ACh and noradrenaline release in the rat urinary bladder. J Physiol 499: 645–654.

22. Orallo F, Salaices M, Alonso MJ, Marin J, Sanchez-Garcia P (1992) Effects of several calcium channels modulators on the [³H]noradrenaline release and ⁴⁵Ca influx in the rat vas deferens. Gen Pharmacol 23: 257–262.

23. Wang R, Karpinski E, Pang PK (1989) Two types of calcium channels in isolated smooth muscle cells from rat tail artery. Am J Physiol 256: H1361–1368.

24. Petkov GV, Fusi F, Saponara S, Gagov HS, Sgaragli GP, et al. (2001) Characterization of voltage-gated calcium currents in freshly isolated smooth muscle cells from rat tail main artery. Acta Physiol Scand 173: 257–265.

25. Garcha RS, Hughes AD (1997) Action of ryanodine on neurogenic responses in rat isolated mesenteric small arteries. Br J Pharmacol 122: 142–148.

26. Bultmann R, von Kugelgen I, Starke K (1993) Effects of nifedipine and ryanodine on adrenergic neurogenic contractions of rat vas deferens: evidence for a pulse-to-pulse change in Ca^{2+} sources. Br J Pharmacol 108: 1062–1070.

27. Laporte R, Hui A, Laher I (2004) Pharmacological modulation of sarcoplasmic reticulum function in smooth muscle. Pharmacol Rev 56: 439–513.

28. van Breemen C, Chen Q, Laher I (1995) Superficial buffer barrier function of smooth muscle sarcoplasmic reticulum. Trends Pharmacol Sci 16: 98–105.

29. Thakali KM, Kharade SV, Sonkusare SK, Rhee SW, Stimers JR, et al. (2010) Intracellular Ca^{2+} silences L-type Ca^{2+} channels in mesenteric veins: mechanism of venous smooth muscle resistance to calcium channel blockers. Circ Res 106: 739–747.

30. Pitt GS, Zuhlke RD, Hudmon A, Schulman H, Reuter H, et al. (2001) Molecular basis of calmodulin tethering and Ca^{2+}-dependent inactivation of L-type Ca^{2+} channels. J Biol Chem 276: 30794–30802.

31. Erickson MG, Alseikhan BA, Peterson BZ, Yue DT (2001) Preassociation of calmodulin with voltage-gated Ca^{2+} channels revealed by FRET in single living cells. Neuron 31: 973–985.

32. Yeoh M, McLachlan EM, Brock JA (2004) Chronic decentralization potentiates neurovascular transmission in the isolated rat tail artery, mimicking the effects of spinal transection. J Physiol 561: 583–596.

33. Maiorov DN, Weaver LC, Krassioukov AV (1997) Relationship between sympathetic activity and arterial pressure in conscious spinal rats. Am J Physiol 272: H625–631.

34. Quintas LE, Cunha VM, Scaramello CB, da Silva CL, Caricati-Neto A, et al. (2005) Adaptive expression pattern of different proteins involved in cellular calcium homeostasis in denervated rat vas deferens. Eur J Pharmacol 525: 54–59.

35. Schulte L, Peters D, Taylor J, Navarro J, Kandarian S (1994) Sarcoplasmic reticulum Ca^{2+} pump expression in denervated skeletal muscle. Am J Physiol 267: C617–622.

36. Tripovic D, Pianova S, McLachlan EM, Brock JA (2010) Transient supersensitivity to α-adrenoceptor agonists, and distinct hyper-reactivity to vasopressin and angiotensin II after denervation of rat tail artery. Br J Pharmacol 159: 142–153.

8

Subacute Intranasal Administration of Tissue Plasminogen Activator Promotes Neuroplasticity and Improves Functional Recovery following Traumatic Brain Injury in Rats

Yuling Meng[1]**, Michael Chopp**[2,3]**, Yanlu Zhang**[1]**, Zhongwu Liu**[2]**, Aaron An**[1]**, Asim Mahmood**[1]**, Ye Xiong**[1]*****

1 Department of Neurosurgery, Henry Ford Hospital, Detroit, Michigan, United States of America, **2** Department of Neurology, Henry Ford Hospital, Detroit, Michigan, United States of America, **3** Department of Physics, Oakland University, Rochester, Michigan, United States of America

Abstract

Traumatic brain injury (TBI) is a major cause of death and long-term disability worldwide. To date, there are no effective pharmacological treatments for TBI. Recombinant human tissue plasminogen activator (tPA) is the effective drug for the treatment of acute ischemic stroke. In addition to its thrombolytic effect, tPA is also involved in neuroplasticity in the central nervous system. However, tPA has potential adverse side effects when administered intravenously including brain edema and hemorrhage. Here we report that tPA, administered by intranasal delivery during the subacute phase after TBI, provides therapeutic benefit. Animals with TBI were treated intranasally with saline or tPA initiated 7 days after TBI. Compared with saline treatment, subacute intranasal tPA treatment significantly 1) improved cognitive (Morris water maze test) and sensorimotor (footfault and modified neurological severity score) functional recovery in rats after TBI, 2) reduced the cortical stimulation threshold evoking ipsilateral forelimb movement, 3) enhanced neurogenesis in the dentate gyrus and axonal sprouting of the corticospinal tract originating from the contralesional cortex into the denervated side of the cervical gray matter, and 4) increased the level of mature brain-derived neurotrophic factor. Our data suggest that subacute intranasal tPA treatment improves functional recovery and promotes brain neurogenesis and spinal cord axonal sprouting after TBI, which may be mediated, at least in part, by tPA/plasmin-dependent maturation of brain-derived neurotrophic factor.

Editor: Hubert Vaudry, University of Rouen, France

Funding: The research presented herein was supported by National Institute of Neurological Disorders and Stroke RO1 NS062002 (YX), and National Institute on Aging RO1 AG037506 (MC). The funders had no role in study design, data collection and analysis, decision to publish, or preparation of the manuscript.

Competing Interests: The authors have declared that no competing interests exist.

* Email: yxiong1@hfhs.org

Introduction

Traumatic brain injury (TBI) remains a leading cause of mortality and morbidity worldwide [1,2]. To date, there is no effective pharmacological therapy available for TBI. For decades, significant efforts have been devoted to the development of neuroprotective agents in an attempt to prevent neural cell death or salvage damaged neurons in the injured brain; however, all these efforts have failed to demonstrate efficacy in clinical trials of TBI [1,3]. Until recently, it was believed that once the brain was damaged, there was little, if any, capability for regeneration of axons and formation of new synapses. However, it has been discovered that the central nervous system (CNS) is indeed capable of significant (though limited) plasticity and regeneration that may contribute to spontaneous functional recovery and can be pharmacologically or otherwise enhanced [4–8].

Recombinant human tissue plasminogen activator (tPA) is the only U.S. Food and Drug Administration approved drug for the treatment of acute ischemic stroke [9]. In addition to its well established thrombolytic effect, tPA also participates in synaptic plasticity, dendritic remodeling and axonal outgrowth in the developing and injured CNS [10]. Our previous studies have demonstrated that upregulated endogenous tPA mediates bone marrow stromal cell-induced functional recovery in animal models of stroke [11] and TBI [12]. tPA is able to convert the pro-brain-derived neurotrophic factor (proBDNF) to the mature BDNF by activating the extracellular protease plasmin, and that such conversion is critical for brain neuroplasticity and function [13–17]. However, tPA has potential adverse side effects when administered intravenously including brain edema and hemorrhagic transformation in rats after stroke [9] and increased brain lesion and hemorrhage in rats after TBI [18]. Intranasal delivery of agents has been demonstrated to directly target the brain and spinal cord [19]. Although the exact mechanisms of this intranasal delivery are not yet fully understood, extensive evidence demonstrates that olfactory nerve pathways, trigeminal nerve pathways, vascular pathways and lymphatic pathways are involved [19]. Our previous study demonstrates that tPA administrated intranasally during the subacute phase of experimental stroke in rats provides beneficial effects on stroke recovery by promoting neuroplasticity [20]. However, there is no study of subacute intranasal tPA as a potential treatment of TBI. Whether and how intranasal tPA administration after TBI regulates BDNF is unknown.

In the present study, we investigated the therapeutic effect of tPA administered intranasally on cognitive and sensorimotor functional recovery in rats during the subacute phase of experimental TBI. We performed intracortical microstimulation (ICMS) that evoked right or left forelimb movement to validate the establishment of functional neuronal connections from the right intact cortex to bilateral forelimbs 5 weeks after TBI. We examined the effects of tPA treatment on neurogenesis in the dentate gyrus (DG) and axonal sprouting of the corticospinal tract (CST) originating from the intact cortex into the denervated side of the spinal cord after TBI to investigate the neuronal substrate of the functional recovery. To elucidate the mechanisms that underlie the beneficial effects of tPA, we investigated expression of proBDNF and BDNF in the injured brain and denervated cervical spinal cord in TBI rats treated with tPA. Here we report that subacute intranasal tPA treatment improves functional recovery and promotes brain neurogenesis and spinal cord axonal sprouting after TBI in rats, which is likely associated with tPA/plasmin-dependent maturation of BDNF.

Materials and Methods

Ethics Statement

All experimental procedures were carried out in accordance with the NIH Guide for the Care and Use of Laboratory Animals. The study protocol was approved by the Institutional Animal Care and Use Committee of Henry Ford Hospital.

TBI Model

A controlled cortical impact (CCI) model of TBI in the rat was utilized for the present study [21]. Young adult male Wistar rats (323 ± 13 g) were anesthetized with chloral hydrate (350 mg/kg body weight), intraperitoneally. Rectal temperature was maintained at $37°C$ using a feedback-regulated water-heating pad. Rats were placed in a stereotactic frame. Two 10-mm-diameter craniotomies were performed adjacent to the central suture, midway between lambda and bregma. The second craniotomy allowed for lateral movement of cortical tissue. The dura mater was kept intact over the cortex. To verify the neuroanatomical substrate of sensorimotor functional recovery after TBI and tPA treatment, we injected an anterograde neuronal tracer biotinylated dextran amine (BDA) into the contralesional right sensorimotor cortex [5,22]. In brief, 10% solution of BDA (10,000 MW; Molecular Probes, Eugene, OR) in phosphate-buffered saline (PBS) was injected through a finely drawn glass capillary into 4 points in the right cortex (100 nl per injection; stereotaxic coordinates: 1 and 2 mm posterior to the bregma, 3 and 4 mm lateral to the midline, at a depth of 1.5 to 1.7 mm from the cortical surface) to anterogradely label the CST originating from this area. The micropipette remained in place for 4 min after completion of the injection. Immediately after BDA injection, cortical injury was delivered by impacting the left cortex (ipsilateral cortex) with a pneumatic piston containing a 6-mm-diameter tip at a rate of 4 m/s and 2.5 mm of compression. Velocity was measured with a linear velocity displacement transducer [5].

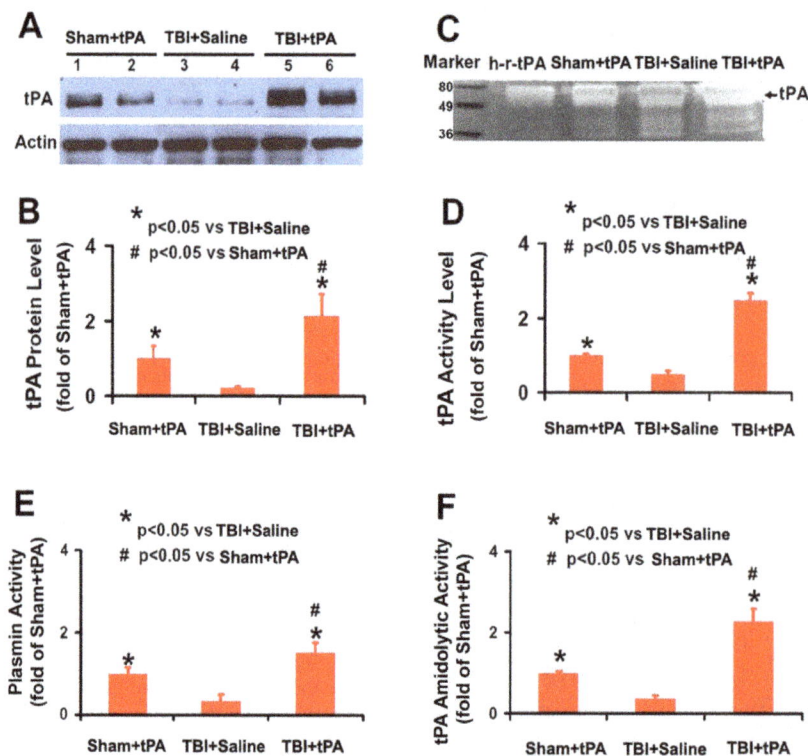

Figure 1. tPA protein level and activity as well as plasmin activity in rat brain. Western blot analysis of tPA protein levels in the rat brain 24 hr after intranasal administration of tPA (A). Bar graph (B) shows the tPA protein level. Of note, Sham+tPA rats received the same amount of intranasal tPA administration as TBI+tPA rats did. Representative zymographic assay (C) shows an increase in tPA activity in the Sham+tPA rats and TBI+tPA rats compared to TBI+Saline rats. h-r-tPA: human recombinant tPA (15 ng, Genentech). Bar graph (D) shows the tPA activity. Bar graph (E) shows amidolytic activity of plasmin assayed with D-Val-Leu-Lys-p-Nitroanilide Dihydrochloride (S-2251) as its specific substrate. Bar graph (F) shows tPA amidolytic activity with S-2251 as the substrate in the presence of added plasminogen compared to Sham. *$p<0.05$ vs TBI+Saline. #$p<0.05$ vs Sham+tPA. Data represent mean $\pm$ SD. n = 4 (rats/group, in graphs D, E, and F).

Experimental Groups and Treatment

Young adult male Wistar rats subjected to TBI were randomly divided into 2 groups: TBI+Saline group ($n = 8$) and TBI+tPA group ($n = 8$). TBI was induced by CCI over the left parietal cortex. Sham+tPA rats ($n = 8$) underwent surgery without injury but received the same dose of intranasal tPA as did the TBI+tPA rats. tPA at a dose of 600 μg/rat (Genentech, San Francisco, CA) was administered intranasally at Days 7 and 14 post TBI or sham-operation. Although our pilot study did not show any significant effect of intranasal delivery of tPA (600 μg/rat) on functional outcomes in sham-operated rats, all the sham animals received intranasal tPA (600 μg/rat) post sham-operation for functional tests, Western blot, enzymatic and immunostaining analyses. The starting dose of tPA was selected based on our previous stroke study in rats [20]. Intranasal delivery does not involve delivery to the bloodstream throughout the body where the body weight is a significant factor, but rather targets the brain and spinal cord [23]. Thus throughout the proposal, we used micrograms (i.e., μg) to express drug dosage administered to the rats. Animals in the saline-treated group received an equal volume of saline. Briefly, under isoflurane anesthesia, the animals were placed in a supine position with rolled 2×2 inch gauze under the neck to maintain a horizontal head position [20]. Ten 6-μl drops for a total volume of 60 μl of saline or tPA solution in saline were placed alternately onto each nostril with a 3-min interval between drops and naturally sniffed in by the rat. The animals were kept in supine position for an additional 10 min. For labeling proliferating cells, 5-bromo-2′-deoxyuridine (BrdU, 100 mg/kg; Sigma, St. Louis, MO, USA) was injected intraperitoneally into rats daily for 10 days, starting 1 day after TBI. All rats were sacrificed at 35 days after TBI.

To investigate the molecular mechanisms by which tPA promotes neuroplasticity and functional recovery, we examined expression level of proBDNF and BDNF proteins in the injured brain cortex and denervated cervical spinal cord in rats after TBI treated with tPA ($n = 8$). The animals were treated intranasally with saline or one dose of 600 μg tPA administered at day 7 after TBI or sham-operation and sacrificed 24 hr later after tPA treatment for immunostaining and Western blot analysis of proBDNF and BDNF expression. To determine the efficiency of intranasal delivery and avoid the interference of endogenous tPA with the assay, we delivered 300 μg recombinant human tPA (ten 3-μl drops) intranasally into tPA knockout mice (Jackson Laboratory, Bar Harbor, ME). The mice were euthanized at 30 min or 120 min (n = 3/group) after the start of intranasal treatment, and their brains were then frozen in liquid nitrogen and stored at −

80°C until use. Brain tissue samples were extracted with 50 mM phosphate-buffered saline (pH 7.4) containing 1% Triton X-100 and centrifuged at 14,000×g for 20 min. The supernatant was collected, and the protein concentration was measured bicinchoninic acid (BCA) protein assay (Pierce, Rockford, IL). The tPA content in the brain was quantitated with equal amounts of lysates from tissue samples using a human tPA total antigen enzyme-linked immunosorbent assay (ELISA) kit (Molecular Innovations, Novi, MI).

Morris Water Maze (MWM) Test

All functional tests were performed by investigators blinded to the treatment status. To detect spatial learning impairments, a recent version of the MWM test was used [24]. The procedure was modified from previous versions [25] and has been found to be useful for spatial memory assessment in rodents with brain injury [24]. Animals were tested during the last 5 days (that is, 31–35 days after TBI) before sacrifice. Data collection was automated using the HVS Image 2020 Plus Tracking System (US HVS Image), as described previously [26]. The advantage of this version of the water maze is that each trial takes on the key characteristics of a probe trial because the platform is not in a fixed location within the target quadrant. In the traditional version of the MWM test, the position of the hidden platform is always fixed and is relatively easy for rodents to locate. With the modified MWM test we used in the present study, the platform is relocated randomly within the target quadrant (that is, Northeast) with each training trial. The rodents must spend more time searching within the target quadrant; therefore each trial effectively acts as a probe trial. The advantage of this protocol is that rodents should find the platform purely and extensively by reference to extra-maze spatial cues, which improves the accuracy of spatial performance in the MWM [24].

Foot Fault Test

To evaluate sensorimotor function, the foot fault test was carried out before TBI and at 1, 7, 14, 21, 28 and 35 days after TBI. The rats were allowed to walk on a grid. With each weight-bearing step, a paw might fall or slip between the wires and, if this occurred, it was recorded as a foot fault [27]. A total of 50 steps were recorded for right forelimbs.

Modified Neurological Severity Score (mNSS) Test

Neurological functional measurement was performed using the mNSS test [28]. The test was carried out on all rats preinjury and

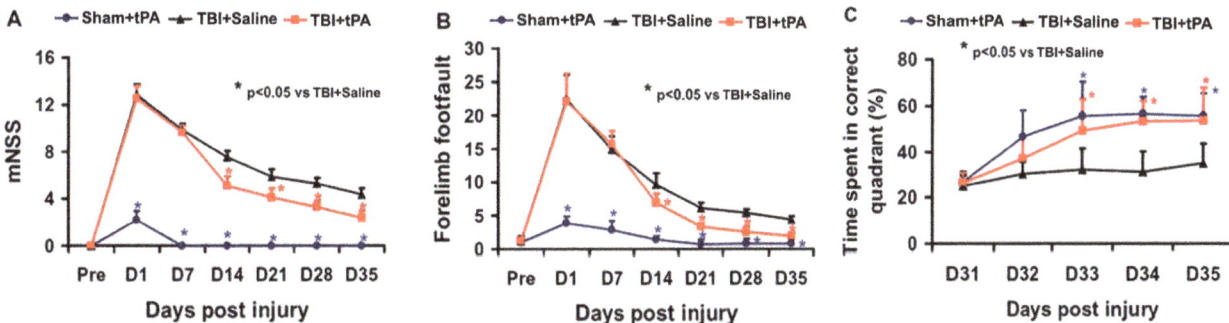

Figure 2. tPA effect on functional outcome. tPA significantly lowered the mNSS scores (A) and reduced frequency of foot faults (B) from Day 14 to 35 after TBI compared to the saline group. tPA treatment significantly improved spatial learning performance from Day 33 to 35 after TBI compared with the saline group (C). *$p < 0.05$ vs TBI+Saline. Data represent mean ± SD. n = 8 (rats/group).

at 1, 7, 14, 21, 28 and 35 days after TBI. The mNSS is a composite of the motor (muscle status, abnormal movement), sensory (visual, tactile, and proprioceptive), and reflex tests and has been used in previous studies [29]. Neurological function was graded on a scale of 0 to 18 (normal score 0; maximal deficit score 18). In the severity scores of injury one point is awarded for each abnormal behavior or for lack of a tested reflex, thus, the higher the score, the more severe the injury.

Electrophysiology

To validate the establishment of functional neuronal connections from the right intact cortex to bilateral forelimbs, intracortical microstimulation (ICMS) and electromyograms (EMG) were performed 5 weeks after TBI [30]. Rats were anesthetized with ketamine hydrochloride (100 mg/kg, intraperitoneally) and xylazine (5 mg/kg, intraperitoneally), and ketamine (20 mg/kg, intraperitoneally) as supplementary injections when needed. The animal rectal temperature was controlled at $37-C$ throughout the experiment. The animal was restricted in a Kopf stereotaxic apparatus and the craniotomy was performed over the right frontal motor cortex. The exposed cerebral cortex surface was covered with warm silicone oil. A pargylinecoated tungsten stimulating microelectrode (2.0 Megaohms, type TM33A20; WPI, Inc., Sarasota, FL) was descended into the forelimb motor cortex to a depth of 1.5 to 1.7 mm from the cortical surface to evoke movement at the lowest threshold at 4 points (stereotaxic coordinates: 1 and 2 mm rostral to the bregma, 2.5 and 3.5 mm lateral to the midline). The electrical stimulus consisted of 20 monophasic cathodal train pulses (60-ms duration at 333 Hz, 0.5-ms pulse duration) of a maximum of 100 μA. For every stimulating point, the lowest threshold value of ICMS that evoked right or left forelimb movement was measured. If no movements were evoked with 100 μA, the current threshold of this point was recorded as 100 μA without additional stimulation at a higher level to avoid cerebral tissue damage. If cortical vessels were encountered at the intended incision site, the site was moved immediately rostral or caudal to avoid the cortical vessel. The average threshold values evoking right or left forelimb movement were calculated from data of 4 stimulation points in each individual animal.

Tissue Preparation

Rats were anesthetized at 8 or 35 days post TBI with chloral hydrate administered intraperitoneally and perfused transcardially with saline solution, followed by 4% paraformaldehyde in 0.1 M PBS, pH 7.4. Rat brains and cervical spinal cords were removed and immersed in 4% paraformaldehyde for 4 days. Using a rat brain matrix (Activational Systems, Inc., Warren, MI), each forebrain was cut into 2-mm-thick coronal blocks for a total of 7 blocks from bregma 5.2 mm to bregma −8.8 mm per animal [31]. For lesion volume measurement, one 6-μm-thick section from each of 7 coronal blocks was traced by a microcomputer imaging device (MCID) (Imaging Research, St. Catharine's, Ontario, Canada), as described previously [32]. The volumes of the ipsilateral and contralateral cortices were computed by integrating the area of each cortex measured at each coronal level and the distance between two sections. The cortical lesion volume was expressed as a percentage calculated by [(contralateral cortical volume − ipsilateral cortical volume)/(contralateral cortical volume) ×100% [33–35]. This method has been widely used to measure lesion volume after TBI [34,36–40] and after stroke [33,35,41,42].

To visualize the BDA-labeled CST, the cervical spinal cord segments were processed for vibratome traverse sections (100 μm). Sections were incubated with 0.5% H_2O_2 for 20 min followed with avidin-biotin-peroxidase complex (Vector

Laboratories Inc., Burlingame, CA) at 4°C for 48 h, and BDA-labeled axons were visualized with 3,3′-diaminobenzidine-nickel (Vector) for light microscopy examination [30]. For measuring axons crossing the midline of cervical spinal cord, the central canal and dorsal median fissure were used as landmarks with the number of labeled axons projecting into the denervated TBI-impaired side of the ventral gray matter. For each animal, the CST remodeling was estimated by the total BDA-labeled axonal length on 40 consecutive cervical cord sections (C4–7), as previously described [30].

Immunohistochemistry

To examine the effect of tPA on neuroblasts, proBDNF and BDNF, immunostaining was performed in five brain coronal sections and cervical spinal cord transverse sections. Briefly, 6-μm paraffin-embedded sections were deparaffinized and rehydrated. Antigen retrieval was performed by boiling sections in 10-mM citrate buffer (pH 6.0) for 10 min. After washing with PBS, sections were incubated with 0.3% H_2O_2 in PBS for 10 min, blocked with 1% BSA containing 0.3% Triton-X 100 for 1 h at room temperature, and incubated with mouse anti-DCX (1:200; Santa Cruz Biotechnology, Santa Cruz, CA) or rabbit anti-proBDNF (1:200; AbCam, Cambridge, MA) or rabbit anti-BDNF (1:200; Santa Cruz Biotechnology, CA) at 4°C overnight. For negative controls, primary antibodies were omitted. After washing, sections were incubated with biotinylated anti-mouse or anti-rabbit antibodies (1:200; Vector Laboratories, Inc., Burlingame, CA) for 30 min at room temperature. After an additional washing, sections were incubated with an avidin-biotin-peroxidase system (ABC kit, Vector Laboratories, Inc.), visualized with diaminobenzidine (Sigma, St. Louis, MO), and counterstained with hematoxylin.

Immunofluorescent Staining

Newly generated neurons in the DG were identified by double labeling for BrdU and NeuN after TBI [43]. Briefly, after being deparaffinized and rehydrated, tissue sections were boiled in 10 mM citric acid buffer (pH 6) for 10 min. After washing with PBS, sections were incubated in 2.4 N HCl at 37°C for 20 min. Sections were incubated with 1% BSA containing 0.3% Triton-X-100 in PBS. Sections were then incubated with mouse anti-NeuN antibody (1:200; Chemicon, Temecula, CA) at 4°C overnight. For negative controls, primary antibodies were omitted. FITC-conjugated anti-mouse antibody (1:400; Jackson ImmunoResearch, West Grove, PA) was added to sections at room temperature for 2 h. Sections were then incubated with rat anti-BrdU antibody (1:200; Dako, Glostrup, Denmark) at 4°C overnight. Sections were then incubated with Cy3-conjugated anti-rat antibody (1:400; Jackson ImmunoResearch, West Grove, PA) at room temperature for 2 h. Each of the steps was followed by three 5-min rinses in PBS. Tissue sections were mounted with Vectashield mounting medium (Vector laboratories, Burlingame, CA).

Cell Counting and Quantitation

Although we did not use unbiased stereology to count cells in the present study, previous studies from us and other investigators have shown that the method used provides a meaningful comparison of differences in cell counting among groups after TBI and treatment [39,44–51] and stroke [52]. Cell counts were performed by observers blinded to the individual treatment status of the animals. For quantitative measurements of immunostaining positive cells in brain, 5 coronal brain slides from each rat were employed, with each slide containing 5 fields of view from the lesion boundary zone from the epicenter of the injury cavity (bregma −3.3 mm), 3 fields of view from the ipsilateral CA3 and 9 fields of view from the ipsilateral DG in the same section. For quantitative measurements of immunostaining positive cells in cervical spinal cord (C4–7), 10 transverse sections from each rat were used. For analysis of proBDNF⁺ and BDNF⁺ cells, we focused on the ventral horn of the denervated cervical spinal cord and on the injured boundary zone of ipsilateral cortex. For analysis of neurogenesis, we focused on the ipsilateral DG and its subregions, including the subgranular zone, granular cell layer, and the molecular layer. The number of BrdU⁺ cells (red stained) and NeuN/BrdU-colabeled cells (yellow after merge) were counted in the DG. The percentage of NeuN/BrdU-colabeled cells over the total number of BrdU⁺ cells in the DG was estimated and used as a parameter to evaluate neurogenesis [53]. The fields of interest were digitized under the light microscope (Nikon, Eclipse 80i, Melville, NY) at a magnification of either 200 or 400 using CoolSNAP color camera (Photometrics, Tucson, AZ) interfaced with MetaMorph image analysis system (Molecular Devices, Downingtown, PA). The immunopositive cells were calculated and divided by the measured areas, and presented as numbers per square mm. All the counting was performed on a computer monitor to improve visualization and in one focal plane to avoid oversampling [54].

Western Blot Analyses

Animals were sacrificed on Day 8 after TBI (24 hr later after tPA treatment). The ipsilateral cortical tissues from lesion boundary zone and denervated cervical spinal cord (right side of C1–7) were dissected, frozen in liquid nitrogen and stored at −80°C. Brain and spinal cord tissues were thawed and lysed in lysis buffer containing 20 mM Tris pH 7.6, 100 mM NaCl, 1% Nonidet P-40, 0.1% SDS, 1% deoxycholic acid, 10% glycerol, 1 mM EDTA, 1 mM NaVO₃, and 50 mM NaF (Calbiochem, San Diego, CA). After sonication, soluble protein was obtained by centrifugation at 13,000×g for 15 min at 4°C. Total protein

concentrations were determined with bicinchoninic acid (BCA) protein assay (Pierce, Rockford, IL). Equal amounts of lysate were subjected to SDS-polyacrylamide electrophoresis on Novex tris-glycine pre-cast gels (Life Technologies, Grand Island, NY) and separated proteins were then electrotransferred to polyvinylidene fluoride (PVDF) membranes (Millipore, Bedford, MA). After exposure to various antibodies, specific proteins were visualized using SuperSignal West Pico chemiluminescence substrate system (Pierce Rockford, IL). Antibodies used for Western blot included anti-proBDNF (1:1000; AbCam, Cambridge, MA), anti-BDNF (1:1000; Santa Cruz Biotechnology, Santa Cruz, CA), anti-tPA (1:2000; H-90: sc-15364, Santa Cruz Biotechnology, Santa Cruz, CA), and anti-Actin (1:5000, Santa Cruz Biotechnology, Santa Cruz, CA). The band intensity was analyzed using Scion image software (Scion, Frederick, MD) [55].

ELISA Assay of Human tPA

To determine the efficiency of intranasal delivery, tPA knockout mice weighing 22–25 g (n = 3/group, Jackson Laboratory, Bar Harbor, ME) were treated with 300 μg recombinant human tPA (ten 3-μl drops) intranasally. The mice were euthanized at 30 min or 120 min after the start of intranasal and brain extracts prepared for human tPA total antigen assay. The human tPA content in the brain of tPA knockout mice was quantitated using a Human tPA Total Antigen ELISA Assay kit (Molecular Innovations, Novi, MI) according to the manufacturer's recommendations. Free and complexed human tPA were detected by the assay. This kit does not cross react with mouse or rat tPA. Brain extract samples were performed with the 96-well strip format ELISA kit. Human tPA bound to the capture antibody coated on the microtiter plate. After appropriate washing steps, anti-human tPA primary antibody bound to the captured protein. Excess primary antibody was washed away and bound antibody was reacted with the secondary antibody conjugated to horseradish peroxidase. Following an additional washing step, tetramethylbenzidine chromogenic substrate was used for color development at 450 nm. Color

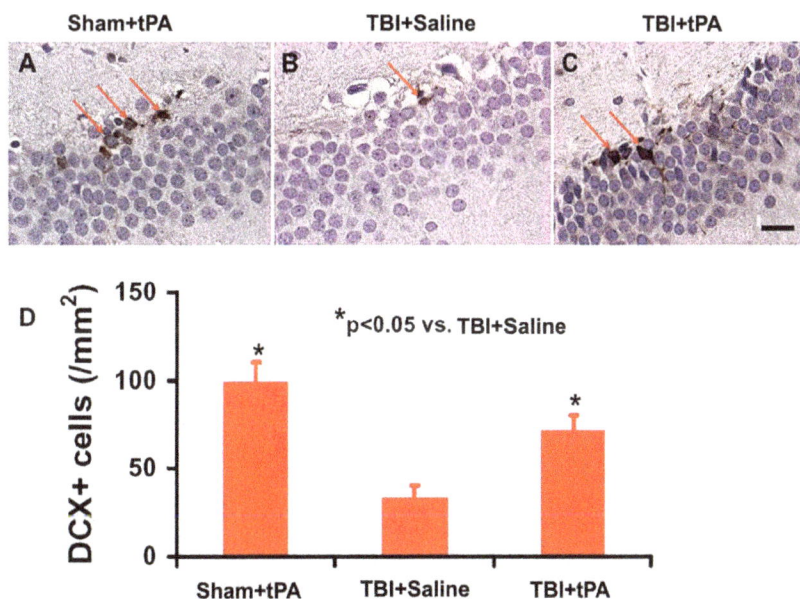

Figure 3. tPA effect on immature neurons after TBI. DCX staining (A–C). tPA significantly increased immature neurons identified with DCX-positive staining in the DG in rats examined 35 days after injury compared with the saline-treated group. The bar graph shows the number of DCX-positive cells. Scale bar = 25 μm. *p<0.05 vs TBI+Saline. Data represent mean ± SD. n = 8 (rats/group).

development was proportional to the concentration of human tPA in the brain samples. A standard calibration curve was prepared in blocking buffer using dilutions of purified human tPA and was measured along with the test samples. The human tPA content was represented as ng/g wet brain tissue.

Amidolytic Assay for Plasmin Activity

We performed colorimetric assays of plasmin in the lysates of brain tissues using D-Val-Leu-Lysp-Nitroanilide Dihydrochloride (S-2251) (Sigma-Aldrich, Saint Louis, MO) as a specific substrate for plasmin [56]. At the time of assay, the frozen brain tissues were thawed on ice, minced in sample buffer containing 50 mM Tris (pH 7.7), 0.2% (v/v) Triton X-100, 50 mM NaCl and 3 mM EDTA. Brain homogenates were prepared as described above for Western blot. To 5 μl of brain total protein extracts (23–50 μg protein), we added 55 μl of assay medium including 1.2 mM S-2251 according to the manufacture's instructions. The samples were incubated at 37°C in flat-bottomed 96-well microtiter plates and monitored the release of para-nitroaniline (pNA) in each well at 405 nm with a micro-ELISA auto reader (Fusion TM AFUSO model, Perkins Elmer Inc, Shelton, CT, USA). Each sample was measured in duplicate. Plasmin enzymatic activity was calculated based on the change of optical density over time, then normalized by protein content, and data were expressed as percentage of increase as compared to sham values.

Indirect Amidolytic Assay for tPA Activity

We performed indirect measurement of tPA activity in the lysates of brain tissues, based on an amidolytic assay with addition of plasminogen to the assay system where tPA cleaves plasminogen to plasmin, by assessing plasmin activity on S-2251, as described previously based on an amidolytic assay that detects the activation of plasminogen to plasmin that cleaves S-2251 to form pNA, as described previously [56–58]. The change in absorbance of the pNA in the reaction solution at 405 nm is directly proportional to the enzymatic activity of plasmin generated by tPA through cleavage of plasminogen. Measurements were performed on brain total protein extracts prepared as above described for plasmin activity assay. To 5 μl of brain extracts, we added 55 μl of assay medium including 1.2 mM S-2251 and plasminogen (4 μg/ml). The samples were incubated at 37°C in flat-bottomed microtiter plates and monitored the release of pNA in each well at 405 nm with a micro-ELISA auto reader (Fusion TM AFUSO model; Perkins Elmer Inc, Shelton, CT, USA). Each sample was measured in duplicate. tPA enzymatic activity was calculated based on the change of optical density over time, then normalized by protein content and data were expressed as percentage of increase as compared to sham values.

Direct Zymography Assay for tPA Activity

Using a human recombinant tPA (h-r-tPA) as a positive control to distinguish tPA from uPA, we measured tPA activity by direct zymography, as described previously by us [11,55,59] and others [60,61]. Briefly, 25 μg protein samples were mixed with the sample loading buffer without β-mercaptoethanol, and heating was omitted. The mixture of the lower gel (10% acrylamide) contained casein (1 mg/ml, Sigma) and plasminogen (13 μg/ml, American Diagnostica, Greenwich, CT) as substrates for plasmin and tPA, respectively. The gel was then washed for 30 min with 2.5% Triton X-100 to remove SDS and further washed for 10 min with 0.1 M Tris buffer, pH 8. The new Tris buffer was replaced and the gel was incubated for 4 hrs at 37°C to allow caseinolysis occur. On the darkly stained casein background, tPA activity was visualized as light bands resulting from casein degradation. To

verify tPA and distinguish from uPA, human recombinant tPA (15 ng, Genentech) was used a positive control. To verify loading variations, duplicate samples were used in gel electrophoresis. After electrophoresis, the gel was stained with Coomassie Blue R-250 and destained with 40% methanol as well as 10% acetic acid.

Statistical Analyses

All data are presented as the means + standard deviation. Data were analyzed by analysis of variance (ANOVA) for repeated measurements of functional tests (spatial performance and sensorimotor function). For lesion volume, cell counting, axonal sprouting, Western blot data, plasmin and tPA activities, a one-way ANOVA followed by post hoc Student-Newman-Keuls tests was used to compare the difference between the tPA-treated, saline-treated and sham groups. Pearson's correlation coefficients were calculated between functional recovery and anatomic reorganization. Statistical significance was set at $p < 0.05$.

Results

tPA Protein Level and Activity in Brain Extracts after Intranasal Administration of tPA

In this study, to avoid potential interference of endogenous tPA with the assay, we first administered human recombinant tPA intranasally into tPA knockout mice. The concentrations of total human tPA were 307 ± 10 ng/g and 228 ± 67 ng/g in brain tissue at 30 and 120 min, respectively after tPA delivered intranasally, indicating that intranasal delivery is an efficacious method to deliver tPA into the brain and a considerable amount of tPA remains in the brain at least up to 2 h after intranasal administration. Our data further demonstrated that brain tPA protein level determined by Western blot was significantly higher in tPA-treated sham rats and tPA-treated TBI rats 24 hr after intranasal administration than that in the saline-treated TBI rats (Fig. 1A and 1B, $p < 0.05$). This result is consistent with the zymographic assay of tPA activity (Fig. 1C and 1D, $p < 0.05$), showing a significantly higher tPA activity in the brain extracts 24 hr after tPA administration relative to the saline group. We

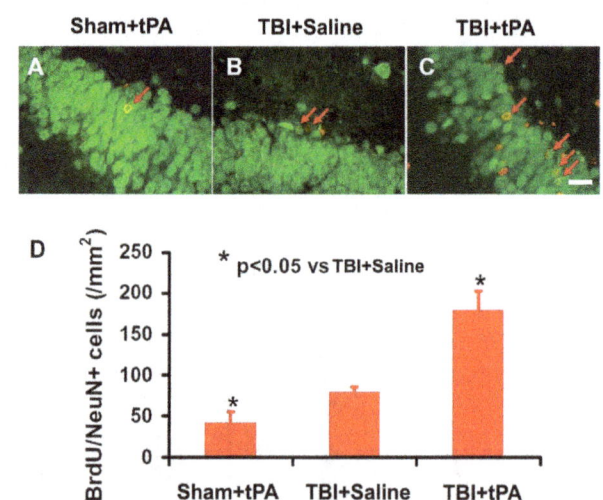

Figure 4. tPA effect on neurogenesis after TBI. Compared to the TBI+Saline group (B), tPA treatment (C) significantly increased newborn mature neurons identified with BrdU/NeuN double immunofluorescent staining in the DG 35 days post injury. The bar graph (D) shows the number of DCX-positive cells. Scale bar = 25 μm. *$p < 0.05$ vs TBI+Saline. Data represent mean ± SD. n = 8 (rats/ group).

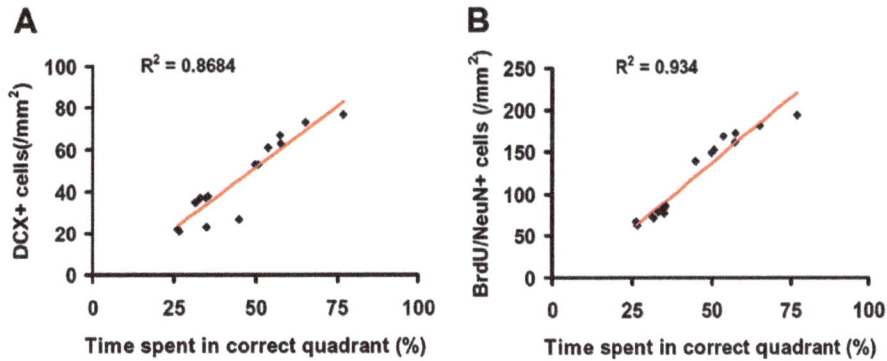

Figure 5. Correlation of the number of neuroblasts (A), and newborn neurons (B) with spatial learning. The line graph shows that spatial learning is significantly correlated with the number of DCX-positive cells (A) and to the number of newborn mature neurons (B) in the DG of the ipsilateral hippocampus in rats examined at 35 days after TBI and tPA treatment ($p<0.05$).

measured plasmin activity of brain extracts with S-2251 (without addition of plasminogen in the assay system), demonstrating that plasmin activity was higher in tPA-treated animals than that in the saline-treated group at 2 days after TBI (Fig. 1E, $p<0.05$). Furthermore, the tPA activity measured by indirect amidolytic assay (Fig. 1F) is in line with that detected by direct zymography assay (Fig. 1C and 1D). Interestingly, the tPA protein level and activity in the injured brain were significantly higher than those in the sham brain although these animals received the same dose of tPA (Fig. 1 and 2, $p<0.05$).

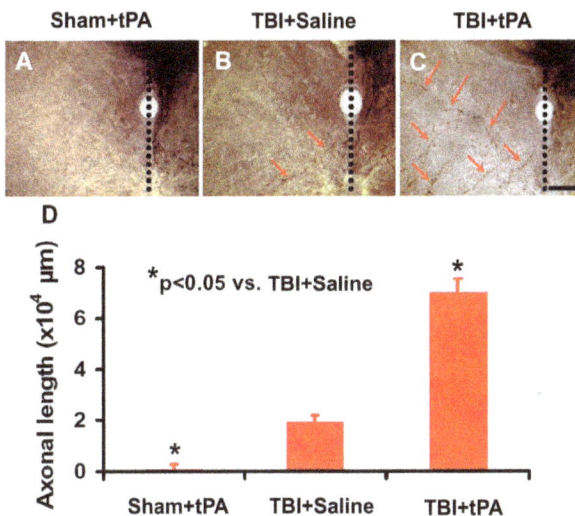

Figure 6. BDA-labeling of CST originating from the contralesional intact hemisphere. Representative images from the cervical spinal cord show BDA-labeled CST axons crossing the midline (arrows in B) and sprouting into the denervated side of the ventral gray matter in a rat after TBI. tPA treatment significantly increased the axon midline crossing (arrows in C). There were no obvious BDA-labeled axons observed in the opposite side of the cervical spinal cord in sham rats (A). Quantitative data (D) show that the number of contralesional CST in the denervated cervical gray matter was increased significantly by traumatic injury ($p<0.05$ vs. Sham+tPA) and tPA treatment ($p<0.05$ vs. TBI+Saline). Scale bar =50 μm. Data represent mean ± SD. n =8 (rats/group).

Subacute Intranasal tPA Administration Significantly Reduced Sensorimotor Deficits after TBI

The modified neurological severity score (mNSS) score was close to 12 in TBI rats (both the vehicle and tPA group) on Day 1 post controlled cortical impact (CCI)-induced TBI, indicating neurological functional deficits were comparable in all TBI rats (Fig. 2A). Spontaneous functional recovery occurred in the saline-treated animals. However, significantly improved functional recovery (that is, reduced mNSS score) was observed after TBI in the tPA group compared to the saline-treated group ($p<0.05$ on Days 14–35). tPA treatment also significantly reduced the frequency of right forelimb foot fault occurrence as compared to saline controls (Fig. 2B, $p<0.05$ on Days 14–35).

Subacute Intranasal tPA Administration Significantly Improved Spatial Learning after TBI

Spatial learning was performed during the last five days (31–35 days post injury) prior to sacrifice using the modified Morris water maze (MWM) test, which is very sensitive to the hippocampal injury [24]. The greater the percentage of time the animals spend in the correct quadrant (i.e., Northeast, where the hidden platform was located) in the water maze, the better the spatial learning function. The percentage of time spent by sham rats in the correct quadrant increased significantly from 32–35 days after sham operation, as compared to time spent in the correct quadrant at Day 31 (Fig. 2C, $p<0.05$). The spatial learning function in the vehicle-treated TBI rats was significantly impaired compared to sham rats at 33–35 days after TBI ($p<0.05$). TBI rats treated with tPA showed significant improvement in spatial learning at 33–35 days when compared to the TBI rats treated with saline ($p<0.05$).

Subacute Intranasal tPA Administration Significantly Increased Neuroblasts and Neurogenesis in the Dentate Gyrus after TBI

Immature newborn neurons in the DG were identified by doublecortin (DCX) staining. tPA significantly increased the number of DCX-positive cells compared to saline (Fig. 3, $p<0.05$). Double immunostaining for BrdU (proliferating marker) and NeuN (mature neuronal marker) was performed to identify newly generated neurons in the DG. tPA treatment significantly increased the number of newborn neurons in the DG compared to vehicle controls (Fig. 4, $p<0.05$). Our data further show that

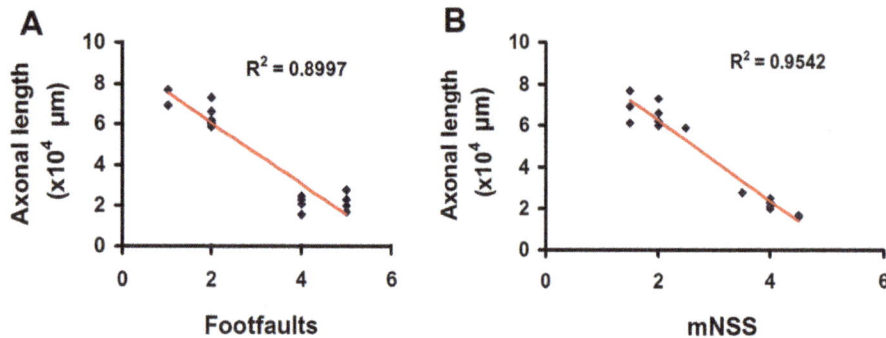

Figure 7. Correlation of the total length of axons crossing the midline at the cervical spinal cord with the right forelimb foot fault (A) and the mNSS score (B). The line graph shows that the total length of axonal crossing at the midline of the cervical level of the spinal cord is significantly reversely correlated with the incidence of forelimb footfault (A) and mNSS score (B) in rats examined at 35 days after TBI and tPA treatment ($p<0.05$).

spatial learning was highly correlated to the number of DCX-positive cells (Fig. 5A, $R^2 = 0.8684$, $p<0.05$) and to the number of newborn mature neurons (Fig. 5B, $R^2 = 0.934$, $p<0.05$) in the DG of the ipsilateral hippocampus examined at Day 35 after TBI.

Subacute Intranasal tPA Administration Significantly Promoted Midline-Crossing CST Axon Sprouting into the Denervated Side of the Cervical Spinal Cord after TBI

To verify the neuroanatomical substrate of sensorimotor functional recovery after TBI, we injected an anterograde neuronal tracer biotinylated dextran amine (BDA) into the contralesional sensorimotor cortex to label the CST originating from this area. Our data showed that tPA treatment significantly increased CST axonal sprouting originating from the contralesional cortex crossing the midline to innervate the TBI-impaired cervical spinal cord (Fig. 6). Our data further show that the total length of axons crossing the midline at the cervical spinal cord was highly and inversely correlated to the incidence of forelimb footfaults examined at Day 35 after TBI (Fig. 7A, $R^2 = 0.8997$, $p<0.05$). Furthermore, the total length of axons crossing the midline at cervical spinal cord was highly and inversely correlated to the mNSS score assessed at Day 35 after TBI (Fig. 7B, $R^2 = 0.9542$, $p<0.05$).

Electrophysiological Assessment of Functional Reorganization in the Contralesional Hemisphere after TBI

In this study, we performed ICMS on the right cortex and electromyogram (EMG) recording of the forelimb extensor muscles to test the contribution of the contralesional cortex to functional recovery in rats after TBI. The current threshold evoking movement in both forelimbs simultaneously was measured at 4 stimulation points. Current thresholds were at low levels to evoke left forelimb movement, and were comparable in all normal and TBI animals (Fig. 8, mean range 19–22 μA). In normal animals, threshold values evoking right forelimb movements were much higher than those required to evoke movement in the left forelimb (mean range 69–97 μA). However, 5 weeks after TBI the mean threshold in the contralesional right cortex eliciting movement in right-sided TBI-impaired forelimbs was significantly decreased (mean range 47–78 μA, $p<0.05$ vs Sham). tPA further reduced the mean threshold in the contralesional right cortex

eliciting movement in the right-sided TBI-impaired forelimbs (mean range 45–63 μA, $p<0.05$ vs saline controls).

Subacute Intranasal tPA Administration Reduced ProBDNF and Increased Mature BDNF Protein Level after TBI

To investigate the molecular mechanisms by which tPA promotes neuroplasticity and functional recovery, we examined the protein levels of proBDNF and BDNF in the cortex of injured brain and denervated cervical spinal cord in rats after TBI treated with tPA. TBI significantly increased ProBDNF protein level and decreased BDNF level in the cortex of injured brain and denervated cervical spinal cord while delayed intranasal tPA treatment significantly reduced the proBDNF protein level and increased BDNF level, as shown by immunostaining (Fig. 9) and Western blot analyses of pro/mature BDNF (Fig. 10), respectively. In the present study, although 4 rats were used for immunostaining, the statistical analysis using a one-way ANOVA followed by post hoc Student-Newman-Keuls tests reveals a significant difference in BDNF+ and ProBDNF+ cell density in brain cortex and spinal cord between the saline and tPA treatments. The number of animals used in this study is in agreement with previous studies in TBI using a minimal number of animals (n = 4 or less) for immunostaining by us [62] and many other investigators [63–67].

Subacute Intranasal tPA Administration Did Not Alter Cortical Lesion Volume after TBI

Lesion volume was measured 35 days post TBI. Delayed intranasal tPA treatment initiated at 7 days post injury did not alter lesion volume compared to vehicle controls (Fig. 11, $12.8\pm2.4\%$ for TBI+Saline rats vs $11.9\pm1.6\%$ for TBI+tPA rats, $p>0.05$).

Discussion

The present study demonstrates that subacute intranasal administration of tPA initiated 7 days after injury and repeated once at 14 days did not alter lesion size but significantly promoted neurological functional recovery in rats after TBI compared to treatment with saline. The subacute intranasal tPA treatment significantly increased immature and mature neurons in the DG of the ipsilateral hippocampus, which was significantly correlated with spatial learning detected by the MMW test. tPA also

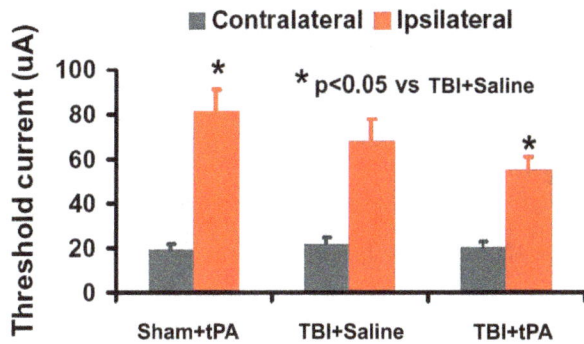

Figure 8. Mean threshold current levels needed to evoke forelimb movements on stimulation of the right cerebral motor cortex. For each animal, the threshold average was calculated from 4 stimulation points. ICMS of the motor cortex in normal adult rats evoked low threshold contralateral forelimb movements and high threshold ipsilateral movements. After TBI, the contralateral movement threshold (for left normal forelimb) was unchanged, whereas the ipsilateral movement threshold was decreased significantly at 5 weeks postinjury compared to sham ($p<0.05$). tPA treatment further reduced the threshold current needed for ipsilateral forelimb movement compared to the saline controls ($p<0.05$). Data represent mean ± SD. n = 8 (rats/group).

significantly enhanced axonal sprouting from the intact CST into the denervated side of the cervical spinal cord, which was significantly correlated with sensorimotor functional recovery assessed by the footfault and mNSS tests. ICMS on the right cortex and EMG recording from the forelimb extensor muscles imply that new neuronal connections were established between the intact cerebral hemisphere and the impaired forelimb after TBI. Our findings further indicate that tPA reduced proBDNF and increased BDNF protein level in the injured brain and denervated cervical spinal cord. Our data demonstrated that levels of tPA protein and activity in the brain extracts 24 hr after intranasal administration of tPA in the tPA-treated animals were significantly

higher than those in the saline-treated group. Taken together, our data suggest that subacute intranasal tPA treatment improves functional recovery, at least in part, by enhancing endogenous brain neurogenesis and CST axonal sprouting, which is associated with tPA/plasmin-dependent maturation of BDNF.

Neuroprotective approaches have historically been dominated by targeting neuron-based injury mechanisms as the primary or even exclusive focus of the therapeutic strategy [68]. The failure of all recent clinical trials for TBI targeting neuroprotection suggests that we need to consider new approaches to the study and development of therapeutic agents. The aim of this study was to test whether intranasal tPA administration would be a new noninvasive neurorestorative treatment for subacute TBI. A wide distribution of tPA biosynthesis in the brain is associated with different actions of tPA, such as facilitating synaptic plasticity [69] and axonal regeneration [70], which may contribute to neural repair after injury. After acute ischemic stroke, the thrombolytic effect of intravenous tPA administration in the intravascular space is beneficial, whereas its extravascular effect on ischemic neurons may be deleterious. It was documented that direct intracerebral perfusion of the tPA solution (15 and 30 µmol/L) via a microdialysis probe caused brain tissue damage in normal rats [71]. Interestingly, acute (10 min post injury) intracortical injection of the t-PA: plasminogen activator inhibitor 1 complex promotes neurovascular injury in mouse models of TBI by upregulating matrix metalloproteinase-3 [72]. The tPA dose, administration time, and route used in our present study was chosen based on our previous study in stroke rats [20], which shows robust therapeutic effects in rats after stroke. In the present study, we focused on the efficacy of delayed (7 days post TBI) intranasal administration of tPA in an animal model of TBI. Reduction in lesion volume after a cortical controlled impact injury is often used to imply recovery of function in animal models of TBI after neuroprotective treatment [1]. The finding from the present study shows that delayed intranasal tPA therapy without reduction of the lesion is capable of improving functional recovery. However, high concentrations of tPA via direct intracerebral perfusion of the tPA solution cause brain tissue damage in normal

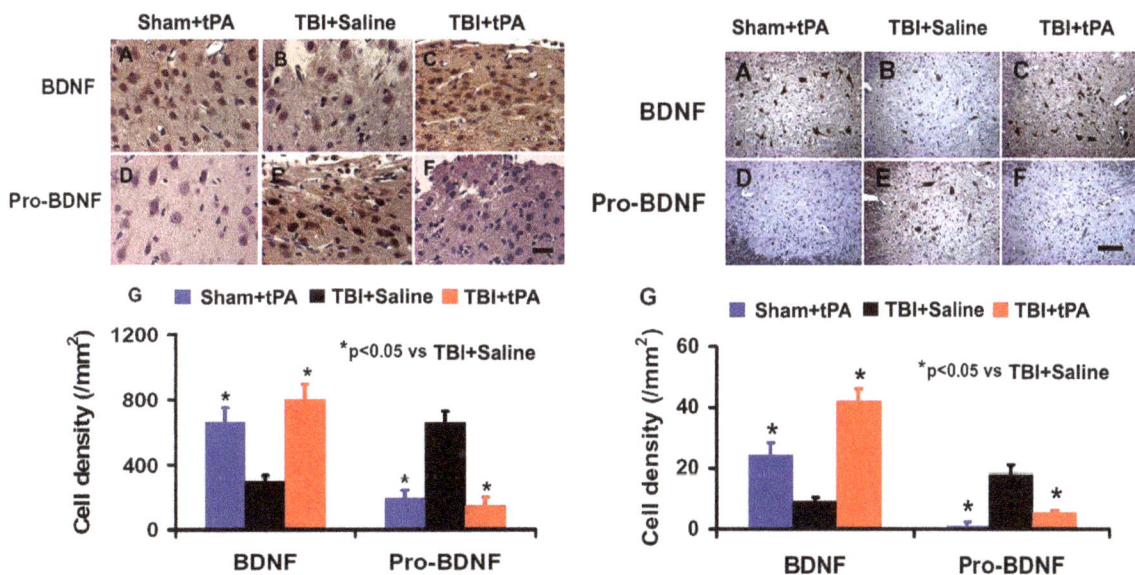

Figure 9. Immunostaining analysis of ProBDNF and mature BDNF-positive cells in the brain and spinal cord. Left panel: ipsilateral brain cortex; Right panel: denervated cervical spinal cord. *$p<0.05$ vs TBI+Saline. Scale bar = 25 µm. Data represent mean ± SD. n = 4 (rats/group).

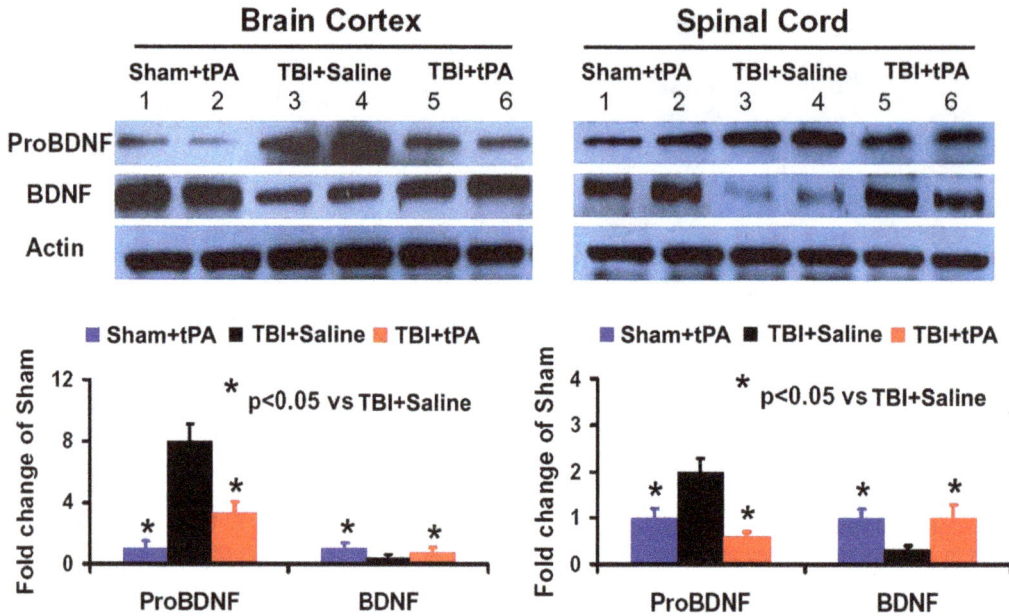

Figure 10. Western blot analysis of ProBDNF and mature BDNF protein levels in the brain and spinal cord. Left panel (ipsilateral brain cortex): Sham+tPA (1, 2), TBI+Saline (3, 4); 3: TBI+tPA (5, 6); Right panel (denervated cervical spinal cord): Sham+tPA (1, 2), TBI+Saline (3, 4), TBI+tPA (5, 6). *$p<0.05$ vs TBI+Saline. Data represent mean ± SD. $n=4$ (rats/group).

rats [71]. Here, we take advantage of intranasal tPA delivery during the subacute phase after TBI. We demonstrated that intranasal administration of h-r-tPA increases brain tPA protein level and tPA activity as measured by Western blot, ELISA, amidolytic assay, and zymography although the exact amount of active h-r-tPA entering the brain via the intranasal route is actually unknown. We do not expect that a vast amount of active tPA was delivered intranasally to the brain after TBI. It is possible that only small amounts of active tPA are needed to produce the beneficial effects as reported in this study. Interestingly, the tPA protein level

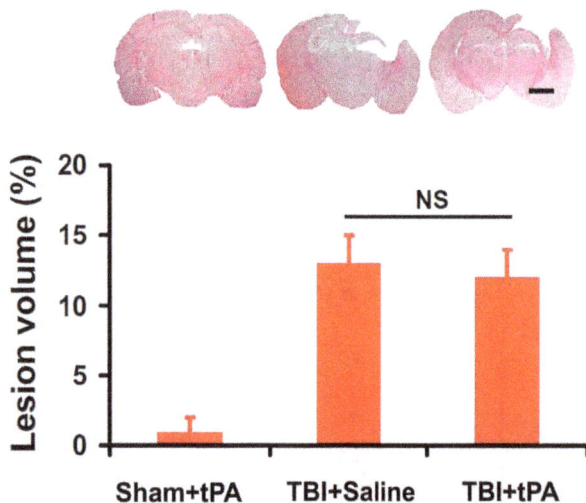

Figure 11. Cortical lesion volume after TBI and tPA treatment. The bar graph shows no significance (NS) in the cortical lesion volume between the TBI+Saline and TBI+tPA groups examined at 35 days post injury ($p>0.05$). Scale bar $=2$ mm. Data represent mean ± SD. $n=8$ (rats/group).

and activity in the injured brain (TBI+tPA group) were significantly higher than those in the Sham+tPA rat brain although these animals received the same dose of tPA. The reason for this difference remains unclear. Although we did not determine the amount of tPA administered which actually entered rat brain, the increase in brain tPA level was not attributed to endogenous tPA after TBI because the tPA level in the injured rat without tPA treatment (TBI+Saline group) was low. We cannot exclude the possibilities that the difference in brain tPA activity may result from the more tPA delivery to the injured brain than to the normal brain or likely reduced levels of specific tPA inhibitors including plasminogen activator inhibitor-1 (PAI-1) and neuroserpin [73], investigation of which is warranted. Our data provide a proof-of-principle supporting the hypothesis that intranasal tPA administration in rats during the subacute phase after TBI provides neurorestorative effects by promoting neuroplasticity (neurogenesis and axonal sprouting) and enhancing neurological recovery, while not reducing the lesion volume.

The role of tPA after brain injury is not fully understood. It is known that tPA plays a detrimental role in acute TBI [18,72,74–76]. For example, a previous study demonstrated that acute intravenous injection of free tPA into rats 15 min after TBI caused significantly larger cortical injuries and greater cerebral hemorrhage [18]. However, 30 min after TBI, intravenous injection of a mutant tPA protein tPA-S481A lacking the catalytic activity but maintaining other functions of the wild type tPA reduced neurotoxicity caused by untoward NMDA-receptor activation mediated by increased tPA and glutamate [74,75,77]. Further investigation of the beneficial effects of mutant tPA on functional recovery is warranted in animal models of TBI. Our present study differs from acute studies in that we deliver tPA initially at 7 days post TBI, intranasally. Although we did not directly measure cerebral hemorrhage, our delayed intranasal tPA administration did not alter lesion size but promoted neuroplasticity including increased brain neurogenesis and CST axonal sprouting. In our previous stroke study, we have shown that intranasal tPA administration in the subacute phase starting 7 days after ischemic stroke in rats and repeated 14 days significantly enhances sensorimotor functional recovery by promoting axonal sprouting into the denervated side of the spinal cord [20]. No adverse effects or hemorrhage were observed in the intranasally delivered tPA-treated stroke animals. In addition, increased endogenous tPA has been implicated to promote brain repair and functional recovery with neurorestorative therapies in rats after subacute brain injuries including stroke [11,78] and TBI [12]. These results indicate that tPA is beneficial if given intranasally at the subacute stage after TBI. In the present study, tPA was administered at 7 and 14 days postinjury (DPI); however, the critical period for functional recovery (Fig. 1A, 1B) was clearly between 7 and 14 DPI. After that period, the slopes of the functional recovery of TBI +Saline and TBI +tPA rats are similar, suggesting that administration at 14 DPI may not be necessary and that the first administration at 7 DPI is sufficient to significantly enhance neurological recovery.

Our ICMS-EMG data indicate that new neuronal connections are established between the intact cerebral hemisphere and the impaired side of the body after TBI and these neuronal connections are further enhanced by tPA treatment. ICMS has been used to define movement representations in motor cortex [79] and to evaluate changes in plasticity in the motor cortex following motor system lesion [80] by applying stimulative current on cortical pyramidal neurons through efferent connections to the spinal motoneurons to elicit limb movement. In the present study, we performed ICMS on the right contralesional cortex and EMG recording of the bilateral forelimb extensor muscles. The lower threshold current evoking ipsilateral forelimb movement suggested an increased neuronal coupling between the intact motor cortex and the spinal motor neurons in the denervated side of the ventral horn. Our ICMS-EMG data are consistent with increased BDA-labeled CST axonal sprouting originating from the contralesional hemisphere at the cervical level. In the present study, using BDA labeling and ICMS-EMG recording, we have found that intranasal tPA facilitates the structural and functional links between the denervated cervical spinal cord and intact motor cortex after subacute TBI. However, other descending pathways in the spinal cord such as the corticorubral tract may also undergo remodeling, which may be beneficial to functional recovery. We cannot exclude this possibility.

Continuous generation of new neurons from neural stem/progenitor cells in the subgranular zone of the DG is essential for hippocampus-dependent learning and memory [81]. Increased neurogenesis occurs in the hippocampus of adult animals and humans after TBI, which may contribute to spontaneous hippocampus-dependent functional recovery [6,82,83]. Preclinical data from us and others have shown that a large proportion of newly generated cells in the DG die within one month in rodents after TBI [82,84]. In the present study, compared to saline controls, tPA treatment increased the number of immature neurons (DCX$^+$ cells) and mature neurons (BrdU/NeuN$^+$ cells) in the DG examined at 35 days after TBI, suggesting that tPA treatment stimulates and supports adult neurogenesis in the hippocampus following TBI. Previous studies show that adult newborn neurons in the DG display typical features of mature granule cells within 4 weeks of their birth [85,86]. At 1 month, these cells have the morphological and physiological characteristics of granule cells, and their full maturation and incorporation into functional circuits appears to be a prolonged process [87]. Indeed, newborn neuron physiology, plasticity, and circuitry may continually evolve for at least 3 months [87]. Thus, further investigation of the long-term effects of tPA treatment is

warranted. Taken together, these results suggest that tPA has therapeutic potential as a noninvasive neurorestorative agent to improve functional recovery during the subacute phase after brain injury.

The molecular mechanisms underlying tPA-mediated brain and spinal cord neuroplasticity associated with functional recovery after subacute TBI remain unclear. Our present study demonstrates that tPA reduces proBDNF level and increases mature BDNF level in the injured brain and denervated cervical spinal cord, indicating a potential conversion of proBDNF to BDNF after tPA treatment. Our previous study indicates that intranasal delivery is an efficacious method to deliver tPA into the rodent brain [20]. tPA is able to activate plasminogen to plasmin, which converts the precursor proBDNF to the mature BDNF, and this conversion is critical for neuroplasticity and neuronal function [14,16,17,58,88,89]. Acute application of mature BDNF facilitates long-term potentiation (LTP) in the hippocampus [90], while inhibition of BDNF activity (by gene knockout or functional blocking using BDNF antibody) attenuates hippocampal LTP [90,91]. BDNF is involved in regulating the survival of adult-born immature neurons in the hippocampus following TBI [92]. Conversely, proneurotrophins often have biological effects that oppose those of mature neurotrophins [93,94]. For example, proBDNF has an opposing role in neurite outgrowth to that of mature BDNF, proBDNF collapses neurite outgrowth of primary neurons [14] and negatively regulates neuronal remodeling and synaptic plasticity in the hippocampus [95]. Increasing evidence indicates that dysregulation of BDNF occurs after TBI, and induction of BDNF and activation of its intracellular receptors promotes neural regeneration, reconnection, and dendritic sprouting, and improves synaptic efficacy [96]. BDNF is unable to cross the intact blood brain barrier in vivo, and it is not effective when given intravenously [97]. Treatment approaches including exercises that enhance endogenous BDNF have the potential to restore neural connectivity and functional recovery [96,98]. In addition, chondroitin sulfate proteoglycans (CSPGs) play a pivotal role in many neuronal growth mechanisms following injury to the spinal cord or brain [99]. tPA/plasmin degrades CSPGs including neurocan and phosphacan in the brain and promotes neurite reorganization after seizures [100]. tPA knockout mice exhibit attenuated neurite outgrowth and blunted sensory and motor recovery after spinal cord injury despite chondroitinase ABC (ChABC) treatment, which degrades the sugar chains of CSPGs and allows for synaptic plasticity [101]. The tPA/plasmin system specifically degrades NG2 and phosphacan after ChABC cleavage in vivo [101]. These findings show that the tPA/plasmin cascade may act downstream of ChABC to allow for synaptic plasticity improvement which enhances functional recovery after neural injury. We cannot exclude the effect of tPA/plasmin on CSPG degradation [101]. Additional studies of tPA/plasmin/CSPG interactions are warranted in TBI after tPA treatment.

Plasmin represents the critical enzyme that drives axonal plasticity and regeneration via BDNF effects and/or by degrading CSPGs [101]. Our current findings demonstrate that tPA enters the brain after intranasal administration and remains active 24 hr after the treatment, which indicates that the tPA/plasmin system is an important pathway responsible for maturation of BDNF likely by converting pro-BDNF to BDNF, suggested by our Western blot and immunostaining data. However, we did not investigate other possible pathways for BDNF maturation in the present study, and cannot exclude the tPA/plasmin-independent pathway. tPA is capable of regulating brain BDNF synthesis through a plasmin-independent effect mediating by N-methyl-D-aspartate (NMDA) receptor signaling [102]. For example, intravenous administration of recombinant tPA (10 mg/kg) induced an increase in hippo-campal recombinant tPA and mature BDNF expression in normal adult male Wistar rats 2 hr and 24 hr after tPA administration but did not increase hippocampal plasmin activity; while MK801 an NMDA receptor antagonist completely abolished the rise in mature BDNF expression induced by tPA [102]. Their data strongly suggest that exogenous tPA increases mature BDNF expression in the hippocampus through NMDA receptor activa-tion, which is independent of plasmin activity. In contrast, our data suggest that intranasal administration of tPA increased plasmin activity in the brain measured by amidolytic assay. Intranasal administration of tPA targeting the tPA/BDNF system opens a new avenue for subacute treatment of TBI. In addition, plasmin formation can also be generated by urokinase-type plasminogen activator (uPA) [103]. It is warranted to compare the effects of intranasal treatment with uPA with those of tPA after subacute TBI.

Conclusion

The present study demonstrates that intranasal administration of tPA at the subacute phase after TBI significantly improves sensorimotor and cognitive functional recovery and enhances brain neurogenesis and CST compensatory axonal remodeling, which is likely associated with tPA/plasmin-dependent maturation of BDNF. These findings suggest that tPA holds potential for a noninvasive neurorestorative treatment for subacute TBI. How-ever, further studies are warranted to discover the optimal dose and therapeutic window of intranasal tPA administration after TBI, and to investigate the molecular mechanisms underlying the therapeutic effects as well as potential side effects including brain hemorrhage.

Acknowledgments

The authors would like to thank Susan MacPhee-Gray for editorial assistance.

Author Contributions

Conceived and designed the experiments: YX MC AM. Performed the experiments: YM YZ ZL AA YX. Analyzed the data: YM YZ AA YX. Contributed reagents/materials/analysis tools: YX MC AM. Wrote the paper: YM YX MC.

References

1. Xiong Y, Mahmood A, Chopp M (2013) Animal models of traumatic brain injury. Nat Rev Neurosci 14: 128–142.
2. Gean AD, Fischbein NJ (2010) Head trauma. Neuroimaging Clin N Am 20: 527–556.
3. Narayan RK, Michel ME, Ansell B, Baethmann A, Biegon A, et al. (2002) Clinical trials in head injury. J Neurotrauma 19: 503–557.
4. Xiong Y, Zhang Y, Mahmood A, Meng Y, Zhang ZG, et al. (2012) Neuroprotective and neurorestorative effects of thymosin beta4 treatment initiated 6 hours after traumatic brain injury in rats. J Neurosurg 116: 1081–1092.
5. Zhang Y, Xiong Y, Mahmood A, Meng Y, Liu Z, et al. (2010) Sprouting of corticospinal tract axons from the contralateral hemisphere into the denervated side of the spinal cord is associated with functional recovery in adult rat after traumatic brain injury and erythropoietin treatment. Brain Res 1353: 249–257.
6. Richardson RM, Sun D, Bullock MR (2007) Neurogenesis after traumatic brain injury. Neurosurg Clin N Am 18: 169–181, xi.
7. Levin HS (2003) Neuroplasticity following non-penetrating traumatic brain injury. Brain Inj 17: 665–674.
8. Garcia AN, Shah MA, Dixon CE, Wagner AK, Kline AE (2011) Biologic and plastic effects of experimental traumatic brain injury treatment paradigms and their relevance to clinical rehabilitation. PM R 3: S18–27.
9. Adibhatla RM, Hatcher JF (2008) Tissue plasminogen activator (tPA) and matrix metalloproteinases in the pathogenesis of stroke: therapeutic strategies. CNS Neurol Disord Drug Targets 7: 243–253.
10. Yepes M, Lawrence DA (2004) New functions for an old enzyme: nonhemostatic roles for tissue-type plasminogen activator in the central nervous system. Exp Biol Med (Maywood) 229: 1097–1104.
11. Shen LH, Xin H, Li Y, Zhang RL, Cui Y, et al. (2011) Endogenous tissue plasminogen activator mediates bone marrow stromal cell-induced neurite remodeling after stroke in mice. Stroke 42: 459–464.
12. Mahmood A, Qu C, Ning R, Wu H, Goussev A, et al. (2011) Treatment of TBI with collagen scaffolds and human marrow stromal cells increases the expression of tissue plasminogen activator. J Neurotrauma 28: 1199–1207.
13. Je HS, Yang F, Ji Y, Nagappan G, Hempstead BL, et al. (2012) Role of pro-brain-derived neurotrophic factor (proBDNF) to mature BDNF conversion in activity-dependent competition at developing neuromuscular synapses. Proc Natl Acad Sci U S A 109: 15924–15929.
14. Sun Y, Lim Y, Li F, Liu S, Lu JJ, et al. (2012) ProBDNF collapses neurite outgrowth of primary neurons by activating RhoA. PLoS One 7: e35883.
15. Greenberg ME, Xu B, Lu B, Hempstead BL (2009) New insights in the biology of BDNF synthesis and release: implications in CNS function. J Neurosci 29: 12764–12767.
16. Koshimizu H, Kiyosue K, Hara T, Hazama S, Suzuki S, et al. (2009) Multiple functions of precursor BDNF to CNS neurons: negative regulation of neurite growth, spine formation and cell survival. Mol Brain 2: 27.
17. Pang PT, Teng HK, Zaitsev E, Woo NT, Sakata K, et al. (2004) Cleavage of proBDNF by tPA/plasmin is essential for long-term hippocampal plasticity. Science 306: 487–491.
18. Stein SC, Ganguly K, Belfield CM, Xu X, Swanson EW, et al. (2009) Erythrocyte-bound tissue plasminogen activator is neuroprotective in experi-mental traumatic brain injury. J Neurotrauma 26: 1585–1592.
19. Dhuria SV, Hanson LR, Frey WH 2nd (2010) Intranasal delivery to the central nervous system: mechanisms and experimental considerations. J Pharm Sci 99: 1654–1673.
20. Liu Z, Li Y, Zhang L, Xin H, Cui Y, et al. (2012) Subacute intranasal administration of tissue plasminogen activator increases functional recovery and axonal remodeling after stroke in rats. Neurobiol Dis 45: 804–809.
21. Dixon CE, Clifton GL, Lighthall JW, Yaghmai AA, Hayes RL (1991) A controlled cortical impact model of traumatic brain injury in the rat. J Neurosci Methods 39: 253–262.
22. Liu Z, Li Y, Qu R, Shen L, Gao Q, et al. (2007) Axonal sprouting into the denervated spinal cord and synaptic and postsynaptic protein expression in the spinal cord after transplantation of bone marrow stromal cell in stroke rats. Brain Res 1149: 172–180.
23. Thorne RG, Pronk GJ, Padmanabhan V, Frey WH 2nd (2004) Delivery of insulin-like growth factor-I to the rat brain and spinal cord along olfactory and trigeminal pathways following intranasal administration. Neuroscience 127: 481–496.
24. Choi SH, Woodlee MT, Hong JJ, Schallert T (2006) A simple modification of the water maze test to enhance daily detection of spatial memory in rats and mice. J Neurosci Methods 156: 182–193.
25. Morris RG, Garrud P, Rawlins JN, O'Keefe J (1982) Place navigation impaired in rats with hippocampal lesions. Nature 297: 681–683.
26. Mahmood A, Lu D, Qu C, Goussev A, Chopp M (2007) Treatment of traumatic brain injury with a combination therapy of marrow stromal cells and atorvastatin in rats. Neurosurgery 60: 546–553; discussion 553–544.
27. Baskin YK, Dietrich WD, Green EJ (2003) Two effective behavioral tasks for evaluating sensorimotor dysfunction following traumatic brain injury in mice. J Neurosci Methods 129: 87–93.
28. Chen J, Sanberg PR, Li Y, Wang L, Lu M, et al. (2001) Intravenous administration of human umbilical cord blood reduces behavioral deficits after stroke in rats. Stroke 32: 2682–2688.
29. Lu D, Mahmood A, Qu C, Hong X, Kaplan D, et al. (2007) Collagen scaffolds populated with human marrow stromal cells reduce lesion volume and improve functional outcome after traumatic brain injury. Neurosurgery 61: 596–602; discussion 602–593.
30. Liu Z, Li Y, Zhang X, Savant-Bhonsale S, Chopp M (2008) Contralesional axonal remodeling of the corticospinal system in adult rats after stroke and bone marrow stromal cell treatment. Stroke 39: 2571–2577.
31. Paxinos G, Watson C (1986) The rat brain in stereotaxic coordinates. Sydney; Orlando: Academic Press. xxvi, 237 p. of plates p.
32. Chen J, Zhang C, Jiang H, Li Y, Zhang L, et al. (2005) Atorvastatin induction of VEGF and BDNF promotes brain plasticity after stroke in mice. J Cereb Blood Flow Metab 25: 281–290.
33. Swanson RA, Morton MT, Tsao-Wu G, Savalos RA, Davidson C, et al. (1990) A semiautomated method for measuring brain infarct volume. J Cereb Blood Flow Metab 10: 290–293.
34. Thau-Zuchman O, Shohami E, Alexandrovich AG, Leker RR (2010) Vascular endothelial growth factor increases neurogenesis after traumatic brain injury. J Cereb Blood Flow Metab 30: 1008–1016.
35. Lin TN, He YY, Wu G, Khan M, Hsu CY (1993) Effect of brain edema on infarct volume in a focal cerebral ischemia model in rats. Stroke 24: 117–121.

36. Fox GB, Fan L, Levasseur RA, Faden AI (1998) Sustained sensory/motor and cognitive deficits with neuronal apoptosis following controlled cortical impact brain injury in the mouse. J Neurotrauma 15: 599–614.

37. Marklund N, Morales D, Clausen F, Hanell A, Kiwanuka O, et al. (2009) Functional outcome is impaired following traumatic brain injury in aging Nogo-A/B-deficient mice. Neuroscience 163: 540–551.

38. Qu C, Mahmood A, Ning R, Xiong Y, Zhang L, et al. (2010) The treatment of traumatic brain injury with velcade. J Neurotrauma 27: 1625–1634.

39. Xiong Y, Mahmood A, Meng Y, Zhang Y, Qu C, et al. (2010) Delayed administration of erythropoietin reducing hippocampal cell loss, enhancing angiogenesis and neurogenesis, and improving functional outcome following traumatic brain injury in rats: comparison of treatment with single and triple dose. J Neurosurg 113: 598–608.

40. Zhang C, Raghupathi R, Saatman KE, Smith DH, Stutzmann JM, et al. (1998) Riluzole attenuates cortical lesion size, but not hippocampal neuronal loss, following traumatic brain injury in the rat. J Neurosci Res 52: 342–349.

41. Zhang RL, Chopp M, Zhang ZG, Divine G (1998) Early (1 h) administration of tissue plasminogen activator reduces infarct volume without increasing hemorrhagic transformation after focal cerebral embolization in rats. J Neurol Sci 160: 1–8.

42. Wang Y, Zhang ZG, Rhodes K, Renzi M, Zhang RL, et al. (2007) Post-ischemic treatment with erythropoietin or carbamylated erythropoietin reduces infarction and improves neurological outcome in a rat model of focal cerebral ischemia. Br J Pharmacol 151: 1377–1384.

43. Xiong Y, Mahmood A, Meng Y, Zhang Y, Zhang ZG, et al. (2011) Treatment of traumatic brain injury with thymosin beta(4) in rats. J Neurosurg 114: 102–115.

44. Xiong Y, Lu D, Qu C, Goussev A, Schallert T, et al. (2008) Effects of erythropoietin on reducing brain damage and improving functional outcome after traumatic brain injury in mice. J Neurosurg 109: 510–521.

45. Meng Y, Xiong Y, Mahmood A, Zhang Y, Qu C, et al. (2011) Dose-dependent neurorestorative effects of delayed treatment of traumatic brain injury with recombinant human erythropoietin in rats. J Neurosurg 115: 550–560.

46. Ning R, Xiong Y, Mahmood A, Zhang Y, Meng Y, et al. (2011) Erythropoietin promotes neurovascular remodeling and long-term functional recovery in rats following traumatic brain injury. Brain Res 1384: 140–150.

47. Xiong Y, Mahmood A, Qu C, Kazmi H, Zhang ZG, et al. (2010) Erythropoietin improves histological and functional outcomes after traumatic brain injury in mice in the absence of the neural erythropoietin receptor. J Neurotrauma 27: 205–215.

48. Zhang Y, Xiong Y, Mahmood A, Meng Y, Qu C, et al. (2009) Therapeutic effects of erythropoietin on histological and functional outcomes following traumatic brain injury in rats are independent of hematocrit. Brain Res 1294: 153–164.

49. Singleton RH, Yan HQ, Fellows-Mayle W, Dixon CE (2010) Resveratrol attenuates behavioral impairments and reduces cortical and hippocampal loss in a rat controlled cortical impact model of traumatic brain injury. J Neurotrauma 27: 1091–1099.

50. Han X, Tong J, Zhang J, Farahvar A, Wang E, et al. (2011) Imipramine treatment improves cognitive outcome associated with enhanced hippocampal neurogenesis after traumatic brain injury in mice. J Neurotrauma 28: 995–1007.

51. Barha CK, Ishrat T, Epp JR, Galea LA, Stein DG (2011) Progesterone treatment normalizes the levels of cell proliferation and cell death in the dentate gyrus of the hippocampus after traumatic brain injury. Exp Neurol 231: 72–81.

52. Zhang R, Wang Y, Zhang L, Zhang Z, Tsang W, et al. (2002) Sildenafil (Viagra) induces neurogenesis and promotes functional recovery after stroke in rats. Stroke 33: 2675–2680.

53. Xiong Y, Mahmood A, Lu D, Qu C, Kazmi H, et al. (2008) Histological and functional outcomes after traumatic brain injury in mice null for the erythropoietin receptor in the central nervous system. Brain Res 1230: 247–257.

54. Zhang R, Wang Y, Zhang L, Zhang Z, Tsang W, et al. (2002) Sildenafil (Viagra) induces neurogenesis and promotes functional recovery after stroke in rats. Stroke 33: 2675–2680.

55. Xin H, Li Y, Shen LH, Liu X, Hozeska-Solgot A, et al. (2011) Multipotent mesenchymal stromal cells increase tPA expression and concomitantly decrease PAI-1 expression in astrocytes through the sonic hedgehog signaling pathway after stroke (in vitro study). J Cereb Blood Flow Metab 31: 2181–2188.

56. Friberger P, Knos M, Gustavsson S, Aurell L, Claeson G (1978) Methods for determination of plasmin, antiplasmin and plasminogen by means of substrate S-2251. Haemostasis 7: 138–145.

57. Festoff BW, Reddy RB, VanBecelaere M, Smirnova I, Chao J (1994) Activation of serpins and their cognate proteases in muscle after crush injury. J Cell Physiol 159: 11–18.

58. Ding Q, Ying Z, Gomez-Pinilla F (2011) Exercise influences hippocampal plasticity by modulating brain-derived neurotrophic factor processing. Neuroscience 192: 773–780.

59. Ahn MY, Zhang ZG, Tsang W, Chopp M (1999) Endogenous plasminogen activator expression after embolic focal cerebral ischemia in mice. Brain Res 837: 169–176.

60. Miskin R, Soreq H (1981) Sensitive autoradiographic quantification of electrophoretically separated proteases. Anal Biochem 118: 252–258.

61. Nagai T, Yamada K, Yoshimura M, Ishikawa K, Miyamoto Y, et al. (2004) The tissue plasminogen activator-plasmin system participates in the rewarding effect of morphine by regulating dopamine release. Proc Natl Acad Sci U S A 101: 3650–3655.

62. Wu H, Lu D, Jiang H, Xiong Y, Qu C, et al. (2008) Simvastatin-mediated upregulation of VEGF and BDNF, activation of the PI3K/Akt pathway, and increase of neurogenesis are associated with therapeutic improvement after traumatic brain injury. J Neurotrauma 25: 130–139.

63. Glover LE, Tajiri N, Lau T, Kaneko Y, van Loveren H, et al. (2012) Immediate, but not delayed, microsurgical skull reconstruction exacerbates brain damage in experimental traumatic brain injury model. PLoS One 7: e33646.

64. Khan M, Im YB, Shunmugavel A, Gilg AG, Dhindsa RK, et al. (2009) Administration of S-nitrosoglutathione after traumatic brain injury protects the neurovascular unit and reduces secondary injury in a rat model of controlled cortical impact. J Neuroinflammation 6: 32.

65. Hall ED, Sullivan PG, Gibson TR, Pavel KM, Thompson BM, et al. (2005) Spatial and temporal characteristics of neurodegeneration after controlled cortical impact in mice: more than a focal brain injury. J Neurotrauma 22: 252–265.

66. Cutler SM, Cekic M, Miller DM, Wali B, VanLandingham JW, et al. (2007) Progesterone improves acute recovery after traumatic brain injury in the aged rat. J Neurotrauma 24: 1475–1486.

67. Tamas A, Zsombok A, Farkas O, Reglodi D, Pal J, et al. (2006) Postinjury administration of pituitary adenylate cyclase activating polypeptide (PACAP) attenuates traumatically induced axonal injury in rats. J Neurotrauma 23: 686–695.

68. Loane DJ, Faden AI (2010) Neuroprotection for traumatic brain injury: translational challenges and emerging therapeutic strategies. Trends Pharmacol Sci 31: 596–604.

69. Samson AL, Medcalf RL (2006) Tissue-type plasminogen activator: a multifaceted modulator of neurotransmission and synaptic plasticity. Neuron 50: 673–678.

70. Minor K, Phillips J, Seeds NW (2009) Tissue plasminogen activator promotes axonal outgrowth on CNS myelin after conditioned injury. Journal of neurochemistry 109: 706–715.

71. Goto H, Fujisawa H, Oka F, Nomura S, Kajiwara K, et al. (2007) Neurotoxic effects of exogenous recombinant tissue-type plasminogen activator on the normal rat brain. J Neurotrauma 24: 745–752.

72. Sashindranath M, Sales E, Daglas M, Freeman R, Samson AL, et al. (2012) The tissue-type plasminogen activator-plasminogen activator inhibitor 1 complex promotes neurovascular injury in brain trauma: evidence from mice and humans. Brain 135: 3251–3264.

73. Vivien D, Buisson A (2000) Serine protease inhibitors: novel therapeutic targets for stroke? J Cereb Blood Flow Metab 20: 755–764.

74. Armstead WM, Bohman LE, Riley J, Yarovoi S, Higazi AA, et al. (2013) tPA-S(481)A Prevents Impairment of Cerebrovascular Autoregulation by Endogenous tPA after Traumatic Brain Injury by Upregulating p38 MAPK and Inhibiting ET-1. J Neurotrauma 30: 1898–1907.

75. Armstead WM, Riley J, Yarovoi S, Cines DB, Smith DH, et al. (2012) tPA-S481A prevents neurotoxicity of endogenous tPA in traumatic brain injury. J Neurotrauma 29: 1794–1802.

76. Mori T, Wang X, Kline AE, Siao CJ, Dixon CE, et al. (2001) Reduced cortical injury and edema in tissue plasminogen activator knockout mice after brain trauma. Neuroreport 12: 4117–4120.

77. Armstead WM, Kiessling JW, Riley J, Cines DB, Higazi AA (2011) tPA contributes to impaired NMDA cerebrovasodilation after traumatic brain injury through activation of JNK MAPK. Neurol Res 33: 726–733.

78. Xin H, Li Y, Shen LH, Liu X, Wang X, et al. (2010) Increasing tPA activity in astrocytes induced by multipotent mesenchymal stromal cells facilitate neurite outgrowth after stroke in the mouse. PLoS One 5: e9027.

79. Neafsey EJ, Bold EL, Haas G, Hurley-Gius KM, Quirk G, et al. (1986) The organization of the rat motor cortex: a microstimulation mapping study. Brain research 396: 77–96.

80. Kartje-Tillotson G, Neafsey EJ, Castro AJ (1985) Electrophysiological analysis of motor cortical plasticity after cortical lesions in newborn rats. Brain research 332: 103–111.

81. Zhao C, Deng W, Gage FH (2008) Mechanisms and functional implications of adult neurogenesis. Cell 132: 645–660.

82. Lu D, Mahmood A, Zhang R, Copp M (2003) Upregulation of neurogenesis and reduction in functional deficits following administration of DEtA/NONOate, a nitric oxide donor, after traumatic brain injury in rats. J Neurosurg 99: 351–361.

83. Zheng W, Zhuge Q, Zhong M, Chen G, Shao B, et al. (2013) Neurogenesis in adult human brain after traumatic brain injury. J Neurotrauma 30: 1872–1880.

84. Sun D, Colello RJ, Daugherty WP, Kwon TH, McGinn MJ, et al. (2005) Cell proliferation and neuronal differentiation in the dentate gyrus in juvenile and adult rats following traumatic brain injury. J Neurotrauma 22: 95–105.

85. Toni N, Teng EM, Bushong EA, Aimone JB, Zhao C, et al. (2007) Synapse formation on neurons born in the adult hippocampus. Nat Neurosci 10: 727–734.

86. Zhao C, Teng EM, Summers RG Jr, Ming GL, Gage FH (2006) Distinct morphological stages of dentate granule neuron maturation in the adult mouse hippocampus. J Neurosci 26: 3–11.

87. Vivar C, van Praag H (2013) Functional circuits of new neurons in the dentate gyrus. Front Neural Circuits 7: 15.

88. Obiang P, Maubert E, Bardou I, Nicole O, Launay S, et al. (2011) Enriched housing reverses age-associated impairment of cognitive functions and tPA-dependent maturation of BDNF. Neurobiol Learn Mem 96: 121–129.

89. Barnes P, Thomas KL (2008) Proteolysis of proBDNF is a key regulator in the formation of memory. PLoS One 3: e3248.

90. Korte M, Carroll P, Wolf E, Brem G, Thoenen H, et al. (1995) Hippocampal long-term potentiation is impaired in mice lacking brain-derived neurotrophic factor. Proc Natl Acad Sci U S A 92: 8856–8860.

91. Figurov A, Pozzo-Miller LD, Olafsson P, Wang T, Lu B (1996) Regulation of synaptic responses to high-frequency stimulation and LTP by neurotrophins in the hippocampus. Nature 381: 706–709.

92. Gao X, Chen J (2009) Conditional knockout of brain-derived neurotrophic factor in the hippocampus increases death of adult-born immature neurons following traumatic brain injury. J Neurotrauma 26: 1325–1335.

93. Lu B, Pang PT, Woo NH (2005) The yin and yang of neurotrophin action. Nat Rev Neurosci 6: 603–614.

94. Mast TG, Fadool DA (2012) Mature and precursor brain-derived neurotrophic factor have individual roles in the mouse olfactory bulb. PLoS One 7: e31978.

95. Yang J, Harte-Hargrove LC, Siao CJ, Marinic T, Clarke R, et al. (2014) proBDNF negatively regulates neuronal remodeling, synaptic transmission, and synaptic plasticity in hippocampus. Cell Rep 7: 796–806.

96. Kaplan GB, Vasterling JJ, Vedak PC (2010) Brain-derived neurotrophic factor in traumatic brain injury, post-traumatic stress disorder, and their comorbid conditions: role in pathogenesis and treatment. Behav Pharmacol 21: 427–437.

97. Zhang Y, Pardridge WM (2006) Blood-brain barrier targeting of BDNF improves motor function in rats with middle cerebral artery occlusion. Brain Res 1111: 227–229.

98. Griesbach GS, Hovda DA, Molteni R, Wu A, Gomez-Pinilla F (2004) Voluntary exercise following traumatic brain injury: brain-derived neurotrophic factor upregulation and recovery of function. Neuroscience 125: 129–139.

99. Yi JH, Katagiri Y, Susarla B, Figge D, Symes AJ, et al. (2012) Alterations in sulfated chondroitin glycosaminoglycans following controlled cortical impact injury in mice. J Comp Neurol 520: 3295–3313.

100. Wu YP, Siao CJ, Lu W, Sung TC, Frohman MA, et al. (2000) The tissue plasminogen activator (tPA)/plasmin extracellular proteolytic system regulates seizure-induced hippocampal mossy fiber outgrowth through a proteoglycan substrate. J Cell Biol 148: 1295–1304.

101. Bukhari N, Torres L, Robinson JK, Tsirka SE (2011) Axonal regrowth after spinal cord injury via chondroitinase and the tissue plasminogen activator (tPA)/plasmin system. J Neurosci 31: 14931–14943.

102. Rodier M, Prigent-Tessier A, Bejot Y, Jacquin A, Mossiat C, et al. (2014) Exogenous t-PA Administration Increases Hippocampal Mature BDNF Levels. Plasmin- or NMDA-Dependent Mechanism? PLoS One 9: e92416.

103. Cho E, Lee KJ, Seo JW, Byun CJ, Chung SJ, et al. (2012) Neuroprotection by urokinase plasminogen activator in the hippocampus. Neurobiol Dis 46: 215–224.

9

Spinal fMRI Reveals Decreased Descending Inhibition during Secondary Mechanical Hyperalgesia

Torge Rempe[1,2]*, **Stephan Wolff**[1], **Christian Riedel**[1], **Ralf Baron**[2,3], **Patrick W. Stroman**[4], **Olav Jansen**[1], **Janne Gierthmühlen**[1,3]

1 Dept of Neuroradiology, University Hospital of Kiel, Arnold-Heller-Strasse 3, Haus 41, 24105 Kiel, Germany, 2 Dept of Neurology, University Hospital of Kiel, Arnold-Heller-Strasse 3, Haus 41, 24105 Kiel, Germany, 3 Division of Neurological Pain Research and Therapy, University Hospital of Kiel, Arnold-Heller-Strasse 3, Haus 41, 24105 Kiel, Germany, 4 Centre for Neuroscience Studies, Dept of Diagnostic Radiology, Dept of Physics, 228 Botterell Hall, Queen's University, Kingston, Ontario, Canada

Abstract

Mechanical hyperalgesia is one distressing symptom of neuropathic pain which is explained by central sensitization of the nociceptive system. This sensitization can be induced experimentally with the heat/capsaicin sensitization model. The aim was to investigate and compare spinal and supraspinal activation patterns of identical mechanical stimulation before and after sensitization using functional spinal magnetic resonance imaging (spinal fMRI). Sixteen healthy subjects (6 female, 10 male, mean age 27.2 ± 4.0 years) were investigated with mechanical stimulation of the C6 dermatome of the right forearm during spinal fMRI. Testing was always performed in the area outside of capsaicin application (i.e. area of secondary mechanical hyperalgesia). During slightly noxious mechanical stimulation before sensitization, activity was observed in ipsilateral dorsolateral pontine tegmentum (DLPT) which correlated with activity in ipsilateral spinal cord dorsal gray matter (dGM) suggesting activation of descending nociceptive inhibition. During secondary mechanical hyperalgesia, decreased activity was observed in bilateral DLPT, ipsilateral/midline rostral ventromedial medulla (RVM), and contralateral subnucleus reticularis dorsalis, which correlated with activity in ipsilateral dGM. Comparison of voxel-based activation patterns during mechanical stimulation before/after sensitization showed deactivations in RVM and activations in superficial ipsilateral dGM. This study revealed increased spinal activity and decreased activity in supraspinal centers involved in pain modulation (SRD, RVM, DLPT) during secondary mechanical hyperalgesia suggesting facilitation of nociception via decreased endogenous inhibition. Results should help prioritize approaches for further in vivo studies on pain processing and modulation in humans.

Editor: Theodore J. Price, University of Texas at Dallas, United States of America

Funding: The study was supported by the German Federal Ministry of Education and Research (BMBF, 01EM05/04). However, the authors received no specific funding for this work. The funders had no role in study design, data collection and analysis, decision to publish, or preparation of the manuscript.

Competing Interests: Ralf Baron reported grant/research support by: Pfizer, Genzyme, Grünenthal. Member of the IMI "Europain" collaboration and industry members of this are: Astra Zeneca, Pfizer, Esteve, UCB-Pharma, Sanofi Aventis, Grünenthal, Eli Lilly and Boehringer Ingelheim. German Federal Ministry of Education and Research (BMBF): German Research Network on Neuropathic Pain, Modelling Pain Switches. German Research Foundation (DFG). He received honoraria as a speaker from Pfizer, Genzyme, Grünenthal, Mundipharma, Sanofi Pasteur, Medtronic, Eisai, UCB BioSciences, Lilly, Boehringer Ingelheim, Astellas, Desitin and as a consultant from Pfizer, Genzyme, Grünenthal, Mundipharma, Allergan, Sanofi Pasteur, Medtronic, Eisai, UCB BioSciences, Lilly, Boehringer Ingelheim, Astellas, Novartis, Bristol-Myers Squibb, Biogenidec, AstraZeneca. Olav Jansen received honoraria as a speaker from Penumbra and as a consultant from Strykker, Philips and Boehringer Ingelheim. Janne Gierthmühlen received honoraria as a speaker from Pfizer and travel grants from Grünenthal. There are no conflicts of interests relevant to this article and none of the competing interests.

* Email: t.rempe@neurologie.uni-kiel.de

Introduction

Mechanical pinprick hyperalgesia is a very distressing symptom presented by approximately 29% of neuropathic pain patients [1]. During a state of hyperalgesia, an already nociceptive stimulus is perceived as even more painful [1]. Secondary hyperalgesia develops in the uninjured area surrounding a nerve injury and is caused by central sensitization, i.e. by modulation of the spinal and supraspinal nociceptive system [2,3]. It can be induced experimentally in healthy humans by the heat/capsaicin model [4].

Anatomically, the vast majority of the nociceptive second order neurons is located in the dorsal gray matter (dGM) of the spinal cord. From there they project to supraspinal nuclei in the brainstem and the thalamus before these afferent nociceptive impulses are transferred to further subcortical and cortical structures [5]. The nociceptive neurons in the spinal cord and in the brainstem have an important contribution in the transmission and modulation of pain. This knowledge is based mostly on animal experiments, observation of the effects of injury and disease as well as postmortem anatomical studies [3,6,7].

With the emergence of functional magnetic resonance imaging of the brain (fMRI) [8] and, to a lesser extent, of the brainstem [9,10], non-invasive methods have become available to provide insight into human pain processing in vivo. To investigate pain processing on the spinal level and in the brainstem, spinal fMRI is of great interest, however, its utilization is limited because of significant technical challenges such as cerebro-spinal fluid-pulsations, breathing/swallowing-motions, and the spinal cord's small cross-sectional dimension.

In order to address these challenges, recent spinal fMRI studies use a turbo spin-echo sequence with a relatively short echo time rather than the more conventional gradient echo imaging sequence sensitive to the blood oxygenation level-dependent (BOLD) effect [11–14]. It demonstrates BOLD contrast but also reveals a second contrast mechanism and important source of neuronal activity-related signal change in spinal fMRI termed "signal enhancement by extravascular water protons" (SEEP). This functionally induced signal is thought to originate from cellular swelling and thus changed extravascular water content due to increased intravascular pressure at sites of activity. This new technique is believed to localize sites of neuronal activity more precisely than conventional T_2*-weighted gradient echo imaging sequences, which have rather poor field homogeneity [11–14].

However, spinal fMRI studies of human pain processing are still rare [15–17]. While spinal fMRI has recently been used successfully to demonstrate signal intensity changes in the spinal cord and brainstem during innocuous and noxious thermal stimulation and heat allodynia/hyperalgesia [18], there is still no spinal fMRI study that examines spinal and supraspinal changes in activity during secondary mechanical hyperalgesia up to this point.

Therefore, the aims were (A) to investigate spinal and supraspinal processes occurring as a consequence of mechanical stimulation and (B) to compare activation patterns of identical mechanical stimuli before and after induction of sensitization with the heat/capsaicin model in healthy subjects in order to investigate the specific pain-related components of secondary mechanical hyperalgesia. Within this study we could successfully demonstrate (A) increased activity in ipsilateral dGM after induction of hyperalgesia, (B) decreased activity in nociceptive regions of the brainstem and (C) a correlation between these supraspinal deactivations and activations of ipsilateral dGM during secondary mechanical hyperalgesia suggesting a facilitation of nociception via decreased descending endogenous inhibition.

Materials and Methods

Subjects

Sixteen right-handed [19] healthy volunteers (6 females, 10 males, mean age 27.2±4.0 years, range 23–32 years) were included in the study. All subjects were free of any acute or chronic pain conditions. Comorbidities such as diseases of the peripheral or central nervous system were ruled out. None of the subjects were on drugs that might have interfered with itch or pain sensations and flare responses. The study was in accordance with the Declaration of Helsinki and was approved by the Ethical Committee of the Faculty of Medicine at Christian-Albrechts-University of Kiel. Written informed consent was obtained from all participants.

Psychophysics

On the right (= ipsilateral) lateral volar forearm approximately 3 cm distal to the elbow in the C6 dermatome a 3×3 cm square area [area A, site of sensitization] and an adjacent 2×5 cm area directly distal to it [area B, for mechanical stimulation] were marked (figure 1).

Experimental set-up

All subjects underwent two identical MRI sessions back-to-back on the same day with mechanical stimulation in the same area before and after sensitization.

fMRI data acquisition. All scans were performed in a 3T human MRI scanner (Philips Achieva 3T). For acquisition of functional image data, a half-Fourier, single-shot turbo spin-echo sequence with a phased-array head-neck receiver coil (TE = 38 ms, TR = 9000 ms, 288×144×20 mm FOV, 192×96 matrix) was used [17,21]. At TE = 38 ms, this sequence is about equally sensitive to contributions of both BOLD and SEEP [14,22,23]. With this configuration 10 contiguous 2 mm thick sagittal slices were acquired, spanning from above the thalamus to below the C7/T1 intervertebral disc with a resulting voxel size of $1.5 \times 1.5 \times 2$ mm^3. To reduce sources of motion artefacts (e.g. heart, lungs and throat), a spatial saturation pulse was applied to the region anterior to the vertebral column.

Mechanical stimulation. In order to enable the stimulation of a larger dermatomal area (possibly leading to a higher signal in the spinal cord) mechanical stimulation was performed using a self-made brush consisting of 15 stiff von-Frey-hairs (166 mN). Care was taken that the site of stimulation was always within the area of secondary hyperalgesia [area B]. The mechanical stimulation paradigms consisted of 8 stimulation periods of 40 seconds alternating with eight baseline periods (64 volumes). After each session, subjects were asked to rate the stimulus intensity on the numerical rating scale (NRS, ranging from 0 to 10 with 0 representing "no pain" and 10 being the "maximum pain that can be imagined") by verbal response.

Heat/Capsaicin sensitization model. The heat/capsaicin sensitization model was used to induce secondary mechanical hyperalgesia [4]. Therefore, area A was stimulated with a computer-controlled Peltier thermode (Medoc TSA-2001, Haifa, Israel) at 45°C for 5 minutes. Afterwards a gauze pad with 1 ml solution of 0.6% capsaicin in 45% ethanol was placed on area A for 30 minutes. During capsaicin-application, the subjects were asked once a minute for NRS ratings of perceived pain intensity and temperature sensation at the application site. The temperature sensation was quantified on the NRS with 0 representing "neutral temperature" and −10/+10 representing "the maximum cold/ warmth that can be imagined". After patch removal and at the end of the second fMRI block the borders of the area of punctate mechanical hyperalgesia were assessed by a stiff von-Frey-hair (166 mN). The dimensions of flare and mechanical hyperalgesia were then determined by the calculation: $(D/2) \times (d/2) \times \pi$ (D = horizontal diameter, d = vertical diameters of the area) to assess the stability of the pain model throughout the experiment.

Analysis and Statistics

For the analysis of the resulting 3D fMRI image data a general linear model (GLM) was used. The basis set consists of a boxcar model paradigm convolved with the tissue response function [12] and models of cardiac-related spinal cord motion as confounds [17,21]. Its results demonstrate the weighting factors β1 (magnitude of the pattern matching the stimulation paradigm convolved with the tissue response function) and β0 (average voxel intensity). Corrections for bulk motion and a normalization to a consistent coordinate space of the brainstem and spinal cord were then performed as described previously [21]. A random-effects analysis by McGonigle et al. was used to determine combined group results [24]. This consists of the calculation of the mean and standard deviation of the ratio of β1/β0 representing the relative signal intensity response across studies. T values of >2.5 or <−2.5 were assumed as significant activity as they correspond with p<0.0075 [17]. Contrast calculations between mechanical stimulation before and after sensitization were performed on a voxel-by-voxel basis by the partial least squares (PLS) method [25]. A bootstrap ratio of

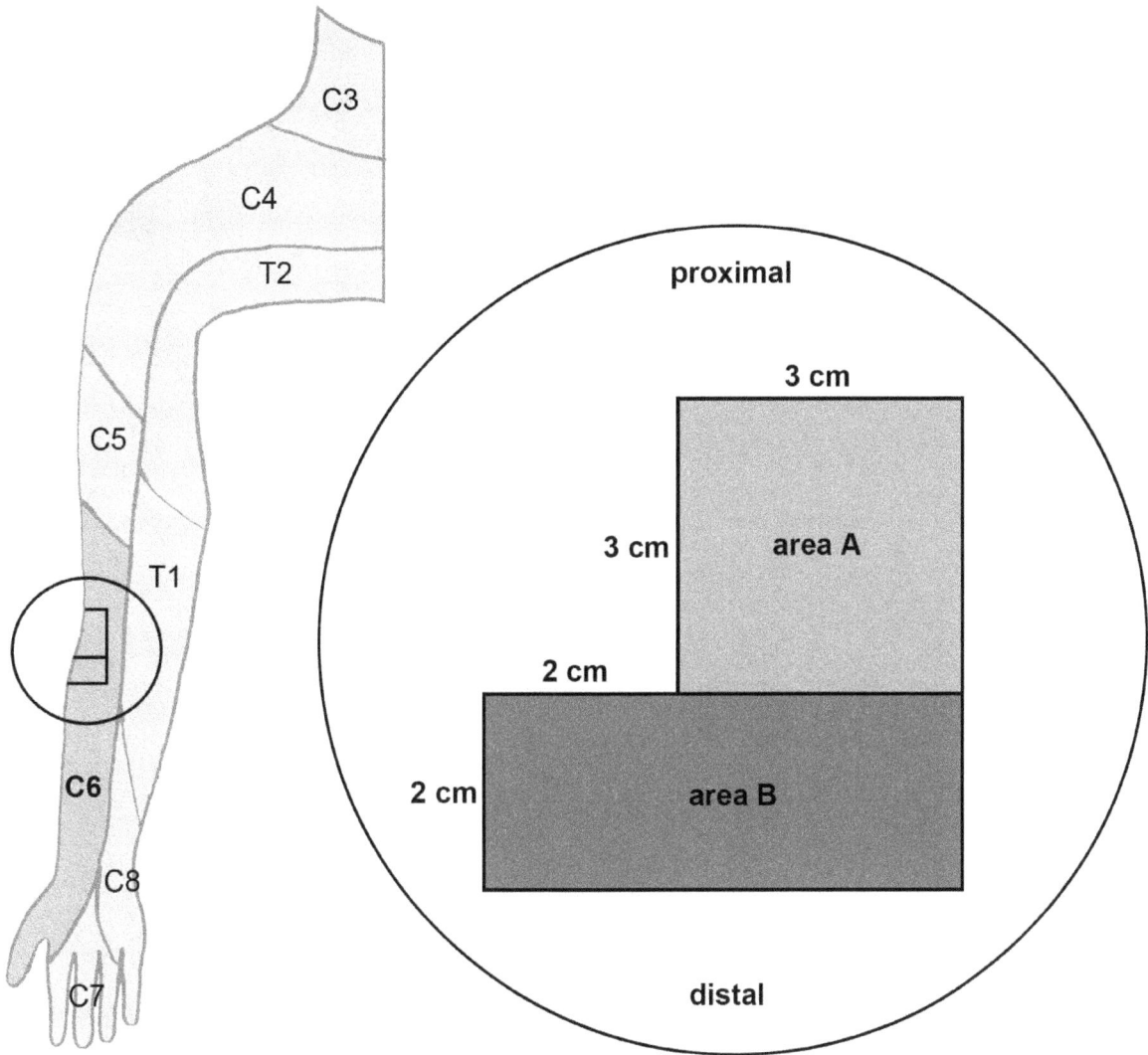

Figure 1. Areas of sensitization and stimulation on the right lateral volar forearm. For orientation, the schematic drawing on the left shows a dermatome map of the right upper extremity (redrawn and modified from [20]). The area of testing (marked by the circle) is situated on the right lateral volar forearm in the C6 dermatome. *Area A:* Site of sensitization with the heat/capsaicin model (3×3 cm square area 3 cm distal to the elbow in the C6 dermatome). *Area B:* Site of mechanical stimulation corresponding to the area of secondary mechanical hyperalgesia (2×5 cm area distal to area A).

≥5 was chosen for differences between two contrasted responses to be significant [17].

Spinal cord segments adjacent to C6 were included in the analysis since (A) primary afferent fibers split up into longitudinal collaterals innervating the bordering segments and (B) slightly individual anatomical dermatome-borders with a coincidental stimulation of surrounding dermatomes (i.e. C5, T1) were respected.

Psychophysical data are presented as mean ± standard deviation (SD) unless otherwise specified. Wilcoxon matched pairs test was used for calculation of psychophysical intragroup differences and Spearman rank test for correlation calculations using the numbers of voxels $(n_{(v)})$, signal change $(\Delta_{(S)})$ and % signal change $(\Delta_{(S/S)})$ across all volunteers provided by the fMRI data. P values <0.05 were considered to be statistically significant.

Results

Psychophysics

Capsaicin-application induced painful and warm sensations in all subjects (figure 2A). The capsaicin-induced flare decreased in size throughout testing (82.0 ± 18.8 cm^2 after patch removal vs. 67.0 ± 16.8 cm^2 at the end of testing, p = 0.002). However, the dimension of secondary mechanical hyperalgesia was stable (77.1 ± 24.5 cm^2 after removal of capsaicin vs. 89.5 ± 35.7 cm^2 at the end of scanning, p = 0,125) and included the area of stimulation [area B] at all times, thus ensuring the stability of the pain model throughout the experiment. Corresponding to mechanical hyperalgesia, the subjects' mean ratings of pain intensity for the mechanical stimulus were higher compared to those before sensitization (3.4 ± 2.2 vs. 2.1 ± 1.8, p = 0.003; figure 2B).

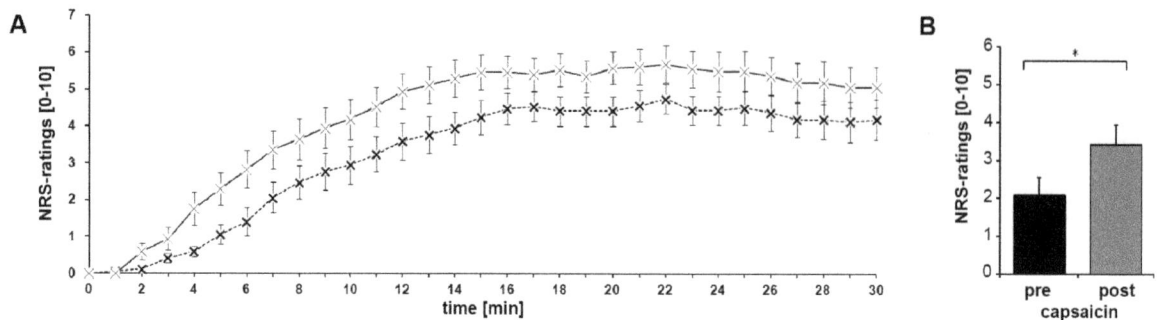

Figure 2. Psychophysical data. (A) Mean ratings of pain intensity (dashed line) and temperature perception (solid line) during capsaicin application. Capsaicin was applied at time 0. Mean ± standard error of the mean (SEM). (B) Mean pain ratings for the mechanical stimulus before and after application of capsaicin. Capsaicin induced secondary mechanical hyperalgesia. Mean ± SEM. *: p<0.05.

fMRI

Spinal group activation patterns and contrast maps. During mechanical stimulation prior to sensitization, spinal deactivations i.e. decreased signal intensity during stimulation were observed in deep dGM layers of C6 and C8 bilaterally and C7 contralaterally. After capsaicin exposure, mechanical stimulation in the area of secondary hyperalgesia lead to activations (increased signal intensity during stimulation) in T1 and deactivations in C7 in ipsilateral superficial dGM. Ventral activations were observed in ipsilateral ventral gray matter (vGM) of C4 before and after sensitization (figures 3, 4).

Activations in ipsilateral vGM of C7 correlated positively to the subjects' NRS-ratings before ($\Delta_{(S)}$: R = 0.513; p = 0.042) and after sensitization ($\Delta_{(S)}$: R = 0.533; p = 0.041), i.e. the higher the perceived pain intensity, the higher were activations in vGM of C7.

Contrast calculations between mechanical stimulation before and after sensitization with the heat/capsaicin model revealed activations in superficial ipsilateral (C7, C8) dGM. The observed lateral deviation of superficial dGM-activations might arise from BOLD-contributions in signal change located in superficial draining veins [14]. Contralateral activations were observed in deep dGM of C8 and vGM of C7. Deactivations were found in C4 in ipsilateral vGM and contralateral dGM (figures 3, 4).

Supraspinal group activation patterns and contrast maps. Prior to sensitization, supraspinal activity was observed in the ipsilateral dorsolateral pontine tegmentum (DLPT) (figure 5A). The activity in the ipsilateral dorsal pons correlated positively to activity in ipsilateral dGM of C4 ($n_{(v)}$: R = 0.611; p = 0.012) and C5 ($n_{(v)}$: R = 0.613; p = 0.012).

In contrast to measurements prior to sensitization, deactivations in contralateral DLPT were observed during secondary mechanical hyperalgesia (figure 5A). These deactivations correlated with activations in ipsilateral dGM of C5 ($n_{(v)}$: R = 0.546; p = 0.035) and T1 ($n_{(v)}$: R = 0.621; p = 0.012). Deactivations in the ipsilateral pons correlated with activations in ipsilateral dGM of C4 ($n_{(v)}$: R = 0.595; p = 0.019) and T1 ($n_{(v)}$: R = 0.555; p = 0.039; $\Delta_{(S/S)}$: R = −0.538; p = 0.047), i.e. the higher the deactivations in the dorsal pons, the higher were activations in ipsilateral dGM (note that R in $n_{(v)}$ is positive because $n_{(deactivated\ voxels)}$ correlates positively to $n_{(activated\ voxels)}$ while $\Delta_{(S/S)}$ is negative because activations, i.e. positive $\Delta_{(S/S)}$-values are correlating to deactivations, i.e. negative $\Delta_{(S/S)}$-values).

After sensitization, deactivations were also visible in the ipsilateral and median caudal pons/rostral medulla most likely corresponding to the area of the rostral ventromedial medulla (RVM, figure 5A). Deactivations in the ipsilateral rostral ventral medulla correlated with ipsilateral dGM activations (C4: $n_{(v)}$: R = 0.699; p = 0.004; $\Delta_{(S)}$: R = −0.827; p<0.001; $\Delta_{(S/S)}$: R = −0.770; p = 0.001; C6: $\Delta_{(S)}$: R = −0.537; p = 0.039). Deactivations in midline RVM correlated with deactivations in ipsilateral dGM (C5: $n_{(v)}$: R = 0.556; p = 0.031; C7 = $n_{(v)}$: R = 0.599; p = 0.018; $\Delta_{(S)}$: R = 0.608; p = 0.016). Visible deactivations in the caudo-dorsal contralateral medulla corresponded to the localization of the subnucleus reticularis dorsalis (SRD, figure 5B) and correlated with spinal activations in ipsilateral dGM (C4: $\Delta_{(S/S)}$: R = −0.560; p = 0.030; C8: $\Delta_{(S/S)}$: R = −0.578; p = 0.024; T1 = $n_{(voxels)}$: R = 0.554; p = 0.040).

Supraspinal calculations of contrast maps showed deactivations in the RVM (figure 5A).

Discussion

The present study shows spinal and supraspinal signal intensity changes during mechanical stimulation and secondary mechanical hyperalgesia in healthy subjects. The main findings are (A) increased activity in ipsilateral dGM after induction of hyperalgesia, (B) decreased activity in supraspinal centers of pain processing and modulation (DLPT, RVM, SRD) and (C) a correlation between supraspinal deactivations and activations of ipsilateral dGM during secondary mechanical hyperalgesia induced by the heat/capsaicin model. Results suggest a facilitation of nociception via decreased descending endogenous inhibition during secondary mechanical hyperalgesia.

Spinal cord

Ipsilateral dGM. Anatomically, the vast majority of primary nociceptive afferent fibers projects to the ipsilateral dGM. Therefore, application of noxious stimuli should lead to activation of projection neurons located in the marginal layer of the dorsal horn [27]. Supportively, this study showed superficial dGM-activations during painful stimulation after sensitization. Animal experiments suggest a higher activation of spinal nociceptive projection neurons by the same noxious stimulus during experimental pain states [3,6]. For example, Simone et al. showed an increase of monkey spinothalamic tract neuron responses to punctate mechanical stimuli during capsaicin-induced secondary hyperalgesia [2]. The current study is now the first one to reproduce such findings from animal experiments in human subjects in vivo as contrast maps revealed activations in superficial dGM that may correspond with increased activity during central sensitization.

Mechanical hyperalgesia and increased dGM activity can also be due to deficient inhibitory interneuron (ININ)-mediated

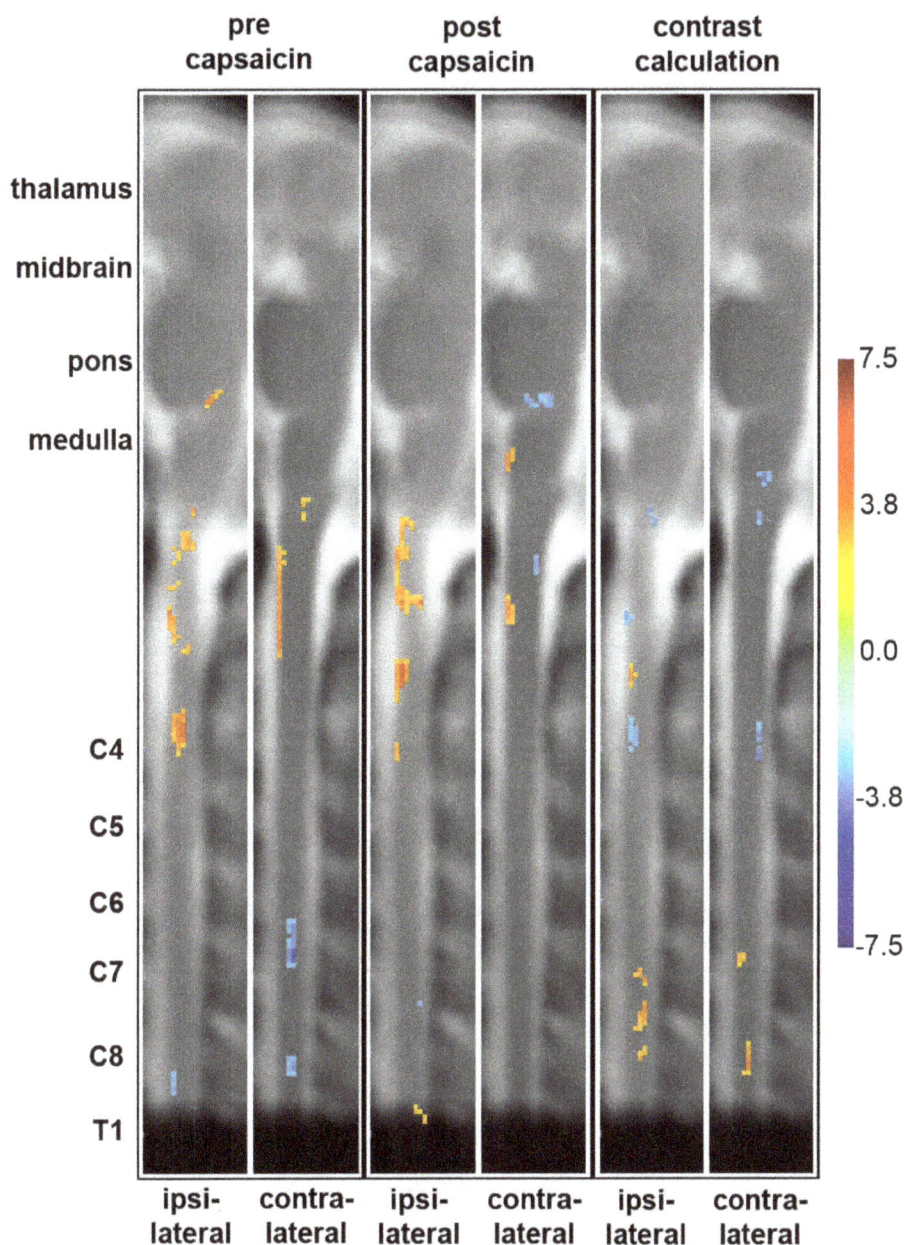

Figure 3. Sagittal slices of group activation patterns and contrast maps. Columns 1 to 4 show areas of activity across brain stem and cervical spinal cord before (1st and 2nd column) and after (3rd and 4th column) sensitization with the heat capsaicin model representing the significance (T-value) of each active voxel across the 16 subjects. Columns 5 and 6 show partial-least squares (PLS) results of contrast calculations on a voxel-by-voxel basis. The left column of each 2 columns (e.g. 1st, 3rd and 5th) corresponds to the ipsilateral side of the stimulus, the right column to the contralateral side. The color bar on the right indicates the corresponding significance, i.e. T-value (columns 1–4) or bootstrap-ratio (columns 5–6) for each color.

inhibition of projection neurons [28,29]. Interestingly, deactivations in deep dGM in C6 and C8 were observed prior to sensitization but disappeared during secondary mechanical hyperalgesia.

Contralateral dGM. Signal intensity changes were also observed in contralateral dGM during both conditions, consistent with a previous study using tactile stimuli [16]. These observations could be explained by primary afferent fibers ending in the contralateral dorsal horn [30] as well as by interneurons of ipsilateral dGM that cross the midline [17]. Our results also show differences during mechanical hyperalgesia compared to mechanical stimulation prior to sensitization suggesting a participation of

the contralateral dGM in the development of central sensitization. It would be important for future studies to focus on such changes in contralateral dGM as contralateral somatosensory abnormalities have been observed in human unilateral neuropathic pain states [31].

vGM. Pain stimuli lead to withdrawal reflexes, i.e. the activation of ipsilateral motor neurons via spinal interneurons or supraspinal reticular nuclei [32]. Because mechanical stimuli were perceived as (slightly) painful, vGM-activity can be expected and was accordingly observed in both fMRI sessions. The positive correlation between the subjects' NRS-ratings and the activity in ipsilateral vGM of C7 suggests that stronger pain stimuli lead to

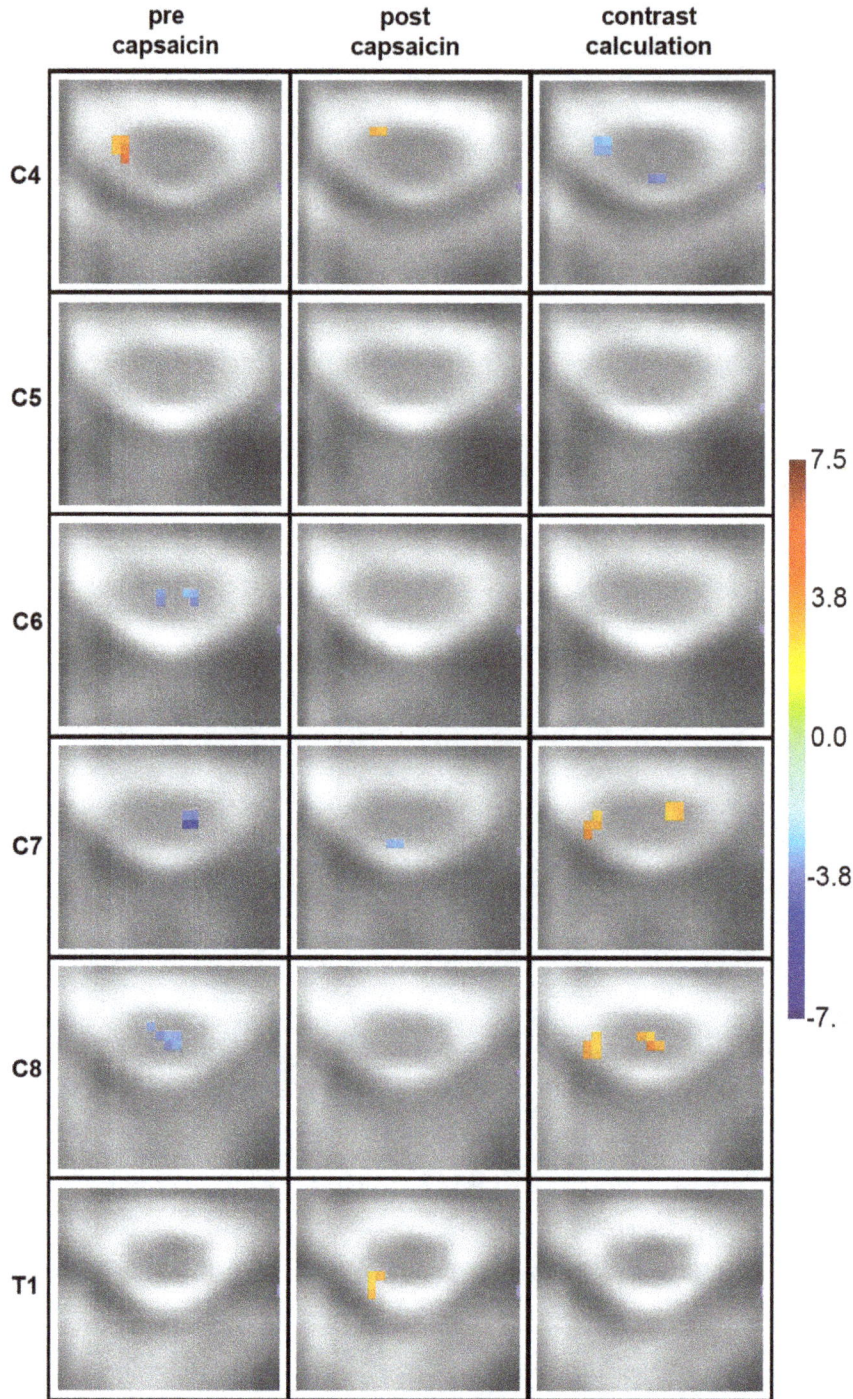

Figure 4. Spinal group activation patterns before (left column) and after (middle column) sensitization and contrast maps (right column). The transverse slices are in radiological orientation with the left side corresponding to the right body side and approximate the corresponding spinal cord segment for a rostral-caudal span from C4 to T1. They show spinal regions of signal intensity change before (left column) and after (middle column) sensitization with the heat/capsaicin model representing the significance (T-value) of each active voxel across the 16 subjects. The right column shows partial-least squares (PLS) results of contrast calculations on a voxel-by-voxel basis. The color bar in figure 3 indicates the corresponding significance, i.e. T-value (left and middle column) or bootstrap-ratio (right column) for each color. *Left Column:* Activations in ipsilateral vGM of C4. Deactivations in bilateral deep dGM of C6 and C8 and contralateral deep dGM of C7. *Middle column:* Ipsilateral activations in superficial dGM of T1 and vGM of C4. Deactivations in ipsilateral superficial dGM of C7. *Right column:* Activations in ipsilateral superficial dGM (C7, C8) and in contralateral vGM (C7) and deep dGM (C8). Deactivations in ipsilateral vGM and contralateral dGM of C4.

higher reflex answers. The C7 segment innervates both M. pronator teres and M. pronator quadratus. As the arm was held in

a supine position throughout noxious stimulation, the activation of these muscles would be needed to escape the stimulus.

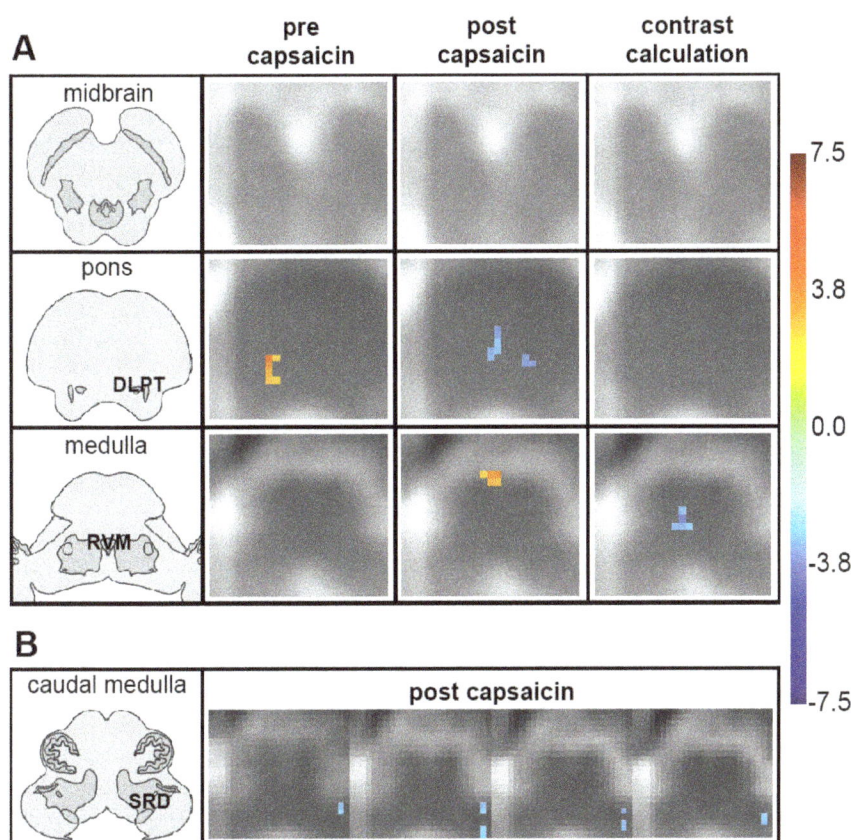

Figure 5. Supraspinal group activation patterns and contrast maps. Slices are in radiological orientation with the left side corresponding to the right body side. The color bar in figure 3 indicates the corresponding significance, i.e. T-value (combined group results pre/post capsaicin) or bootstrap-ratio (contrast calculation) for each color. Anatomical transverse sections on the left were modified from [26]. (A) The transverse slices approximate the corresponding brainstem region (midbrain, pons, medulla) for a rostral-caudal span. They show supraspinal regions of signal intensity change before (left column) and after (middle column) sensitization with the heat/capsaicin model representing the significance (T-value) of each active voxel across the 16 subjects. The right column shows partial-least squares (PLS) results of contrast calculations on a voxel-by-voxel basis. *Left column:* Activations in the ipsilateral DLPT (dorsolateral pontine tegmentum) during mechanical stimulation prior to application of capsaicin. *Middle column:* Deactivations in the contralateral DLPT and in the RVM (rostral ventromedial medulla) during secondary mechanical hyperalgesia (note that visible medial pontine deactivations are situated in the caudal pons/rostral medulla and therefore most likely correspond to the location of the RVM). *Right column:* Deactivations in the RVM. (B) The adjacent 1 mm thick transverse slices in consecutive arrangement located in the medulla show signal intensity changes during secondary mechanical hyperalgesia. Deactivations are observed in contralateral subnucleus reticularis dorsalis (SRD).

Brainstem

DLPT. Animal testing shows that the DLPT plays a central role in the modulation of nociception. With its noradrenergic fibers to the dGM, it mediates a negative feedback loop triggered by noxious stimuli to prevent excessive pain sensation [7,33]. This descending inhibition is for the most part mediated by the ipsilateral DLPT [34]. Accordingly, this study showed activations in the ipsilateral DLPT during painful mechanical stimulation prior to sensitization. Moreover these activations correlated with activations in ipsilateral dGM, possibly reflecting either an augmented activation of endogenous inhibition by higher activation of projection neurons [7] or a noradrenergic activation of spinal ININs (indirect inhibition of projection neurons) as it has been shown in animal studies [35]. Similarly, previous fMRI studies also showed activations of the DLPT during painful stimuli in healthy humans [15,36].

An absence of this noradrenergic inhibition by the DLPT is thought to be a mechanism for the development of neuropathic pain [3,37]. Interestingly, a bilateral decrease of DLPT-activation was seen during secondary mechanical hyperalgesia which

correlated with ipsilateral dGM-activations. Compatibly, Becerra et al. showed bilaterally decreased DLPT-activity during mechanical hyperalgesia/allodynia in neuropathic pain patients [38]. Our results could thus correspond to a reduced descending noradrenergic inhibition with consecutive higher activation of spinal projection neurons.

Besides decreased inhibition, central sensitization is also thought to be mediated by coexisting excitatory descending facilitation [3,6,39]. Two earlier fMRI studies investigating secondary mechanical hyperalgesia demonstrated activity in rostral brainstem regions (midline-periaqueductal gray, contralateral cuneiform nucleus [10], contralateral mesencephalic pontine reticular formation [9]) that could be a correlate for excitatory nociceptive facilitation. Why did the current study not show these activations? Possible explanations could be overlapping processes of activation and simultaneous suppression of anti-nociceptive descending pathways in the very limited space of these brainstem nuclei or the different experimental set ups (MRI sequences or devices).

RVM. Based on current concepts of pain modulation, OFF-cells, a specific cell-type of the RVM, physiologically mediate antinociception [39,40]. In the condition of central sensitization, this OFF-cell activity is decreased [41]. Compatibly, this study shows decreased activity in the RVM during secondary mechanical hyperalgesia. A deactivation of OFF-cells would lead to a decreased inhibition of spinal projection neurons. Supportingly, this study shows correlations between deactivation of ipsilateral RVM and activations in ipsilateral dGM during secondary mechanical hyperalgesia. However, it has to be kept in mind that spinal inhibition can also be caused by the activation of ININs [29]. The observed correlation between deactivations in median RVM and ipsilateral dGM could therefore correspond to decreased OFF-cell mediated activation of ININs during secondary mechanical hyperalgesia.

SRD. The SRD is believed to play a major role in the mechanism of diffuse noxious inhibitory control (DNIC) [42]. An absence of this control is thought to be a reason for the development of neuropathic pain [39]. Accordingly, this study shows deactivations in contralateral SRD during secondary mechanical hyperalgesia which correlated with activations in the ipsilateral dGM. This could correspond to a facilitation of nociception via decreased endogenous inhibition by SRD and consequently higher dGM-activations - a similar and additional mechanism to nociceptive modulation by DLPT and RVM.

Limitations

Even though spin-echo spinal cord fMRI is a new reliable and non-invasive method to show functional processes in the spinal cord [15–18], its spatial resolution is still limited. Thus, an exact localization of the anatomical area corresponding to the observed activity is extremely difficult and can sometimes be only speculative. Furthermore, interpretation of results is complicated due to interconnections and often dichotomous roles of areas involved in pain processing/modulation, i.e. excitatory and inhibitory roles.

Conclusion

Using spin-echo spinal cord fMRI, it was possible to investigate pain modulatory processes during secondary mechanical hyperalgesia in the brainstem and spinal cord of healthy subjects. This study is the first one to show an increase of ipsilateral dGM-activity during secondary mechanical hyperalgesia in human subjects in vivo. Furthermore, this study succeeds in showing decreased activity in areas of the brainstem that have been proven important for processes of central sensitization in animal experiments (DLPT, RVM, SRD). Moreover, those deactivations correlated with dGM-activity. With these findings, this study gives new insights in human pain processing in vivo. Since findings of animal experiments and results of previous fMRI studies could be reproduced, spin-echo spinal cord fMRI has been shown to be a reliable method for the examination of spinal and supraspinal pain processing and modulation. Herewith, it qualifies for further investigations including treatment of neuropathic pain.

Acknowledgments

We are indebted to the subjects who participated in the study for their consent and co-operation.

Author Contributions

Conceived and designed the experiments: JG. Performed the experiments: TR SW. Analyzed the data: TR PWS JG. Contributed reagents/materials/analysis tools: PWS. Contributed to the writing of the manuscript: TR CR RB PWS OJ JG.

References

1. Baron R, Binder A, Wasner G (2010) Neuropathic pain: diagnosis, pathophysiological mechanisms, and treatment. Lancet Neurol 9: 807–819.
2. Simone DA, Sorkin LS, Oh U, Chung JM, Owens C, et al. (1991) Neurogenic hyperalgesia: central neural correlates in responses of spinothalamic tract neurons. J Neurophysiol 66: 228–246.
3. Westlund KN (2006) The dorsal horn and hyperalgesia. In: Cervero F, Jensen TS, editors. Handbook of Clinical Neurology, Vol 81 (3rd series): Pain. Amsterdam: Elsevier B.V. pp. 178–186.
4. Petersen KL, Rowbotham MC (1999) A new human experimental pain model: the heat/capsaicin sensitization model. Neuroreport 10: 1511–1516.
5. Villanueva L, Lopez-Avila A, Le Bars D (2006) Ascending nociceptive pathways. In: Cervero F, Jensen TS, editors. Handbook of Clinical Neurology, Vol 81 (3rd series): Pain. Amsterdam: Elsevier B.V. pp. 93–102.
6. Ossipov MH, Porreca F (2006) Descending excitatory systems. In: Cervero F, Jensen TS, editors. Handbook of Clinical Neurology, Vol 81 (3rd series): Pain. Amsterdam: Elsevier B.V. pp. 193–210.
7. Pertovaara A, Almeida A (2006) Descending inhibitory systems. In: Cervero F, Jensen TS, editors. Handbook of Clinical Neurology, Vol 81 (3rd series): Pain. Amsterdam: Elsevier B.V. pp. 179–192.
8. Baron R, Baron Y, Disbrow E, Roberts TP (1999) Brain processing of capsaicin-induced secondary hyperalgesia: a functional MRI study. Neurology 53: 548–557.
9. Lee MC, Zambreanu L, Menon DK, Tracey I (2008) Identifying brain activity specifically related to the maintenance and perceptual consequence of central sensitization in humans. J Neurosci 28: 11642–11649.
10. Zambreanu L, Wise RG, Brooks JC, Iannetti GD, Tracey I (2005) A role for the brainstem in central sensitisation in humans. Evidence from functional magnetic resonance imaging. Pain 114: 397–407.
11. Stroman PW (2005) Magnetic resonance imaging of neuronal function in the spinal cord: spinal FMRI. Clin Med Res 3: 146–156.
12. Stroman PW, Kornelsen J, Lawrence J, Malisza KL (2005) Functional magnetic resonance imaging based on SEEP contrast: response function and anatomical specificity. Magn Reson Imaging 23: 843–850.
13. Stroman PW, Krause V, Malisza KL, Frankenstein UN, Tomanek B (2002) Extravascular proton-density changes as a non-BOLD component of contrast in fMRI of the human spinal cord. Magn Reson Med 48: 122–127.
14. Stroman PW, Wheeler-Kingshott C, Bacon M, Schwab JM, Bosma R, et al. (2014) The current state-of-the-art of spinal cord imaging: methods. Neuroimage 84: 1070–1081.
15. Cahill CM, Stroman PW (2011) Mapping of neural activity produced by thermal pain in the healthy human spinal cord and brain stem: a functional magnetic resonance imaging study. Magn Reson Imaging 29: 342–352.
16. Ghazni NF, Cahill CM, Stroman PW (2010) Tactile sensory and pain networks in the human spinal cord and brain stem mapped by means of functional MR imaging. AJNR Am J Neuroradiol 31: 661–667.
17. Stroman PW (2009) Spinal fMRI investigation of human spinal cord function over a range of innocuous thermal sensory stimuli and study-related emotional influences. Magn Reson Imaging 27: 1333–1346.
18. Rempe T, Wolff S, Riedel C, Baron R, Stroman PW, et al. (2014) Spinal and supraspinal processing of thermal stimuli: An fMRI study. J Magn Reson Imaging DOI:10.1002/jmri.24627.
19. Oldfield RC (1971) The assessment and analysis of handedness: the Edinburgh inventory. Neuropsychologia 9: 97–113.
20. Trepel M (2008) Neuroanatomie: Struktur und Funktion. Munich: Elsevier GmbH, Urban & Fischer Verlag.
21. Stroman PW, Figley CR, Cahill CM (2008) Spatial normalization, bulk motion correction and coregistration for functional magnetic resonance imaging of the human cervical spinal cord and brainstem. Magn Reson Imaging 26: 809–814.
22. Figley CR, Stroman PW (2012) Measurement and characterization of the human spinal cord SEEP response using event-related spinal fMRI. Magn Reson Imaging 30: 471–484.
23. Stroman PW, Bosma RL, Beynon M, Dobek C (2012) Removal of synergistic physiological motion and image artefacts in functional MRI of the human spinal cord. 20th Annual Meeting of the International Society for Magnetic Resonance in Medicine. Melbourne, Australia.
24. McGonigle DJ, Howseman AM, Athwal BS, Friston KJ, Frackowiak RS, et al. (2000) Variability in fMRI: an examination of intersession differences. Neuroimage 11: 708–734.
25. McIntosh AR, Lobaugh NJ (2004) Partial least squares analysis of neuroimaging data: applications and advances. Neuroimage 23 Suppl 1: S250–263.
26. Naidich TP, Duvernoy HM, Delman BN, Sorensen AG, Kollias SS, et al. (2009) Duvernoy's Atlas of the Human Brain Stem and Cerebellum. Wien New York: Springer. pp. 53–93.

27. Millan MJ (1999) The induction of pain: an integrative review. Prog Neurobiol 57: 1–164.
28. Meisner JG, Marsh AD, Marsh DR (2010) Loss of GABAergic interneurons in laminae I–III of the spinal cord dorsal horn contributes to reduced GABAergic tone and neuropathic pain after spinal cord injury. J Neurotrauma 27: 729–737.
29. Millan MJ (2002) Descending control of pain. Prog Neurobiol 66: 355–474.
30. Light AR, Perl ER (1979) Spinal termination of functionally identified primary afferent neurons with slowly conducting myelinated fibers. J Comp Neurol 186: 133–150.
31. Huge V, Lauchart M, Forderreuther S, Kaufhold W, Valet M, et al. (2008) Interaction of hyperalgesia and sensory loss in complex regional pain syndrome type I (CRPS I). PLoS One 3: e2742.
32. Morgan MM (1998) Direct comparison of heat-evoked activity of nociceptive neurons in the dorsal horn with the hindpaw withdrawal reflex in the rat. J Neurophysiol 79: 174–180.
33. Fields HL, Basbaum AI (1994) Central nervous system mechanisms of pain modulation. In: Wall PD, Melzack R, editors. Textbook of Pain. 3 ed. Edinburgh: Churchill Livingstone. pp. 243–257.
34. Clark FM, Proudfit HK (1991) The projection of noradrenergic neurons in the A7 catecholamine cell group to the spinal cord in the rat demonstrated by anterograde tracing combined with immunocytochemistry. Brain Res 547: 279–288.
35. Gassner M, Ruscheweyh R, Sandkuhler J (2009) Direct excitation of spinal GABAergic interneurons by noradrenaline. Pain 145: 204–210.
36. Dunckley P, Wise RG, Fairhurst M, Hobden P, Aziz Q, et al. (2005) A comparison of visceral and somatic pain processing in the human brainstem using functional magnetic resonance imaging. J Neurosci 25: 7333–7341.
37. Xu M, Kontinen VK, Kalso E (1999) Endogenous noradrenergic tone controls symptoms of allodynia in the spinal nerve ligation model of neuropathic pain. Eur J Pharmacol 366: 41–45.
38. Becerra L, Morris S, Bazes S, Gostic R, Sherman S, et al. (2006) Trigeminal neuropathic pain alters responses in CNS circuits to mechanical (brush) and thermal (cold and heat) stimuli. J Neurosci 26: 10646–10657.
39. Ossipov MH, Dussor GO, Porreca F (2010) Central modulation of pain. J Clin Invest 120: 3779–3787.
40. Gebhart GF (2004) Descending modulation of pain. Neurosci Biobehav Rev 27: 729–737.
41. Kincaid W, Neubert MJ, Xu M, Kim CJ, Heinricher MM (2006) Role for medullary pain facilitating neurons in secondary thermal hyperalgesia. J Neurophysiol 95: 33–41.
42. Villanueva L, Bouhassira D, Le Bars D (1996) The medullary subnucleus reticularis dorsalis (SRD) as a key link in both the transmission and modulation of pain signals. Pain 67: 231–240.

β1-Integrin and Integrin Linked Kinase Regulate Astrocytic Differentiation of Neural Stem Cells

Liuliu Pan[1]*, Hilary A. North[1], Vibhu Sahni[1], Su Ji Jeong[1], Tammy L. Mcguire[1], Eric J. Berns[2], Samuel I. Stupp[3,4,5], John A. Kessler[1]

1 Department of Neurology, Northwestern University, Chicago, Illinois, United States of America, 2 Department of Biomedical Engineering, Northwestern University, Evanston, Illinois, United States of America, 3 Department of Materials Science and Engineering, Northwestern University, Evanston, Illinois, United States of America, 4 Department of Chemistry, Northwestern University, Evanston, Illinois, United States of America, 5 Department of Medicine and Institute for BioNanotechnology in Medicine, Northwestern University, Chicago, Illinois, United States of America

Abstract

Astrogliosis with glial scar formation after damage to the nervous system is a major impediment to axonal regeneration and functional recovery. The present study examined the role of β1-integrin signaling in regulating astrocytic differentiation of neural stem cells. In the adult spinal cord β1-integrin is expressed predominantly in the ependymal region where ependymal stem cells (ESCs) reside. β1-integrin signaling suppressed astrocytic differentiation of both cultured ESCs and subventricular zone (SVZ) progenitor cells. Conditional knockout of β1-integrin enhanced astrogliogenesis both by cultured ESCs and by SVZ progenitor cells. Previous studies have shown that injection into the injured spinal cord of a self-assembling peptide amphiphile that displays an IKVAV epitope (IKVAV-PA) limits glial scar formation and enhances functional recovery. Here we find that injection of IKVAV-PA induced high levels of β1-integrin in ESCs in vivo, and that conditional knockout of β1-integrin abolished the astroglial suppressive effects of IKVAV-PA in vitro. Injection into an injured spinal cord of PAs expressing two other epitopes known to interact with β1-integrin, a Tenascin C epitope and the fibronectin epitope RGD, improved functional recovery comparable to the effects of IKVAV-PA. Finally we found that the effects of β1-integrin signaling on astrogliosis are mediated by integrin linked kinase (ILK). These observations demonstrate an important role for β1-integrin/ILK signaling in regulating astrogliosis from ESCs and suggest ILK as a potential target for limiting glial scar formation after nervous system injury.

Editor: Michael Fehlings, University of Toronto, Canada

Funding: This project was supported by National Institutes of Health Grants R01 NS 20013 and R01 NS 20778. The funders had no role in study design, data collection and analysis, decision to publish, or preparation of the manuscript.

Competing Interests: The authors have declared that no competing interests exist.

* Email: liuliupan2012@u.northwestern.edu

Introduction

After injury to the nervous system, astrocytes undergo a series of morphologic and molecular changes that facilitate sealing of the blood brain barrier and functional recovery [10,11,42]. However, there is also an increase in the number of astrocytes and formation of a glial scar that significantly impedes axonal regeneration [10,48,50,54]. New astrocytes are generated after spinal cord injury (SCI) both by ependymal stem cells (ESCs) as well as by preexisting astrocytes [2]. Several signaling pathways are known to be involved in the generation of astrocytes after SCI [18,37], but the precise molecular mechanisms regulating astrogliosis are not known.

Injection into an injured spinal cord of a self-assembling peptide amphiphile (PA) that contains an IKVAV epitope (IKVAV-PA) markedly reduced glial scar formation after SCI [54]. IKVAV-PA also profoundly suppressed astrocytic differentiation of cultured neural stem/progenitor cells (NSCs) [47]. The IKVAV sequence is an important neuroactive site on the laminin A chain that can mimic the effects of laminin-1 on neurite outgrowth [36,46,53]. Some of the effects of the IKVAV epitope are mediated via the β1-

integrin receptor subunit [14] which is the most ubiquitously expressed integrin subunit. This suggested the possibility that β1-integrin signaling might be involved in astrogliosis after SCI.

The integrin family of cell surface receptors is an important link between cells and the extracellular matrix (ECM) and acts both to anchor the cell surface to the ECM and to initiate a variety of intracellular signaling events. Integrin signaling is complex. Integrin heterodimer formation can be induced both by extracellular ligand binding and by cytoplasmic signaling [45], resulting in a conformational change into an activated form. Integrin activation eventually induces intracellular signaling through assembly of a signaling complex at its cytoplasmic tail [7]. Integrins play multiple roles during the development of the nervous system [34]. β1-integrin is highly expressed by neural stem/progenitor cells (NSCs) and in fact has been used as a cell surface marker for NSC enrichment [15,40]. β1-integrin signaling is an important pathway by which NSCs respond to cues from the ECM to regulate both survival and proliferation [25]. Higher levels of β1-integrin expression by cultured NSCs correlate with a higher capability for self-renewal mediated via the MAPK cascade [8].

Although β1-integrin signaling influences astrocytic morphology and gene expression, it does not alter astrocyte proliferation [43]. We therefore asked whether the effects of IKVAV-PA in limiting the glial scar might be mediated by interactions with β1-integrin expressed by ESCs, and what downstream signaling pathways might be involved. We report a series of observations that demonstrate an important role for β1-integrin/ILK signaling in regulating astrocytic differentiation of ESCs and suggest ILK as a potential target for limiting glial scar formation after nervous system injury.

Materials and Methods

Animals

Timed pregnant CD1 mice, 129 SvJ mice and Long Evans rats were supplied by Charles River Laboratories (Wilmington, MA). β1 integrin floxed mice were supplied by Jackson Laboratory (strain name: B6;129-Itgb1tm1Efu/J).

Cell Culture reagents

Neurosphere growth media were made from supplementing DMEM/F12 (Gibco/Invitrogen) with N2 Supplement (Gibco/Invitrogen) and B27 Supplement (Gibco/Invitrogen), along with Pen/Strap/Glut 100x Mix (Gibco/Invitrogen). ILK inhibitor Cpd 22 was purchased from Millipore and dissolved in DMSO. IKVAV-PA and VVIAK-PA were made by the laboratory of Dr. Samuel Stupp (Northwestern University, IL, US).

Generation of progenitor cell neurospheres and differentiation cultures

To isolate NSCs from spinal cord, the spinal cord of postnatal day 1 mice were mechanically dissociated using razor blades along with pipetting and grown in serum-free neurosphere growth medium with EGF (20 ng/ml, human recombinant, BD) plus bFGF (20 ng/ml, human recombinant, Millipore) supplemented with Heparin (Sigma) for 7 days, to generate neurospheres. Primary spheres were grown for 7 days in vitro (DIV), and then passaged by dissociating with 0.05% trypsin (Invitrogen) for 2 minutes followed by incubation with a soybean trypsin inhibitor (Sigma), a 5- minute spin, and repeated trituration. Secondary spheres were grown for an additional 5–7 DIV and used for subsequent studies.

To isolate NSCs from SVZ, the lateral ganglionic eminences of postnatal day 1 mice were dissociated and grown in serum-free neurosphere growth medium with EGF (20 ng/ml, human recombinant, BD) for 5 days, as previously described, to generate neurospheres [30,56]. Primary spheres were grown for 3–4 days in vitro (DIV), and then passaged by dissociating with 0.05% trypsin (Invitrogen) for 2 minutes followed by incubation with a soybean trypsin inhibitor (Sigma), a 5 minute spin, and repeated trituration. Secondary spheres were grown for an additional 3–4 DIV and used for subsequent studies.

For differentiation studies, neurospheres were dissociated and plated at a density of 1×10^4 cells/cm^2 onto poly-D-lysine-coated (PDL, Sigma) coverslips additionally coated with Laminin (Roche) within 24-well culture plates, and then grown for 7 DIV in neurosphere growth medium with low concentration EGF(1 ng/ml or 0.2 ng/ml).

Immunochemistry of cultures

Prior to PFA fixation, O4 antibody (mouse IgM, Chemicon) was added to cells for 30 minutes at 4°C. 10 μM thymidine analog 5-Ethyl-2′-deoxyuridine (EdU, invitrogen) was added to the cells for 12 hours. Fixed coverslips were incubated with primary antibodies at 4°C overnight in blocking media (0.2% Triton with 1% BSA in PBS). Antibodies were as follows: GFAP (Rabbit, Dako); βIII-tubulin (mouse IgG2b, Sigma); β1 integrin (Rat, Millipore); β1 integrin, activated, HUTS-4 (Mouse IgG2b, Millipore); phosphore-ILK, Ser246 (Rabbit, Millipore); ILK (Rabbit, Millipore); Sox2 (Goat, Santa Cruz). Primary antibodies were visualized with Alexa 647- (infrared) Alexa 555/594- (red), Alexa 488- (green) and Alexa 350- (blue) conjugated secondary antibodies (Invitrogen). Cells were counted in 26 alternate fields of each coverslip and verified in a minimum of three independent experiments.

Western Blot analysis

Cells were lysed in T-PER Tissue Protein Extraction Reagent (Pierce, Thermo Scientific), supplemented with complete protease and phosphatase inhibitor cocktail (Roche). After removal of cellular debris by centrifugation at 13200 g for 5 min at 4°C, the protein concentration of the lysate was determined using the Bio-Rad Protein Assay standardized to bovine serum albumin. The indicated amounts of cell lysate were resolved by sodium dodecyl sulfate–polyacrylamide gel electrophoresis (SDS–PAGE) and electro-transferred onto nitrocellulose membranes (Bio-Rad). The following primary antibodies were used at 1:1000 dilution unless otherwise noted: pFAK (Rabbit, Cell Signaling); FAK (Rabbit, Cell Signaling); GFAP (Rabbit, Dako); ILK (Rabbit, Millipore); GAPDH (Mouse IgG, Millipore); pAkt (Rabbit, Cell Signling); Akt (Rabbit, Cell Signaling). Horseradish peroxidases (HRP)-conjugated secondary antibodies (Santa Cruz) were used at 1:2000 dilutions. Detection was carried out using SuperSignal West Femto Maximum Sensitivity Substrate detection system (Pierce). Immunoblots were stripped and re-probed using Restore Western Blot Stripping Buffer (Pierce).

RT-qPCR (reverse transcriptase-quantitative polymerase chain reaction)

RNA was harvested from plated cells using Trizol (Invitrogen) and RNAqueous-Micro kit (Ambion). 500 ng of RNA was used to generate cDNA using oligo-dT primers (Thermoscript RT-PCR kit, Invitrogen). Real-time PCR was performed using SybrGreen Master Mix (Applied Biosystems). Three replicates were run for each cDNA sample with the test and control primers. An amplification plot showing cycle number versus the change in fluorescent intensity was generated by the Sequence Detector program (Applied Biosystems).

Retrovirus production and infection

The β1 integrin constructs were cloned into the pCLE-IRES-EGFP retroviral vector and the retrovirus production is as previously described [4]. 293 FT cells were transfected with pCLE retroviral and pCMV-VSVG helper plasmids using Lipofectamine 2000 transfection reagent (Invitrogen). The supernatant from the cells was collected on day 2, 4 and 7 post transfection, concentrated, tittered and then $\sim 10^7$ viral particles were used to infect 2.5 million cells for 48 hours in sphere forming media (containing 20 ng/ml EGF). Cells were then FACS sorted for GFP and then either used immediately for RNA isolation or plated on PDL-laminin as described above.

Thymidine analog labeling

For 5-ethynyl-2′-deoxyuridine (EdU) (Invitrogen) labeling of neurospheres in culture, cells were incubated in neurospheres media containing 10 μM EdU for 12 h and then processed for

EdU detection according to the protocol of the manufacturer (Click-IT Flow Cytometry Assay kit; Invitrogen).

Generation of mutated ILK, b1integrin constructs

Constitutive active ILK expressing construct ILK_S343D were generated by point mutation using QuikChange II XL Site-Directed Mutagenesis Kit (Agilent Technologies). Mutation backbone template was mouse ilk expressing vector ordered from OriGene (ilk (NM_010562) Mouse cDNA ORF Clone). Mutation primers were designed as follows: 5′-GGCTGATGTTAAGTTT-GATTTCCAGTGCCCTGGG-3′ and 5′-CCCAGGGCACTG-GAAATCAAACTTAACATCAGCC-3′. Kinase dead ILK expressing construct ILK_S343A were generated using mutation primers designed as follows:

5′-GCTGATGTTAAGTTTGCTTTCCAGTGCCCTG-3′.

5′-CAGGGCACTGGAAAGCAAACTTAACATCAGC-3′.

Mouse spinal cord injury and PA injection

All animal procedures were performed in accordance with the Public Health Service Policy on Humane Care and Use of Laboratory Animals and all procedures were approved by the Northwestern University Institutional Animal Care and Use Committee. Female 129 SvJ mice (10 weeks of age) or female Longs Evans Rats (8 weeks of age) were anesthetized by inhalation of 2.5% isoflurane anesthetic in 100% oxygen administered by a VetEquip Rodent anesthesia machine. A T11 vertebral laminectomy was performed to expose the spinal cord. The spinal cord was injured using an IH-0400 Spinal Cord impactor (Precision Systems) with a 1.25 mm tip with 70 Kdynes of force and 60 s of dwell time for mice and with a 2.50 mm tip with 185 Kdynes of force and 60 s of dwell time for rats. Skin was sutured using AUTOCLIPs (9 mm; BD Biosciences). For postoperative care, animals were kept on a heating pad for 24 h to maintain body temperature. Both mice and rats were given Buprenex (2.5 mg/kg, s.c.) and Baytril (5 mg/kg, s.c.) to minimize discomfort and infection. Bladders were manually expressed twice daily. A 5d Baytril treatment course (5 mg/kg daily, s.c.) was started in the event of hematuria.

PA (1% aqueous solution) or vehicle was injected 48 h after SCI using borosilicate glass capillary micropipettes (Sutter Instruments, Novato, CA) (outer diameter, 100 μm). The capillaries were loaded onto a Hamilton syringe using a female luer adaptor (World Precision Instruments, Sarasota, FL) controlled by a Micro4 microsyringe pump controller (World Precision Instruments). The amphiphile was diluted 1:1 with a 580 μM solution of glucose just before injection and loaded into the capillary. Under Avertin anesthesia, the autoclips were removed and the injury site was exposed. The micropipette was inserted to a depth of 750 μm measured from the dorsal surface of the cord for mice and a depth of 1250 μm measured for rats, and 2.5 μl for mice or 5.0 μl for rats of the diluted amphiphile solution or vehicle was injected at 1 μl/min. The micropipette was withdrawn at intervals of 250 μm to leave a trail (ventral to dorsal) of the PA in the cord. At the end of the injection, the capillary tip was left in the cord for an additional 1 min, after which the pipette was withdrawn and the wound closed. For all experiments, the experimenters were kept blinded to the identity of the animals.

Animal perfusions, tissue processing and immunohistochemistry

Animals were killed using an overdose of halothane anesthesia and transcardially perfused with 4% paraformaldehyde in PBS. The spinal cords were dissected and fixed for 2 h with 4% paraformaldehyde and subsequently overnight in 30% sucrose in PBS. The spinal cords were then frozen in Tissue-Tek embedding compound and sectioned on a Leica (Deerfield, IL) CM3050S cryostat.

20 μm thick frozen sections were cut on a leica (CM3050S) Cryostat and collected on Superfrost Bond Rite slides (Richard Allen Scientific). Every fifth section was placed on the same slide such that each adjacent section was 80 μm away from its neighbor. Four sections were placed on each slide and hence the width of the frozen cord spanned on each slide was 240 μm. We roughly averaged about 20 slides per cord. Sections were processed for immunohistochemistry in the same manner as described for the cells. Primary antibodies used were: GFAP (Sigma, mouse IgG1 1:500), β1integrin (Millipore, rat IgG, 1:500), HUTS-4 (Millipore, mouse IgG1 1:500).

Statistical analyses

Student's unpaired t test was used for all two group comparisons. Analysis of variance (ANOVA) with the Bonferroni post hoc test was used for all multiple group experiments. P values<0.05 were deemed significant. Values in graphs are shown are Mean ±S.E.M.

Results

Knockout of β1-integrin from cultured ESCs increases astrocytic differentiation

Immunocytochemical examination of adult spinal cord revealed that β1-integrin is expressed predominantly in the ependymal zone (Figure 1A) where ESCs reside [32]. ESCs are able to form neurospheres and can generate all three neural lineages, neurons, astrocytes and oligodendrocytes (Figure 1B and Meletis et al, 2008 [32]). To assess the role of β1-integrin signaling in this process, we isolated and cultured ependymal cells from β1-integrin$^{flx/flx}$ mice and ablated out β1-integrin by infecting cells with Adeno-Cre-GFP virus or a control Adeno-GFP virus. Two days after virus infection, neurospheres were dissociated, sorted by fluorescence activated cell sorting (FACS) to select virus infected cells, and grown again as neurospheres. Western blot analysis confirmed the depletion of β1-integrin in the Adeno-Cre-GFP treated cells (Figure 1C). One week later the cells were dissociated, plated in differentiating conditions for 7 days, and analyzed immunocytochemically (Figure 1B, 1D, 1E). The total number of cells did not differ between control and β1 integrin null cultures (Figure 1D). Control ESCs generated a large number of GFAP-expressing astrocytes (35.3±3.3%of the cells) and smaller numbers of βIIItubulin-immunoreactive neurons (3.3±0.1%) and CNPase-expressing oligodendrocytes (~3.0±1.3%) (Figure 1B, 1E). The remainder of the cells remained undifferentiated. Knockout of β1 integrin significantly increased the number of GFAP+ cells by 67% (to a total amount of 59.1±3.7% of the cells; p≤0.004) without altering the numbers of neurons or oligodendroglia (Figure 1B, 1E). This suggests that β1-integrin signaling suppresses astrocytic differentiation by ESCs.

To determine whether this regulatory process is unique to the ependymal population of NSCs, we repeated the experiment using SVZ-derived NSCs with strikingly similar results. The total number of cells did not differ between control and β1 integrin null cultures (Figure 2C). Control SVZ-derived NPCs generated 37.3±3.1% astrocytes, 3.4±0.1% neurons, and 3.1±0.5% oligodendrocytes (Figure 2A, 2D). Knockout of β1-integrin (Figure 2B) did not alter neuronal or oligodendroglial lineage differentiation but significantly increased the number of GFAP+ astrocytes generated to more than 55% (55.65±7.8%) of the cells (p≤

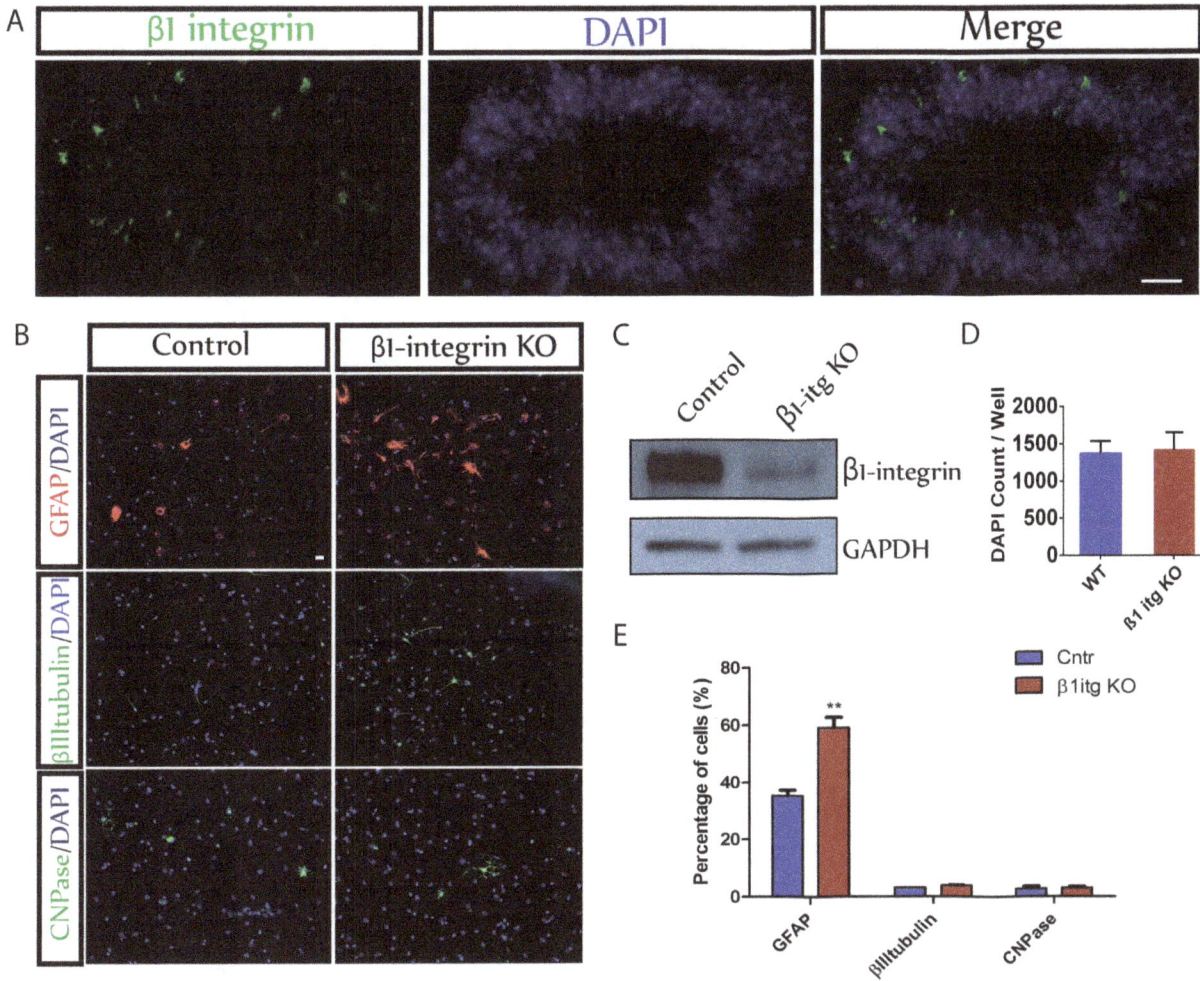

Figure 1. β1-integrin suppresses generation of astrocytes by NSCs derived from the spinal cord. A. Ependymal NSCs in adult mouse spinal cord express β1-integrin. B. NSCs derived from spinal cord are able to differentiate into astrocytes (GFAP -red), neurons (βIIItubulin-green) and oligodendrocytes (CNPase-green). β1-integrin Knock-Out (KO) increases astrocyte differentiation without altering neuronal or oligodendroglial differentiation. *Scale bar = 20 µm.* C. Western blot analysis shows depletion of β1 integrin protein levels in β1-itg KO NSCs derived from the spinal cord. D. Quantification of total cell numbers (DAPI) in the cultures of control and β1-integrin null cells analyzed for lineage commitment (E). There was no difference in overall cell numbers (n = 12, p = 0.89). Values are means ± SEM. E. Quantification of cell numbers of different lineages shows a significant increase (**p≤0.004) in astrocytes (67% of increase) in cultures of β1 integrin null cells at 7DIV without any change in neuronal or oligodendroglial differentiation.

0.046). Knockout of β1-integrin had an even greater effect on levels of GFAP mRNA which increased more than 2-fold compared to control, but levels of βIIItubulin and CNPase mRNAs were unchanged (Figure 2E). Thus the astrocyte-suppressive effects of β1-integrin are comparable in ESCs and in SVZ NSCs (Figure1E, 2D).

Inhibition of β1 integrin signaling by a dominant negative construct increases astrocytic differentiation

After binding to ligands, integrin receptors trigger an intracellular signaling cascade mediated predominantly via a small cytoplasmic domain of the β subunit [12]. This domain can cross talk with multiple intracellular signal transduction systems [28], thereby altering progenitor cell responses to extrinsic factors [13]. Specifically the cytoplasmic domain of β1 integrin mediates the majority of its intracellular signaling [12], and mutant forms of β1 integrin that lack this domain act as a dominant negative form of the receptor [20,22,41]. We misexpressed this form of β1 integrin,

hereafter referred to as β1ΔC, in NSCs using retroviral mediated gene transfer. Cultured NSCs were transduced with either control pCLE-IRES-GFP or β1ΔC-IRES-GFP retroviruses, FAC-sorted 48 hours later for the positively transfected cells, and plated in differentiating conditions. Seven days after plating, the percentages of neurons (βIII tubulin), astrocytes (GFAP) and oligodendrocytes (O4) were assayed. Expression of β1ΔC increased the number of GFAP⁺ astrocytes more than 2.5-fold (p≤0.005) compared to control pCLE cultures (Figure 3A, 3B), without altering numbers of neurons or oligodendrocytes (Figure 3B). This further supports the conclusion that β1-integrin signaling suppresses astrocytic differentiation.

IKVAV-PA increases β1-integrin expression in cultured NSCs and suppresses astrocytic differentiation

We next tried to overexpress β1-integrin in cultured NSCs using techniques identical to those used to overexpress β1ΔC. Since the overexpressed cDNA lacked the 3′UTR, we could design PCR

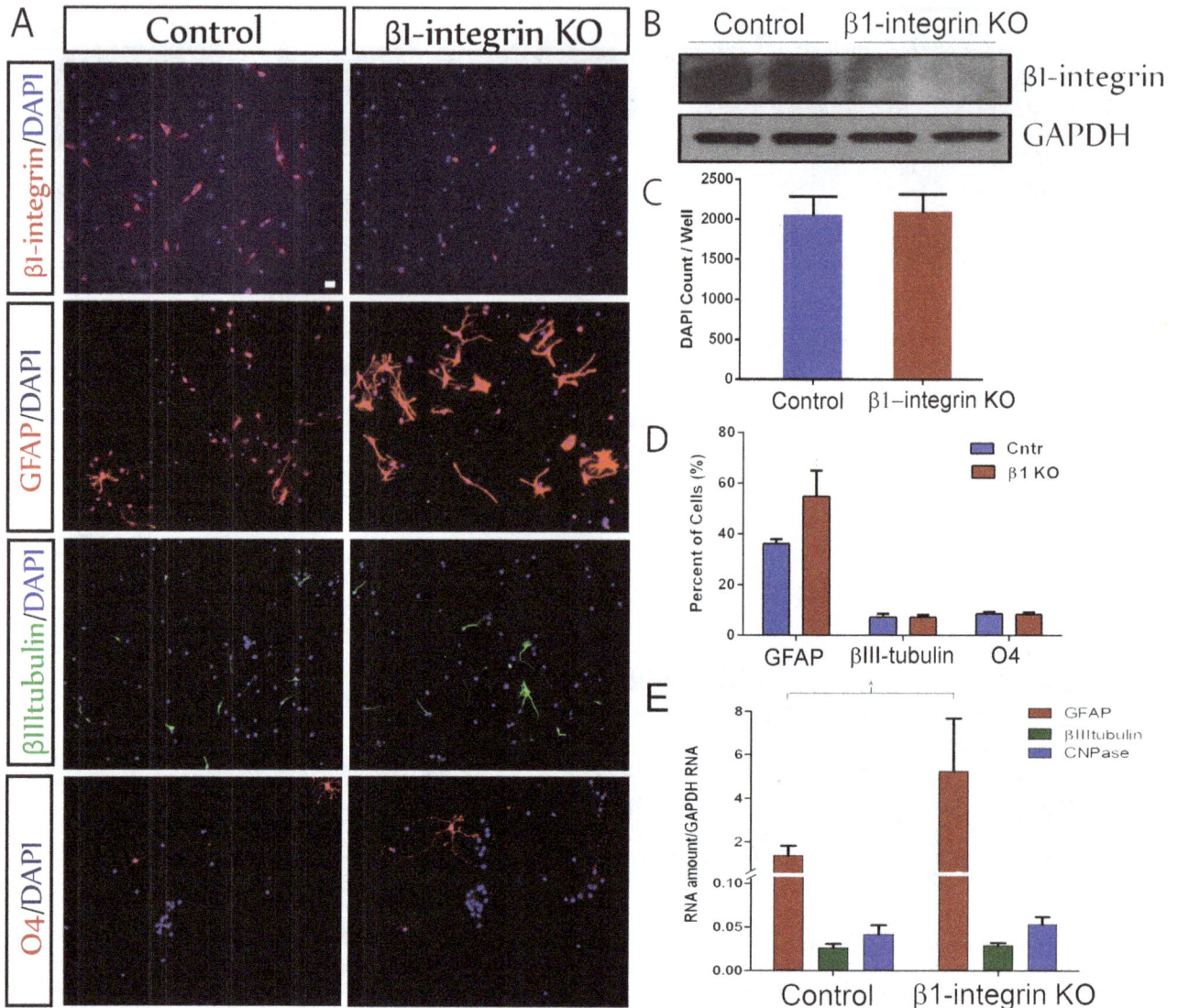

Figure 2. β1-integrin suppresses generation of astrocytes by NSCs derived from the SVZ. A. NSCs derived from the SVZ show a similar profile of differentiation as those derived from spinal cord. β1-integrin Knock-Out (KO) increases astrocytic differentiation (GFAP - red) without altering neuronal (βIIItubulin - green) or oligodendroglial (O4 -red) differentiation. *Scale bar = 20* μm. B. Western blot analysis shows depletion of β1-integrin protein in the β1KO derived NSCs compared with control. C. Quantification of total cell numbers (DAPI) in the cultures of control and β1-integrin null cells analyzed for lineage commitment (D). There was no difference in overall cell numbers (n = 20, p = 0.91). Values are means ± SEM. D. Quantification of cell numbers of different lineages shows a significant increase (*p≤0.046) in astrocytes (56% increase) in the β1-integrin KO group compared with control at 7DIV without any change in neuronal or oligodendroglial differentiation. E. Quantification of mRNA levels by qPCR after 7DIV reveals a significant increase in GFAP mRNA in the β1-integrin KO group compared with control. βIIItubulin and CNPase mRNAs were unchanged.

primers that detect the endogenous transcript alone as well ones that detect total β1 integrin. At 2 days post infection, there was a significant (~3 fold) increase in the levels of total β1-integrin. However, even at this time levels of endogenous transcript had already decreased by 60%. At 7 days, we could detect no difference in the levels of β1-integrin between the two groups (not shown). Multiple attempts to overexpress β1-integrin failed, presumably due to a strong feedback loop that maintained β1-integrin expression at a stable level. By contrast, culture of NSCs in the presence of IKVAV-PA markedly increased levels of β1-integrin expression compared to control cells grown in the presence of laminin (Figure 3C, 3D, 3E, 3F). There were

significant increases in expression of both β1-integrin protein (Figure 3C, 3D) and mRNA (Figure 3E, 3F).

We also evaluated the expression of different integrin subunits in cultured NSCs and found significant levels of α5, α6, and αV but no significant levels of β3 or β4 integrins. We then examined the levels of these integrin transcripts in NSCs cultured in IKVAV PA for 7 days using real time RT-PCR. There was a significant (~3 fold) increase in the β1 integrin transcript levels in cells cultured in IKVAV PA as compared to the control (Figure 3E, 3F). However, there were no changes in levels of the α5, α6 or αV subunits and no detectable levels of the β3 or β4 subunits. This suggests that IKVAV-PA is a uniquely effective tool for increasing β1-integrin expression by NSCs.

A
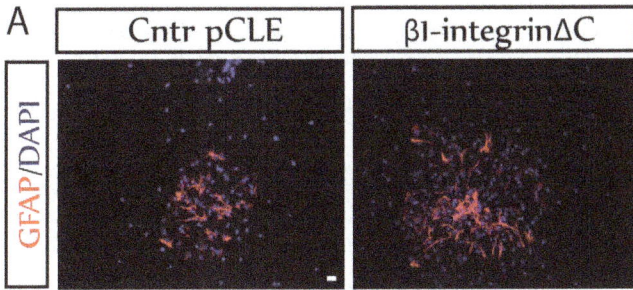

B
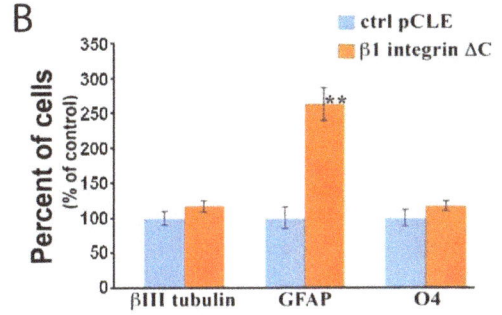

C
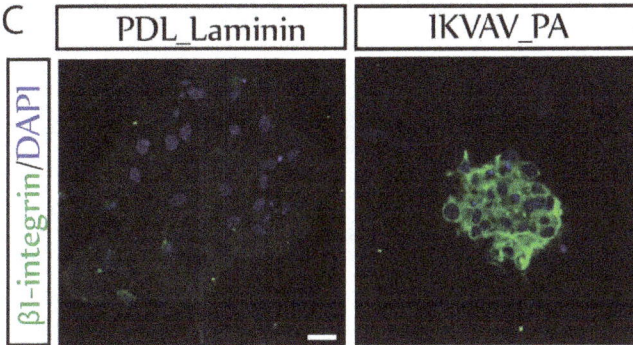

D
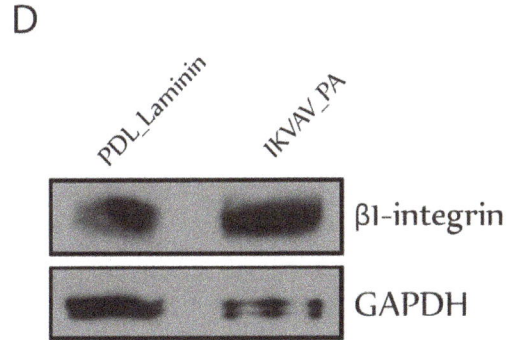

E
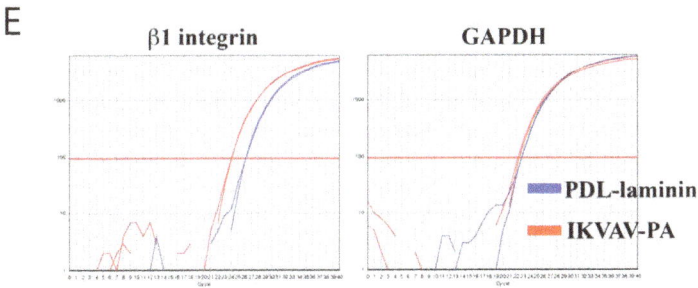

F
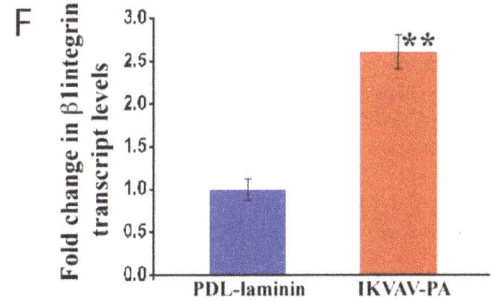

G
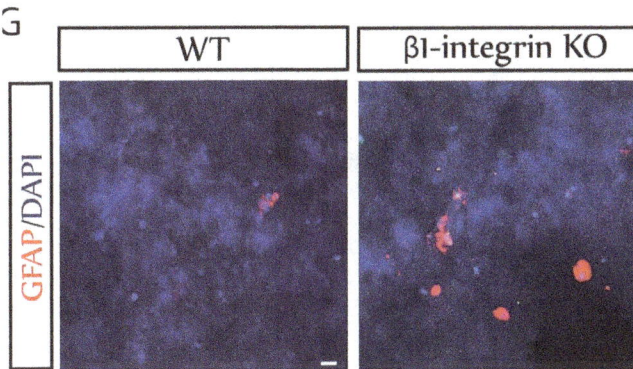

H
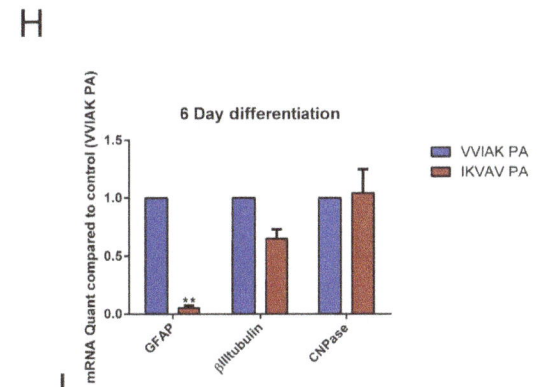

I
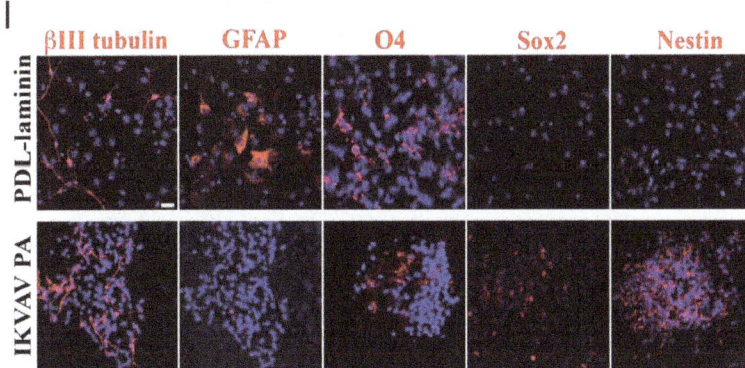

J
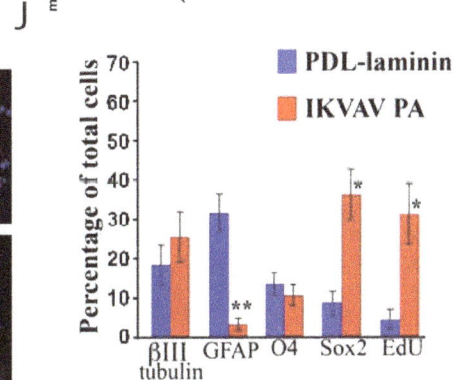

Figure 3. β1-integrin regulates astrocytic differentiation. A. NSCs were infected with retrovirus expressing GFP alone (ctrl pCLE) orβ1-integrinlacking the cytoplasmic domain (β1-integrin ΔC), cultured for 7 days on PDL-laminin and immunostained for GFAP (red) and DAPI (blue). *Scale bar = 20 μm.* B. Astrocytic differentiation (GFAP expression) increased more than 2.5 fold (**p≤0.005) in the β1- integrin ΔC group compared to control while neuronal (βIIItubulin) and oligodendroglial (O4) differentiation were unchanged. C. NSCs were cultured either on PDL-laminin or IKVAV-PA for one day and immunostained with β1- integrin (green) and DAPI (blue). Culture in IKVAV-PA dramatically increased expression of β1- integrin. *Scale bar = 20 μm.* D. Western Blot analysis shows that NSCs express higher levels of β1integrin protein when cultured for one day in IKVAV-PA compared to control (PDL-laminin). E. Real time PCR amplification plots showing that the β1integrin transcripts increase in cells cultured in IKVAV-PA compared to control (PDL-laminin). F. Quantitation of the increase in transcript levels of β1integrin in the IKVAV PA versus PDL-laminin group. (**p≤ 0.0007). G. KO of β1-integrin increases the number of astrocytes (GFAP – red) generated by NSCs cultured in IKVAV PA for 7 DIV. Blue = DAPI. H. NSCs were cultured in either control PA (VVIAK PA) or IKVAV PA for 7DIV, and RNA was extracted for qPCR quantification. The graph represents each lineage marker mRNA level in IKVAV PA normalized to levels in the control PA. Levels of GFAP mRNA were profoundly decreased (**p≤0.0005 in the IKVAV-PA group) without any significant change in levels of βIIItubulin of CNPase mRNAs. I. NPCs were cultured either on PDL-laminin or in IKVAV PA for 7DIV and immunostained with DAPI (blue) and several lineage markers (red). Note the absence of GFAP staining in the IKVAV PA group and the increase in the progenitor markers Sox2 and nestin. *Scale bar = 20 μm.* J. Quantification of the percentages of cells in the conditions described in (i) (*p≤0.017, **p≤0.005).

Culture of NSCs in the presence of IKVAV-PA increased levels of β1-integrin expression and suppressed astrocytic differentiation suggesting a causal relationship [47]. However, to directly test whether the suppressive effects on astrocyte development were due to the expression of β1-integrin, we examined the effects of IKVAV-PA on NSCs in which β1-integrin was knocked out using Adeno-Cre retrovirus as described above (Figure 3G). Culture of control NSCs in IKVAV-PA markedly suppressed astrocytic differentiation (12.5±1.4% of cells) as previously described [48]. However, more than 37% of cells (37.3±5.1%) in which β1-integrin was ablated differentiated into GFAP⁺ astrocytes even in the presence of IKVAV-PA. Thus the suppressive effects of IKVAV-PA on astrogliosis depended upon the presence of β1-integrin in the cells. We next wanted to ascertain that the effects of IKVAV-PA depended upon the integrity of the IKVAV epitope and were not related to other physicochemical properties of the PA. We therefore compared the effects of IKVAV-PA on mRNA expression with those of a PA in which the amino acid sequence of the epitope was scrambled (VVIAK-PA) (Figure 3H). The profound inhibitory effects of IKVAV-PA on expression of GFAP mRNA were lost when the IKVAV epitope was scrambled. However, there were no significant differences in levels of either βIIItubulin or CNPase mRNAs in IKVAV-PA and VVIAK-PA treated cells, indicating the specificity of the effects of the IKVAV epitope on expression of GFAP mRNA.

IKVAV-PA consistently suppressed astrocyte differentiation by cultured NSCs without changing either neuronal or oligodendroglial differentiation. This suggested that the PA maintained cells in an undifferentiated stem/progenitor cell state. To directly test this hypothesis we examined the effects of the PA on expression of the NSC marker, SOX2, as well as incorporation of the thymidine analog EdU. We used the most optimal substratum for control cells, PDL-laminin, for comparison even though it presented to cells a small amount of the IKVAV epitope (Figure 3I, 3J). Again the IKVAV-PA almost completely suppressed astrocytic differentiation (3.2±0.8% of the cells expressed GFAP versus 32.4±4.7% in controls; p≤0.005) without altering neuronal (βIIItubulin) or oligodendroglial (O4) lineage differentiation. However, the decrease in the percentage of GFAP-expressing cells was almost exactly matched by an increase in the percentage of cells that expressed Sox2 and that were proliferative as measured by EdU incorporation. These observations indicate that IKVAV suppressed astrocytic differentiation by maintaining cells in the NSC state.

The ILK pathway mediates suppressive effects of β1-integrin on astrocytic differentiation

We next sought to determine whether IKVAV-PA actually activates β1-integrin and to define the signaling pathways mediating the effects of β1-integrin on astrocytic development by NSCs. Integrins are heterodimeric receptors, and the relationship between the α and β subunits changes after ligand binding resulting in an "activated" protein conformation [29]. This conformational change initiates intracellular signaling and also increases the affinity of ligand binding [9,52]. We used a conformation sensitive β1-integrin antibody, HUTS-4 [29], to detect the activated form of β1-integrin in NSCs one day after plating in either IKVAV-PA or VVIAK-PA (Figure 4A). Almost all cells cultured in IKVAV-PA immunostained for the activated conformation of β1-integrin whereas little immunostaining was detectable in cells culture in VVIAK-PA. This provides evidence that IKVAV-PA rapidly activated β1-integrin.

β1-integrin signals through a variety of different mechanisms including but not limited to associating with other membrane proteins, serving as a binding dock for intracellular signaling molecules to bind and aggregate, and activating a specific set of intracellular domain bound kinases such as focal adhesion kinase (FAK) and integrin-linked kinase (ILK) [1,5]. Integrin-linked kinase (ILK) is a 59kDa serine/threonine protein kinase that associates with the cytoplasmic domain of β-integrins and transduces signaling after activation of the integrin [17]. Western blot analysis showed no difference in levels of FAK in NSCs grown in IKVAV PA compared to cells grown in VVIAK PA (Figure 4B). By contrast, culture of the cells in IKVAV PA resulted in a very large increase in levels of ILK (Figure 4B). Similarly, immunostaining for ILK indicated that most NSCs cultured in IKVAV PA expressed ILK whereas little staining was apparent in cells cultured in VVIAK PA (Figure 4A).

This suggested that ILK might mediate suppressive effects of β1-integrin on astrocytic development. To explore this hypothesis, we designed a rescue experiment to determine whether expression of a constitutively active form of ILK was sufficient to block the effects of knockout of β1-integrin (Figure 4C). We created two functionally mutated ILK expression constructs based on the findings of Hannigan, Troussard et al [16]. We substituted serine 343 of the potential autophosphorylation site with aspartate (S343D), to get a constitutive active form of ILK (ILK_CA), and we substituted serine 343 with Alanine (S343A) to make a kinase-dead ILK (ILK_KD). NSCs were isolated from β1-integrin^flx/flx mice and β1-integrin was knocked out as described above by infecting cells with Adeno-Cre or control virus. The cells were electroporated with either the ILK_CA or the ILK_KD construct, FAC- sorted two days later, and plated on PDL-Laminin for 7

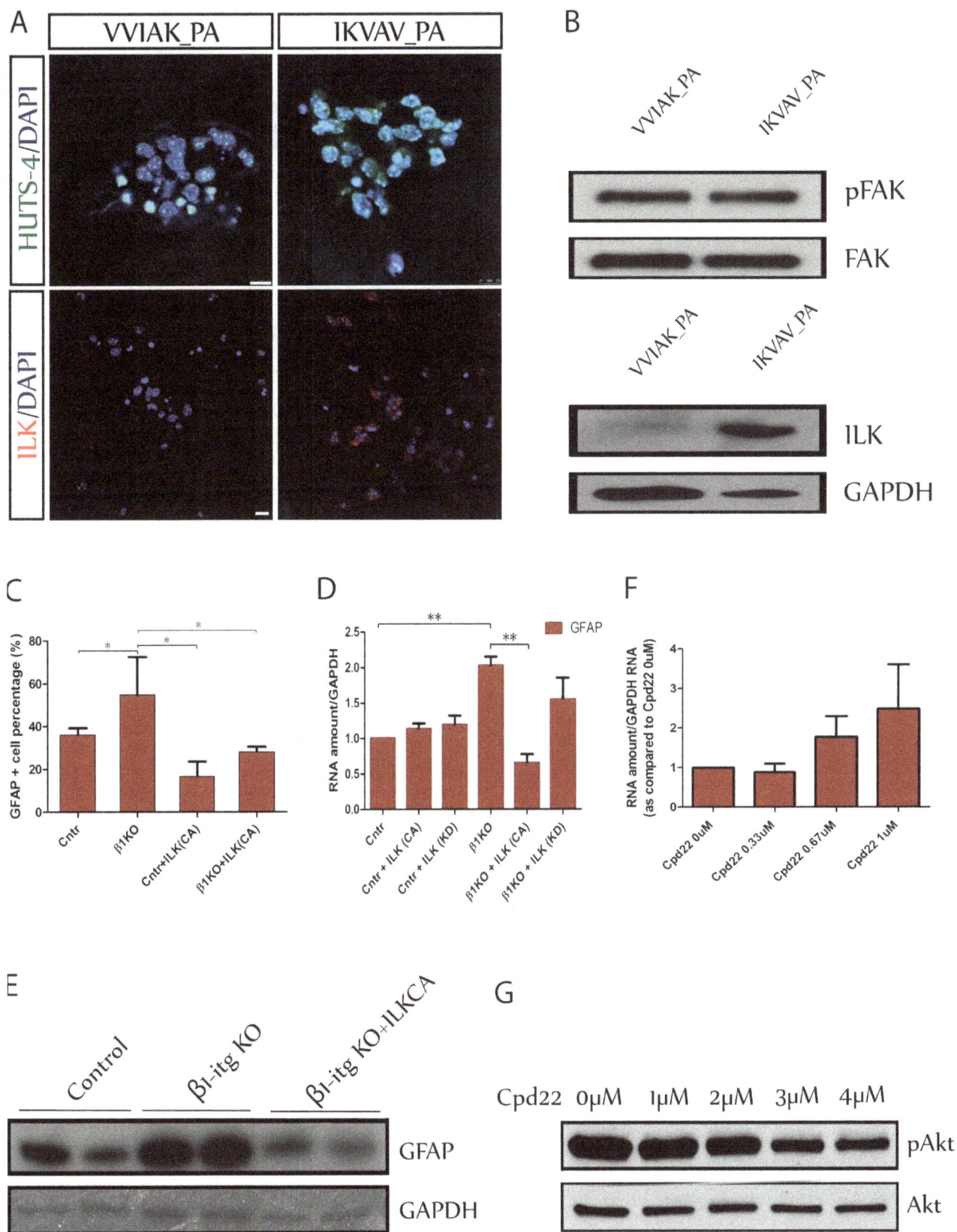

Figure 4. Integrin Linked Kinase (ILK) regulates astrocytic differentiation by NSCs. A. NSCs cultured in either control (scrambled) PA (VVIAK PA) or IKVAV PA for one day, and immunostained with activated β1integrin antibody HUTS-4 (green) or ILK (red). *Scale bar in HUTS-4 staining image = 10 μm, and in the ILK staining image = 20 μm.* B. Western blot analysis of NSCs cultured in either control PA (VVIAK PA) or IKVAV PA for one day. Note that levels of ILK are markedly elevated in the IKVAV-PA group without any change in FAK. C. β1-integrin KO and control NSCs were

transfected with either a control construct or a construct expressing a constitutively active form of ILK (ILK-CA). At 7DIV the cells were immunostained for GFAP and numbers of GFAP$^+$ cells were counted. (*p≤0.05) D. β1-integrin KO and control NSCs were transfected with a control construct, a construct expressing constitutively active ILK (ILK-CA), or a construct expressing kinase-dead ILK (ILK-KD) and cultured for 7DIV. RNA was extracted for qPCR measurement of GFAP mRNA graphed as a ratio compared to the control (**p≤0.004). Note that β1-integrin KO increased levels of GFAP mRNA, but this increase was blocked by expression of ILK-CA. E. Western blot analysis of GFAP expression in control NSCs and in β1-integrin KO NSCs transfected with either with a control construct or ILK-CA. Note that transfection with ILK-CA prevented the increase in GFAP expression in β1-integrin KO NSCs. F. NSCs were treated with different doses of the ILK inhibitor, Cpd22. After 6DIV RNA was extracted for qPCR quantification of GFAP. Note that GFAP expression increased in a dose dependent manner after treatment with Cpd22. H. NSCs were treated with different doses of the ILK inhibitor, Cpd22 for 3h, and protein was extracted for western blot analysis. Note that treatment with the drug reduced levels of phospho-Akt without any change in levels of AKT.

days in differentiating conditions. On day 7 cells were examined immunocytochemically (Figure 4C) and also were examined for levels of mRNAs for βIIItubulin, CNPase, and GFAP (Figure 4D). There were no detectable differences in the number of either βIIItubulin or CNPase immunoreactive cells across the different conditions (not shown). 37.3±3.1% of control cells expressed GFAP, but knockout of β1-integrin increased the percentage of GFAP-immunoreactive cells to 55.65±7.8% (p≤0.05) (Figure 4C). Overexpression of ILK-CA reduced the percentage of GFAP$^+$ cells to 16.7±4.0%, and overexpression of ILK-CA in β1-integrin knockout cells prevented the increase associated with knockout of β1-integrin (GFAP$^+$ cells number dropped to 28.1±1.4%). There were no detectable differences in levels of mRNA encoding either βIIItubulin or CNPase across the different conditions (not shown). Moreover neither construct exerted any effect on GFAP mRNA in control cells. However, knockout of β1-integrin increased levels of GFAP mRNA more than twofold, but expression of the ILK-CA construct prevented this increase and levels of mRNA in these cells actually trended lower than in control cells (Figure 4D). We then examined levels of GFAP protein in these cells by western blot analysis. Knockout of β1-integrin resulted in a very large increase in levels of GFAP protein (Figure 4E). Expression of the ILK-CA construct in β1-integrin knockout cells not only prevented the increase in GFAP but actually reduced it below control levels. There were no differences in proliferation (EdU$^+$ incorporation) among the groups. These observations indicate that ILK signaling suppresses astrogliogenesis, analogous to the effects of β1-integrin, and suggest that ILK mediates at least some of the effects of β1-integrin on astrocytic differentiation. To further test this hypothesis, we examined the effects of a chemical inhibitor of ILK, Cpd22 [23], on differentiation of NSCs. ILK has been shown act directly on Ser473 kinase in Akt [19]. To first verify that the inhibitor actually acted as expected in NSCs, the cells were treated with different concentrations of Cpd22 one day after plating (Figure 4G). 3 hours after drug application, we harvested protein for western blot analysis and found a dose-dependent inhibition of levels of phospho-Akt without any change in the overall levels of Akt. This suggested that the drug was able to penetrate NSCs and exert effects on a known ILK target. We therefore next assessed the effects of Cpd22 treatment on astrocytic differentiation. We chose a dose range that was tolerated well by the cells for a 6 day period of treatment without any evidence of cell death and examined the cells for levels of GFAP mRNA. Treatment of NSCs with the inhibitor resulted in a dose-dependent increase in levels of GFAP mRNA (Figure 4F). These data are supportive of the hypothesis that ILK signaling inhibits astrocytic differentiation.

IKVAV PA activates β1-integrin and suppresses glial scar formation after SCI

Previously we reported that injection of IKVAV-PA into an injured spinal cord suppresses glial scar formation and enhances behavioral outcome [54]. Since our findings *in vitro* suggested that

IKVAV-PA suppresses astrocytic development by activating β1-integrin, we sought to determine whether the PA actually activates β1-integrin signaling in the injured spinal cord. IKVAV-PA and a PA with a bioinert epitope (KKIAV-PA) were injected into the damaged spinal cord 24 hours after a contusion injury. The spinal cords were removed 3 weeks later for immunocytochemical analyses. As previously reported, injection of IKVAV-PA significantly reduced glial scarring as indicated by GFAP immunocytochemistry (Figure 5A, 5B). By contrast, the PA with an inert epitope had no demonstrable effect.

We then examined the spinal cords immunocytochemically using the HUTS-4 antibody to probe for the activated conformation of β1-integrin. IKVAV-PA and control vehicle were injected into the damaged spinal cord 48 hours after a contusion injury. The spinal cords were removed 1 week later for immunocytochemical analyses. Very little HUTS-4 staining was detectable in a vehicle-injected spinal cord (Figure 5C). By contrast, there was abundant HUTS-4 staining in the spinal cord injected with IKVAV-PA, demonstrating that the PA activated β1-integrin signaling *in vivo*.

Injection of IKVAV-PA into the injured spinal cord also consistently improved behavioral outcome [54] as measured by open field testing [3,21], but it was unclear whether the behavioral enhancement was also due to β1-integrin signaling. To help determine this we examined the effects of PAs displaying two different epitopes that are known to interact with β1-integrin, a Tenascin C epitope and the fibronectin epitope RGD [39,55]. The Tenascin C epitope, ADEGVFDNFVLK, is just a small portion of Tenascin C that interacts specifically with β1-integrin [31,33]. We injected these PAs into injured spinal cords of 8 weeks old adult rats two days after a standard impaction injury and followed behavioral outcome for 12 weeks. Similar to prior findings with IKVAV-PA, we found improvements with both Tenascin C-PA and RGD-PA (Figure 5D). Vehicle-injected animals reached an average score of 5.58±0.59 by 12 weeks after the injury. The Tenascin C-PA group reached an average score of 10.20±0.84 (p≤0.002) and the RGD-PA group achieved an average score of 8.5±2.1 (p≤0.024).

Discussion

β1-integrin is a transmembrane receptor protein expressed by stem cells in many organ systems [15,25]. β1-integrin signaling mediates a variety of stem cell functions including pluripotency maintenance, self-renewal, proliferation and regulation of migration [25]. In the present study, we report that β1-integrin signaling inhibits astrocytic differentiation by both spinal cord ependymal stem cells and subventricular zone stem cells and helps to maintain stemness. We further found that these effects are mediated, at least in part, by ILK. In previous studies we found that injection of IKVAV-PA into an injured spinal cord limited glial scar formation and enhanced behavioral outcome. In this present study, we report an underlying mechanism to be a ligand (IKVAV) mediated

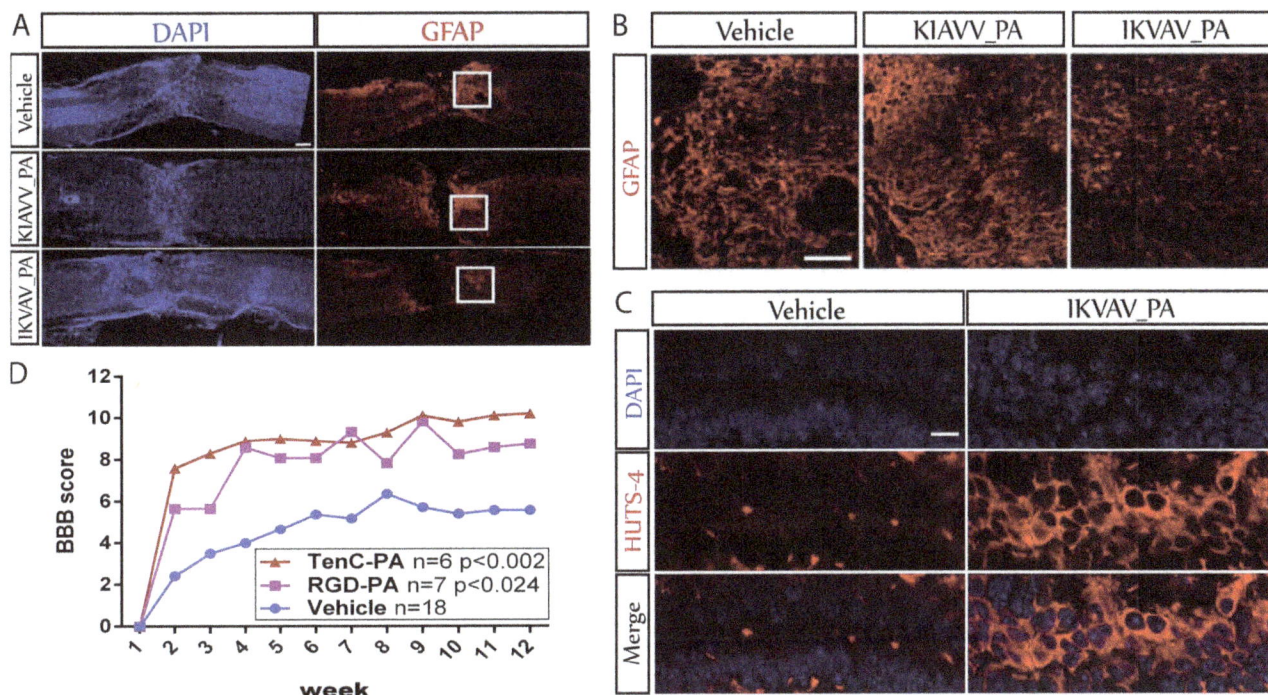

Figure 5. β1-integrin signaling in vivo regulates astrogliogenesis after spinal cord injury (SCI). A. Low magnification (10X) images of representative longitudinal sections of injured mouse spinal cords at 3 weeks post SCI, that were injected with either the IKVAV PA, scrambled KIAVV PA or vehicle injected at 24 hours post injury. Sections are stained with DAPI (blue) and GFAP (red). *Scale bar = 200 µm.* B. Representative confocal Z-stacks taken at higher magnification (20X) of the areas boxed in (a) showing reduced gliosis in the IKVAV PA injected animals at 3 weeks post SCI. *Scale bar = 100 µm.* C. High magnification (63x) confocal images of the ependymal regions stained with activated β1integrin antibody HUTS-4 (red) and DAPI (blue). Injured mouse spinal cords were injected either with IKVAV PA or vehicle 2 days post injury. *Scale bar = 20 µm.* D. Spinal cord injured rats were injected with either Tenascin-C epitope presenting PA, RGD epitope presenting PA or vehicle 2 days post injury, and monitored with BBB scoring for 12 weeks. Both PA groups showed significant improvement compared to the vehicle group.

increase of β1 integrin signaling in ependymal cells which suppresses astrogliosis.

Astrogliosis after SCI has both beneficial and detrimental effects on recovery. Astrocytic hypertrophy is necessary for repairing the damaged blood-brain barrier, and it is a beneficial process that limits inflammatory damage and restores homeostasis [10,27,38]. However, astrocytic hyperplasia leads to formation of a dense glial scar that inhibits axonal regeneration [48]. Therapeutic approaches to limiting glial scar formation after SCI must therefore seek to limit the detrimental effects of astrocytic hyperplasia while maintaining the beneficial effects of the initial reactive astrocytes. In previous studies we found that injection into an injured spinal cord of IKVAV-PA limited astrocytic hyperplasia without altering the early hypertrophic response to the injury [54]. However, the reason for these divergent effects was unclear. In the present study we found that ESCs expressed high levels of β1-integrin after SCI whereas levels of the protein were not demonstrably increased in resident astrocytes after the injury. Further, our findings suggested that the effects of the PA reflected limitation of ESC differentiation into astrocytes. By contrast, β1-integrin signaling does not alter astrocyte proliferation although it exerts effects on reactive gliosis [43]. Thus injection of IKVAV-PA into a damaged spinal cord was able to limit astrogliosis by limiting ESC differentiation into astrocytes without altering the beneficial responses of resident astrocytes to the injury. Our findings indicate a causal relationship between IKVAV PA application and β1-intregrin signaling activation in vivo. This conclusion is supported by our observation that ablation of β1-intregrin in ESCs significantly worsens behavioral outcome after SCI (unpublished observation).

Identification of the molecular mechanisms underlying the beneficial effects of the PA should enable design of new targeted molecules that are even more effective in promoting recovery after SCI. For example, we found that PAs displaying two other epitopes known to interact with β1-integrin, a Tenascin C epitope and the RGD epitope of fibronectin, facilitated behavioral recovery after SCI. Ultimately it should be possible to design molecules that are even more effective therapeutically. For example, PAs can be created that incorporate more than one β1-integrin-interacting epitope and that also include epitopes targeting other signaling molecules such BMP receptors [44] or cytokines that activate JAK-STAT signaling [37] that have been implicated in astrocytic responses after SCI.

The increase in GFAP expression after ablation of β1-integrin in NSCs was accompanied by an increase in the number of GFAP+ astrocytes detected by immunocytochemistry suggesting an increase in astrocyte lineage commitment. Because this comparison was done under differentiation conditions with very low levels of EGF, proliferation was limited. However it is possible that the increase in GFAP expression simply allowed detection of preexisting astrocytes with previously undetectable levels of GFAP. In either case, our findings support our hypothesis that β1-integrin signaling suppresses astrocytic differentiation, and is consistent with our finding *in vivo* that increased β1-integrin signaling leads to reduced glial scar formation. It should also be noted that the increase in GFAP+ cells *in vitro* in the presence of IKVAV-PA was matched by a decrease in the number of Sox2+ stem cells suggesting an effect on lineage commitment.

Our observations indicate that at least some of the effects of β1-integrin signaling on astrocytic differentiation are mediated by ILK, but the precise mechanisms mediating the effects of ILK remain unclear. ILK is a serine/threonine protein kinase that directly affects numerous other signaling pathways [17,24]. For example, in dendritic formation ILK directly phosphorylates GSK-3beta thus inhibiting its signaling [35]. However, in addition to its kinase activity, ILK can initiate signal transduction through its function as a scaffolding protein. For example, in mouse kidney development, the auto-phosphorylation site of ILK is dispensable, whereas the alpha-parvin binding ability of ILK is critical for normal development [49]. In both cases the effects of ILK reflect modulation of other important signaling pathways in the cell. Possible candidates include the PI3K/Akt and PI3K/RhoA pathways, that are known downstream targets of ILK and that have been implicated in reducing the potential for astrocytic differentiation [6]. However in other systems ILK signaling has also been linked to BMP and JAK-STAT signaling which are the major pathways involved in astrocytic differentiation [26,51]. Delineation of the set of pathways that mediate the effects of ILK on astrogliosis will ultimately be required to design effective interventions for limiting gliosis after injury to the nervous system.

It is noteworthy that the effects of β1-integrin signaling on astrocytic development were almost identical in ESCs isolated from the adult spinal cord and NSCs isolated from the adult SVZ. In turn this suggests that this signaling system may be an important target for regulating astrogliosis after brain injury as well as after SCI. Although this study did not examine the responses of subgranular zone stem cells to β1-integrin signaling, we find that the molecule is expressed abundantly in the SGZ. Thus it is likely that β1-integrin signaling an important regulator of stem cell proliferation and differentiation throughout the adult nervous system.

Acknowledgments

We thank Mark Benton for his critical reading of this manuscript.

Author Contributions

Conceived and designed the experiments: LP HAN VS JAK. Performed the experiments: LP HAN VS SJ TLM EJB. Analyzed the data: LP VS JAK. Contributed reagents/materials/analysis tools: EJB SIS JAK. Contributed to the writing of the manuscript: LP VS JAK.

References

1. Anthis NJ, Campbell ID (2011) The tail of integrin activation. Trends Biochem Sci, 36(4): p. 191–8.
2. Barnabe-Heider F, Goritz C, Sabelstrom H, Takebayashi H, Pfrieger FW, et al. (2010) Origin of new glial cells in intact and injured adult spinal cord. Cell Stem Cell, 7(4): p. 470–82.
3. Basso DM, Beattie MS, Bresnahan JC, Anderson DK, Faden AI, et al. (1996) MASCIS evaluation of open field locomotor scores: effects of experience and teamwork on reliability. Multicenter Animal Spinal Cord Injury Study. J Neurotrauma, 13(7): p. 343–59.
4. Bonaguidi MA, McGuire T, Hu M, Kan L, Samanta J, et al. (2005) LIF and BMP signaling generate separate and discrete types of GFAP-expressing cells. Development, 132(24): p. 5503–14.
5. Brakebusch C, Fassler R (2005) beta 1 integrin function in vivo: adhesion, migration and more. Cancer Metastasis Rev, 24(3): p. 403–11.
6. Brozzi F, Arcuri C, Giambanco I, Donato R (2009) S100B Protein Regulates Astrocyte Shape and Migration via Interaction with Src Kinase: IMPLICATIONS FOR ASTROCYTE DEVELOPMENT, ACTIVATION, AND TUMOR GROWTH. J Biol Chem, 284(13): p. 8797–811.
7. Campbell ID, Humphries MJ (2011) Integrin structure, activation, and interactions. Cold Spring Harb Perspect Biol, 3(3)
8. Campos LS, Leone DP, Relvas JB, Brakebusch C, Fassler R, et al. (2004) Beta1 integrins activate a MAPK signalling pathway in neural stem cells that contributes to their maintenance. Development, 131(14): p. 3433–44.
9. Casar B, Rimann I, Kato H, Shattil SJ, Quigley JP, et al. (2012) In vivo cleaved CDCP1 promotes early tumor dissemination via complexing with activated beta1 integrin and induction of FAK/PI3K/Akt motility signaling. Oncogene.
10. Dusart I, Marty S, Peschanski M (1991) Glial changes following an excitotoxic lesion in the CNS–II. Astrocytes. Neuroscience, 45(3): p. 541–9.
11. Fawcett JW, Asher RA (1999) The glial scar and central nervous system repair. Brain Res Bull, 49(6): p. 377–91.
12. Giancotti FG (1997) Integrin signaling: specificity and control of cell survival and cell cycle progression. Curr Opin Cell Biol, 9(5): p. 691–700.
13. Giancotti FG, Ruoslahti E (1999) Integrin signaling. Science, 285(5430): p. 1028–32.
14. Hall DE, Reichardt LF, Crowley E, Holley B, Moezzi H, et al. (1990) The alpha 1/beta 1 and alpha 6/beta 1 integrin heterodimers mediate cell attachment to distinct sites on laminin. J Cell Biol, 110(6): p. 2175–84.
15. Hall PE, Lathia JD, Miller NG, Caldwell MA, ffrench-Constant C (2006) Integrins are markers of human neural stem cells. Stem Cells, 24(9): p. 2078–84.
16. Hannigan G, Troussard AA, Dedhar S(2005) Integrin-linked kinase: a cancer therapeutic target unique among its ILK. Nat Rev Cancer, 5(1): p. 51–63.
17. Hannigan GE, Leung-Hagesteijn C, Fitz-Gibbon L, Coppolino MG, Radeva G, et al. (1996) Regulation of cell adhesion and anchorage-dependent growth by a new beta 1-integrin-linked protein kinase. Nature, 379(6560): p. 91–6.
18. Herrmann JE, Imura T, Song B, Qi J, Ao Y, et al. (2008) STAT3 is a critical regulator of astrogliosis and scar formation after spinal cord injury. J Neurosci, 28(28): p. 7231–43.
19. Hill MM, Feng J, Hemmings BA (2002) Identification of a plasma membrane Raft-associated PKB Ser473 kinase activity that is distinct from ILK and PDK1. Curr Biol, 12(14): p. 1251–5.
20. Hynes RO (1992) Integrins: versatility, modulation, and signaling in cell adhesion. Cell, 69(1): p. 11–25.

21. Joshi M, Fehlings MG (2002) Development and characterization of a novel, graded model of clip compressive spinal cord injury in the mouse: Part 1. Clip design, behavioral outcomes, and histopathology. J Neurotrauma, 19(2): p. 175–90.
22. Lee KK, de Repentigny Y, Saulnier R, Rippstein P, Macklin WB, et al. (2006) Dominant-negative beta1 integrin mice have region-specific myelin defects accompanied by alterations in MAPK activity. Glia, 53(8): p. 836–44.
23. Lee SL, Hsu EC, Chou CC, Chuang HC, Bai LY, et al. (2011) Identification and characterization of a novel integrin-linked kinase inhibitor. J Med Chem, 54(18): p. 6364–74.
24. Legate KR, Montanez E, Kudlacek O, Fassler R (2006) ILK, PINCH and parvin: the tIPP of integrin signalling. Nat Rev Mol Cell Biol, 7(1): p. 20–31.
25. Leone DP, Relvas JB, Campos LS, Hemmi S, Brakebusch C, et al. (2005) Regulation of neural progenitor proliferation and survival by beta1 integrins. J Cell Sci, 118(Pt 12): p. 2589–99.
26. Leung-Hagesteijn C, Hu MC, Mahendra AS, Hartwig S, Klamut HJ, et al. (2005) Integrin-linked kinase mediates bone morphogenetic protein 7-dependent renal epithelial cell morphogenesis. Mol Cell Biol, 25(9): p. 3648–57.
27. Liberto CM, Albrecht PJ, Herx LM, Yong VW, Levison SW (2004) Pro-regenerative properties of cytokine-activated astrocytes. J Neurochem, 89(5): p. 1092–100.
28. Liu S, Calderwood DA, Ginsberg MH (2000) Integrin cytoplasmic domain-binding proteins. J Cell Sci, 113 (Pt 20): p. 3563–71.
29. Luque A, Gomez M, Puzon W, Takada Y, Sanchez-Madrid F, et al. (1996) Activated conformations of very late activation integrins detected by a group of antibodies (HUTS) specific for a novel regulatory region (355–425) of the common beta 1 chain. J Biol Chem, 271(19): p. 11067–75.
30. Mehler MF, Mabie PC, Zhu G, Gokhan S, Kessler JA (2000) Developmental changes in progenitor cell responsiveness to bone morphogenetic proteins differentially modulate progressive CNS lineage fate. Dev Neurosci, 22(1–2): p. 74–85.
31. Meiners S, Nur-e-Kamal MS, Mercado ML (2001) Identification of a neurite outgrowth-promoting motif within the alternatively spliced region of human tenascin-C. J Neurosci, 21(18): p. 7215–25.
32. Meletis K, Barnabe-Heider F, Carlen M, Evergren E, Tomilin N, et al. (2008) Spinal cord injury reveals multilineage differentiation of ependymal cells. PLoS Biol, 6(7): p. e182.
33. Mercado ML, Nur-e-Kamal A, Liu HY, Gross SR, Movahed R, et al. (2004) Neurite outgrowth by the alternatively spliced region of human tenascin-C is mediated by neuronal alpha7beta1 integrin. J Neurosci, 24(1): p. 238–47.
34. Milner R, Campbell IL (2002) The integrin family of cell adhesion molecules has multiple functions within the CNS. J Neurosci Res, 69(3): p. 286–91.
35. Naska S, Park KJ, Hannigan GE, Dedhar S, Miller FD, et al. (2006) An essential role for the integrin-linked kinase-glycogen synthase kinase-3 beta pathway during dendrite initiation and growth. J Neurosci, 26(51): p. 13344–56.
36. Nomizu M, Weeks BS, Weston CA, Kim WH, Kleinman HK, et al. (1995) Structure-activity study of a laminin alpha 1 chain active peptide segment Ile-Lys-Val-Ala-Val (IKVAV). FEBS Lett, 365(2–3): p. 227–31.
37. Okada S, Nakamura M, Katoh H, Miyao T, Shimazaki T, et al. (2006) Conditional ablation of Stat3 or Socs3 discloses a dual role for reactive astrocytes after spinal cord injury. Nat Med, 12(7): p. 829–34.

38. Pekny M, Nilsson M (2005) Astrocyte activation and reactive gliosis. Glia, 50(4): p. 427–34.

39. Pfaff M, Gohring W, Brown JC, Timpl R (1994) Binding of purified collagen receptors (alpha 1 beta 1, alpha 2 beta 1) and RGD-dependent integrins to laminins and laminin fragments. Eur J Biochem, 225(3): p. 975–84.

40. Pruszak J, Ludwig W, Blak A, Alavian K, Isacson O (2009) CD15, CD24, and CD29 define a surface biomarker code for neural lineage differentiation of stem cells. Stem Cells, 27(12): p. 2928–40.

41. Relvas JB, Setzu A, Baron W, Buttery PC, LaFlamme SE, et al. (2001) Expression of dominant-negative and chimeric subunits reveals an essential role for beta1 integrin during myelination. Curr Biol, 11(13): p. 1039–43.

42. Robel S, Berninger B, Gotz M(2011) The stem cell potential of glia: lessons from reactive gliosis. Nat Rev Neurosci, 12(2): p. 88–104.

43. Robel S, Mori T, Zoubaa S, Schlegel J, Sirko S, et al. (2009) Conditional deletion of beta1-integrin in astroglia causes partial reactive gliosis. Glia, 57(15): p. 1630–47.

44. Sahni V, Mukhopadhyay A, Tysseling V, Hebert A, Birch D, et al. (2010) BMPR1a and BMPR1b signaling exert opposing effects on gliosis after spinal cord injury. J Neurosci, 30(5): p. 1839–55.

45. Sanchez-Mateos P, Cabanas C, Sanchez-Madrid F (1996) Regulation of integrin function. Semin Cancer Biol, 7(3): p. 99–109.

46. Sephel GC, Tashiro KI, Sasaki M, Greatorex D, Martin GR, et al. (1989) Laminin A chain synthetic peptide which supports neurite outgrowth. Biochem Biophys Res Commun, 162(2): p. 821–9.

47. Silva GA, Czeisler C, Niece KL, Beniash E, Harrington DA, et al. (2004) Selective differentiation of neural progenitor cells by high-epitope density nanofibers. Science, 303(5662): p. 1352–5.

48. Silver J, Miller JH (2004) Regeneration beyond the glial scar. Nat Rev Neurosci, 5(2): p. 146–56.

49. Smeeton J, Zhang X, Bulus N, Mernaugh G, Lange A, et al. (2010) Integrin-linked kinase regulates p38 MAPK-dependent cell cycle arrest in ureteric bud development. Development, 137(19): p. 3233–43.

50. Stirling DP, Liu S, Kubes P, Yong VW (2009) Depletion of Ly6G/Gr-1 leukocytes after spinal cord injury in mice alters wound healing and worsens neurological outcome. J Neurosci, 29(3): p. 753–64.

51. Tabe Y, Jin L, Tsutsumi-Ishii Y, Xu Y, McQueen T, et al. (2007) Activation of integrin-linked kinase is a critical prosurvival pathway induced in leukemic cells by bone marrow-derived stromal cells. Cancer Res, 67(2): p. 684–94.

52. Tadokoro S, Shattil SJ, Eto K, Tai V, Liddington RC, et al. (2003) Talin binding to integrin beta tails: a final common step in integrin activation. Science, 302(5642): p. 103–6.

53. Tashiro K, Sephel GC, Weeks B, Sasaki M, Martin GR, et al. (1989) A synthetic peptide containing the IKVAV sequence from the A chain of laminin mediates cell attachment, migration, and neurite outgrowth. J Biol Chem, 264(27): p. 16174–82.

54. Tysseling-Mattiace VM, Sahni V, Niece KL, Birch D, Czeisler C, et al. (2008) Self-assembling nanofibers inhibit glial scar formation and promote axon elongation after spinal cord injury. J Neurosci, 28(14): p. 3814–23.

55. Yokosaki Y, Monis H, Chen J, Sheppard D (1996) Differential effects of the integrins alpha9beta1, alphavbeta3, and alphavbeta6 on cell proliferative responses to tenascin. Roles of the beta subunit extracellular and cytoplasmic domains. J Biol Chem, 271(39): p. 24144–50.

56. Zhu Y, Li H, Zhou L, Wu JY, Rao Y (1999) Cellular and molecular guidance of GABAergic neuronal migration from an extracortical origin to the neocortex. Neuron, 23(3): p. 473–85.

11

Spinal Cord Transection-Induced Allodynia in Rats – Behavioral, Physiopathological and Pharmacological Characterization

Saïd M'Dahoma[1,2]*, **Sylvie Bourgoin**[1,2], **Valérie Kayser**[1,2], **Sandrine Barthélémy**[1,2], **Caroline Chevarin**[1,2], **Farah Chali**[3], **Didier Orsal**[3], **Michel Hamon**[1,2]

1 Centre de Psychiatrie et Neurosciences, Institut National de la Santé et de la Recherche Médicale, INSERM U894, Université Paris Descartes, Paris, France, **2** Neuropsychopharmacologie, Faculté de Médecine Pierre et Marie Curie, site Pitié-Salpêtrière, Paris, France, **3** Laboratoire de Neurobiologie des Signaux Intercellulaires, Centre National de la Recherche Scientifique, CNRS UMR 7101, Université Pierre et Marie Curie, Paris, France

Abstract

In humans, spinal cord lesions induce not only major motor and neurovegetative deficits but also severe neuropathic pain which is mostly resistant to classical analgesics. Better treatments can be expected from precise characterization of underlying physiopathological mechanisms. This led us to thoroughly investigate (i) mechanical and thermal sensory alterations, (ii) responses to acute treatments with drugs having patent or potential anti-allodynic properties and (iii) the spinal/ganglion expression of transcripts encoding markers of neuronal injury, microglia and astrocyte activation in rats that underwent complete spinal cord transection (SCT). SCT was performed at thoracic T8–T9 level under deep isoflurane anaesthesia, and SCT rats were examined for up to two months post surgery. SCT induced a marked hyper-reflexia at hindpaws and strong mechanical and cold allodynia in a limited (6 cm^2) cutaneous territory just rostral to the lesion site. At this level, pressure threshold value to trigger nocifensive reactions to locally applied von Frey filaments was 100-fold lower in SCT- versus sham-operated rats. A marked up-regulation of mRNAs encoding ATF3 (neuronal injury) and glial activation markers (OX-42, GFAP, P2×4, P2×7, TLR4) was observed in spinal cord and/or dorsal root ganglia at T6-T11 levels from day 2 up to day 60 post surgery. Transcripts encoding the proinflammatory cytokines IL-1β, IL-6 and TNF-α were also markedly but differentially up-regulated at T6–T11 levels in SCT rats. Acute treatment with ketamine (50 mg/kg i.p.), morphine (3–10 mg/kg s.c.) and tapentadol (10–20 mg/kg i.p.) significantly increased pressure threshold to trigger nocifensive reaction in the von Frey filaments test, whereas amitriptyline, pregabalin, gabapentin and clonazepam were ineffective. Because *all* SCT rats developed *long lasting, reproducible and stable* allodynia, which could be alleviated by drugs effective in humans, thoracic cord transection might be a reliable model for testing innovative therapies aimed at reducing spinal cord lesion-induced central neuropathic pain.

Editor: Mohammed Shamji, Toronto Western Hospital, Canada

Funding: This research has been supported by grants from Institut National de la Santé et de la Recherche Médicale (INSERM), University Pierre and Marie Curie (UPMC), Agence Nationale de la Recherche (Contract ANR 11BSV4 017 04, TrkBDNFarmod), and Institut pour la Recherche sur la Moelle Epinière et l'Encéphale (IRME, Contract "M.Hamon, 2010–2011"). Saïd M'Dahoma was supported by fellowships from the Ministère de la Recherche et de l'Enseignement Supérieur (France) during performance of this work. The funders had no role in study design, data collection and analysis, decision to publish, or preparation of the manuscript.

Competing Interests: The authors have declared that no competing interests exist.

* Email: said.mdahoma@yahoo.fr

Introduction

Spinal cord injury (SCI) is a debilitating state which causes not only severe motor dysfunctions, loss of bladder control and impairment of sexual function, but also chronic pain, especially neuropathic pain [1,2]. Pain can be so severe that some SCI patients would be ready to privilege pain relief at the expense of further deficits in bladder control or sexual function. SCI-induced central neuropathic pain can be localized above-, at- or below- the level of injury and is mostly characterized by allodynia refractory to conventional treatments [2,3].

Several animal models of SCI-induced neuropathic pain have been developed (through spinal cord contusion, compression, ischemia, section; see [4]), each of them displaying different characteristics in terms of localization, duration, type of pain and

even responses to drugs. Although some studies did provide relevant data regarding treatment efficacy and underlying molecular mechanisms [5–7], they focused mostly on pain below the lesion produced by contusion or clip compression of the spinal cord. Yet, despite the fact that these SCI models reproduce adequately some types of spinal cord injuries seen in humans, they suffer from limitations because of unavoidable, large, interindividual variations in the extent and severity of evoked lesions [8,9]. Furthermore, lesion-induced neuroinflammatory processes could be highly variable among SCI rats which underwent the very same lesion procedure [10], so that characterization of actual physiopathological mechanisms underlying neuropathic pain might be a real challenge in, at least, some SCI models.

In contrast to these models, complete transection of the spinal cord would be cleared of such limitations due to unavoidable interindividual variations in the extent and severity of the lesion. Indeed, spinal cord transection (SCT) has already been widely used to study the mechanisms of subsequent locomotor recovery [11–13] and reorganization of the somatosensory system [14–15] in medullary lesioned rats. However, to date, only few studies showed that the SCT model could be used to investigate spinal lesion-induced neuropathic pain [16], and, indeed, some authors even reported that no neuropathic pain develops in rats with complete SCT [17,18].

These discrepant data led us to reinvestigate whether or not the rat model consisting of complete SCT at the thoracic level could be a relevant model of central neuropathic pain, allowing studies of underlying physiopathological mechanisms and responses to drugs with patent or potential alleviating properties. Nocifensive responses to mechanical and thermal stimulations were assessed using the validated von Frey filaments test and the paw immersion and acetone drop tests, respectively. We then investigated whether responses to these tests could be affected by acute treatments with various drugs (opioids, antidepressants, anticonvulsants and others) known to alleviate neuropathic pain in SCI patients. Finally, we analyzed by real time quantitative RT-PCR, at different times after thoracic cord transection, the expression of mRNAs encoding proteins implicated in neuroinflammation and neuroplasticity, with particular focus on markers of microglia and astrocyte activation, pro- and anti-inflammatory cytokines (Interleukins IL-1β, IL-6 and IL-10, Tumor Necrosis Factor alpha,TNF-α), Brain-Derived Neurotrophic Factor (BDNF) and nociceptive signaling pathways in dorsal root ganglia (DRG) and spinal cord tissues, for comparison with previous studies aimed at unveiling physiopathological mechanisms associated with neuropathic pain in other SCI models.

Materials and Methods

Animals and Ethics Statements

Male Sprague–Dawley rats, weighing 225–250 g (7–8 weeks old) on arrival in the laboratory, were purchased from Janvier Breeding Center (53940 Le Genest Saint Isle, France). They were housed under standard controlled environmental conditions ($22\pm1°C$, 60% relative humidity, 12:12 h light–dark cycle, lights on at 7:00 am), on ground corn cobs (GM-12, SAFE, 89290, Augy, France), with complete diet for rats/mice/hamster (105, SAFE, 89290, Augy) and tap water available *ad libitum*. Before surgery, rats were housed 5 per cage (40×40 cm, 20 cm high) and allowed to habituate to the housing facilities without any handling for at least 1 week before being used. After surgery, all efforts were made to minimize suffering. In particular, SCT rats were housed under the very same conditions, except that each cage was for only two operated rats, so as to avoid as much as possible allodynic contacts between them. All animals were thoroughly examined each day, and in case of any sign of abnormal physiological alterations or suffering appeared, they were immediately sacrificed by a lethal dose of pentobarbital (150 mg/kg i.p.), strictly following the recommendations of the Ethical Committee of the French Ministry of Research and High Education (articles R.214–124, R.214–125). Both the Ethics and Scientific Committee of the French *Institut pour la Recherche sur la Moelle Epinière et l'Encéphale* (IRME; contract to M.H., 2010–2011) and the national (French) Committee for Animal Care and Use for Scientific Research (registration nb.01296.01; official authorization B75-116 to M.H., 31 December 2012) specifically approved the study.

In addition, the Ethical Guidelines of the Committee for Research and Ethical Issues of the International Association for the Study of Pain [19] and the Institutional Guidelines in compliance with French and international laws and policies (Council directive 87–848, October 19, 1987, *Ministère de l'Agriculture et de la Forêt, Service vétérinaire de la santé et de la protection animale*, permissions nb A752128 to S.M., 006228 to S.B., nb 00482 to V.K.) were strictly followed.

Spinal Cord Transection

Animals underwent surgery under deep isoflurane anaesthesia (3%). Paravertebral muscles were cut bilaterally and the T8 vertebra was opened using a gouge-forceps. Local anaesthesia was made by cooling the spinal cord with cryoflurane (Promedica, France) a few seconds before the lesion. Complete transverse section with ophthalmic scissors at the T8–T9 spinal cord segments level was performed following the procedure described by Antri et al. [11], then sterile absorbable haemostatic gel foam (Surgicel; Ethicon, Somerville, NJ, USA) was inserted into the lesion. Sham-operated animals underwent laminectomy only. At the last step of surgery, muscles were sutured and the skin was closed up by skin clips. Both SCT and sham-operated rats then received antibiotic treatments to prevent staphylococcic infection (oxacillin, Bristol Myers Squibb S.P.A., Italy, 0.3 mg/100 g s.c. once a day during 7 days) and urinary infection (gentamicin, Panpharma, France, 0.2 mg/100 g s.c., immediately after the surgery). No further treatment was administered to operated animals, to avoid potential interference with the development of allodynia and hyperalgesia. For recovery, SCT and sham rats were housed two per cage. The bladder of SCT rats was emptied manually once daily until reappearance of the voiding reflex (usually before the 10th day post surgery) (see Results).

Tests with Von Frey Filaments

Assessment of At-Level Mechanical Allodynia. For assessment of SCT-induced neuropathic-like pain in the cutaneous territory bordering surgery scar, rats were placed individually into a plastic cage ($42\times24\times15$ cm) and allowed to adapt to this environment for 1 hour before any stimulation. Tactile allodynia was then looked for with a graded series of von Frey filaments (Bioseb, 92370 Chaville, France) producing a bending force ranging between 0.008 g and 100 g. The threshold pressure to trigger a response (see below) was determined using the "up-down" method [20]. The stimuli were applied 3 times (3 seconds apart) for each filament, within a cutaneous territory of about 6 cm^2 just rostral to the lesion (see Results). When positive nociceptive behaviors, consisting of either a shake, an attack (filament biting), or an escape reaction [5,20], occurred, the next lower pressure-von Frey filaments were tested down to the filament producing no response. Then, the next higher pressure-filaments were applied back to the one triggering a response. The minimal force filament causing at least one of these responses (usually biting) allowed determination of the mechanical pressure threshold value. The 100 g filament, chosen as cut-off to prevent tissue injury, induced no nociceptive behavior in the majority (> 90%) of naïve rats. To avoid nonspecific responses, only these "non-reactive" rats were selected for surgery and included in the study.

Assessment of Mechanical Sensitivity in Body Territories Outside the Allodynic Area. SCT and sham-operated rats were also subjected to mechanical stimulation with von Frey filaments to assess evoked responses at the level of forepaws, hindpaws, vibrissae pad and other body territories outside the allodynic 6 cm^2 area just rostral to the surgery scar. For these tests, each rat was placed on a wire grid platform (5×5 mm mesh) under a small plastic ($35\times20\times15$ cm) cage for 2 hours, and mechanical sensitivity was determined with a graded series of 9 von Frey filaments (bending force of 4, 6, 8, 10, 12, 15, 26, 60 and 100 g). The "up-down" method [20] was also used at all of these sites. At paw level, stimuli were applied onto the lateral plantar surface of the right forepaw or hindpaw 3 times (3 seconds apart) for each filament. The minimal force filament for which animals presented either a brisk paw withdrawal and/or an escape attempt allowed determination of the mechanical pressure threshold [21]. Usually, the mechanical pressure threshold value to trigger a (non nocifensive) response in naïve healthy rats was around 60 g. Because SCT rats presented large time-dependent changes in mechanical sensitivity (see Fig. 1), higher pressures were also tested, with cut-off fixed at 100 g to avoid any tissue injury.

Assessment of Thermal Sensitivity

Paw Immersion Test. Because variations in skin temperature can affect the responses in nociceptive tests [22], we systematically performed control experiments that consisted of measuring hindpaw skin temperature just before the paw immersion test. The rat was left in its cage and a thermistor probe (Thermocouple thermometer Digi-Sense, Model N°8528-10; Cole-Parmer Instrument Company, Chicago, IL; 15 mm in diameter) was applied onto the plantar surface of hindpaw. Stable

temperature readings were obtained after 10 sec with a precision measure of 0.1°C [23].

Thermal sensitivity at the hindpaw level was determined using the paw immersion test in both SCT and sham-operated rats [24]. Briefly, the right hindpaw was immersed into a water bath maintained at 46°C (Polystat, Bioblock Scientific, Illkirch-Graffenstaden, France) for heat stimulation or at 10°C (Ministat, Bioblock Scientific) for cold stimulation, and the latency to struggle reaction (paw withdrawal) was measured to the nearest 0.1 sec.

At-Level Cold Allodynia. Cold allodynia in SCT rats was assessed at day 15 post-surgery using a procedure slightly adapted from the acetone drop test described by Baastrup et al. [5]. Four drops of 10 µL acetone were gently deposited within two seconds all around the surgery scar in SCT and sham-operated rats. The number of trunk shakes and the time spent in escape or licking behavior were determined for one min after acetone drops application.

Pharmacological Treatments

Gabapentin and pregabalin were purchased from Sequoia (Pangbourne, UK). Amitriptyline, baclofen, ketamine and 8-OH-DPAT [(±)-8 hydroxy-2-dipropylamino-tetralin] were from Sigma-Aldrich (Saint-Quentin Fallavier, France). Other compounds

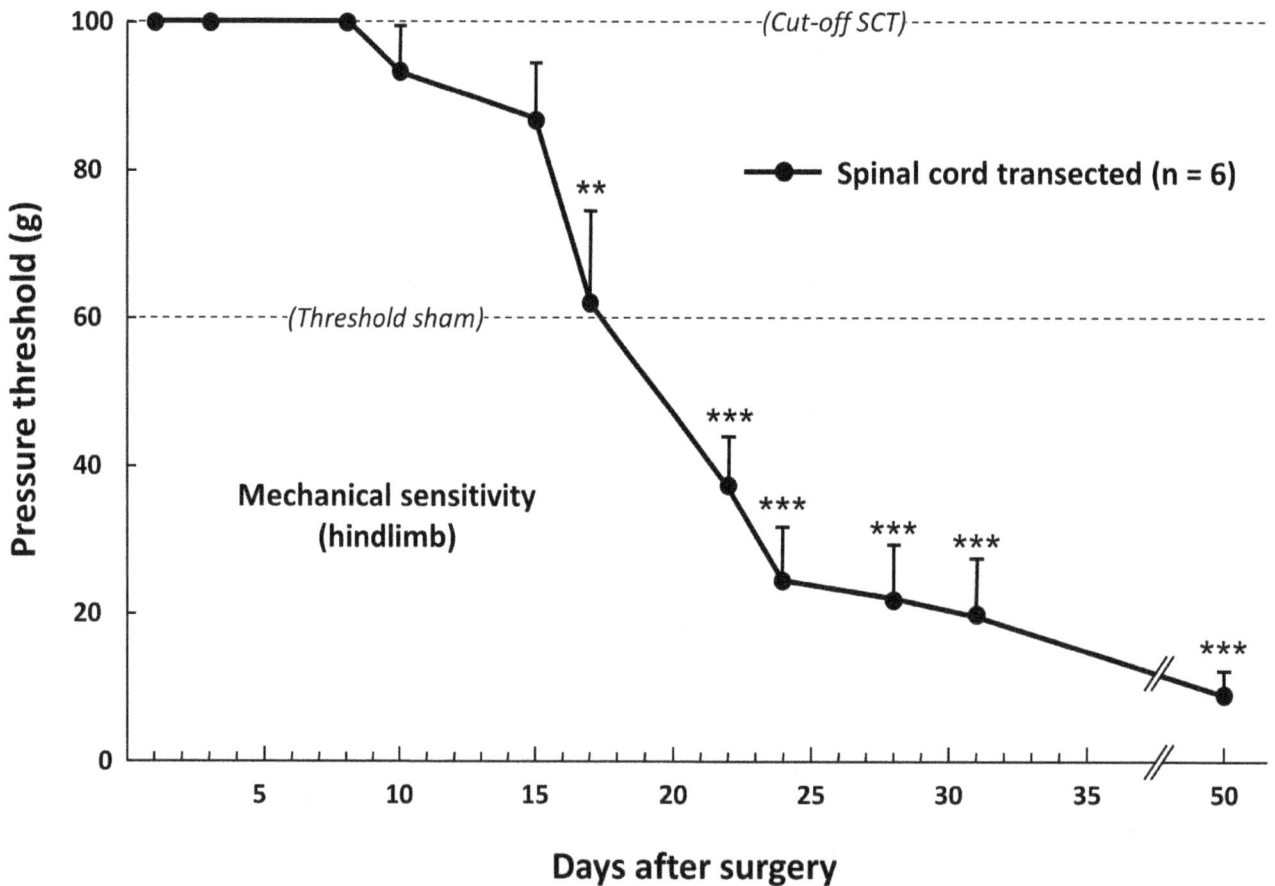

Figure 1. Time-course changes in the pressure threshold value to trigger hindpaw withdrawal in spinal cord-transected rats.
Pressure threshold values were determined using a graded series of von Frey filaments applied onto hindpaw. Each point is the mean + S.E.M. of independent determinations in 6 rats. « Cut-off SCT » corresponded to the maximal pressure tested in spinal cord-transected rats; even at this high pressure level (100 g), no response of hindpaws was evoked for the first 9 days post-surgery. The « Threshold sham » corresponded to the minimal pressure (60 g) to which sham-operated animals start to respond by hindpaw withdrawal. ** P<0.01, *** P<0.001, significantly different from 100 g « cut-off SCT » value. One-way ANOVA for repeated measures followed by Dunnett's test.

were clonazepam (Roche, Basel, Switzerland), cyclotraxin B (BIO S&T, Montreal, Canada), morphine (Pharmacie Centrale des Hôpitaux de Paris, France), tapentadol (Grünenthal, Aachen, Germany), naratriptan and ondansetron (Glaxo Wellcome, Harlow, UK).

All treatments were administered between 2 pm and 4 pm. Routes of administration and doses (as free bases; see Table 1) were chosen according to previous data in the literature (see appropriate references in sections of Results and Discussion). All drugs were dissolved in saline (0.9% NaCl) except baclofen which was dissolved in dimethyl-sulfoxide (DMSO):0.9% NaCl (50:50) and clonazepam in ethanol:water (50:50). Drugs or their vehicles were injected acutely 30 days after thoracic cord transection, when mechanical allodynia had fully developed in the 6 cm^2 area just rostral to the lesion (see Results). For intrathecal injections (of ondansetron), rats were briefly anaesthetized with isoflurane (3% in air), and the needle (26 G) was inserted into the lumbar space between the L5 and L6 vertebrae [25] for administration of the appropriate dose in 20 µL of saline. Von Frey filaments test was then applied (by a skilled experimenter blind to treatments) at various times after acute drugs administration to determine the time course of drug-induced changes in pressure threshold value to trigger nocifensive response (biting of the filament, see Results), until the drug effect completely disappeared. In all experiments, only one treatment was administered per rat.

Real Time Quantitative RT-PCR Measurements

SCT- and sham-operated rats were decapitated at various times, from 2 to 60 days, after surgery. DRG, thoracic cord segments below (T9–T11) and above (T6–T8) the lesion, along with cervical and lumbar enlargements, were rapidly dissected out at 0–4°C, and immediately frozen in liquid nitrogen to be stored at −80°C. In some experiments, spinal cord samples were further sectioned by a medio-vertical cut to separate dorsal and ventral halves. Total RNA was extracted using the NucleoSpin RNA II extraction kit (Macherey-Nagel, 67722 Hoerdt, France) and quantified using NanoDrop. First-stranded cDNA synthesis (from 660 ng total RNA per 20 µL reaction mixture) was carried out using High Capacity cDNA reverse transcription kit (Applied Biosystems, Courtaboeuf, France). PCR amplification, in triplicate for each sample, was performed using ABI Prism 7300 (Applied Biosystems), TaqMan Universal PCR Master Mix No AmpErase UNG (Applied Biosystems) and Assays-on-Demand Gene Expression probes (Applied Biosystems) for targets'genes: *ATF3* (assay ID Rn00563784_m1), *GFAP* (Rn01460868_m1), *OX-42* (Rn00709342_m1), *IL-1β* (Rn00580432_m1), *IL-6* (Rn00561420_m1), *TNF-α* (Rn00562055_m1), *IL-10* (Rn00563409_m1), *BDNF* (Rn02531967_s1), *TLR4* (Rn00569848_m1), *P2×4* (Rn00580949_m1), *P2×7* (Rn00570451_m1). mRNA determinations were made with reference to the reporter gene encoding glyceraldehyde 3-phosphate dehydrogenase (*GaPDH*; Rn99999916_s1). The polymerase activation step at 95°C for 15 min was followed by 40 cycles of 15 s at 95°C and 60 s at 60°C. The validity of the results was checked by running appropriate negative controls (replacement of cDNA by water for PCR amplification; omission of reverse transcriptase for cDNA synthesis). Specific mRNA levels were calculated after normalizing from *GaPDH* mRNA in each sample. Data are presented as relative mRNA units compared to control (sham) values (see [21]).

Statistical Analyses

All values are expressed as means ± S.E.M. For von Frey filaments tests, the data were analyzed by one-way ANOVA for repeated measures (effect of a drug over time) followed by Dunnett's test. Statistical evaluations of SCT-induced changes in behavioral responses to thermal stimulations were made using the Student's t test. For qRT-PCR data, the $2^{-\Delta\Delta Ct}$ method [26] was used for analysis of the relative changes in specific mRNA levels and for graphic representations (RQ Study Software 1.2 version; Applied Biosystems). For analysis of the time course expression of the targets'genes, a two-way ANOVA was performed, followed by Bonferroni test for comparison of SCT rats versus respective

Table 1. Pharmacological treatments tested for potential anti-allodynic effects in spinal cord-transected rats.

Drugs	Pharmacological effect	Dose	Efficacy on biting behavior
Morphine	Opioid receptor agonist	1, 3, 10 mg/kg s.c.	+++
Tapentadol	Opioid receptor agonist and noradrenaline reuptake inhibitor	10, 20 mg/kg i.p.	+++
Ketamine	NMDA receptor antagonist	50 mg/kg i.p.	++
Baclofen	GABA B receptor agonist	10 mg/kg i.p.	+
Clonazepam	Benzodiazepine (agonist)	0.25, 2 mg/kg i.p.	-
Gabapentin	Blockade of calcium channel α2δ subunit	30, 100, 300 mg/kg i.p.	-
Pregabalin	Blockade of calcium channel α2δ subunit	30 mg/kg i.p.	-
Amitriptyline	Tricyclic antidepressant	10 mg/kg i.p.	-
Amitriptyline + Gabapentin	Tricyclic antidepressant + Blockade of calcium channel α2δ subunit	10 mg/kg i.p. +100 mg/kg i.p.	-
Cyclotraxin B	TrkB receptor blocker	20 mg/kg i.p.	-
Naratriptan	5-HT$_{1B/D}$ receptor agonist	0.1 mg/kg i.p.	-
Ondansetron	5-HT$_3$ receptor antagonist	20 µg i.t.	-
8-OH-DPAT	5-HT$_{1A/7}$ receptor agonist	0.25 mg/kg i.p.	-

+++: potent anti-allodynic effect (complete recovery of control mechanical sensitivity);
++: potent but short lasting anti-allodynic effect;
+: modest but significant anti-allodynic effect; -: inactive treatment.

(sham) controls at each time. The critical level of statistical significance was set at $P < 0.05$.

Results

Physiological State of Spinal Cord Transected Rats

After full recovery from anaesthesia, SCT rats first showed hindlimb paralysis and flabbiness. Although they moved in their cage without major difficulty and could access food and water as readily as before the surgery, SCT rats stopped gaining weight for the first week after surgery (-6.3 ± 3.8 g, mean $\pm$ S.E.M., n = 8), in contrast to sham-operated animals (+43$\pm$2 g, mean $\pm$ S.E.M., n = 8); but, afterwards, weight gain was parallel in both SCT- and sham-operated rats (+175.4$\pm$28.3 g and +171.2$\pm$12.5 g from day 7 to day 30 post-surgery, respectively, means $\pm$ S.E.M., n = 8 in each group).

Most striking symptoms were urinary retention and/or hematuria. Hematuria disappeared after 3 or 4 days without any specific treatment. To deal with urinary retention, we had to trigger off the miction reflex by rubbing the bladder once a day during 8–9 days on average. Then, the reflex recovered completely. It also happened that some SCT rats had an accelerated gut transit with diarrhea for the first 3 days post surgery. Later on, such gut disorders were only exceptionally observed. On the other hand, SCT rats had their fur a little bit more tousled than sham animals, but it stayed very clean in areas located both rostrally and caudally of the lesion site, most probably through grooming (that we regularly noted) by their cage mate. Abnormal suffering (with signs such as skin scratching) and/or autotomy were never observed when SCT rats were housed two per cage, as always used for these studies.

Immediately after the surgery and during usually 9–10 days, SCT rats showed paraplegia, first characterized by a total absence of reaction when hindlimbs were mechanically stimulated with von Frey filaments exerting pressure up to the cut-off value (100 g) (Fig. 1). This was followed by a hypo-reflexia which progressively vanished up to normal-like response (as in control unoperated rats) to mechanical stimulation which was usually recovered two weeks post surgery. Later on, SCT rats developed a hyper-reflexia with a pressure threshold value to trigger brisk hindpaw withdrawal strikingly lower (-80%) than that determined in sham rats up to at least 7 weeks post-surgery (Fig. 1). All along the observation period, SCT rats had paralyzed hindlimbs with spasticity, rigidity and tonicity. They also had frequent spontaneous movements of the tail and hindlimbs (shaking), and developed uncoordinated flexion and extension movements.

Development and Localization of Mechanical Allodynia

Among all the body areas tested, only the lesion site on the back and the hindlimbs (see above) showed altered behavioral responses in the von Frey filaments test in SCT- compared to sham-operated rats.

Within a few days after SCT, supersensitivity to mechanical stimulation appeared at the lesion site. From day 2 to day 9, such supersensitivity was mostly rostro-lateral to the lesion site within small areas on both sides (Fig. 2). Then, the supersensitive territory extended medially and laterally to cover an approximately 6 cm^2 cutaneous area just rostral to the thoracic cord transection. In contrast, no supersensitivity was detected behind the transection, and, indeed, SCT rats did not react even to a 100 g pressure exerted by von Frey filament applied within the cutaneous territory on the back, caudal to the transection.

Further assessment of supersensitivity to application of von Frey filaments within the 6 cm^2 area just rostral to the lesion led to identify three different aversive reactions: biting, shaking and escape (Fig. 3), in agreement with previous observations in SCI rats [5]. Determinations of pressure threshold values to trigger each of these behaviors showed parallel time-course decreases, down to very low levels that were reached 10–14 days after surgery and remained unchanged for the 7-weeks-observation period (Fig. 3).

Thermal Sensitivity

To make sure that no bias due to possible changes in skin temperature occurred in SCT- versus sham-operated rats, we first measured hindpaw skin temperature just prior performance of the paw immersion test, two weeks post surgery. Under controlled environmental conditions (with ambient temperature at $22 \pm 1°C$; see Materials and Methods), hindpaw skin temperature was of $30.1 \pm 1.0°C$ and $29.8 \pm 0.5°C$ (means $\pm$ S.E.M. of 8 independent determinations in each group) in SCT- and sham-operated rats, respectively, indicating the lack of incidence of SCT on this parameter. However, clear-cut differences between SCT- and sham-operated rats were noted in withdrawal latencies after hindpaw immersion in cold ($10°C$) as well as hot ($46°C$) water. As shown in Figure 4A, SCT rats reacted with much shorter latencies compared to sham-operated animals, as expected of increased sensitivity to both cold and hot stimulation two weeks post SCT.

Further evaluation of cold hypersensitivity was made using the acetone drop test applied at the lesion site, where SCT rats developed mechanical allodynia (Fig. 2). As illustrated in Figure 4B, both the number of trunk shakes and the time spent in back licking and escape attempts for the first min after acetone drops application were significantly increased in SCT- compared to sham-operated animals (+67% and +400%, respectively).

Pharmacological Studies

Effects of Opioïdergic Drugs (Morphine and Tapentadol) on At-Level Mechanical Allodynia. As treatments with opioids were shown to reduce pain in humans with spinal cord lesions [27,28], we investigated whether morphine (1, 3 and 10 mg/kg s.c.) was effective to reduce at-level mechanical allodynia in SCT-rats. Acute treatment was performed 30 days after the surgery, when pressure threshold to elicit biting behavior in response to von Frey filament application had reached its minimum value (Fig. 3). As illustrated in Figure 5A, morphine exerted a dose-dependent effect: it was inactive at 1 mg/kg s.c., but increased pressure threshold value at higher doses, with complete suppression of allodynia-like response 30 and 60 min after administration of the highest dose tested (10 mg/kg s.c.). Confirmation of the anti-allodynic efficacy of opiate receptor activation was made with tapentadol, a mixed mu opioid receptor agonist and noradrenaline reuptake inhibitor with potent antalgic properties [29], which also reversed SCT-induced mechanical allodynia in a dose-dependent manner. As shown in Figure 5B, tapentadol at 10 mg/kg i.p. slightly increased the pressure threshold value, but the dose of 20 mg/kg i.p. completely suppressed allodynia-like response 30 and 60 min after its administration to SCT rats.

Effects of Ketamine on At-Level Mechanical Allodynia. Ketamine is well known to reduce pain in humans suffering from spinal cord injury, and its pain alleviating efficacy has also been reported in rat models of SCI, such as the one obtained by spinal cord contusion [30]. In SCT rats, acute administration of ketamine (50 mg/kg i.p.) induced a significant increase in pressure threshold value to trigger nocifensive response to von Frey filament application within the allodynic cutaneous area (Fig. 5C). At its maximum, 30 min after treatment, pressure threshold value reached 77.3 ± 17.6 g (from 0.96 g$\pm$0.39 g before

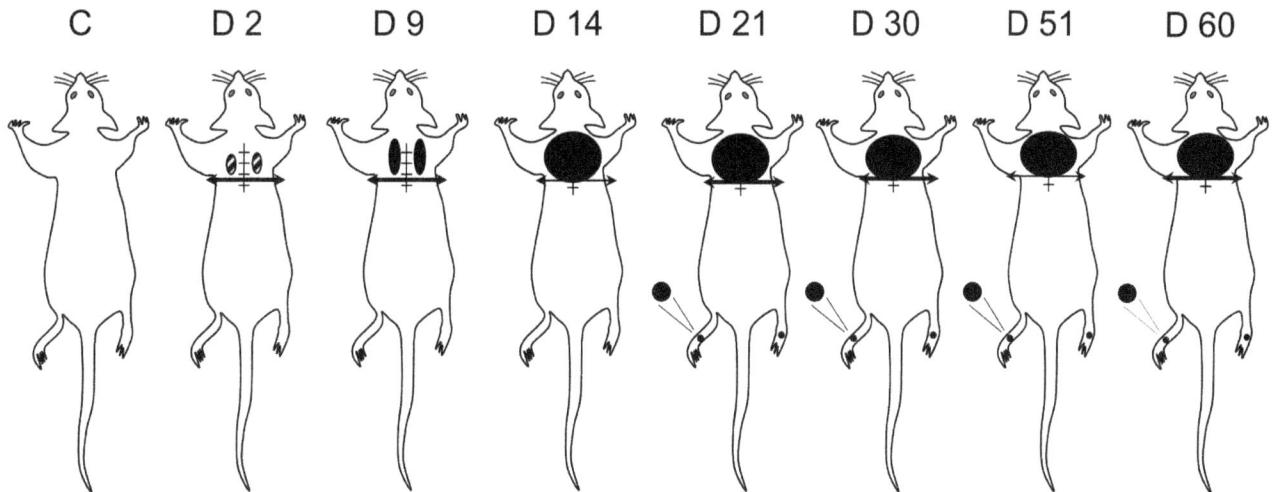

Figure 2. Body territories with increased mechanical sensitivity in spinal cord-transected rats. Pressure threshold values to trigger nocifensive responses were determined using a graded series of von Frey filaments applied throughout the body. Comparison with sham-operated rats (C) showed that pressure threshold values differed in SCT rats only in a limited territory (6 cm²) bordering rostrally the spinal cord section (at T8–T9, horizontal bar with arrow heads) and in hindpaws (black areas tested), where reactions were obtained for pressure values significantly less than in controls. Time course (day 2 to day 60) changes in spinal cord transected rats showed that supersensitivity (allodynia) in the at-level area just rostral to the lesion was already detected at day 2 (D2) post-surgery, then extended and increased up to a plateau reached at D14 post-surgery. At hindpaw level, supersensitivity developed much later (from D21 post-surgery). Data were obtained in 8–14 rats at each time.

treatment, means ± S.E.M. of 6 determinations), which was not significantly different from the cut-off value corresponding to the non-allodynic state (in naïve rats, before surgery). However, this effect vanished rapidly because mechanical allodynia was completely restored 90 min after ketamine administration (Fig. 5C).

Effects of Baclofen on At-Level Mechanical Allodynia. Because baclofen, a GABA B receptor agonist, is often prescribed to reduce SCI-induced spasticity in humans, and is endowed with anti-neuropathic pain properties [31], we investigated whether this drug could reduce at-level mechanical allodynia in SCT rats. Indeed, baclofen induced a limited and transient increase (p<0.05) in pressure threshold value, from 0.6±0.4 g before treatment to 5.0±2.1 g 30 min after i.p. administration of this drug at 10 mg/kg (Fig. 5D).

Effects of Anticonvulsant Drugs on At-Level Mechanical Allodynia. The calcium channel blockers gabapentin and pregabalin and the benzodiazepine clonazepam are anticonvulsants endowed with anti-neuropathic pain properties both in humans [3,27] and in rodent models [32,33], and we tested whether these drugs also exerted anti-allodynic effects in SCT rats. In fact, acute treatments with either gabapentin (30 mg/kg i.p.), pregabalin (30 mg/kg i.p.) or clonazepam (0.25 mg/kg i.p.), at doses devoid of any inhibitory effect on locomotor coordination (as assessed using the rotarod test; not shown), had no significant effect on pressure threshold to trigger nocifensive response in SCT rats (Table 1). Some increase in pressure threshold values was noted with higher doses of clonazepam (2 mg/kg i.p.) and gabapentin

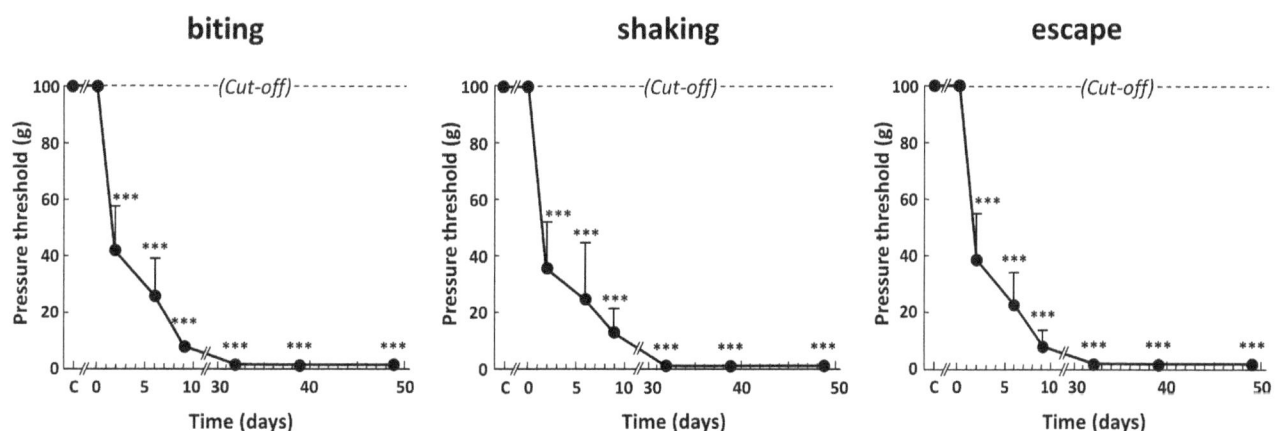

Figure 3. Time-course changes in nocifensive reactions to von Frey filaments application in the « at-level » allodynic territory rostral to the lesion in spinal cord-transected rats. Pressure threshold values to trigger biting (of the filament), shaking or escape were determined using the "up-down" method with a graded series of von Frey filaments applied onto the allodynic at-level area on the back at various times (in days) after surgery (0 on abscissa). Each bar is the mean + S.E.M. of independent determinations in 8 rats. *** P<0.001 compared to control (intact) rats (C on abscissa). One-way ANOVA for repeated measures followed by Dunnett's test.

A

10° C   46° C

Sham-operated rats (n = 5)

SCT rats (n = 9)

B

Shaking   Escape/licking

Sham-operated rats (n = 7)

SCT rats (n = 8)

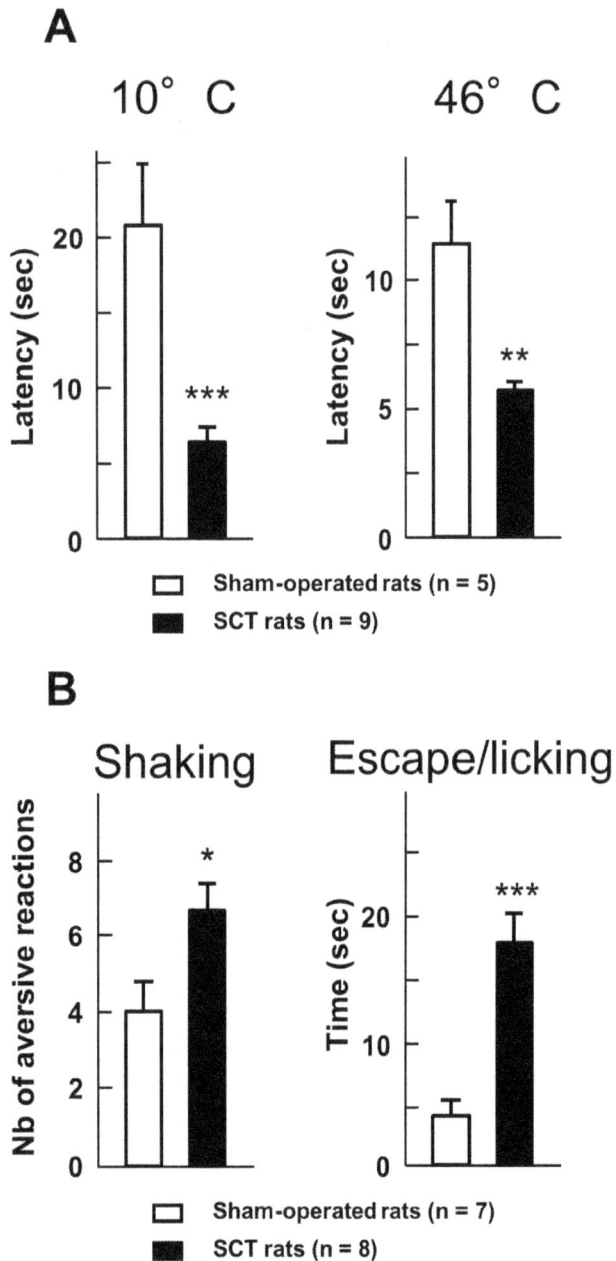

Figure 4. Hyper-responsiveness to thermal stimulation in spinal cord-transected rats. A – Latency (in sec) to hindpaw withdrawal was determined after paw immersion into a bath of hot (46°C) or cold (10°C) water, two weeks after the surgery. Each bar is the mean + S.E.M. of independent determinations in 9 SCT rats and 5 sham-operated rats. ** P<0.01, *** P<0.001 compared to respective values in sham-operated rats. Student's t test. **B** – Behavioral responses to the acetone drop test applied at the surgical scar two weeks after surgery. The number of shakes and the time (in sec) spent in escape attempts and licking of the back were measured for one minute after acetone drops application. Each bar is the mean + S.E.M. of independent determinations in 8 SCT rats and 7 sham-operated rats. * P<0.05, ** P< 0.01 compared to respective values in sham-operated rats. Student's t test.

(100 and 300 mg/kg i.p.), but rats presented profound ataxia after such treatments (not shown).

Effects of Other Drugs on At-Level Mechanical Allodynia. As detailed in Table 1, the antidepressant amitriptyline, alone or combined with gabapentin, the anti-migraine drug naratriptan, the 5-HT$_{1A/7}$ receptor agonist 8-OH-DPAT, the 5-HT$_3$ receptor antagonist ondansetron, the BDNF-Trk B receptor blocker cyclotraxin B, at effective doses to reduce pain in validated neuropathic models in rodents [34–39], exerted no anti-allodynic effects up to 3 hours after acute administration in SCT rats.

Neuroinflammatory and Neuroplasticity Markers in Spinal Cord and DRG of SCT rats

Spinal Cord. A first series of determinations consisted of measuring the tissue concentrations of transcripts encoding the neuronal injury marker ATF3, the macrophage-microglial activation marker OX-42 and the astrocytic marker GFAP [21] in the dorsal and ventral halves of spinal cord segments just above (T6–T8) and just below (T9–T11) the surgery level in SCT- compared to sham-operated rats. Measurements were made at day 17 post surgery, when both mechanical (Fig.3) and thermal (Fig.4) allodynia had fully developed. As shown in Figure 6, expression of these three genes was markedly upregulated in both dorsal and ventral halves in segments above and below the section compared to sham-operated rats. Upregulation of ATF3 mRNA was slightly larger in dorsal spinal cord above and below SCT (×20.8- and ×21.1-fold, respectively) than in the corresponding ventral spinal cord segments (×15.7 and ×15.1-fold, respectively). On the other hand, no significant differences were noted between SCT-induced elevation of OX-42 mRNA and GFAP mRNA levels in the dorsal versus the ventral halves of spinal segments above and below SCT. Accordingly, no further distinction between the dorsal and ventral halves was made in subsequent experiments, and whole spinal cord segments were dissected out and processed for investigating the time-course changes in neuroinflammatory and neuroplasticity markers after thoracic cord transection.

As shown in Figure 7, already on day 2 post-surgery, ATF3 mRNA levels were 16.0- and 21.0-fold higher in thoracic spinal cord segments just caudal and rostral to the section, respectively, than in corresponding tissues from sham-operated rats. This upregulation was long lasting as it persisted, but to a lower extent, up to the last observation day (×7.0 and 6.7 on day 60 post-surgery) (Fig. 7A). As illustrated in Figure 7A, a long lasting up regulation of ATF3 mRNA was also detected in both the cervical and lumbar enlargements of the spinal cord in SCT rats. However, this change was of much lower amplitude than in thoracic segments. OX42 mRNA levels were also markedly increased in thoracic segments of the spinal cord just caudal and rostral to the section on day 2 post-surgery (×6.2 and 4.8, respectively), and remained significantly elevated until day 60 (×2.8 and 2.5, respectively) (Fig. 7B). A long lasting up-regulation of OX-42 mRNA was also noted in both the cervical and lumbar enlargements of the spinal cord. However, it was of lower amplitude than in thoracic segments (Fig. 7B). The time course of SCT-induced changes in GFAP mRNA levels differed from those of the former two transcripts, as the observed up-regulation was delayed and relatively less pronounced (×3 at maximum) (Fig. 7C). However, these changes persisted to similar extents up to the last observation day (day 60 post surgery). In cervical and lumbar enlargements, only slight, generally non significant, increases in GFAP mRNA levels were observed in SCT rats, but they were also of long duration (Fig. 7C).

Concerning pro-inflammatory cytokines, a massive increase in IL-6 mRNA levels was observed as soon as 2 days after the section in thoracic segments bordering caudally (x 76.8 as compared to

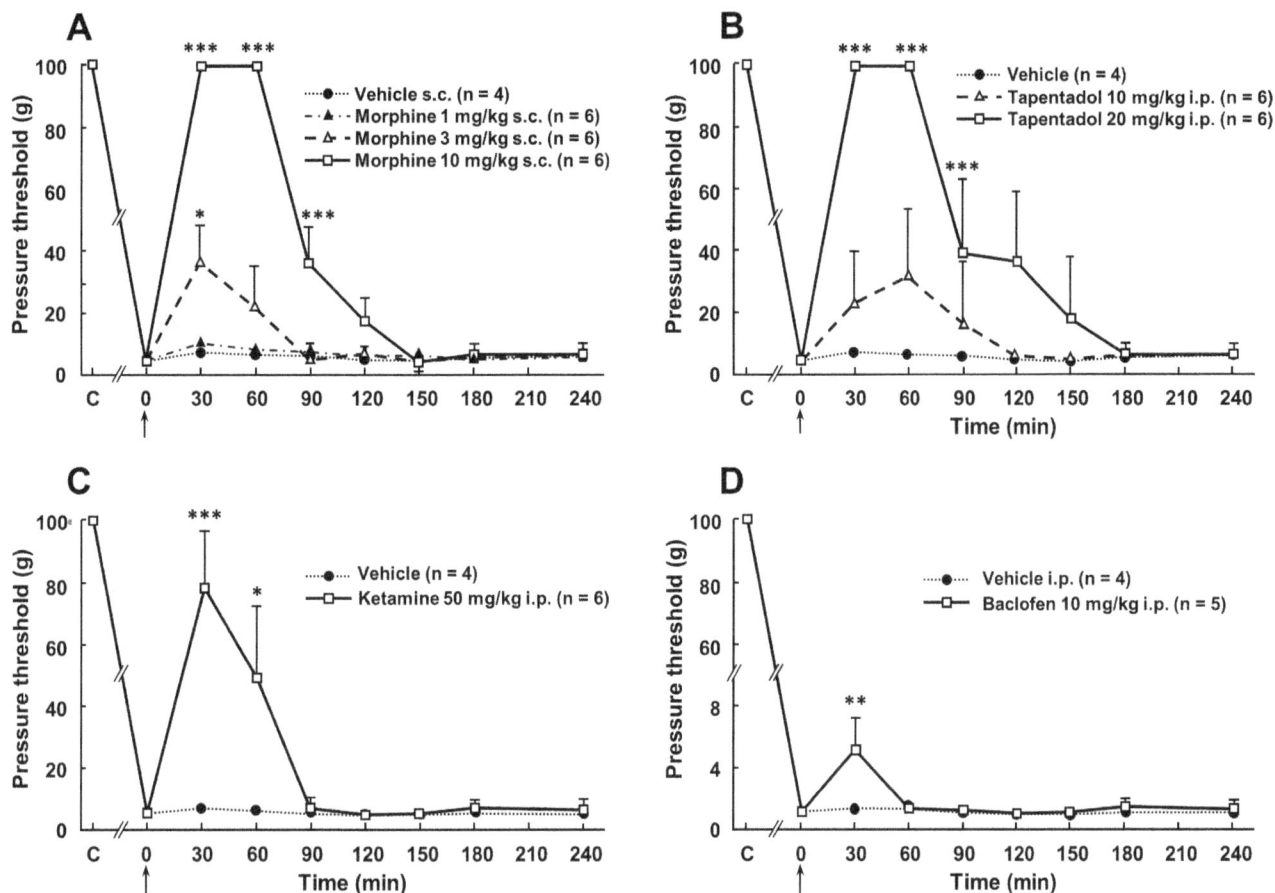

Figure 5. Anti-allodynic effects of acute administration of morphine (A), tapentadol (B), ketamine (C) or baclofen (D) in spinal cord-transected rats. Acute administration of morphine (1, 3 or 10 mg/kg s.c.), tapentadol (10 or 20 mg/kg i.p.), ketamine (50 mg/kg i.p.), baclofen (10 mg/kg i.p.) or their respective vehicle was performed (0 on abscissa, arrow) in rats whose spinal cord had been transected at T8–T9 level one month before. Pressure threshold values to trigger nocifensive biting were determined using von Frey filaments applied within the at-level allodynic territory at various times after treatment. Each point is the mean + S.E.M. of independent determinations in n rats. C on abscissa: Control (naive) rats (prior to surgery). P<0.05, ** P<0.01, *** P<0.001 compared to respective values in vehicle-treated rats. One-way ANOVA for repeated measures followed by Dunnett's test.

sham-operated rats) and rostrally (x 66.4) the section (Fig. 8A). A modest up-regulation was still observed on day 15 but not on day 60 post surgery. In contrast, no significant changes in IL-6 mRNA levels were detected in both the cervical and lumbar enlargements of the spinal cord at any time after SCT as compared to transcript levels measured in the same tissues of sham-operated rats (not shown).

The levels of IL-1β mRNA were also markedly increased 2 days after surgery in thoracic segments bordering caudally (x 172.2 as compared to sham-operated rats) and rostrally (x 98.6) the transection (Fig. 8B). Significant increases in IL-1β mRNA levels still persisted in caudal- and rostral-level segments on day 60 post-surgery, but to a much lower extent than on day 2. Similar but less pronounced changes in TNF-α mRNA levels were noted with a significant up-regulation in thoracic segments on day 2 post surgery (×3.0 caudally and ×1.9 rostrally to the section, respectively) (Fig. 8C). On day 60, a significant increase in TNF-α mRNA levels was still detected principally in thoracic segments rostral to the transection (x 1.9) (Fig. 8C). Finally, tissue concentrations of mRNA encoding the anti-inflammatory cytokine IL-10 were also markedly increased on day 2 after transection in both caudal-level (x 36.3) and rostral-level (x 38.7) thoracic

segments, and an up-regulation of much lower amplitude was still detected on day 60 post surgery (Fig. 8D).

In contrast with the aforementioned transcripts, BDNF mRNA levels were reduced in spinal cord tissues of SCT rats, both on days 2 (−49% as compared to sham-operated rats, P<0.05) and 60 (−38%, P<0.05) post surgery in thoracic segments caudal to the section and on day 60 (−23%, P≤0.05) post surgery in thoracic segments rostral to the section (not shown). On the other hand, mRNAs encoding P2×4, P2×7 and TLR4 were upregulated in thoracic segments bordering caudally (×3.2, ×1.8 and ×3.8, respectively) and rostrally (×2.6, ×1.5 and ×3.6, respectively) the transection on day 2 post-surgery. This up-regulation was even more pronounced on post-surgery day 60 (×3.6, ×2.9 and ×4.5 caudal to the section, ×3.8, ×2.9 and ×5.6 rostral to the section, respectively) (Fig. 9A, 9B, 9C).

Dorsal Root Ganglia. Like that observed at spinal level, ATF3 mRNA was strongly up-regulated in DRG at T9–T11 caudal level as well as T6–T8 rostral level for the first two weeks after thoracic cord transection (Fig. 7A). Then, significant increases persisted up to the last observation day, two months after surgery, but to a lower extent, only in T6–T8 DRG (Fig. 7A). Transcripts encoding OX-42 (macrophages) and GFAP (satellite

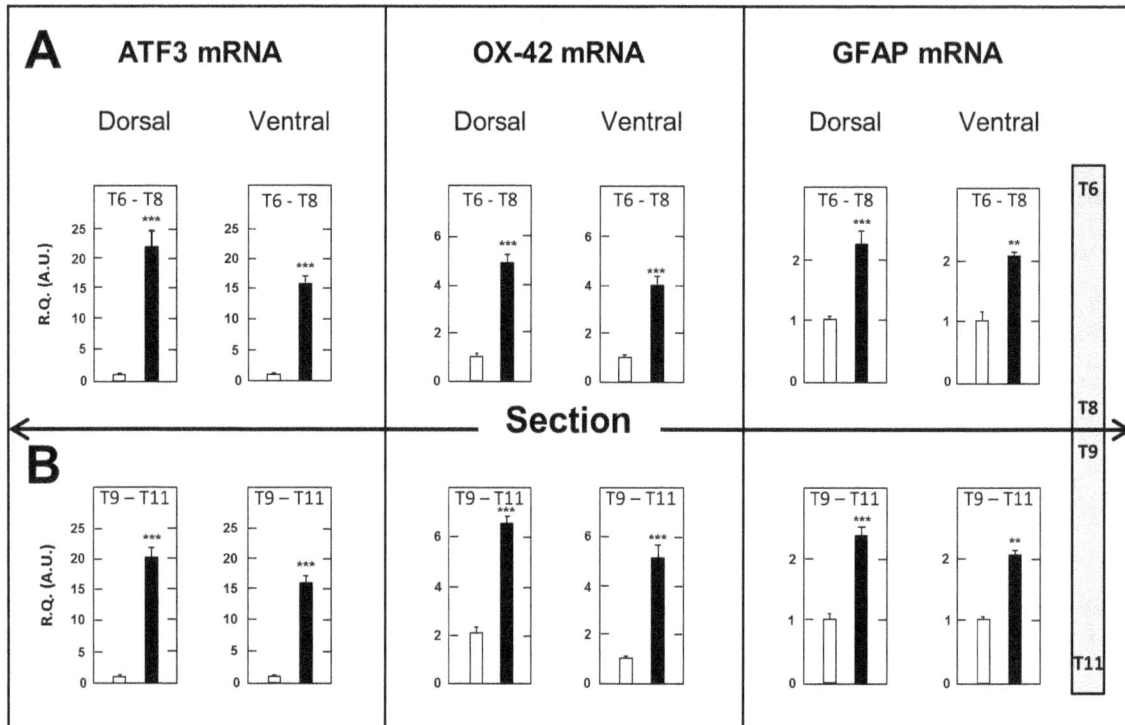

Figure 6. Increased expression of ATF3, OX-42 and GFAP mRNAs in the dorsal and ventral halves of spinal cord segments just above (T6–T8) and below (T9–T11) the surgery level in spinal cord-transected rats. Real time RT-qPCR determinations were made at day 17 after surgery. Data are expressed as the ratio of specific mRNA over GaPDH mRNA [R.Q.(A.U.)]. Each bar is the mean + S.E.M. of 10 independent determinations in both SCT (black bars) and sham-operated (empty bars) rats. *** P<0.001 compared to respective values in sham-operated rats. Two-way ANOVA followed by Bonferroni test.

glial cells) were also markedly up regulated in DRG at spinal cord segments caudal (T9–T11) and rostral (T6–T8) to the transection. However, this effect was transient, especially at rostral level (T6–T8) where significant increases in OX-42 and GFAP transcripts were noted on days 2–4 and up to day 9 post-surgery, respectively. At caudal level (T9–T11), up regulation of these transcripts lasted a few days more, but three weeks post-surgery, both OX-42 and GFAP transcripts no longer differed in thoracic DRG of SCT-versus sham-rats (Figs 7B,7C).

As illustrated in Figure 8A, mRNA encoding IL-6 also showed a dramatic up-regulation (x 65.6) in T9-T11 DRG at day 2 post surgery. Its levels then decreased rapidly, but remained significantly higher than in sham-operated rats up to day 9 post surgery (x 4.4; not shown). Interestingly, up-regulation of IL-6 mRNA was even larger at day 2 (x 145.0) and remained significant for a longer period (up to day 50 post surgery: ×1.6) in rostral level T6–T8 DRG (Fig. 8A, and data not shown). An up regulation of IL-1β mRNA was also noted in thoracic DRG at day 2 post-surgery (but not at day 60) in SCT rats (Fig. 8B), but this change was of much lower amplitude than that noted at spinal level. Also in sharp contrast with that previously noted at spinal level, TNF-α mRNA was not up-regulated in thoracic DRG of SCT rats, neither at day 2 nor at day 60 post-surgery (Fig. 8C). Finally, the levels of mRNA encoding the anti-inflammatory cytokine IL-10 were found to be slightly increased (x 3.1), but only in DRG caudal to the section (T9–T11) on day 2 post surgery, and at a markedly lower extent than in thoracic cord segments (Fig. 8D).

Further transcripts quantifications confirmed the existence of marked differences between DRG and spinal cord tissues. In particular, BDNF mRNA levels were significantly increased in

caudal level T9–T11 DRG at both days 2 (×5.6, P<0.01) and 55 (×1.6, P≤0.05) post-surgery, but only at day 2 (×4.3, P<0.01) in rostral level T6–T8 DRG (not shown). On the other hand, mRNAs encoding P2×4, P2×7 and TLR4, which are all expressed by activated macrophages and satellite glial cells [40–42], showed no modification of their expression levels in T9–T11 DRG of SCT rats whatever the time after surgery. Similar negative results were noted in T6–T8 DRG except a modest but significant increase in P2×7 mRNA levels observed on day 2 post surgery (Fig. 9A, 9B, 9C).

Discussion

Spinal cord transection is a model widely used for the study of induced spasticity, hyper-reflexia and subsequent functional and structural plasticity underlying locomotor recovery under the control of the Central Pattern Generator [11–13]. Although neuropathic pain concerns a high proportion of SCI patients, only few investigations have been dedicated to alterations in pain signaling mechanisms in rats with complete SCT. Indeed, a large body of data has already been generated from studies in rodents with partial spinal cord lesion, but unavoidable interindividual variations in the severity and extent of lesion constitute serious limitations of such models (see Introduction). These considerations led us to thoroughly characterize the homogeneous model of complete transection of the spinal cord at thoracic level with regard to its possible relevance for studying central neuropathic pain, associated neuroplasticity changes and responses to drugs used to alleviate pain in SCI patients.

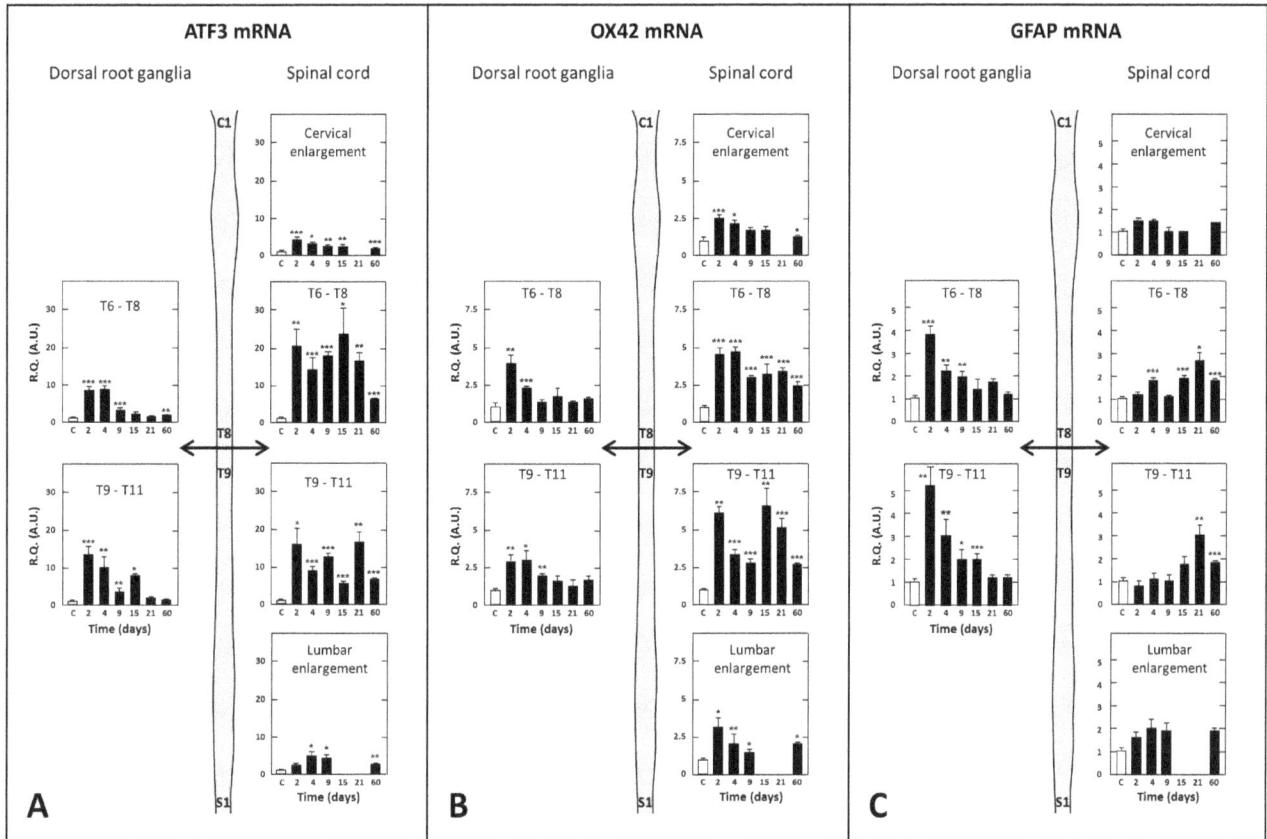

Figure 7. Time-course changes in tissue levels of transcripts encoding ATF3 (A), OX-42 (B) or GFAP (C) in dorsal root ganglia and spinal cord at various times after spinal cord transection. Real-time RT-qPCR determinations were made in T6–T8 and T9–T11 dorsal root ganglia, T6–T8 and T9–T11 spinal cord segments and the cervical and lumbar enlargements at various times (in days, D, abscissa) after spinal cord transection at T8–T9 level. Data are expressed as the ratio of specific mRNA over GaPDH mRNA [R.Q.(A.U.)]. Each bar is the mean + S.E.M. of n independent determinations (D2, D4, D9, D15, D21: n = 6; D60: n = 12). Sham values at every postoperative time are pooled under "C" (control) on abscissa. * P<0.05, * P<0.01, *** P<0.001 compared to respective values in sham-operated rats (C).Two-way ANOVA followed by Bonferroni test.

Clinical State of Spinal Cord Transected Rats

Despite complete transection of the spinal cord, rats showed a relatively good physiological state. The lack of micturition reflex and the hematuria, which are commonly encountered in paraplegic patients [43], usually resolved within 9 days post-surgery. Otherwise, their fur was clean, and very probably because they shared their cage with a congener, autotomia never occurred. Although rats lose weight for the first week after surgery, as a consequence of hindlimb muscles atrophy, they subsequently gained weight at the same rate as sham-operated rats, as expected from animals in good health [44].

Effects of Spinal Cord Transection on Hindlimb Sensitivity

Just after the lesion, hindlimbs no longer responded by a reflex motor reaction to cutaneous mechanical stimulation at high intensity (with the 100 g von Frey filament). Motor reaction then reappeared progressively up to a level corresponding to that found in control (unoperated) animals around the second week post-surgery. A marked hyper-reflexivity subsequently developed, along with spasticity, which reached their maximum approximately 7 weeks post-surgery and were still fully present on the last day (60) of our study. Marked alterations of motor reflexes also occur in humans with complete spinal cord transection, as evidenced by the exacerbated response in the H reflex of hindlimb muscles [45,46]. Such facilitated reflex responses may be due to α-motoneurons

hyperexcitability [47]. Indeed, spinal cord transection causes an up-regulation of constitutively active 5-HT$_{2C}$ receptors expressed by motoneurons, and the reinforcement of their membrane depolarizing influence has been demonstrated to contribute to motoneuron hyperexcitability in lesioned rats [48]. On the other hand, spasticity could also be accounted for by a down regulation of the potassium-chloride cotransporter KCC2 within the lumbar spinal cord below transection [12]. Although spasticity can be painful in humans, and below-level pain exists in patients with extensive spinal cord injury [2,49], hyper-reflexivity and spasticity at hindlimb level could not be related to pain behavior in SCT rats because completeness of the lesion prevented the nociceptive messages to reach the sensory cortex where they can generate pain sensation.

Along with mechanical hypersensitivity, SCT rats also developed heat and cold hypersensitivity as shown by the reduced latency of hindpaw withdrawal after immersion in water at 46°C or 10°C (Fig.4). Heat hypersensitivity has already been described in mice after spinal cord contusion and transection [50], and cold hypersensitivity at hindpaw level has been well documented in rats with contused spinal cord [51]. Whether or not similar neuroplasticity mechanisms underlay thermal and mechanical hypersensitivity at hindpaw level in SCT rats is a pending question to be addressed in future studies. In particular, because thermal hypersensitivity was evidenced from a motor response (hindpaw

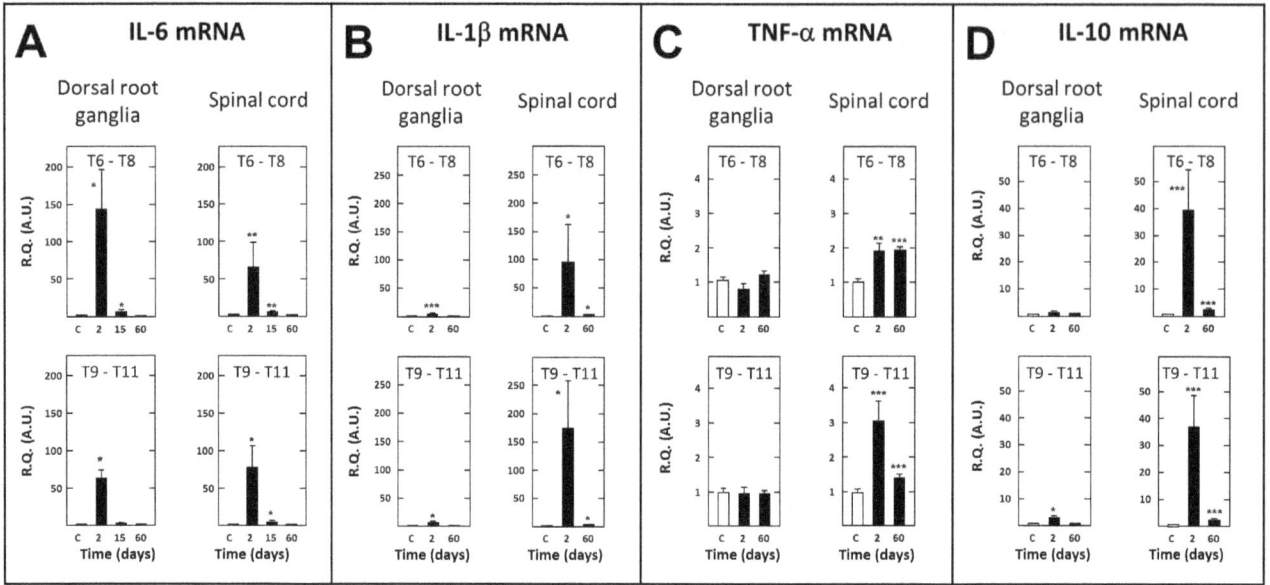

Figure 8. Short- and long-term changes in levels of transcripts encoding IL-6 (A), IL-1β (B), TNF-α (C) and IL-10 in dorsal root ganglia and spinal tissues in spinal cord-transected rats. Real-time RT-qPCR determinations were made in T6–T8 and T9–T11 dorsal root ganglia and T6–T8 and T9–T11 spinal segments at day (D) 2, 15 or 60 (abscissa) after spinal cord transection at T8–T9 level. Data are expressed as the ratio of specific mRNA over GaPDH mRNA [R.Q.(A.U.)]. Each bar is the mean + S.E.M. of n independent determinations (D2, D15: n = 6; D60: n = 12). Sham values at every postoperative time are pooled under "C" (control) on abscissa. * P<0.05, * P<0.01, *** P<0.001 compared to respective values in sham-operated rats (C). Two-way ANOVA followed by Bonferroni test.

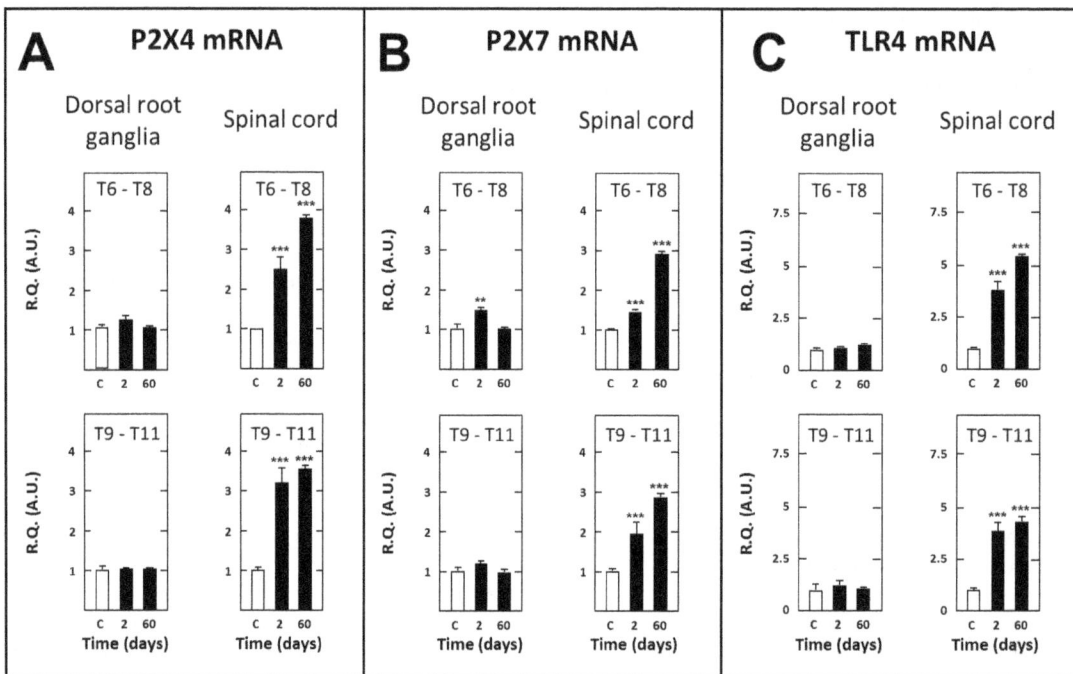

Figure 9. Short- and long-term changes in levels of transcripts encoding P2×4 (A), P2×7 (B) and TLR4 (C) in dorsal root ganglia and spinal tissues in spinal cord-transected rats. Real-time RT-qPCR determinations were made in T6–T8 and T9–T11 dorsal root ganglia and T6–T8 and T9–T11 spinal segments at day 2 or 60 (abscissa) after spinal cord transection at T8–T9 level. Data are expressed as the ratio of specific mRNA over GaPDH mRNA [R.Q.(A.U.)]. Each bar is the mean + S.E.M. of n independent determinations (D2: n = 6; D60: n = 12). Sham values at every postoperative time are pooled under "C" (control) on abscissa. ** P<0.01, *** P<0.001 compared to respective levels in sham-operated rats (C). Two-way ANOVA followed by Bonferroni test.

withdrawal), it might have also involved – at least in part - some α-motoneuron hyperexcitability as discussed above about SCT-induced mechanical hypersensitivity.

At-Level Allodynia

Whereas no behavioral reaction to the application of von Frey filaments within the trunk caudal to the lesion could be elicited in SCT rats, at-level allodynia-like reactions appeared relatively rapidly and reached a maximum 2–3 weeks after surgery. In particular, biting, which is considered as a brainstem response, and escape as a cortical response, were very probably associated with pain in SCT rats [5]. Since sham-operated rats did not develop such behaviors, we can exclude that they might have corresponded to musculoskeletal pain. Instead, at-level mechanical allodynia pain was very probably caused by spinal cord injury itself, as expected of neuropathic pain of central (spinal) origin [2]. Interestingly, 100% of SCT rats developed at-level allodynia, contrary to humans with spinal cord lesion and rats with spinal cord contusion as only a fraction of lesioned subjects suffer from such pain symptoms. Indeed, the prevalence for the rat/human to develop at-level pain depends on the extent of the lesion [52]. Such homogeneous data in SCT rats support the idea that the SCT model might be especially useful to assess the potential effects of drugs aimed at reducing centrally-evoked neuropathic pain and to investigate underlying physiopathological mechanisms.

Even though at-level cold allodynia is frequently seen in SCI patients [53], only few studies have reported this symptom in spinal cord lesioned rodents [5,54]. Indeed, according to Baastrup et al. [5], only 3% of the rats with contusion of the spinal cord exhibit clear-cut cold allodynia. In contrast, in our study, 100% of SCT rats presented at-level cold allodynia further emphasizing the usefulness of this model for improving experimental group homogeneity. A potential at-level heat allodynia could not be assessed in our studies because of the unavailability of appropriate equipment. Nevertheless, it can be recalled that using a Peltier device, Gao et al. [54] were unable to detect any heat allodynia in spinal cord contused rats.

Pharmacological Sensitivity of At-Level Mechanical Allodynia in SCT Rats

Only a few drugs among those tested were found to efficiently reduce at-level allodynia when injected acutely in SCT rats. The efficacy of morphine and tapentadol was probably underlain by the capacity of mu opioid receptor activation to inhibit the activity of wide dynamic range neurons in the dorsal horn of the spinal cord [55]. Interestingly, tapentadol had a somewhat more prolonged effect than morphine, may be because of its additional capacity to inhibit noradrenaline reuptake as this monoamine has been shown to be implicated in descending inhibitory control of neuropathic pain [56].

Ketamine also reversed at-level allodynia in SCT rats, in consistence with human data that demonstrated that this NMDA receptor antagonist is especially efficient to reduce allodynia in SCI patients [57]. This marked effect of ketamine, that may be sustained by a temporary inhibition of astrocyte activation, further supports the key role played by glutamate receptors, particularly NMDA receptors, in physiopathological mechanisms underlying neuropathic pain [58].

Finally, the last drug of the series tested which was found to exert some (but modest) anti-allodynic effects in SCT rats was the GABA B receptor agonist, baclofen, commonly used to suppress spasticity in spinal cord injured patients [59]. Spinal cord injury is known to be associated with a decreased tone of inhibitory GABAergic neurotransmission [7], and it can be proposed that

baclofen transiently compensated for this deficit, thereby reducing allodynia in SCT rats. In contrast, clonazepam, which is used to alleviate SCI patients from neuropathic pain [27], was inefficient suggesting that GABA A receptor activation was ineffective to inhibit at-level allodynia in SCT rats.

Serotonin is known to play a major role in pain control via the activation of several receptor types [36]. Thus, F13640, a potent and selective 5-HT$_{1A}$ receptor agonist, appeared to be especially effective to suppress allodynia in spinal cord lesioned rats [60]. In our hands, the prototypical 5-HT$_{1A}$ receptor agonist, 8-OH-DPAT, did not reduce allodynia in SCT rats. Yet, this molecule is also an agonist at 5-HT$_7$ receptors, whose activation can result in effects opposite to that expected from 5-HT$_{1A}$ receptor activation [61]. Further studies with selective 5-HT$_{1A}$ and 5-HT$_7$ receptor ligands have therefore to be performed in order to reach a clear-cut conclusion regarding the potential modulations of at-level allodynia by serotonin acting at these receptors.

Because allodynia-like sensory dysfunctions are associated with migraine [62], we also investigated whether the anti-migraine drug, naratriptan, with potent 5-HT$_{1B/1D}$ receptor agonist properties [36], could alleviate at-level allodynia in SCT rats. Indeed, no effect was observed, possibly because triptans were found to selectively reduce neuropathic pain at cephalic level but not in extra-cephalic territories [35]. Finally, the last 5-HT receptor that we selected for our pharmacological investigations was the 5-HT$_3$ type whose implication in modulatory controls of neuropathic pain has been firmly established [63]. In contrast to the capacity of i.t. injection of ondansetron to attenuate neuropathic pain caused by spinal cord compression [64], this treatment was inactive in SCT rats, probably because complete transection of the spinal cord had suppressed the bulbo-spinal connections involved in 5-HT$_3$ receptor-mediated effects [38].

Under our acute treatment conditions, neither the antidepressant amitriptyline nor the anticonvulsants gabapentin and pregabalin, which are commonly used to reduce neuropathic pain in SCI patients [3], exerted any significant anti-allodynic effect in SCT rats (Table 1). Indeed, numerous studies showed that these drugs are effective only under chronic treatment conditions [39,65], and further experiments consisting of repeated administrations of antidepressants and anticonvulsants have to be performed before concluding about their effectiveness or ineffectiveness in the SCT rat model.

Finally, because BDNF and its receptor TrkB play key roles in physiopathological mechanisms underlying neuropathic pain [66,67], we investigated whether acute TrkB blockade by cyclotraxin B could affect allodynia in SCT rats. Indeed, Constandil et al. [34] reported that this drug can prevent and reverse neuropathic pain caused by peripheral nerve ligation in rats. In contrast, we found that cyclotraxin B was unable to reduce allodynia in SCT rats (Table 1), in line with RT-qPCR determinations which suggested that spinal BDNF expression would not be upregulated (in contrast to that observed in peripheral neuropathic pain models [66,67]) but rather downregulated after thoracic cord transection, as previously reported after other types of SCI in rats [68,69].

Neuroinflammation and Glial Activation in SCT Rats

The transcription factor ATF3 is induced when neurons are injured, and implicated in regeneration and plasticity [21]. Its role in the *maintenance* of central neuropathic pain is the matter of controversy, as it is no longer expressed when pain is still present after spinal cord injury [70]. However, ATF3 implication in the *induction* of central neuropathic pain is supported by data showing that it promotes the expression of the microglial/macrophage marker OX-42 and the astrocyte/satellite glial cell marker GFAP [71,72], two factors closely associated with neural lesion-evoked neuropathic pain [21,70,73–75]. Because ATF3 activation is triggered by cellular damages, and this transcription factor is able to repress its own promoter [71], the long lasting up-regulation of ATF3 transcript that occurred after SCT might reflect an ongoing neuronal damage associated with microglia activation. Convergent data in the literature showed that microglia activation is mediated, among others, by purinergic receptors [76] and Toll-Like Receptors [77]. Consistently, we observed, in thoracic cord segments just caudal (T9–T11) and rostral (T6–T8) to the transection, a long lasting (up to 60 days post-surgery) increase in the expression of mRNAs encoding P2XA, P2×7 and TLR4 receptors.

Numerous reports in the literature ascribe to activated microglia an important role in neuropathic pain consecutive to spinal cord injury [70,73,78], and the marked induction of OX42 mRNA in SCT rats is congruent with these data. In fact, IL-6, IL-1β, and TNF-α cytokines released from activated microglia can induce, by themselves, central (spinal) sensitization, thus maintaining neuropathic pain [79,80]. The huge induction of IL-6 and IL-1β that occurred on day 2 post-surgery suggests that these cytokines were involved more in the *induction* than in the *maintenance* of SCT-evoked neuropathic pain. In contrast, TNF-α would be more concerned by pain *maintenance* as SCT-induced up-regulation of its transcript in spinal T6–T8 segments was as pronounced at day 60 as at day 2 post-surgery. The strong increase in IL-10 mRNA that occurred shortly after the lesion might be linked to some inhibitory control of neuropathic pain for the first days after SCT, through the anti-inflammatory potency of this cytokine [81] and/or its neuroprotective effects in spinal cord injured models [82]. Overall, in contrast to that found in spinal tissues, none of the 11 genes studied were up-regulated beyond two weeks post-surgery in DRG above the lesion, supporting the idea that SCT-induced long lasting at-level allodynia did not involve some peripheral hypersensitivity but corresponded mainly, if not exclusively, to central neuropathic pain. Indeed, the short lasting induction of ATF3, OX-42, GFAP and cytokines encoding genes in DRG might have reflected some limited lesion of T8–T9 dorsal roots possibly occurring during surgery for thoracic cord transection. As a matter of fact, it has to be emphasized that our RT-qPCR determinations of time-course changes in mRNA levels will have

to be completed by measurements of corresponding proteins in order to validate the inferences made above about the respective implications of pro-inflammatory cytokines and other neuroinflammatory markers in neuropathic pain-inducing mechanisms in SCT rats.

Within the spinal cord, GFAP mRNA up-regulation after SCT was delayed compared to that of transcripts encoding the pro-inflammatory cytokines IL-1β, IL-6 and TNF-α, in line with the idea that early production and release of these cytokines from microglial activation [83] leads to secondary induction of astrogliosis after injury [84]. That astrogliosis with an up-regulation of GFAP [74] - like that found in SCT rats - contributes to neuropathic pain after spinal cord injury is supported by the fact that pharmacological blockade of astroglia activation reduced pain in spinal cord-lesioned rats [73,85].

Conclusion

Spinal cord transection at thoracic level in rats appeared to generate a highly reproducible model of at-level neuropathic pain, mainly of central origin, suitable for pharmacological studies aimed at testing innovative treatments targeted specifically on spinal lesion-evoked neuropathic pain. Time course changes in mRNA levels of neuroinflammatory markers induced by the lesion supported the idea that both activated microglia and activated astroglia contributed to neuropathic pain in spinally transected rats. However, further investigations of these markers have to be made at protein level in order to determine more precisely the respective roles of both cell types in mechanisms underlying central allodynia in SCT rats.

Acknowledgments

We are grateful to pharmaceutical companies (Glaxo-Wellcome, Grünenthal) for generous gifts of drugs, and to Pr Guglielmo Foffani (Toledo, Spain) for helpful discussions.

Author Contributions

Conceived and designed the experiments: SM S. Bourgoin MH. Performed the experiments: SM S. Bourgoin VK S. Barthélémy CC FC DO. Analyzed the data: SM S. Bourgoin DO MH. Wrote the paper: SM MH.

References

1. Finnerup NB, Johannesen IL, Sindrup SH, Bach FW, Jensen TS (2001) Pain and dysesthesia in patients with spinal cord injury: A postal survey. Spinal Cord 39: 256–262.

2. Bryce TN, Biering-Sørensen F, Finnerup NB, Cardenas DD, Defrin R, et al. (2012) International spinal cord injury pain classification: part I. Background and description. March 6–7, 2009. Spinal Cord 50: 413–417.

3. Attal N, Cruccu G, Baron R, Haanpaa M, Hansson P, et al. (2010) EFNS guidelines on the pharmacological treatment of neuropathic pain: 2010 revision. Eur J Neurol 17: 1113–e1188.

4. Nakae A, Nakai K, Yano K, Hosokawa K, Shibata M, et al. (2011) The animal model of spinal cord injury as an experimental pain model. J Biomed Biotechnol 2011: 939023.

5. Baastrup C, Maersk-Moller CC, Nyengaard JR, Jensen TS, Finnerup NB (2010) Spinal-, brainstem- and cerebrally mediated responses at- and below-level of a spinal cord contusion in rats: evaluation of pain-like behavior. Pain 151: 670–679.

6. Baastrup C, Jensen TS, Finnerup NB (2011) Pregabalin attenuates place escape/avoidance behavior in a rat model of spinal cord injury. Brain Res 1370: 129–135.

7. Yezierski RP (2000) Pain following spinal cord injury: pathophysiology and central mechanisms. Prog Brain Res 129: 429–449.

8. Basso DM, Beattie MS, Bresnahan JC (1996) Graded histological and locomotor outcomes after spinal cord contusion using the NYU weight-drop device versus transection. Exp Neurol 139: 244–256.

9. Onifer SM, Rabchevsky AG, Scheff SW (2007) Rat models of traumatic spinal cord injury to assess motor recovery. ILAR J 48: 385–395.

10. Crown ED, Ye Z, Johnson KM, Xu GY, McAdoo DJ, et al. (2006) Increases in the activated forms of ERK 1/2, p38 MAPK, and CREB are correlated with the expression of at-level mechanical allodynia following spinal cord injury. Exp Neurol 199: 397–407.

11. Antri M, Barthe JY, Mouffle C, Orsal D (2005) Long-lasting recovery of locomotor function in chronic spinal rat following chronic combined pharmacological stimulation of serotonergic receptors with 8-OHDPAT and quipazine. Neurosci Lett 384: 162–167.

12. Boulenguez P, Liabeuf S, Bos R, Bras H, Jean-Xavier C, et al. (2010) Down-regulation of the potassium-chloride cotransporter KCC2 contributes to spasticity after spinal cord injury. Nat Med 16: 302–307.

13. Rossignol S, Frigon A (2011) Recovery of locomotion after spinal cord injury: some facts and mechanisms. Annu Rev Neurosci 34: 413–440.

14. Graziano A, Foffani G, Knudsen EB, Shumsky J, Moxon KA (2013) Passive exercise of the hind limbs after complete thoracic transection of the spinal cord promotes cortical reorganization. PLoS ONE 8(1):e54350.

15. Humanes-Valera D, Aguilar J, Foffani G (2013) Reorganization of the intact somatosensoty cortex immediately after spinal cord injury. PLoS ONE 8(7):e69655.

16. Santos-Nogueira E, Redondo Castro E, Mancuso R, Navarro X (2012) Randall-Selitto test: a new approach for the detection of neuropathic pain after spinal cord injury. J Neurotrauma 29: 898–904.

17. Hubscher CH, Kaddumi EG, Johnson RD (2008) Segmental neurtopathic pain does not develop in male rats with complete spinal transections. J Neurotrauma 25: 1241–1245.

18. Densmore VS, Kalous A, Keast JR, Osborne PB (2010) Above-level mechanical hyperalgesia in rats develops after incomplete spinal cord injury but not after cord transection, and is reversed by amitriptyline, morphine and gabapentin. Pain 151: 184–193.

19. Zimmermann M (1983) Ethical guidelines for investigations of experimental pain in conscious animals. Pain 16: 109–110.

20. Chaplan SR, Bach FW, Pogrel JW, Chung JM, Yaksh TL (1994) Quantitative assessment of tactile allodynia in the rat paw. J Neurosci Methods 53: 55–63.

21. Latrémolière A, Mauborgne A, Masson J, Bourgoin S, Kayser V, et al. (2008) Differential implication of proinflammatory cytokine interleukin-6 in the development of cephalic versus extracephalic neuropathic pain in rats. J Neurosci 28: 8489–8501.

22. Hole K, Tjølsen A (1993) The tail-flick and formalin tests in rodents: changes in skin temperature as a confounding factor. Pain 53: 247–254.

23. Kayser V, Elfassi IE, Aubel B, Melfort M, Julius D, et al. (2007) Mechanical, thermal and formalin-induced nociception is differentially altered in 5-HT1A-/-, 5-HT1B-/-, 5-HT2A-/-, 5-HT3A-/- and 5-HTT-/- knock-out male mice. Pain 130: 235–248.

24. Attal N, Jazat F, Kayser V, Guilbaud G (1990) Further evidence for 'pain-related' behaviours in a model of unilateral peripheral mononeuropathy. Pain 41: 235–251.

25. Mestre C, Pelissier T, Fialip J, Wilcox G, Eschalier A (1994) A method to perform direct transcutaneous intrathecal injection in rats. J Pharmacol Toxicol Methods 32: 197–200.

26. Schmittgen TD, Livak KJ (2008) Analyzing real-time PCR data by the comparative C(T) method. Nat Protoc 3: 1101–1108.

27. Fenollosa P, Pallares J, Cervera J, Pelegrin F, Inigo V, et al. (1993) Chronic pain in the spinal cord injured: statistical approach and pharmacological treatment. Paraplegia 31: 722–729.

28. Norrbrink C, Lundeberg T (2009) Tramadol in neuropathic pain after spinal cord injury: a randomized, double-blind, placebo-controlled trial. Clin J Pain 25: 177–184.

29. Tzschentke TM, Christoph T, Kogel B, Schiene K, Hennies HH, et al. (2007) (-)-(1R,2R)-3-(3-dimethylamino-1-ethyl-2-methyl-propyl)-phenol hydrochloride (tapentadol HCl): a novel mu-opioid receptor agonist/norepinephrine reuptake inhibitor with broad-spectrum analgesic properties. J Pharmacol Exp Ther 323: 265–276.

30. Bennett AD, Everhart AW, Hulsebosch CE (2000) Intrathecal administration of an NMDA or a non-NMDA receptor antagonist reduces mechanical but not thermal allodynia in a rodent model of chronic central pain after spinal cord injury. Brain Res 859: 72–82.

31. Gwak YS, Tan HY, Nam TS, Paik KS, Hulsebosch CE, et al. (2006) Activation of spinal GABA receptors attenuates chronic central neuropathic pain after spinal cord injury. J Neurotrauma 23: 1111–1124.

32. Yasuda T, Iwamoto T, Ohara M, Sato S, Kohri H, et al. (1999) The novel analgesic compound OT-700 (5-n-butyl-7-(3,4,5-trimethoxybenzoyl-amino)pyr-azolo[1,5-a]pyrimidine) attenuates mechanical nociceptive responses in animal models of acute and peripheral neuropathic hyperalgesia. Jpn J Pharmacol 79: 65–73.

33. Wallin J, Cui JG, Yakhnitsa V, Schechtmann G, Meyerson BA, et al. (2002) Gabapentin and pregabalin suppress tactile allodynia and potentiate spinal cord stimulation in a model of neuropathy. Eur J Pain 6: 261–272.

34. Constandil L, Goich M, Hernàndez A, Bourgeais L, Cazorla M, et al. (2012) Cyclotraxin-B, a new TrkB antagonist, and glial blockade by propentofylline, equally prevent and reverse cold allodynia induced by BDNF or partial infraorbital nerve constriction in mice. J Pain 13: 579–589.

35. Kayser V, Aubel B, Hamon M, Bourgoin S (2002) The antimigraine 5-HT1B/1D receptor agonists, sumatriptan, zolmitriptan and dihydroergotamine, attenuate pain-related behavior in a rat model of trigeminal neuropathic pain. Br J Pharmacol 137: 1287–1297.

36. Kayser V, Bourgoin S, Viguier F, Michot B, Hamon M (2010) Toward deciphering the respective roles of multiple 5-HT receptors in the complex serotonin-mediated control of pain. In: Beaulieu P, Lussier D, Porreca F, Dickenson AH, editors. Pharmacology of pain. Seattle: IASP Press. pp. 185–206.

37. Kayser V, Latrémolière A, Hamon M, Bourgoin S (2011) N-methyl-D-aspartate receptor-mediated modulations of the anti-allodynic effects of 5-HT1B/1D receptor stimulation in a rat model of trigeminal neuropathic pain. Eur J Pain 15: 451–458.

38. Suzuki R, Rahman W, Hunt SP, Dickenson AH (2004) Descending facilitatory control of mechanically evoked responses is enhanced in deep dorsal horn neurons following peripheral nerve injury. Brain Res 1019: 68–76.

39. Vanelderen P, Rouwette T, Kozicz T, Heylen R, Van Zundert J, et al. (2013) Effects of chronic administration of amitriptyline, gabapentin and minocycline on spinal brain-derived neurotrophic factor expression and neuropathic pain behavior in a rat chronic constriction injury model. Reg Anesth Pain Med 38: 124–130.

40. Fellner L, Irschick R, Schanda K, Reindl M, Klimaschewski L, et al. (2013) Toll-like receptor 4 is required for α-synuclein dependent activation of microglia and astroglia. Glia 61: 349–360.

41. Inoue K (2002) Microglial activation by purines and pyrimidines. Glia 40: 156–163.

42. Inoue K (2006) The function of microglia through purinergic receptors: neuropathic pain and cytokine release. Pharmacol Ther 109: 210–226.

43. Singh R, Rohilla RK, Sangwan K, Siwach R, Magu NK, et al. (2011) Bladder management methods and urological complications in spinal cord injury patients. Indian J Orthop 45: 141–147.

44. Ramsey JB, Ramer LM, Inskip JA, Alan N, Ramer MS, et al. (2010) Care of rats with complete high-thoracic spinal cord injury. J Neurotrauma 27: 1709–1722.

45. Lotta S, Scelsi R, Alfonsi E, Saitta A, Nicolotti D, et al. (1991) Morphometric and neurophysiological analysis of skeletal muscle in paraplegic patients with traumatic cord lesion. Paraplegia 29: 247–252.

46. Calancie B, Broton JG, Klose KJ, Traad M, Difini J, et al. (1993) Evidence that alterations in presynaptic inhibition contribute to segmental hypo- and hyperexcitability after spinal cord injury in man. Electroencephalogr Clin Neurophysiol 89: 177–186.

47. Garrison MK, Yates CC, Reese NB, Skinner RD, Garcia-Rill E (2011) Wind-up of stretch reflexes as a measure of spasticity in chronic spinalized rats: The effects of passive exercise and modafinil. Exp Neurol 227: 104–109.

48. Murray KC, Nakae A, Stephens MJ, Rank M, D'Amico J, et al. (2010) Recovery of motoneuron and locomotor function after spinal cord injury depends on constitutive activity in 5-HT2C receptors. Nat Med 16: 694–700.

49. L, Budh CN, Hultling C, Molander C (2004) Neuropathic pain after traumatic spinal cord injury - relations to gender, spinal level, completeness, and age at the time of injury. Spinal Cord 42: 665–673.

50. Hoschouer EL, Basso DM, Jakeman LB (2009) Aberrant sensory responses are dependent on lesion severity after spinal cord contusion injury in mice. Pain 148: 328–342.

51. Jung JI, Kim J, Hong SK, Yoon YW (2008) Long-term follow-up of cutaneous hypersensitivity in rats with a spinal cord contusion. Korean J Physiol Pharmacol 12: 299–306.

52. Hulsebosch CE, Hains BC, Crown ED, Carlton SM (2009) Mechanisms of chronic central neuropathic pain after spinal cord injury. Brain Res Rev 60: 202–213.

53. Finnerup NB, Norrbrink C, Trok K, Piehl F, Johannesen IL, et al. (2014) Phenotypes and predictors of pain following traumatic spinal cord injury: a prospective study. J Pain 15: 40–48.

54. Gao T, Hao JX, Wiesenfeld-Hallin Z, Xu XJ (2013) Quantitative test of responses to thermal stimulation in spinally injured rats using a Peltier thermode: a new approach to study cold allodynia. J Neurosci Methods 212: 317–321.

55. Wang J, Kawamata M, Namiki A (2005) Changes in properties of spinal dorsal horn neurons and their sensitivity to morphine after spinal cord injury in the rat. Anesthesiology 102: 152–164.

56. Millan MJ (2002) Descending control of pain. Prog Neurobiol 66: 355–474.

57. Kim K, Mishina M, Kokubo R, Nakajima T, Morimoto D, et al. (2013) Ketamine for acute neuropathic pain in patients with spinal cord injury. J Clin Neurosci 20: 804–807.

58. Niesters M, Dahan A (2012) Pharmacokinetic and pharmacodynamic considerations in the treatment of chronic neuropathic pain. Exp Opin Drug Metab Toxicol 8: 1409–1417.

59. Rekand T (2010) Clinical assessment and management of spasticity: a review. Acta Neurol Scand Suppl. 190: 62–66.

60. Colpaert FC, Wu WP, Hao JX, Royer I, Sautel F, et al. (2004) High-efficacy 5-HT1A receptor activation causes a curative-like action on allodynia in rats with spinal cord injury. Eur J Pharmacol 497: 29–33.

61. Amaya-Castellanos E, Pineda-Farias JB, Castaneda-Corral G, Vidal-Cantu GC, Murbartian J, et al. (2011) Blockade of 5-HT7 reduces tactile allodynia in the rat. Pharmacol Biochem Behav 99: 591–597.

62. Aguggia M, Saracco MG, Cavallini M, Bussone G, Cortelli P (2013) Sensitization and pain. Neurol Sci 34 (Suppl 1): S37–40.

63. McCleane GJ, Suzuki R, Dickenson AH (2003) Does a single intravenous injection of the 5-HT3 receptor antagonist ondansetron have an analgesic effect in neuropathic pain? A double-blinded, placebo-controlled cross-over study. Anesth Analg 97: 1474–1478.

64. Chen Y, Oatway MA, Weaver LC (2009) Blockade of the 5-HT3 receptor for days causes sustained relief from mechanical allodynia following spinal cord injury. J Neurosci Res 87: 418–424.

65. Tzellos TG, Papazisis G, Amaniti E, Kouvelas D (2008) Efficacy of pregabalin and gabapentin for neuropathic pain in spinal-cord injury: an evidence-based evaluation of the literature. Eur J Clin Pharmacol 64: 851–858.

66. Merighi A, Salio C, Ghirri A, Lossi L, Ferrini F, et al. (2008) BDNF as a pain modulator. Progr Neurobiol 85: 297–317.

67. Trang T, Beggs S, Salter MW (2011) Brain-derived neurotrophic factor from microglia: a molecular substrate for neuropathic pain. Neuron Glia Biol 7: 99–108.

68. Hajebrahimi Z, Mowla SJ, Movahedin M, Tavallaei M (2008) Gene expression alterations of neurotrophins, their receptors and prohormone convertases in a rat model of spinal cord contusion. Neurosci Lett 441: 261–266.

69. Ying ZI, Roy RR, Edgerton VR, Gomez-Pinilla F (2005) Exercise restores levels of neurotrophins and synaptic plasticity following spinal cord injury. Exp Neurol 193: 411–419.

70. Carlton SM, Du J, Tan HY, Nesic O, Hargett GL, et al. (2009) Peripheral and central sensitization in remote spinal cord regions contribute to central neuropathic pain after spinal cord injury. Pain 147: 265–276.

71. Hai T, Hartman MG (2001) The molecular biology and nomenclature of the activating transcription factor/cAMP responsive element binding family of

transcription factors: activating transcription factor proteins and homeostasis. Gene 273: 1–11.

72. Block ML, Zecca L, Hong JS (2007) Microglia-mediated neurotoxicity: uncovering the molecular mechanisms. Nat Rev Neurosci 8: 57–69.

73. Gwak YS, Crown ED, Unabia GC, Hulsebosch CE (2008) Propentofylline attenuates allodynia, glial activation and modulates GABAergic tone after spinal cord injury in the rat. Pain 138: 410–422.

74. Gwak YS, Kang J, Unabia GC, Hulsebosch CE (2012) Spatial and temporal activation of spinal glial cells: role of gliopathy in central neuropathic pain following spinal cord injury in rats. Exp Neurol 234: 362–372.

75. Kim JY, Choi GS, Cho YW, Cho H, Hwang SJ, et al. (2013) Attenuation of spinal cord injury-induced astroglial and microglial activation by repetitive transcranial magnetic stimulation in rats. J Korean Med Sci 28: 295–299.

76. Marcillo A, Frydel B, Bramlett HM, Dietrich WD (2012) A reassessment of P2×7 receptor inhibition as a neuroprotective strategy in rat models of contusion injury. Exp Neurol 233: 687–692.

77. Kigerl KA, Lai W, Rivest S, Hart RP, Satoskar AR, et al. (2007) Toll-like receptor (TLR)-2 and TLR-4 regulate inflammation, gliosis, and myelin sparing after spinal cord injury. J Neurochem 102: 37–50.

78. Marchand F, Tsantoulas C, Singh D, Grist J, Clark AK, et al. (2009) Effects of etanercept and minocycline in a rat model of spinal cord injury. Pain 13: 673–681.

79. Chen K, Uchida K, Nakajima H, Yayama T, Hirai T, et al. (2011) Tumor necrosis factor-α antagonist reduces apoptosis of neurons and oligodendroglia in rat spinal cord injury. Spine 36: 1350–1358.

80. Guptarak J, Wanchoo S, Durham-Lee J, Wu Y, Zivadinovic D, et al. (2013) Inhibition of IL-6 signaling: A novel therapeutic approach to treating spinal cord injury pain. Pain 154: 1115–1128.

81. Genovese T, Esposito E, Mazzon E, Di Paola R, Caminiti R, et al. (2009) Absence of endogenous interleukin-10 enhances secondary inflammatory process after spinal cord compression injury in mice. J Neurochem 108: 1360–1372.

82. Zhou Z, Peng X, Insolera R, Fink DJ, Mata M (2009) IL-10 promotes neuronal survival following spinal cord injury. Exp Neurol 220: 183–190.

83. John GR, Lee SC, Brosnan CF (2003) Cytokines: powerful regulators of glial cell activation. Neuroscientist 9: 10–22.

84. Tian DS, Dong Q, Pan DJ, He Y, Yu ZY, et al. (2007) Attenuation of astrogliosis by suppressing of microglial proliferation with the cell cycle inhibitor olomoucine in rat spinal cord injury model. Brain Res 1154: 206–214.

85. Cronin M, Anderson PN, Cook JE, Green CR, Becker DL (2008) Blocking connexin43 expression reduces inflammation and improves functional recovery after spinal cord injury. Mol Cell Neurosci 39: 152–160.

12

Late-Onset of Spinal Neurodegeneration in Knock-In Mice Expressing a Mutant BiP

Hisayo Jin[1], Naoya Mimura[2], Makiko Kashio[1], Haruhiko Koseki[3], Tomohiko Aoe[1,4]*

1 Department of Anesthesiology, Chiba University Graduate School of Medicine, Chiba City, Chiba, Japan, 2 Department of Medicine and Clinical Oncology, Chiba University Graduate School of Medicine, Chiba City, Chiba, Japan, 3 Laboratory for Developmental Genetics, RIKEN Research Center for Allergy and Immunology, Yokohama, Japan, 4 Department of Anesthesiology, Tokyo Women's Medical University, Yachiyo Medical, Center, Yachiyo, Chiba, Japan

Abstract

Most human neurodegenerative diseases are sporadic, and appear later in life. While the underlying mechanisms of the progression of those diseases are still unclear, investigations into the familial forms of comparable diseases suggest that endoplasmic reticulum (ER) stress is involved in the pathogenesis. Binding immunoglobulin protein (BiP) is an ER chaperone that is central to ER function. We produced knock-in mice expressing a mutant BiP that lacked the retrieval sequence in order to evaluate the effect of a functional defect in an ER chaperone in multi-cellular organisms. Here we report that heterozygous mutant BiP mice revealed motor disabilities in aging. We found a degeneration of some motoneurons in the spinal cord accompanied by accumulations of ubiquitinated proteins. The defect in retrieval of BiP by the KDEL receptor leads to impaired activities in quality control and autophagy, suggesting that functional defects in the ER chaperones may contribute to the late onset of neurodegenerative diseases.

Editor: Hiroyasu Nakano, Toho University School of Medicine, Japan

Funding: Grants-in-Aids for Science Research from the Ministry of Education, Culture, Sports, Science and Technology of Japan to T.A. (20059008, http://www.mext.go.jp/english/) The funders had no role in study design, data collection and analysis, decision to publish, or preparation of the manuscript.

Competing Interests: The authors have declared that no competing interests exist.

* Email: taoe@faculty.chiba-u.jp

Introduction

Proteins destined for the secretory pathway are inserted into the ER cotranslationally and subjected to quality control [1]. ER molecular chaperones and folding enzymes such as BiP, calnexin, and protein disulfide isomerase facilitate the correct folding or degradation of these newly synthesized proteins as well as of misfolded proteins [2]. The accumulation of misfolded proteins in the ER beyond the capacity of quality control causes ER stress and induces the unfolded protein response (UPR) [3]. Further ER stress can cause cellular dysfunction and cell death, resulting in diverse human disorders such as neurodegenerative diseases [4].

Mammalian ER luminal chaperones have a carboxyl terminal Lys-Asp-Glu-Leu (KDEL) amino acid sequence, which is recognized by the KDEL receptor in post-ER compartments [5]. ER chaperones and the KDEL receptor are sorted into the transport vesicles coated with coat protein (COP) I complex and retrieved to the ER [6]. Yeast BiP (Kar2p) is essential for survival, while the deletion of the retrieval sequence (in yeast: His-Asp-Glu-Leu, HDEL) is dispensable because the UPR is activated and the loss of the chaperone in the ER is compensated for [7]. The complete depletion of BiP also has lethal effects on mammalian early embryonic cells [8].

In order to elucidate the physiological processes that are sensitive to the retrieval of BiP during development and adulthood in multi-cellular organisms, we previously produced knock-in mice expressing a mutant BiP in which the retrieval sequence was deleted by homologous recombination. The homozygous mutant BiP mice died within several hours after birth due to respiratory failure with impaired biosynthesis of the pulmonary surfactant, especially surfactant protein C, by alveolar type II cells [9]. The heterozygous mutant BiP mice grew up to be apparently normal adults. However, vulnerability to ER stress may exist in the mutant BiP mice, leading to chronic organ injuries. Indeed, some of them displayed motor disabilities in aging. We found a degeneration of some motoneurons in the spinal cord accompanied by accumulations of ubiquitinated proteins. The accumulation of misfolded proteins is one of the most common features in neurodegenerative diseases. Functional defects in the ER chaperones may contribute to the late onset of neurodegenerative diseases.

Results

The mutant BiP mice revealed motor disabilities in aging

The heterozygous mutant BiP mice live as long as the wild type mice (Figure 1A). We could not detect a significant motor disability during their young period, using the Rotarod performance test. At very advanced ages, some of the mutant BiP mice displayed paralysis and tremors after they were more than one year old, although a few wild-type mice show partial paresis (Figure 1B). Some of aged mutant BiP mice displayed loss of righting reflex and suffered from paralysis (Figure 1C, D, and Video S1). The ratio of motor disabilities is significantly higher in the heterozygous mutant BiP mice.

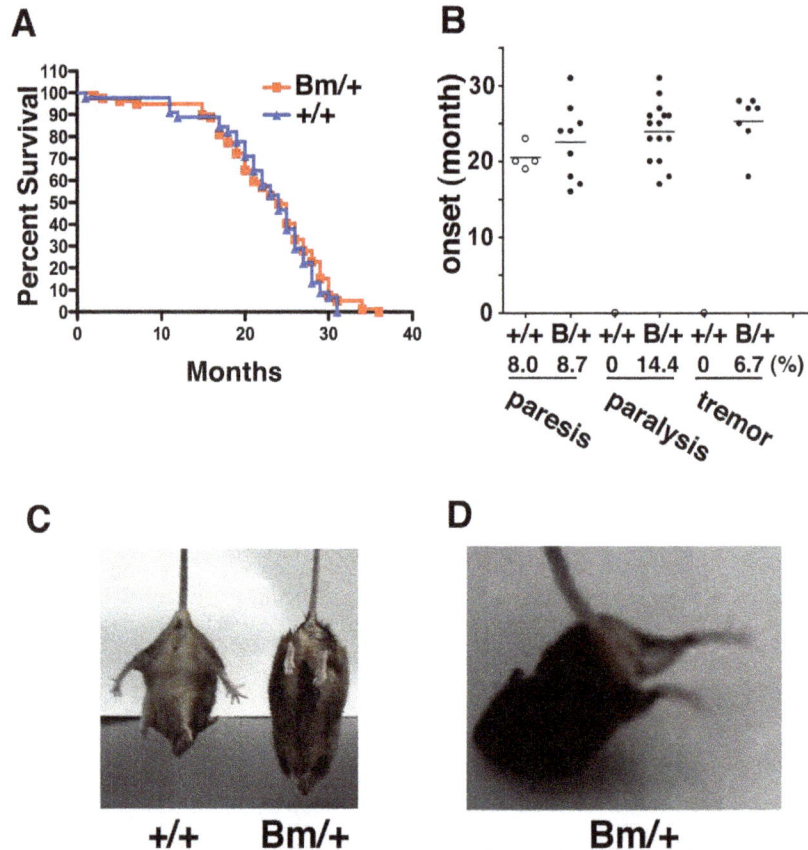

Figure 1. The mutant BiP mice revealed motor disabilities in aging. (A) Kaplan-Meier plots demonstrate that the heterozygous mutant BiP mice (Bm/+, n = 80) live as long as the wild-type mice (+/+, n = 45). (B) Some of the mutant BiP mice displayed paralysis and tremors after they were more than one year old. Heterozygous mutant BiP mice (Bm/+, n = 104) and wild type mice (n = 50) more than 10 months old were observed. No sign of weakness; +/+ 46/50, Bm/+ 73/104, tremor; +/+ 0/50, Bm/+ 9/104, paresis of one hindlimb; +/+ 4/50, Bm/+ 9/104, paralysis of one or both hindlimbs; +/+ 0/50, Bm/+ 15/104. To compare values between two groups, Chi-square and Fisher's exact test was done. Statistical significance was found. P value is 0.0033. (C) A seventeen month-old mutant BiP mouse displayed paralysis and loss of righting reflex. (D) A seventeen month-old mutant BiP mouse displayed paralysis (Video S1).

Motoneurons at the anterior horn of spinal cords of aged mutant BiP mice suffer from ER stress

In order to investigate whether defective retrieval of the mutant BiP may contribute to the pathogenesis of motor disability, we examined the spinal cords of both the wild type and mutant BiP mice. By staining with an anti-KDEL antibody, we found that some large cells expressed BiP and other KDEL-containing chaperones highly at the anterior horn of the spinal cords of 6 month-old mice of both types. Those cells were also stained with an anti-choline acetyltransferase antibody, suggesting that motoneurons at the anterior horn expressed ER chaperones highly (Figure 2A). Then we examined much older mutant BiP mice with motor disability. Motoneurons at the anterior horn of the spinal cord stained with an anti-choline acetyltransferase antibody in a 29 month-old mutant BiP mouse were less than those in the wild type mice (Figure 2B). We found that some large cells at the anterior horn of the spinal cord of the 29 month-old mutant BiP mouse expressed CHOP, a cell death related transcriptional factor during ER stress. The expression of CHOP was less obvious in the wild type littermate (Figure 2C). In accordance with these findings, terminal deoxynucleotidyl transferase dUTP nick end labeling (TUNEL) staining revealed that some apoptotic cells existed in the mutant spinal cord, accompanied by an enhanced gliosis stained with an anti-glial fibrillary acidic protein (GFAP) antibody

(Figure 3A and B). It was difficult to find a TUNEL positive cell in the wild type spinal cord. We counted cells in Figure 3B. The ratio of GFAP positive cells was significantly higher in the mutant BiP spinal cord (Bm/+, 17 m) compared to that in the wild type (+/+, 16 m).

These data suggest that motoneurons at the anterior horn of spinal cords of aged mutant BiP mice suffer from ER stress, resulting in cell death.

Some motoneurons in the spinal cord revealed a degeneration accompanied by accumulations of protein aggregations

Protein aggregation and neuronal cell death are hallmarks of various neurodegenerative diseases [10]. We examined protein aggregation in the mutant spinal cord by staining it with an anti-ubiquitin antibody, which revealed cytoplasmic aggregations in the large cells at the anterior horn of the aged mutant BiP mouse (Figure 3C). One possible candidate for the aggregated proteins is superoxide dismutase (SOD) 1 [11]. Point mutations of the human SOD 1 gene are associated with a familial motoneuron disease (amyotrophic lateral sclerosis, ALS) [12]. While we observed fuzzy perinuclear staining with an anti-SOD1 antibody in large cells at the anterior horn of the spinal cords of wild type mice,

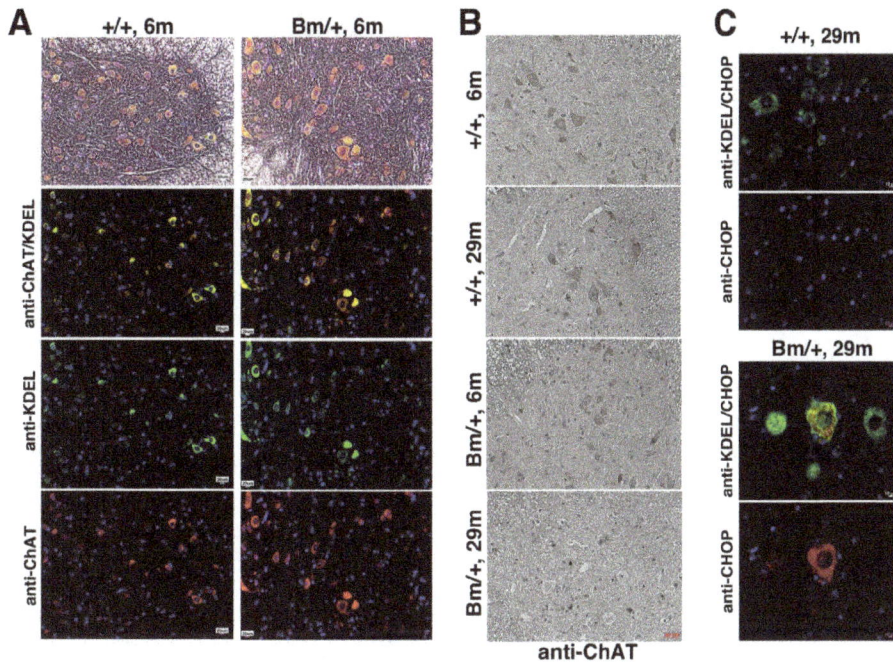

Figure 2. Motoneurons at the anterior horn of spinal cords of aged mutant BiP mice suffer from ER stress. (A) Motoneurons stained by an anti-choline acetyltransferase antibody (red) at the anterior horn in the spinal cord of both a 6 month-old wild type (+/+, 6 m) and a 6 month-old mutant BiP mouse (Bm/+, 6 m) express ER chaperones as well (green). Scale bars, 20 um. (B) The immunoreactivity with an anti-choline acetyltransferase antibody at the anterior horn is reduced in the aged 29 month-old mutant spinal cord (Bm/+, 29 m). Scale bars, 20 um. (C) Large cells at the anterior horn of the aged 29 month-old mutant spinal cord (Bm/+, 29 m) express ER chaperones as well as CHOP. Scale bars, 10 um. The nuclei were stained with Hoechst 33258 (blue, A and C).

aggregations were found instead in the cells of the mutant BiP mice. Those aggregations were much more obvious in the aged 26 month-old mutant BiP mouse (Figure 4, Bm/+, 26 m).

We examined the expression of BiP and the mutant BiP in the brain and spinal cord of the mutant BiP mice by Western blotting in Figure 5. The expression of GRP94, another ER chaperone, seemed to be increased in the aged mutant BiP brain and spinal cord. We also found an accumulation of SOD1 aggregates in the aged mutant BiP spinal cord, which corresponds to the finding in Figure 4.

Deletion of the retrieval signal from BiP may cause aberrant quality control

We examined the effect of ER stress on the distribution of BiP, an endogenous ligand of the KDEL receptor, in the secretory pathway by sucrose gradient analysis in Hela cells (Figure 6A). While most BiP was found in the ER in the resting state, a significant amount could be detected in the post-ER fractions in these cells during ER stress when treated with tunicamycin (2.5 ug/ml for 24 h) which disrupts protein glycosylation in the ER, thereby inducing the UPR (Figure 6B). Then, we examined the effect of deletion of the retrieval signal from BiP. A myc-tagged mutant BiP with the KDEL sequence deleted was transiently expressed in HeLa cells. While some of the mutant BiP were localized in the ER, significant amounts were also found in the post-ER fractions (Figure 6C), suggesting that a certain fraction of BiP was transported from the ER and retrieved from the post-ER by the KDEL receptor [13]. Thus, the deletion of the retrieval signal from BiP may results in mis-sortings of cargo proteins to the secretory pathway out of the ER.

Loss of the retrieval signal may also cause a failure of the activation of the KDEL receptor. Since KDEL receptor activation has been reported to promote autophagy and removal of aggregated proteins, including SOD1 [14], we examined whether autophagy induced in the mutant BiP cells (Figure 6D). We found ER stress caused by tunicamycin treatment induced the expression of BiP in the wild type mouse embryonic cells (MEF) as well as that of the mutant BiP in the mutant MEF, while autophagy was induced only in the wild type MEF accompanying the accumulation of light chain 3AII (LC3AII).

If the lack of the KDEL sequence from BiP affects autophagy, cytosolic aggregates might be accumulated in the homozygous mutant BiP MEF. We over-expressed SOD1-GFP in the wild type and the homozygous mutant BiP MEF. While SOD1 distributed through the cytoplasm in the wild type MEF, it accumulated in the perinuclear space and some aggregations were found in the cytoplasm of the mutant BiP MEF (Figure 7).

Thus, lack of the KDEL sequence from BiP may lead to some functional defects of the ER chaperone in quality control and autophagy, resulting in the late onset of neurodegenerative diseases.

Discussion

Some of the mutant BiP mice revealed motor disabilities in aging. We found a degeneration of some motoneurons in the spinal cord accompanied by the accumulation of ubiquitinated proteins. BiP, also called the 78-kD glucose-regulated protein (GRP78), is a member of the heat shock protein 70 family of proteins and is one of the most abundant ER chaperones, assisting in protein translocation, folding, and degradation [15]. Quality control in the early secretory pathway is a ubiquitous mechanism

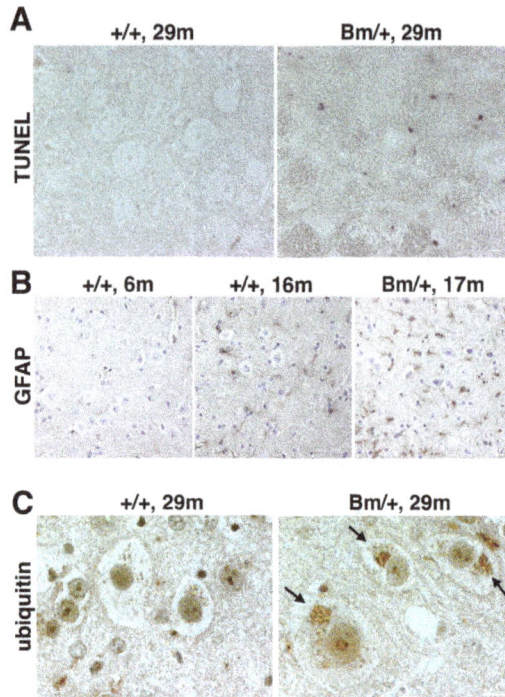

Figure 3. Some motoneurons in the spinal cord revealed a degeneration accompanied by accumulations of ubiquitinated proteins. (A) TUNEL staining revealed some apoptotic cells at the anterior horn in the spinal cord of a 29 month-old mutant BiP mouse (Bm/+, 29 m). Scale bars, 10 um. (B) The immunoreactivity with an anti-GFAP antibody at the anterior horn is increased in a 17 month-old mutant spinal cord (Bm/+, 17 m). Scale bars, 20 um. GFAP positive cells are counted (five fields in each mouse, GFAP positive cells/the number of nucleus). +/+, 16 m; 33/199, 35/174, 34/192, 40/181, 42/207, Bm/+, 17 m; 42/132, 50/140, 59/147, 39/154, 58/143 +/+, 6 m; 5/143, 4/131, 4/141, 0/95, 0/107. The ratio of GFAP positive cells is significantly higher in the mutant BiP spinal cord (Bm/+, 17 m) compared to that in the wild type (+/+, 16 m) by t test (p value is 0.0009). (C) The aggregations were stained by an anti-ubiquitin antibody in the large cells at the anterior horn of the 29 month-old mutant spinal cord (Bm/+, 29 m, arrowheads). Scale bars, 10 um.

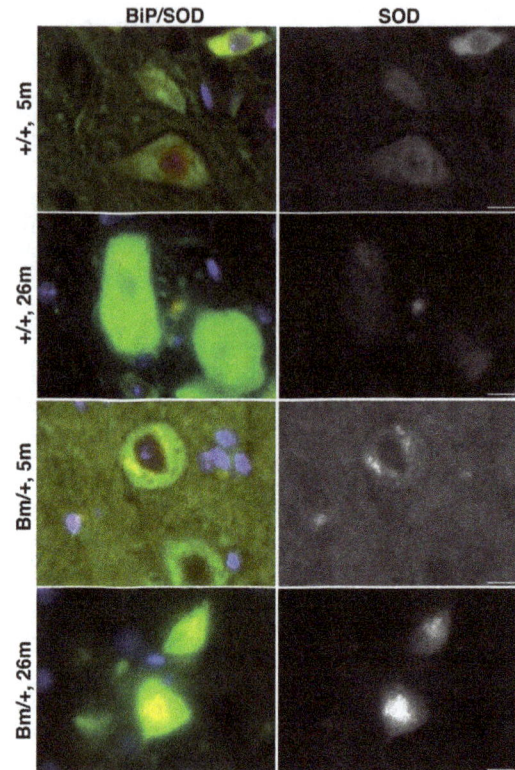

Figure 4. Aggregations were obvious in the aged mutant BiP mouse. The aggregations were evaluated by immunofluorescence microscopy with double labeling by using a rabbit anti-SOD1 antibody (red) and a mouse anti-KDEL mAb for the wild type BiP and other ER chaperones (green, +/+, 5 and 26 month-old), or by using a rabbit anti-SOD1 antibody (red) and a mouse anti-HA mAb (15E6) for the mutant BiP (green, Bm/+, 5 and 26 month-old). Scale bars, 10 um. Aggregations were observed in large cells at the anterior horn of a 26-month-old mutant spinal cord (Bm/+, 26 m).

for adapting to ER stress, and the KDEL receptor and BiP are essential components of this system [13]. Proper ER-to-Golgi transport, and the subsequent retrieval of proteins and lipids to the ER, are thought to contribute to quality control [13,16]. Deletion of the retrieval sequence from the BiP, and the consequent lack of mutant BiP recycling by the KDEL receptor, could have possible effects on protein folding in the ER and post-ER.

Mutant BiP were mostly localized to the ER, and the expression was enhanced by tunicamycin in the mutant BiP MEF [9]. A significant fraction of the mutant BiP was secreted from the cells even in the resting state, reflecting a deletion of the KDEL sequence and an impaired retrieval of mutant BiP [9]. The KDEL proteins are ER chaperones; therefore, their expression is induced extensively upon ER stress, which may cause the saturation of the KDEL receptor-mediated retrieval. A fraction of the wild-type BiP was also secreted into the medium upon ER stress caused by the tunicamycin treatment, indicating that retrieval by the KDEL receptor is saturable [9].

The homozygous mutant BiP mice have defects in some professional secretory cells. They survive only several hours after birth due to impaired pulmonary surfactant biosynthesis by alveolar type II epithelial cells causing respiratory failure [9].

They also have cortical dysplasia in the brain due to impaired synthesis of reelin by Cajal-Retzius cells. Thus, the retrieval function of BiP is essential in vivo. However, mouse embryonic fibroblasts from the homozygous mutant BiP mice are viable. Therefore, living as a whole animal may suffer from various insults from the environment.

The accumulation of misfolded proteins is one of the most common features in neurodegenerative diseases. One possible explanation for the late onset of sporadic forms of neurodegeneration is a decline, with aging, of the cellular machinery to cope with protein overload in the ER. The expression level of BiP decreases, and its chaperone function is progressively reduced due to age-related oxidization reported in rodents [10,17]. The mutant BiP with impaired retrieval seemed to fail the induction of autophagy, which might further limit the capacity of ER quality control.

The heterozygous mutant BiP mice grew up to be adults and showed apparently normal organ development. However, vulnerability to ER stress may exist, and that vulnerability could result in chronic organ injuries with aging such as renal tubular-interstitial injury, as described in our previous work [18]. We are also interested in the relationship between ER stress and neural degeneration due to aging, such as Alzheimer's disease [19], Parkinson's disease [20], and amyotrophic lateral sclerosis [11]. The involvement of impaired BiP function in neurodegenerative

brain

6m 12m 20m 6m 12m 20m

-GRP94
-BiP

-mutant BiP

-CHOP

-tubulin

+/+   Bm/+

spinal cord

2m 2m 24m 24m

-SOD1 X 3

-SOD1 X 2

-SOD1(23kD)

-GRP94

-BiP

-mutant BiP

-tubulin

+/+ Bm/+ +/+ Bm/+

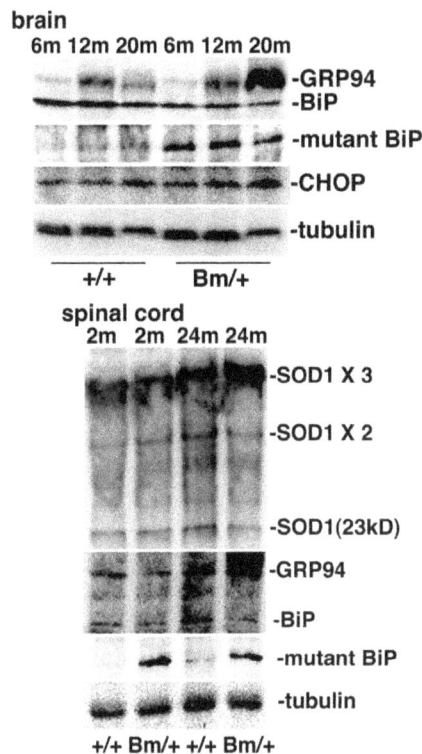

Figure 5. The expressions of chaperones in the mutant BiP mice. The heterozygous mutant BiP mice and the litter mate wild type mice were anesthetized by pentobarbital, and the brains and spinal cords were removed. They were subjected to Western blot analysis with an anti-KDEL mouse mAb for BiP and GRP94, an anti-HA mouse mAb for mutant BiP, an anti-CHOP rabbit antiserum, and an anti-SOD1 rabbit antiserum.

diseases has been reported in a mouse model where the disruption of SIL1, a co-chaperone of BiP, causes protein accumulation and neurodegeneration [21].

Interestingly, we previously found disordered layer formation in the cerebral cortex and cerebellum in the homozygous mutant BiP neonates. Among proteins involved in corticogenesis, we found that the expression of reelin, secreted by Cajal-Retzius cells [22] was markedly reduced in the mutant brain [23]. Several studies have suggested the possible role of reelin in the pathogenesis of human mental disorders such as schizophrenia, autism, bipolar disorder, and Alzheimer's disease [24,25]. Reelin and ApoE share ApoER2 on the cortical neurons [26], and ApoE inhibits reelin signaling by competing for binding to ApoER2. The E4 allele of ApoE increases the risk of developing sporadic forms of Alzheimer's disease. Because reelin signaling through ApoER2 in adult brains modulates synaptic plasticity and memory formation [27], a defective reelin signaling pathway may contribute to the pathogenesis of adult mental disorders. Thus, reelin signaling and ER quality control may be related to the pathogenesis of adult mental disorders, as seen in the reeler mutant–like cerebral malformation in the homozygous mutant BiP neonates [23].

The administration of chemical chaperones that promote protein folding in the ER has been reported to be effective in treating type2 diabetes, which has been shown, in experiments using a mouse model, to be connected to ER stress [28]. We have also shown that a chemical chaperone prevented the development of morphine tolerance caused by ER stress [29]. Our present study

suggests that ER chaperones would be promising therapeutic targets in the treatment of chronic neurodegenerative diseases.

Methods

Cells and reagents

Mouse embryonic fibroblasts (MEFs) were prepared from 13.5-day-old embryos [9]. MEFs and HeLa cells were grown in a complete medium that consisted of Dulbecco's modified Eagle's medium (DMEM; Sigma Chemical Co., Irvine, UK) with 10% fetal bovine serum, 2 mM glutamine, 50 μg/ml streptomycin and 50 U/ml penicillin G at 37°C in a 5% CO_2 incubator.

The following antibodies were used: rabbit antiserum against CHOP/GADD153, rabbit antiserum against ubiquitin, rabbit antiserum against superoxide dismutase 1 (Santa Cruz Biotechnology), rabbit antiserum against choline acetyltransferase (Millipore), rabbit antiserum against glial fibrillary acidic protein (GFAP, DakoCytomation), rabbit antiserum against Derlin-1 (MBL), mouse mAb 9E10 against the myc epitope (ATCC), mouse mAb against g-tubulin, mouse mAb against Golgi p58 (Sigma Chemical), mouse mAb SPA-827 against BiP (KDEL sequence, Stressgen), mouse mAb AF8 against calnexin (kindly provided by MM. Brenner, Boston, MA), mouse mAb 15E6 against HA tag (kindly provided by VW Hsu, Boston, MA). rabbit polyclonal antiserum against light chain (LC) 3A (Cell Signaling), Cy-2-conjugated donkey antibody against rabbit IgG, Cy-3-conjugated donkey antibody against rabbit IgG and Cy-3-conjugated donkey antibody against mouse IgG (Jackson Immunoresearch Laboratories). Tunicamycin was purchased from Nacali tasque. Hoechst 33258 was purchased from Invitrogen. Chloroquine was purchased from Sigma-Aldrich.

Plasmids and transfection

A cDNA for the BiP deleted with the KDEL sequence was obtained by inserting a stop codon into a rat BiP cDNA (a gift from Dr. H.R.B. Pelham, MRC Laboratory of Molecular Biology, UK) just before the region encoding the carboxyl terminal KDEL sequence with a PCR reaction. The PCR product was subcloned into a pcDNA3.1 myc-His vector (Invitrogen). A PCR-generated fragment corresponding to the wild-type human SOD1 cDNA from human cDNA library was cloned into the plasmid pGFP vector (Clontech). The DNA sequences were verified using the Applied Biosystems ABI Prism 310 genetic analyzer. Transfection was performed with Fugene 6 (Roche, Basel, Switzerland).

Mutant BiP mice

All animal experimental procedures were in accordance with a protocol approved by the Institutional Animal Care Committee of Chiba University, Chiba, Japan. A rat BiP cDNA was used as a probe to isolate a genomic clone containing the whole exon of the BiP gene from the 129/SvJ mouse genomic library in lFIXII (Stratagene). A targeting vector was used for electroporation into R1 EScells. We used homologous recombination to establish knock-in mice expressing BiP lacking the carboxyl-terminal KDEL sequence [9]. The missing KDEL sequence was replaced by a hemagglutinin (HA) tag. The resulting male chimeras were mated to C57BL/6 females. The mutant-BiP mice were investigated on the compound genetic background between the 129/SvJ derived from R1 ES cells and C57BL/6J. The heterozygotes were intercrossed to generate homozygous mutants. This hybrid line was maintained by brother-sister mating for at least ten generations.

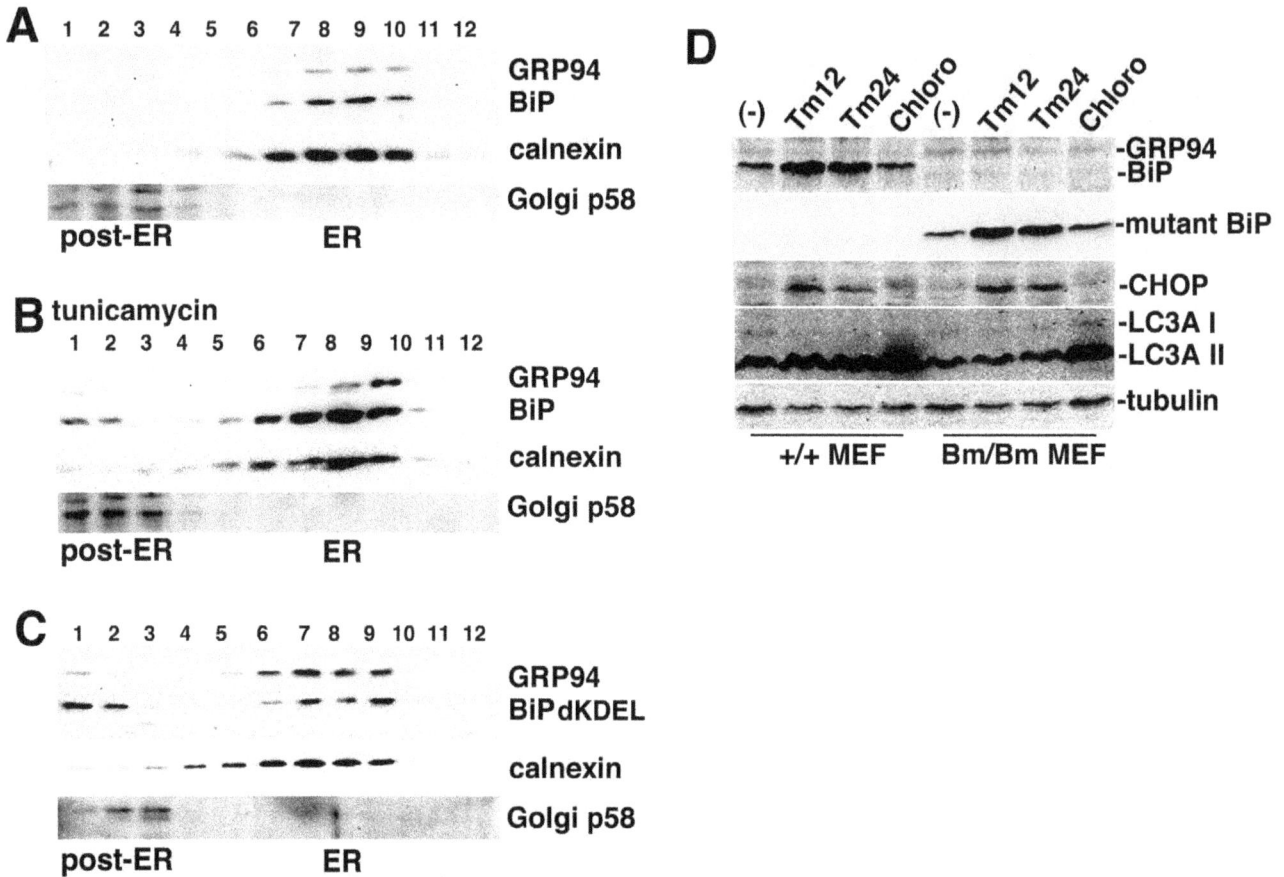

Figure 6. Lack of the KDEL sequence from BiP may lead to some functional defects of the ER chaperone in quality control and autophagy. (A, B) A fraction of BiP is secreted from the ER under stressed conditions. The postnuclear supernatants (PNS) from HeLa cells with (B) or without (A) treatment by tunicamycin 2.5 ug ml^{-1} for 24 h were separated on a continuous sucrose gradient (20% to 50%, fraction 1; top, fraction 12; bottom). An aliquot of each fraction was analyzed by SDS-PAGE. The distributions of GRP94, BiP, Golgi p58 and calnexin were determined by Western blotting. (C) HeLa cells transiently expressing the mutant BiP with the KDEL sequence deleted were collected and homogenized. The PNS from those cells were separated on a continuous sucrose gradient (20% to 50%, fraction 1; top, fraction 12; bottom). An aliquot of each fraction was analyzed by SDS-PAGE. The distributions of the GRP94, myc-tagged mutant BiP, Golgi p58 and calnexin were determined by Western blotting. (D) Wild-type MEFs and BiP MEFs were treated with tunicamycin (2.5 ug ml^{-1} for 12, 24 h) or chloroquine (50 uM for 12 h). Cells were subjected to Western blot analysis with an anti-KDEL mouse mAb for BiP, an anti-HA mouse mAb for mutant BiP, an anti-CHOP rabbit antiserum, an anti-LC3A antiserum, and an anti-tubulin mAb.

Western blotting

Cultured cells were washed twice with ice-cold PBS and then homogenized in a buffer containing 0.4% (w/v) Nonidet P-40, 0.2% N-lauroylsarcosine, 30 mM Tris/HCl pH 8.0, 1 mM EDTA, 10 µg/ml aprotinin, 10 µg/ml leupeptin, 30 µg/ml N-acetyl-L-leucinal-L-lecinal-L-norleucinal (ALLN, Sigma Chemical). The mice were deeply anesthetized with pentobarbital (Dainippon Sumitomo Pharma). Brains and spinal cords were homogenized by sonication (UR-20P, TOMY, Tokyo, Japan) in a buffer containing 0.4% (w/v) Nonidet P-40, 0.2% N-lauroylsarcosine, 30 mM Tris/HCl pH 8.0, 1 mM EDTA, 10 µg/ml aprotinin, 10 µg/ml leupeptin, 30 µg/ml ALLN.

The lysates were centrifuged, and the supernatants were resuspended in SDS-PAGE sample buffer and then separated by SDS-PAGE under reducing conditions. The proteins were transferred from the gels to polyvinylidene fluoride membranes (Immobilon-P, Millipore Corp.), and Western blotting was done as previously described [30]. Imaging was obtained by LAS-1000 and Image Gauge software (Fuji Photo Film Co. Ltd.).

Sucrose gradient experiment

A postnuclear supernatant was obtained and loaded on a continuous sucrose gradient (20–50%), as described previously [13]. Twelve fractions were obtained from each sample. An aliquot of each fraction was separated by SDS-PAGE under reducing conditions, and the distribution of each protein was determined by Western blotting, developed by chemiluminescence (ECL, Amersham Pharmacia Biotech). Imaging was obtained by LAS1000 and Image Gauge software (Fuji Photo Film Co. Ltd., Tokyo, Japan).

Immunohistochemistry

The mice were deeply anesthetized with pentobarbital and fixed by transcardiac perfusion with 4% paraformaldehyde in phosphate-buffered saline (PBS). The spinal cords were further immersion-fixed for 12 h in 4% paraformaldehyde at 4°C. After fixation, they were dehydrated in increasing concentrations of ethanol and embedded in paraffin wax. For the immunofluorescence, the sections (8 µm) were incubated with 10% normal goat or bovine serum in PBS for 30 min to block nonspecific antibody

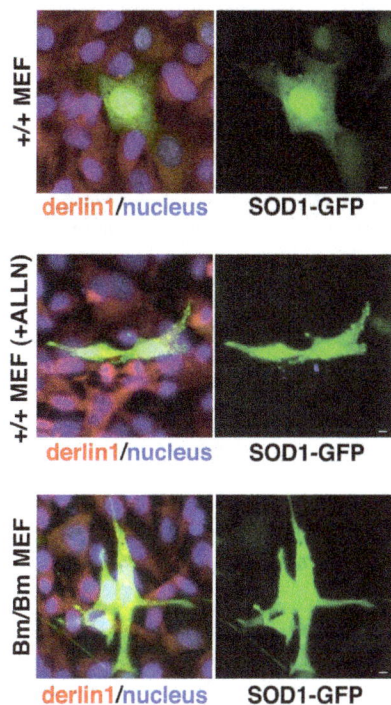

Figure 7. Aggregations were obvious in the mutant BiP MEF. The aggregations by transient expressions of SOD1-GFP were evaluated by immunofluorescence microscopy with labeling by using a rabbit anti-Derlin1 antibody for the ER staining (red) and SOD1-GFP (green) in wild type (+/+) and the homozygous mutant (Bm/Bm) MEF with Hoechst 33342 for nuclear staining. Scale bars, 10 um. Aggregations of SOD1were observed in the mutant BiP MEF as well as in the wild type MEF treated with a proteasome inhibitor, ALLN (10 ug/ml), at 37°C for 12 h.

binding, and then incubated with a primary antibody in PBS for 1 h at room temperature. The sections were rinsed with PBS and then incubated with a mixture of Cy3-conjugated anti-rabbit IgG and Cy2-conjugated anti-mouse IgG in PBS for 1 h at room temperature. Then, the sections were rinsed with PBS and mounted on glass slides with Perma Fluor (Immunon). Immuno-localization was observed with a fluorescence microscope using FITC/rhodamine filters and a Plan-Neofluar 20× and 40× NA 0.75 objective (Axiovert 200 M, Carl Zeiss). The brightness and

contrast were optimized by AxioVision 4.4 software (Carl Zeiss), and the immunofluorescence images were captured with a digital camera (AxioCam MRm, Carl Zeiss). For the immunohistochemistry, the spinal cord sections were incubated with 10% normal goat or bovine serum in PBS for 30 min to block nonspecific antibody binding, and then incubated with a primary antibody in PBS for 12 h at 4°C. The sections were rinsed with PBS, incubated with a secondary antibody in PBS for 2 h at room temperature, and then visualized using the VECTASTAIN Elite ABC kit (Vector Laboratories) with diaminobenzidine (Sigma).

TUNEL staining

The mice were deeply anesthetized with pentobarbital (Dainippon Sumitomo Pharma). The spinal cords were isolated, and apoptotic cells were visualized by TUNEL assay based on the manufacturer's protocol (Roche) as previously described [30]. The TUNEL staining was observed with a microscope using a N-Achroplan 40× NA 0.65 objective (Axio Imager A1, Carl Zeiss). The brightness and contrast were optimized by AxioVision Rel.4.7 software (Carl Zeiss), and the images were captured with a digital camera (AxioCam MRc, Carl Zeiss).

Statistical analysis

To compare values between groups, Chi-square and Fisher's exact test (Figure. 1) and t-test (Figure 3B) were used (GraphPad Prism 4.0, GraphPad Software, San Diego, CA). Statistical significance was accepted at $P<0.05$.

Supporting Information

Video S1   A seventeen month-old heterozygous mutant BiP mouse displayed paralysis.

Acknowledgments

We thank Dr. Shigemasa Goto (National hospital organization Chiba medical center) and Dr. Keita Kimura for helpful aids and critical comments.

Author Contributions

Conceived and designed the experiments: TA HK. Performed the experiments: HJ NM MK HK TA. Analyzed the data: TA. Contributed reagents/materials/analysis tools: TA HJ. Wrote the paper: TA.

References

1. Ellgaard L, Helenius A (2003) Quality control in the endoplasmic reticulum. Nat Rev Mol Cell Biol 4: 181–191.
2. Pfaffenbach KT, Lee AS (2011) The critical role of GRP78 in physiologic and pathologic stress. Curr Opin Cell Biol 23: 150–156.
3. Ron D, Walter P (2007) Signal integration in the endoplasmic reticulum unfolded protein response. Nat Rev Mol Cell Biol 8: 519–529.
4. Roussel BD, Kruppa AJ, Miranda E, Crowther DC, Lomas DA, et al. (2013)Endoplasmic reticulum dysfunction in neurological disease. Lancet Neurol 12: 105–118.
5. Lewis MJ, Pelham HR (1992) Ligand-induced redistribution of a human KDEL receptor from the Golgi complex to the endoplasmic reticulum. Cell 68: 353–364.
6. Orci L, Stamnes M, Ravazzola M, Amherdt M, Perrelet A, et al. (1997) Bidirectional transport by distinct populations of COPI-coated vesicles. Cell 90: 335–349.
7. Beh CT, Rose MD (1995) Two redundant systems maintain levels of resident proteins within the yeast endoplasmic reticulum. Proc Natl Acad Sci U S A 92: 9820–9823.
8. Luo S, Mao C, Lee B, Lee AS (2006) GRP78/BiP is required for cell proliferation and protecting the inner cell mass from apoptosis during early mouse embryonic development. Mol Cell Biol 26: 5688–5697.
9. Mimura N, Hamada H, Kashio M, Jin H, Toyama Y, et al. (2007) Aberrant quality control in the endoplasmic reticulum impairs the biosynthesis of pulmonary surfactant in mice expressing mutant BiP. Cell Death Differ 14: 1475–1485.
10. Gorbatyuk MS, Gorbatyuk OS (2013) The Molecular Chaperone GRP78/BiP as a Therapeutic Target for Neurodegenerative Disorders: A Mini Review. J Genet Syndr Gene Ther 4.
11. Nishitoh H, Kadowaki H, Nagai A, Maruyama T, Yokota T, et al. (2008) ALS-linked mutant SOD1 induces ER stress- and ASK1-dependent motor neuron death by targeting Derlin-1. Genes Dev 22: 1451–1464.
12. Gurney ME, Pu H, Chiu AY, Dal Canto MC, Polchow CY, et al. (1994) Motor neuron degeneration in mice that express a human Cu, Zn superoxide dismutase mutation. Science 264: 1772–1775.
13. Yamamoto K, Fujii R, Toyofuku Y, Saito T, Koseki H, et al. (2001) The KDEL receptor mediates a retrieval mechanism that contributes to quality control at the endoplasmic reticulum. Embo J 20: 3082–3091.
14. Wang P, Li B, Zhou L, Fei E, Wang G (2011) The KDEL receptor induces autophagy to promote the clearance of neurodegenerative disease-related proteins. Neuroscience 190: 43–55.

15. Munro S, Pelham HR (1986) An Hsp70-like protein in the ER: identity with the 78 kd glucose- regulated protein and immunoglobulin heavy chain binding protein. Cell 46: 291–300.

16. Hammond C, Helenius A (1994) Quality control in the secretory pathway: retention of a misfolded viral membrane glycoprotein involves cycling between the ER, intermediate compartment, and Golgi apparatus. J Cell Biol 126: 41–52.

17. Brown MK, Naidoo N (2012) The endoplasmic reticulum stress response in aging and age-related diseases. Front Physiol 3: 263.

18. Kimura K, Jin H, Ogawa M, Aoe T (2008) Dysfunction of the ER chaperone BiP accelerates the renal tubular injury. Biochem Biophys Res Commun 366: 1048–1053.

19. Katayama T, Imaizumi K, Sato N, Miyoshi K, Kudo T, et al. (1999) Presenilin-1 mutations downregulate the signalling pathway of the unfolded-protein response. Nat Cell Biol 1: 479–485.

20. Imai Y, Soda M, Inoue H, Hattori N, Mizuno Y, et al. (2001) An unfolded putative transmembrane polypeptide, which can lead to endoplasmic reticulum stress, is a substrate of Parkin. Cell 105: 891–902.

21. Zhao L, Longo-Guess C, Harris BS, Lee JW, Ackerman SL (2005) Protein accumulation and neurodegeneration in the woozy mutant mouse is caused by disruption of SIL1, a cochaperone of BiP. Nat Genet 37: 974–979.

22. D'Arcangelo G, Miao GG, Chen SC, Soares HD, Morgan JI, et al. (1995) A protein related to extracellular matrix proteins deleted in the mouse mutant reeler. Nature 374: 719–723.

23. Mimura N, Yuasa S, Soma M, Jin H, Kimura K, et al. (2008) Altered quality control in the endoplasmic reticulum causes cortical dysplasia in knock-in mice expressing a mutant BiP. Mol Cell Biol 28: 293–301.

24. Tissir F, Goffinet AM (2003) Reelin and brain development. Nat Rev Neurosci 4: 496–505.

25. Fatemi SH (2005) Reelin glycoprotein: structure, biology and roles in health and disease. Mol Psychiatry 10: 251–257.

26. D'Arcangelo G, Homayouni R, Keshvara L, Rice DS, Sheldon M, et al. (1999) Reelin is a ligand for lipoprotein receptors. Neuron 24: 471–479.

27. Beffert U, Weeber EJ, Durudas A, Qiu S, Masiulis I, et al. (2005) Modulation of synaptic plasticity and memory by Reelin involves differential splicing of the lipoprotein receptor Apoer2. Neuron 47: 567–579.

28. Ozcan U, Yilmaz E, Ozcan L, Furuhashi M, Vaillancourt E, et al. (2006) Chemical chaperones reduce ER stress and restore glucose homeostasis in a mouse model of type 2 diabetes. Science 313: 1137–1140.

29. Dobashi T, Tanabe S, Jin H, Mimura N, Yamamoto T, et al. (2010) BiP, an endoplasmic reticulum chaperone, modulates the development of morphine antinociceptive tolerance. J Cell Mol Med 14: 2816–2826.

30. Hamada H, Suzuki M, Yuasa S, Mimura N, Shinozuka N, et al. (2004) Dilated cardiomyopathy caused by aberrant endoplasmic reticulum quality control in mutant KDEL receptor transgenic mice. Mol Cell Biol 24: 8007–8017.

13

Influence of Delivery Method on Neuroprotection by Bone Marrow Mononuclear Cell Therapy following Ventral Root Reimplantation with Fibrin Sealant

Roberta Barbizan[1], Mateus V. Castro[1], Benedito Barraviera[2], Rui S. Ferreira Jr.[2], Alexandre L. R. Oliveira[1]*

1 Laboratory of Nerve Regeneration, Department of Structural and Functional Biology, University of Campinas - UNICAMP, Campinas, São Paulo, Brazil, 2 Center for the Study of Venoms and Venomous Animals (CEVAP), São Paulo State University (UNESP – Univ Estadual Paulista), Botucatu, São Paulo, Brazil

Abstract

The present work compared the local injection of mononuclear cells to the spinal cord lateral funiculus with the alternative approach of local delivery with fibrin sealant after ventral root avulsion (VRA) and reimplantation. For that, female adult Lewis rats were divided into the following groups: avulsion only, reimplantation with fibrin sealant; root repair with fibrin sealant associated with mononuclear cells; and repair with fibrin sealant and injected mononuclear cells. Cell therapy resulted in greater survival of spinal motoneurons up to four weeks post-surgery, especially when mononuclear cells were added to the fibrin glue. Injection of mononuclear cells to the lateral funiculus yield similar results to the reimplantation alone. Additionally, mononuclear cells added to the fibrin glue increased neurotrophic factor gene transcript levels in the spinal cord ventral horn. Regarding the motor recovery, evaluated by the functional peroneal index, as well as the paw print pressure, cell treated rats performed equally well as compared to reimplanted only animals, and significantly better than the avulsion only subjects. The results herein demonstrate that mononuclear cells therapy is neuroprotective by increasing levels of brain derived neurotrophic factor (BDNF) and glial derived neurotrophic factor (GDNF). Moreover, the use of fibrin sealant mononuclear cells delivery approach gave the best and more long lasting results.

Editor: Graca Almeida-Porada, Wake Forest Institute for Regenerative Medicine, United States of America

Funding: The present work was supported by a grant from Fundação de Amparo a Pesquisa do Estado de São Paulo – FAPESP, Brazil (2010/0986-5). Barbizan R. was supported by Fundação de Amparo a Pesquisa do Estado de Sao Paulo – FAPESP (process number: 2010/00729-2). This work was funded by grants from Coordenação de Aperfeiçoamento de Pessoal de Nível Superior (CAPES), Conselho Nacional de Desenvolvimento Científico e Tecnológico (CNPq) and Fundação de Amparo à Pesquisa do Estado de São Paulo (FAPESP). The funders had no role in study design, data collection and analysis, decision to publish, or preparation of the manuscript.

Competing Interests: The authors have declared that no competing interests exist.

* Email: alroliv@unicamp.br

Introduction

In order to enhance the success of adult stem cell (SC) translational medicine efforts, the source as well as the most effective delivery method has to be considered. The bone marrow contains endothelial progenitor cells and mononuclear cells (MC). The MC fraction corresponds to the totality of hematopoietic and mesenchymal stem cells. MC present clinical advantages over other stem cells, based on the minimally invasive harvesting procedures, which are fast and cost-effective. Also, the possibility of autografting avoids the use of immunosuppressants, present low oncogenic potential and does not raise ethical issues [1] as compared to other SC. Moreover, MCs have similar potential therapeutic outcome for nerve regeneration in comparison to mesenchymal cells [2]. The peripheral nerve regeneration after MC has been connected to the local production of neurotrophic factors [1,3,4]. Relevantly, stem cell therapy may also present an immunomodulatory effect, reducing pro-inflammatory events as well as glial reaction following lesion.

Ventral root avulsion in rats has been used as a model for brachial plexus lesion (BPL). BPL is frequently caused by motorbike accidents in young adults as well as following complicated child-birth delivery [5]. It causes paralysis in the corresponding muscle groups and loss of sensory functions [6]. The degenerative impact on motoneurons is well characterized and is potentiated by pulling out the ventral roots from the CNS/PNS interface at the spinal cord surface [6]. Similarly to BPL, VRA results in extensive loss of neurons in the first weeks after injury [7,8].

Reimplantation of avulsed roots can rescue motoneurons from degeneration, increasing the regenerative capacity of axonal regrowth [9,10]. As a result, anatomical and functional reinnervation of denervated muscles can be obtained [11–13]. As seen in a previous work [10], a snake venom derived fibrin sealant allowed successful and stable ventral root implantation. Nevertheless, additional therapeutic approaches need to be developed, since root reimplantation alone, although neuroprotective, results in insufficient functional sensory-motor recovery [12,14–16].

In order to improve the outcome following VRA, regarding neuronal survival, several attempts have been made to provide neurotrophic molecules at the site of injury. In this regard, the association of the root reimplantation with BDNF and CNTF resulted in rescue of injured motoneurons after avulsion in rabbits [17]. Therefore, the use of neurotrophic factors in combination with root reimplantation is a potential therapy to be used in patients.

The use of recombinant neurotrophic factors, however, present important drawbacks. One of them is the need of relatively large amounts of the purified substance, to reach the target lesioned area. Due to the short biological activity window of such substances, there is also need of constant perfusion, what may contribute to infection and further lesion of the affected spinal cord area. Additionally, it is improbable that a single neurothrophic molecule will be sufficient to provide the necessary conditions for optimal regeneration.

Based on such facts, the advent of stem cell technology brought new insights on cell therapy and local delivery of trophic substances. To date, however, there is not sufficient data on the delivery method to the nervous system, especially following VRA. So far, it is known that mesenchymal stem cells synthesize and possibly release BDNF and GDNF, when grafted to the VRA lesion area [18]. No data, however, indicates that MC exhibit the same properties.

Therefore, the present study investigated two delivery strategies of MC, comparing the local injection to the spinal cord with the possibility of mixing MC with fibrin sealant on the interface of the CNS/PNS. Local production of BDNF and GDNF were evaluated in both situations.

The results herein demonstrate that MC therapy is neroprotective and increases the transcript and protein levels of BDNF and GDNF in the lesioned spinal cord area. Moreover, the administration method significantly influenced treatment outcome, so that the use of fibrin sealant MC delivery approach gave the best and more long lasting results.

Material and Methods

2.1- Experimental animals

Adult female Lewis (LEW/HsdUnib) rats, 7 weeks old, were obtained from the Multidisciplinary Center for Biological Investigation (CEMIB/UNICAMP) and housed under a 12-hour light/dark cycle with free access to food and water. The study was approved by the Institutional Committee for Ethics in Animal Experimentation (Committee for Ethics in Animal Use – Institute of Biology - CEUA/IB/UNICAMP, proc. n° 2073-1). All experiments were performed in accordance with the guidelines of the Brazilian College for Animal Experimentation. The animals were subjected to unilateral avulsion of the L4-L6 lumbar ventral roots and divided into 4 groups: 1) VRA without reimplantation (AV 1 week, n = 5; AV 4 weeks, n = 15 and AV 8 weeks, n = 10); 2) VRA followed by lesioned roots reimplantation with fibrin sealant (AV+S 1 week n = 5, AV+S 4 weeks, n = 15 and AV+S 8 weeks, n = 10); 3) VRA followed by lesioned roots reimplantation with fibrin sealant and MC homogenized to the sealant (AV+S+HC 1 week, n = 5, AV+S+HC 4 weeks, n = 15 and AV+S+HC 8 weeks, n = 10) and 4) VRA followed by lesioned roots reimplantation with fibrin sealant and injection of MC (AV+S+IC 4 weeks, n = 15 and AV+S+IC 8 weeks, n = 10).

The peroneal functional index was calculated weekly up to 8 weeks after injury (n = 10 for each group). Animals were killed 1 week and 4 weeks after injury and their lumbar spinal cords were processed for PCR (n = 5 for each group). The animals were killed after 4 and 8 weeks after avulsion and the lumbar spinal cords were processed for immunohistochemistry (n = 5 for each group) and neuronal survival counting (n = 5 for each group). Each animal's unlesioned, contralateral spinal cord side, served as an internal control.

2.2- Bone Marrow Mononuclear Cells Extraction

MC were extracted from transgenic Lewis rats (LEW-Tg EGFP F455/Rrrc), with the EGFP (Enhanced green fluorescent protein) gene under Ubiquitin C promoter control. The animals were imported from Missouri University (EUA) and were provided by Dr. Alfredo Miranda Góes, Federal University of Minas Gerais – UFMG, Brazil.

The EGFP rats were killed with lethal dose of halothane (Tanohalo, Cristália Chemicals and Pharmaceuticals, Brazil), and the femur and tibia were dissected out from the muscular and connective tissue. The cells were isolated by density gradient centrifugation using Histopaque 1077 following the separation of mononuclear cells methods of Sigma-Aldrich n° 1119 protocol. The cell suspension consists of heterogeneous cell populations (13.2% CD11b, 1.52% CD3, 92.2% CD45, 20.8% CD34 of CD45). After 2 washing steps, cells were immediately transplanted.

2.3- Ventral root avulsion (VRA)

The rats were anesthetized with 50 mg/Kg of Ketamine (Fort Dodge) and 10 mg/Kg of xylasine (Köning) and subjected to unilateral avulsion of the lumbar ventral roots as previously described [19]. Right side avulsion was performed at the L4, L5 and L6 lumbar ventral root after laminectomy. A longitudinal incision was made to open the dural sac, the denticulate ligament was dissected and the ventral roots associated with the lumbar intumescence could be identified and avulsed with fine forceps (No 4). Finally, the musculature, fascia and skin were sutured in layers. Chlorhydrate of tramadol was administered by gavage after the surgical procedures (20 mg/kg) and 2.5 mg/day soluble in water during 5 days.

2.4- Reimplantation of the motor roots

In AV+S, AV+S+MC and AV+S+IC groups, the roots were replaced at the exact point of detachment, on the ventral surface of the lumbar spinal cord at the avulsion site with the aid of a snake venom fibrin sealant [10]. The fibrin sealant was kindly provided by CEVAP/UNESP and is under the scope of the Brazilian Patents BR 10 2014 011432 7 and BR 10 2014 011436 0 [20–22]. The sealant used herein is composed of three separate solutions (1-fibrinogen, 2-calcium chloride and 3-thrombin-like fraction). During surgical repair of the avulsed roots, the first two components were applied and the avulsed roots were returned to their original sites. The third component was then added for polymerization. The reimplanted roots were then gently pulled from the spinal cord, and the stability of the fixation was observed to evaluate the success of the repair.

2.5- Mononuclear cells transplantation

In group 3 (AV+S+HC), 3×10^5 MCs were added to the fibrin sealant in avulsed roots reimplantation at the moment of implantation. In this case, the cells are grouped in the right ventrolateral surface of the spinal cord (Figure 1 A and B). In group 4, 3×10^5 MCs were placed directly into the lateral funiculus on the lesioned side (ipsilateral) in the segments L4–L6 of the spinal cord with the aid of a thick capillary Pasteur pipette coupled to a Hamilton syringe and then the avulsed roots were repaired with sealant. In this group, the cells are at the site of injection (Figure 1 C and D).

2.6- Specimen preparation

The animals were anaesthetized with an overdose of mixture of xylasine and Ketamine, and the vascular system was transcardially perfused with phosphate buffer 0.1 M (pH 7.4). For PCR, the rats

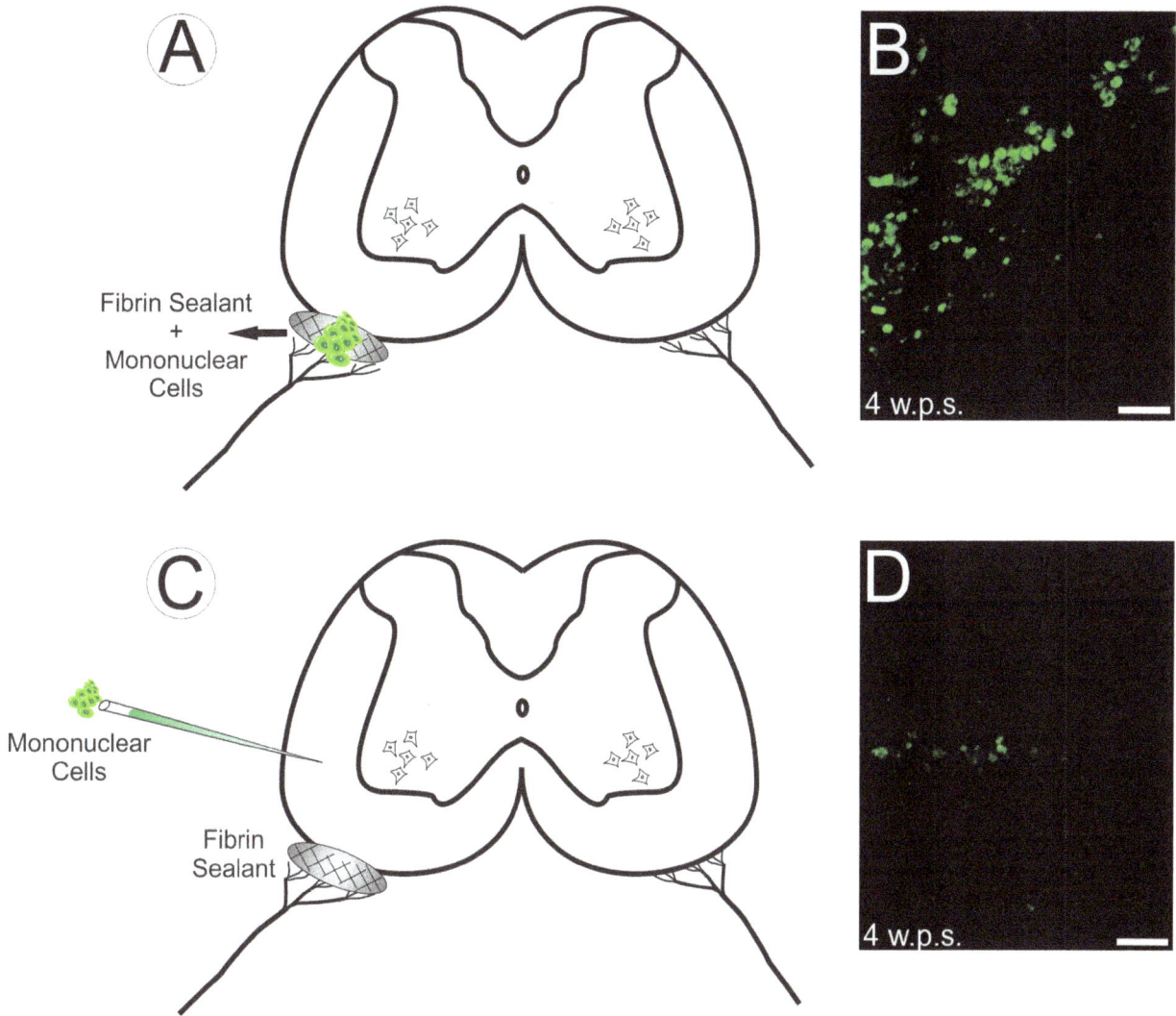

Figure 1. Scheme of the spinal cord subjected to motor root avulsion and reimplantation, with the two different cell delivery locations. A) Scheme of transverse spinal cord section subjected to motor avulsion followed by fibrin sealant reimplantation plus MC. B) MC are grouped in the right ventrolateral surface of the spinal cord (AV+S+HC), four weeks post surgery (4 w.p.s.). C) Scheme of the transverse spinal cord section subjected to motor root avulsion followed by fibrin sealant reimplantation and cell injection in the lateral funiculus. D) The cells are at the site of injection (AV+S+IC), 4 w.p.s. Such cells were E-GFP fluorescent donors. Scale bar = 50 μm.

were killed 1 and 4 weeks after VRA and their lumbar intumescences were frozen in liquid nitrogen. For neuron survival counting and immunohistochemistry the rats were killed 4 and 8 weeks after VRA and fixed by vascular perfusion of 10% formaldehyde in phosphate buffer (pH 7.4). The lumbar intumescence was dissected, post-fixed overnight and then washed in phosphate buffer and stored overnight in sucrose 20% before freezing. Transverse cryostat 12 μm thick sections of spinal cords were obtained and transferred to gelatin-coated slides and dried at room temperature for 30 min before being stored at −20°C.

2.7- Counting of motoneurons survival

Cell counts were performed on sections from the lumbar enlargement. Transverse cryostat sections of the spinal cords were stained for 3 min in aqueous 1% cresyl fast violet solution (Sigma-Aldrich, USA). The sections were then washed in distilled water, dehydrated and mounted with Entellan (Merck, USA). The motoneurons were identified (based on their morphology, size, and location in the dorsolateral lamina IX) and cells with a visible nucleus and nucleolus were counted. The absolute number of motoneurons on the lesioned and non-lesioned side of each section was used to calculate the percentage of surviving cells in each specimen. This percentage was calculated by dividing the number of motoneurons in the ipsilateral (lesioned) side by the number of neurons in the contralateral (non-lesioned) side and multiplying the result by 100. Abercrombie's formula was used to correct for the duplicate counting of neurons [23].

$$N = nt/(t+d)$$

where N is the corrected number of counted neurons, n is the counted number of cells, t is the thickness of the sections (12 μm) and d is the average diameter of the cells. Because differences in cell size can significantly affect cell counts, the value of d was calculated specifically for each experimental group and for both ipsilateral and contralateral neurons. The diameters of 15 randomly chosen neurons from each group were measured by using the ImageTool software (version 3.00, The University of Texas Health Science Center, San Antonio, USA).

2.8- Immunohistochemistry

Transverse sections of spinal cord were incubated with mouse anti-synaptophysin (Dako, 1:250), goat anti-GFAP (Dako, 1:900), and rabbit anti-Iba1 (Wako, 1:800) diluted in a solution containing 1% BSA in TBS-T (Tris-Buffered Saline and Tween) and 2% Triton X-100 in PB 0.1 M (phosphate buffer). All sections were incubated for 6 hours at room temperature in a moist chamber. After rinsing in TBS-T, the sections were incubated according to the primary host antibody (CY-3, Jackson Immunoresearch; 1:250) for 45 minutes in a moist chamber at room temperature. After 3 times washing in TBS-T, the slides were mounted in a mixture of glycerol/PBS (3:1) and observed with a Nikon eclipse TS100 inverted microscope (Nikon, Japan). For quantitative measurements, 3 representative images (with 2 MNs) of the spinal cord (L4–L6 at lamina IX, ventral horn) from each animal were captured at a final magnification of ×200. Double blind quantification was performed in IMAGEJ software (version 1.33 u, National Institute of Health, USA) using the enhanced contrast and density slicing two features [24]. The integrated density of pixels was systematically measured in six representative areas of the motor nucleus from each section, according to [19]. The integrated pixel density was calculated for each section of spinal cord, and then a mean value for each spinal cord was calculated. The data are represented as the mean ± standard error (SE).

2.9- Real time polymerase chain reaction (PCR)

Total RNA was extracted from the ipsilateral and contralateral sides of the frozen lumbar intumescences, 1 and 4 weeks after lesion, using the RNeasy Lipid Tissue Kit (cat n° 74804, Quiagen), according to the manufacturer's recommendations. The RNA was quantified using a NanoDrop Spectrophotometer (A260/280; model 2000, Thermo Scientific). The RNA (1 μg) obtained from five samples was reverse-transcribed using a commercial kit (AffinityScripts QPCR cDNA Synthesis Kit - Agilent Technologies, La Jolla, CA, USA) to achieve a final reaction volume of 20 μL. Real time quantitative PCR was performed on Mx3005P qPCR System (Agilent Technologies, La Jolla, CA, USA), after an initial denaturation for 10 minutes at 95°C, followed by 35 cycles of amplification (95°C for 30 seconds followed by 72°C for one minute). The reactions were carried out with 12.5 μL 2×SYBR Green PCR master mix (Agilent Technologies), 0.2 μM of each forward and reverse primer 100 ng cDNA template, in a final reaction volume of 20 μL. All quantifications were normalized to the house keeping gene β-actin. A non-template control with non-genetic material was included to eliminate contamination or nonspecific reactions. Each sample (n = 5) was tested in triplicate and then used for the analysis of the relative transcription data using the $2^{-\Delta\Delta CT}$ method [25]. The following forward (F) and reverse (R) primers were used: BDNF: (F) 5'-CCACAATGTTC-CACCAGGTG-3', (R) 5'-TGGGCGCAGCCTTCAT-3'; GDNF: (F) 5'-CCACCATCAAAAGACTGAAAAG-3', (R) 5'-CGGTTCCTCTCTCTTCGAGGA-3'; Iba-1 (F) 5'- CCC-CACCTAAGGCCACCAGC-3', (R) 5'-TCCTGTTGGCTTT-CAGCAGTCC-3'; GFAP (F) 5'-TGCTGGAGGGCGAA-GAAAACCG-3' 5'-CCAGGCTGGTTTCTCGGATCTGG-3'; β-actin (F) 5'-GGAGATTACTGCCCTGGCTCCTA-3' (R) 5'-GACTCAICGTACTCCTGCTTGCTG-3'. The BDNF and GDNF were based on [18] and the β-actin was based on [26].

2.10- Functional Analysis

For the gait recovery analysis, the CatWalk system (Noldus Inc., The Netherlands; was used. In this set up, the animal crosses a walkway with an illuminated glass floor. A high-speed video camera Gevicam (GP-3360, USA) equipped with a wide-angle lens (8.5 mm, Fujicon Corp., China) is positioned underneath the walkway and the paw prints are automatically recorded and classified by the software. The paw prints from each animal were obtained before and after the VRA. Post-operative CatWalk data were collected twice a week for 12 weeks. The peroneal functional index (PFI) was calculated as the distance between the third toe and hind limb pads (print length) and the distance between the first and fifth toes (print width). Measurements of these parameters were obtained from the right (lesioned) and left (unlesioned) paw prints, and the values were calculated using the following formula [27].

$$PFI = 174.9 \, x \, ((EPL - NPL)/NPL)) + 80.3x \, ((ETS - NTS)/NTS)) - 13.4$$

Where N: normal, or non-operated side; E: experimental, or operated; PL: print length; TS: total toe spread, or distance between first to fifth toe.

The pressure exerted on the platform by individual paws was also evaluated. The Catwalk data from each day were expressed as an ipsi-/contralateral ratio.

2.11- Statistical analysis

Statistical analysis was performed with Graphpad Prisma 4.0 software. The neuronal survival, immunohistochemistry, and PCR were firstly evaluated with one-way ANOVA. Data from the functional analysis was evaluated with two-way ANOVA. Bonferroni post-test was used to identify intergroup differences. The data are presented as the mean ± SE and the differences between groups were considered significant when the P-value was <0.05 (*), <0.01 (**) and <0.001 (***).

Results

3.1- Neuroprotection after root reimplantation plus MC treatment after VRA

Neuronal survival was assessed as the ipsi-/contralateral ratio of motoneurons present in the lamina IX of the ventral horn. No significant differences between the numbers of motoneurons on the contralateral side in the different experimental conditions were observed. After four weeks, there was severe degeneration of affected motorneurons in the AV group (Fig. 2A). In implanted groups (Fig 2 C, E and G) a higher number of surviving neurons was observed. Such neuroprotection was even more evident in the AV+S+HC group (Fig. 2I) (AV 36.09%±3.67%; AV+S 65.19%±6.93%; AV+S+HC 89.44%±1.89%; AV+S+IC 64.60%±1.33% percentage of survival ipsi-/contralateral ± SEM; p<0.001).

Neuroprotection in the implanted groups remained superior to the avulsion only throughout the time course of the study, i.e. up to 8 weeks post lesion (Fig. 2 D, E and F). Nevertheless, the AV+S+HC group was similar to AV+S. Figure 2I shows the ipsi-/contralateral ratio for the groups where a statistically significant neuroprotective effect was observed (AV 34.58%±4.12%; AV+S 66.46%±3.88%; AV+S+HC 67.11%±4.83%; AV+S+IC 46.81%±5.87% percentage of survival ipsi-/contralateral ± SEM; p<0.001).

Neuronal Counting

Figure 2. Nissl-stained spinal cord transverse sections at lamina IX illustrating the neuroprotective effects of root reimplantation and MC treatment on motoneurons 4 and 8 weeks after VRA. Motoneuron cell bodies of the ipsilateral side of VRA after 4 weeks (A, C, E and G) and after 8 weeks (B, D, F and H). (A and B) AV, (C and D) AV+S, (E and F) AV+S+HC and (G and H) AV+S+IC. Scale bar = 50 μm. (I) Percentage of neuronal survival after ventral root avulsion, reimplantation and reimplantantion with MC. Note a significant rescue of lesioned neurons in the implanted groups with and without cells in two different survival times (4 and 8 weeks). This neuroprotection was even more intense in AV+S+HC 4 weeks after avulsion. (†† p<0.01 and ††† p<0.001 comparing all groups 4 weeks after avulsion, § p<0.05, §§ p<0.01 and §§§ p<0.001 comparing all groups 8 weeks after AV and *p<0.05 comparing AV+S+HC at two different times after avulsion, n = 5).

3.2- Decreased synaptic elimination after VRA followed by implantation and cell treatment

Synaptic network changes after root avulsion were evaluated in the ventral horn by immunohistochemistry with an antibody against synaptophysin. Quantitative measurements of synaptophysin immunoreactivity in the sciatic motor nuclei after avulsion (AV) and after avulsion followed by ventral root implantation (AV+S), implantation with cells homogenized on the sealant (AV+S+HC) and implantation with cell injection (AV+S+IC) were carried out. As shown in Fig. 3, AV only led to a significant decrease in synaptophysin expression four weeks after avulsion, which remained until 8 weeks. Such results indicate a significant decrease of complexity of intraspinal networks following lesion. In contrast, in implanted groups with or without cells, the repair resulted in preservation of synaptophysin immunoreactivity, in the immediate vicinity of the motoneurons. In AV+S+IC group the synaptic inputs decreased when comparing 4 and 8 weeks. Four weeks after avulsion: (AV 0.43±0.01; AV+S 0.66±0.09; AV+S+HC 0.65±0.07; AV+S+IC 0.60±0.01 mean ratio ipsi-/contralateral ± SE with p<0.01) and 8 weeks after avulsion: (AV 0.40±0.05; AV+S 0.72±0.05; AV+S+HC 0.84±0.07; AV+S+IC 0.855±0.03 mean ratio ipsi-/contralateral ± SE, p<0.05).

3.3- Astroglial reactivity is not further enhanced by mononuclear cells around motoneuron vicinity

Immunoreactivity against GFAP was used to analyze the degree of astroglial reactivity after lesion. This demonstrates the presence of GFAP-positive astrocytic processes in the vicinity of the avulsed motoneurons. Figure 4 shows that the astroglial reactivity was not significantly further increased after implantation and cell treatment in both experimental times: Four weeks after avulsion (AV 2.65±0.48; AV+S 2.49±0.60; AV+S+HC 2.62±0.43; AV+S+IC 2.17±0.12 mean ratio ipsi-/contralateral ± SE); eight weeks after avulsion (AV 3.45±0.61; AV+S 2.09±0.26; AV+S+HC 2.58±0.37; AV+S+IC 2.30±0.32 mean ratio ipsi-/contralateral ± SE).

The real-time PCR analysis was performed to measure GFAPmRNA in the RNA in all ventral horn after avulsion. Figure 4 demonstrated that the levels of GFAPmRNA were similar in all groups, 1 week (Fig 4 J) after lesion (AV 1.51±0.38; AV+S 1.20±0.24; AV+S+HC 1.65±0.26 mean ratio ipsi-/contralateral ± SE). However, 4 weeks (Fig 4 K) after avulsion, AV+S group presented a decreased number of transcripts to GFAP (AV 2.64±0.45; AV+S 1.35±0.14; AV+S+HC 2.11±0.12; AV+S+IC 2.00±0.12 mean ratio ipsi-/contralateral ± SE).

3.4- Microglial reactivity is enhanced by mononuclear cells one week after tranplantation

To detect possible changes in the microglial cells close to large motoneurons cell bodies after avulsion, the immunoreactivity against Iba-1 was evaluated in the ventral horn in the different experimental groups. Figure 5 shows that the microglial reactivity was not significantly further increased after implantation and cell treatment in both experimental times. However, the AV+S and

AV+S+IC groups showed decreased microglia reaction in the course of experimental time. Four weeks after avulsion: (AV 4.71±0.41; AV+S 4.73±0.94; AV+S+HC 3.02±0.64; AV+S+IC 5.67±1.34; mean ratio ipsi-/contralateral ±SE with p<0.01) and 8 weeks after avulsion: (AV 2.70±0.51; AV+S 2.18±0.57; AV+S+HC 2.32±0.59; AV+S+IC 2.25±0.35 mean ratio ipsi-/contralateral ± SE, p<0.05).

The real-time PCR analysis was performed to measure Iba-1 mRNA in the in ventral horn RNA after avulsion. Figure 5 demonstrated that the levels of Iba-1 mRNA in AV+S+HC were significantly greater than in the AV and AV+S groups (AV 0.95±0.30; AV+S 1.63±0.60; AV+S+HC 4.15±0.48 mean ratio ipsi-/contralateral ± SE). Nevertheless, 4 weeks (Fig 5 K) after avulsion, Iba-1 mRNA were similar in all groups (AV 2.07±0.26; AV+S 1.07±0.18; AV+S+HC 1.64±0.26; AV+S+IC 1.73±0.03 mean ratio ipsi-/contralateral ± SE).

3.5- Mononuclear cells enhance BDNF and GDNF expression one week after avulsion

Real time PCR was used to detect BDNF and GDNF mRNAs in the lumbar spinal cord after avulsion (Figure 6). The results demonstrated the levels of both neurotrophic factors in the AV+S+HC group were significantly greater, when compared to the other groups, one week after surgery (A and C) (BDNF - AV 1.20±0.29; AV+S 1.33±0.18; AV+S+HC 2.48±0.10 mean ratio ipsi-/contralateral ± SE *p<0.05) and (GDNF - AV 1.71±0.56; AV+S 1.24±0.23; AV+S+HC 2.86±0.34; mean ratio ipsi-/contralateral ± SE *p<0.05). Four weeks after avulsion, BDNF and GDNF mRNA levels were similar in all groups (B and D) (BDNF - AV 2.04±0.18; AV+S 1.45±0.35; AV+S+HC 1.53±0.16; AV+S+IC 1.70±0.17 mean ratio ipsi-/contralateral ± SE) and (GDNF - AV 2.25±0.10; AV+S 1.92±0.43; AV+S+HC 1.72±0.30; AV+S+IC 1.77±0.01 mean ratio ipsi-/contralateral ± SE).

3.6- Functional motor recovery

The recovery of motor function was analysed by the CatWalk System. Post-operative assessments of peroneal function were performed for eight consecutive weeks. The preoperative peroneal functional index mean values (Figure 7A) did not significantly differ between groups. The peroneal functional index drastically declined after avulsion. The three implanted groups presented significantly better peroneal index performance as compared to AV group (AV −228.89±23.0; AV+S −139.75±12.5; AV+S+HC −155.50±17.2; AV+S+IC −205.14±18.6, mean ratio ipsi-/contralateral ± SE, *p<0.05, **p<0.01 and ***p<0.001. These results are consistent with the footprint paw pressure data (Figure 7B), indicating that all three implanted groups presented a better performance as compared to avulsion group (AV 0.20±0.07; AV+S 0.81±0.09726454; AV+S+HC 0.66±0.078; AV+S+IC 0.40±0.11 mean ratio ipsi-/contralateral ± SE with *p<0.05 and ***p<0.001).

Synaptophysin

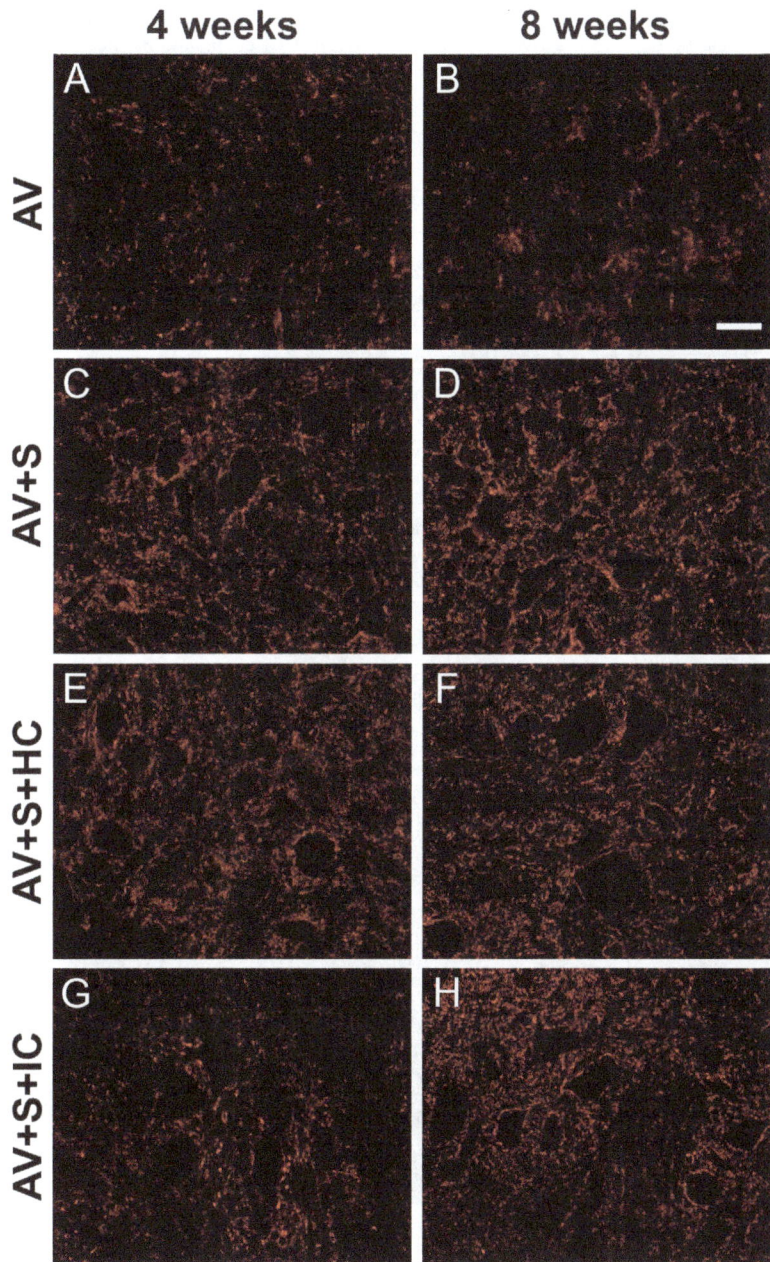

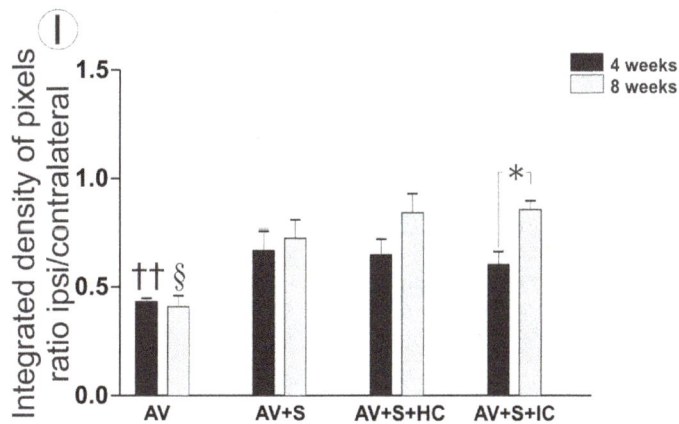

Figure 3. Immunohistochemical analysis of the spinal cord ventral horn stained with anti-synaptophysin 4 and 8 weeks after VRA. Observe the preservation of synaptophysin labeling, especially at the surface of the lesioned motoneurons in implanted group and both implanted with mononuclear cells treatment. After 4 weeks post lesion (A, C, E and G) and after 8 weeks (B, D, F and H). (A and B) AV, (C and D) AV+S, (E and F) AV+S+HC and (G and H) AV+S+IC. Scale bar =50 µm. (I) Quantification of synaptic covering obtained by the ratio ipsi/contralateral sides of the integrated density of pixels at lamina IX four and eight weeks after injury. (†† $p<0.01$ comparing all groups 4 weeks after avulsion, § $p<0.05$ comparing all groups 8 weeks after AV and * $p<0.05$ comparing AV+S+IC at two different times after avulsion, n = 5).

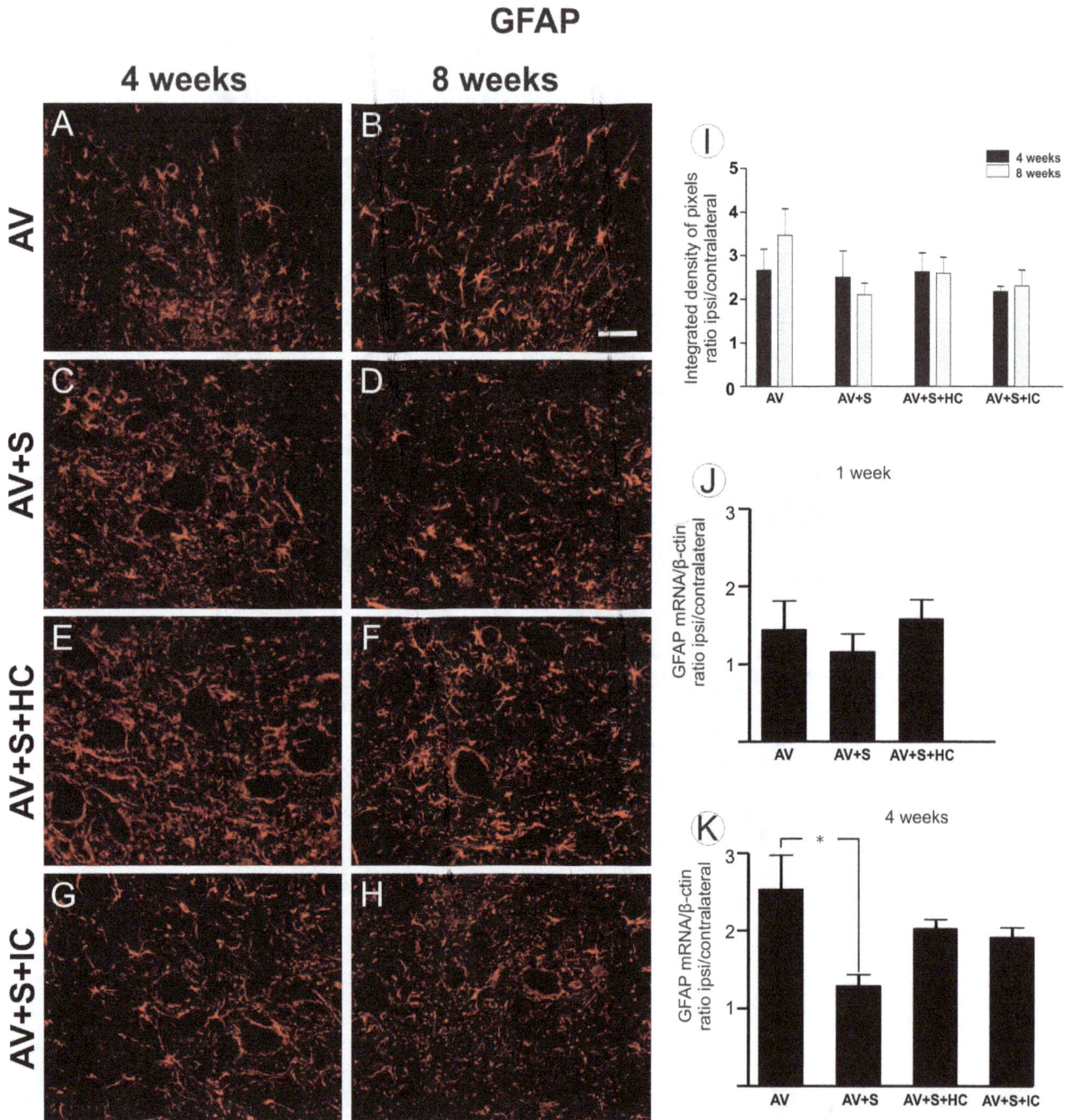

Figure 4. Glial fibrillary acidic protein (GFAP) in the spinal cord ventral horn. Immunohistochemical analysis of the anterior horn of the spinal cord was labeled with anti-GFAP, 4 and 8 weeks after injury to assess the degree of astroglial reactivity after root avulsion (A–H). Representative images of AV, AV+S, AV+S+HC and AV+S+IC. Scale bar =50 µm. Observe that ventral root implantation and cell treatment did not increase astroglial reaction. (I) The mean ratio of the ipsi-/contralateral integrated intensity of pixels of the ipsilateral and contralateral sides in all groups. (* $p<0.05$, n = 5). (J) One week after avulsion, there were no differences between groups by GFAPmRNA analysis. (K) The RT-qPCR performed 4 weeks after avulsion demonstrated significant decrease in the synthesis of GFAP mRNA in AV+S group compared with AV (*$p<0.05$, n = 5).

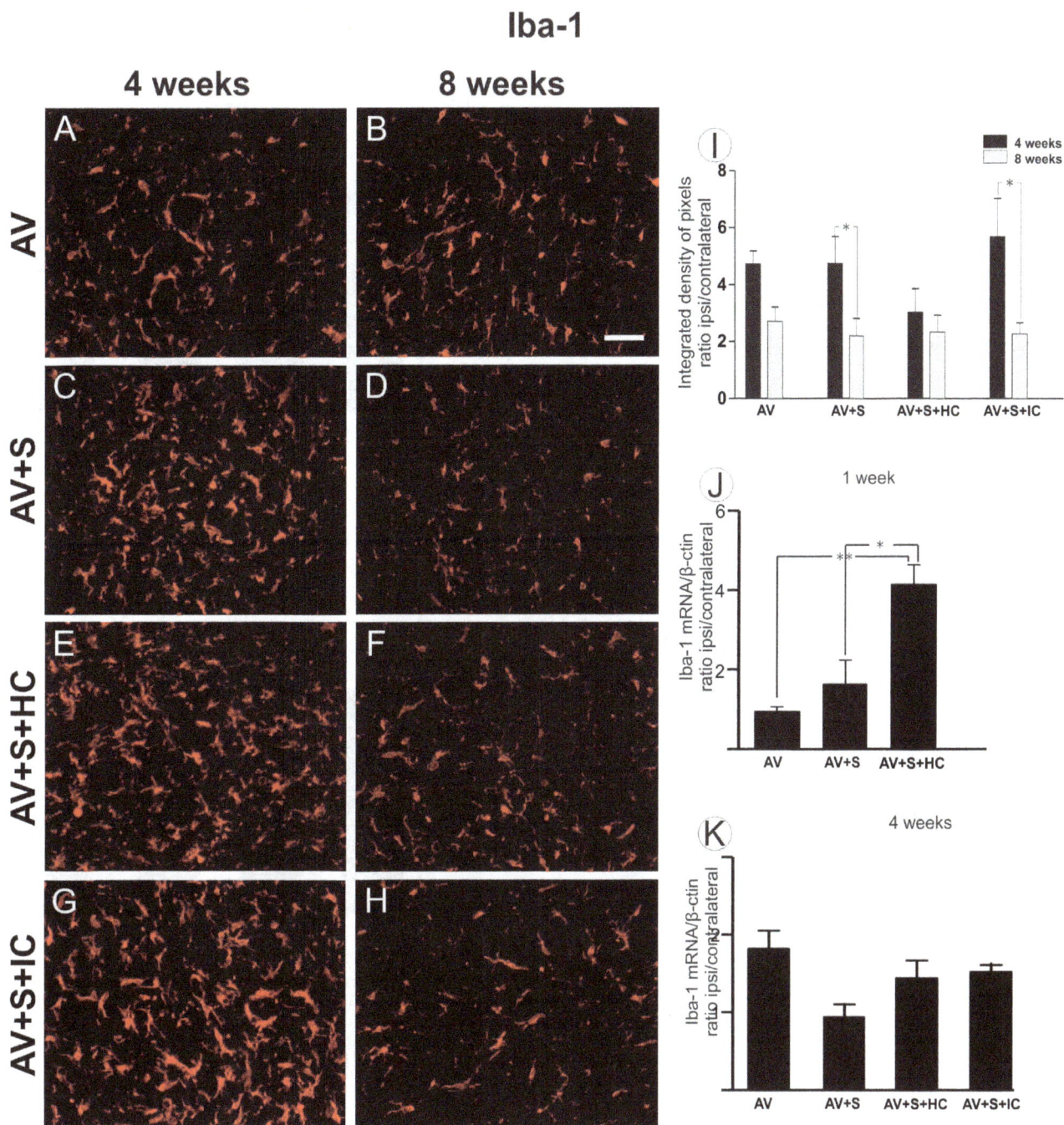

Figure 5. Microglial analysis of the spinal cord ventral horn 4 and 8 weeks after VRA. The quantification analysis on motoneuron cell bodies stained with anti- Iba1 of the ipsilateral side of VRA after 4 weeks (A, C, E and G) and after 8 weeks (B, D, F and H). (A and B) AV, (C and D) AV+S, (E and F) AV+S+HC and (G and H) AV+S+IC. Scale bar =50 μm. (I) The mean ratio of the ipsil-/contralateral integrated intensity of pixels of the ipsilateral and contralateral sides in both groups. Note the decrease in microglial reactivity in AV+S and AV+S+IC as compared 4 and 8 weeks after injury. (J) There were significant increase in the synthesis of Iba-1 mRNA in the lumbar spinal cord one week after avulsion (*p<0.05 and **p<0.01, n=5). (K) The RT-qPCR, performed 4 weeks after avulsion, did not demonstrate significant differences between groups in Iba-1 mRNA.

Discussion

Brachial plexus lesions are particularly debilitating and usually affect young adults. To date, new technological refinements aiming at improving the repair of such traumatic injury are necessary. Although nerve reimplantation has been proposed [7,10] the relatively poor clinical outcome requires further attention. Treatment with neurotrophic factors, following root reimplantation, has proven to be efficient [17]. Importantly, it has been previously shown that mesenchymal stem cells naturally produce BDNF and GDNF when grafted to the VRA lesion area [18]. Considering it, the present study main objective was to compare the root reimplantation regenerative outcome by either injecting or engrafting the mononuclear cells at the wounded area,

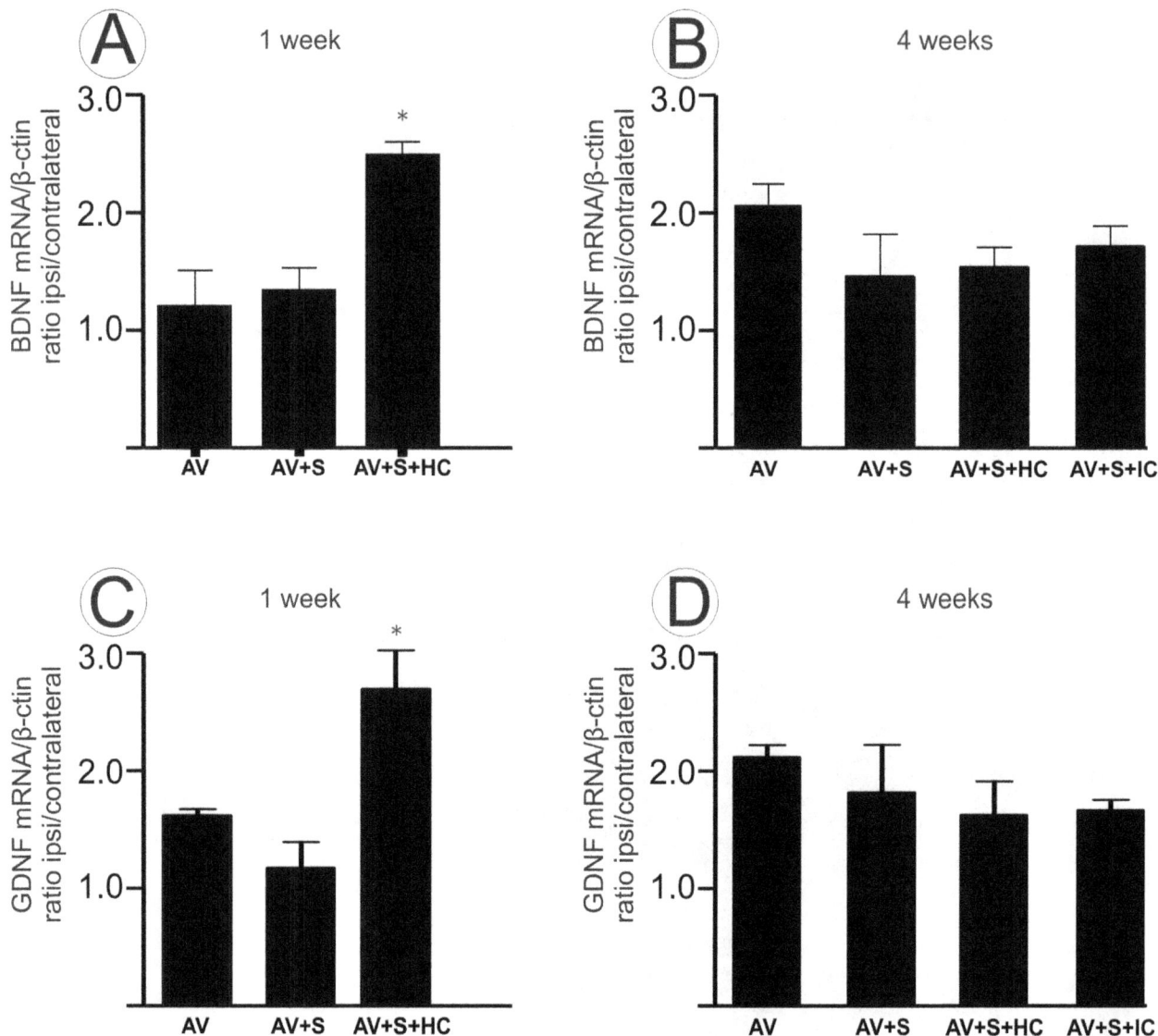

Figure 6. Neurotrophic factor expression (BDNF and GDNF) by RT-qPCR in the ventral horn spinal cord 1 and 4 weeks after avulsion. Expression of mean ratio of the ipsi-/contralateral mRNA for BDNF obtained by RT-qPCR in the lumbar spinal cord one (A) and four (B) weeks after avulsion. Note that one week after avulsion AV+S+HC enhanced the BDNF mRNA production compared to others groups (*p<0.05, n=5). Expression of mean ratio of the ipsi-/contralateral mRNA for GDNF obtained by RT-qPCR in the lumbar spinal cord one (C) and four (D) weeks after avulsion. Note that, one week after avulsion in the AV+S+HC group, there is enhanced GDNF mRNA production as compared to others groups (*p< 0.05, n=5).

with aid of a fibrin sealant scaffold. However, evaluating the perspective of translational studies, the use of bone marrow MC has been preferred instead of mesenchymal stem cells.

The use of MC resulted in neuroprotection following peripheral nervous system lesion [1,3] and following spinal cord injury [28]. Furthermore, the mononuclear fraction is easy to obtain, implicating in lower costs and less processing time, as compared with other cell types [1,29].

An important point to be observed is the best moment for performing the cell therapy. Therefore, in some instances, it has been proposed a late cell transplantation, following the acute phase after injury [30]. However, immediate cell engrafting increases the survival of motoneurons after root avulsion [17].

Based on such observations, the present work was based on cells treatment immediately after avulsion, in order to obtain the best

neuroprotective results possible. This is particularly important following CNS/PNS injuries that cause extensive degeneration of adult motoneurons [31–33]. Such neuronal loss reaches up to 80% of motoneuron degeneration in the first two weeks post injury [7]. Our results showed that both intraspinal administration and fibrin sealant implantation of MC preserved a significant number of motoneurons when compared to the untreated group (avulsion). The neuroprotective effect observed herein reinforces that the combination of root reimplantatio and cell therapy leads to enhancement of axotomized motoneurons. On the contrary, most of the motoneurons degenerated following AV, which reinforces the need of acute neuroprotective treatments following VRA.

Neuronal rescue was highest following root reimplantation and fibrin sealant cell engrafting, 4 weeks after injury. Such effect may be the result of stem cell neurotrophic factor release in the site of

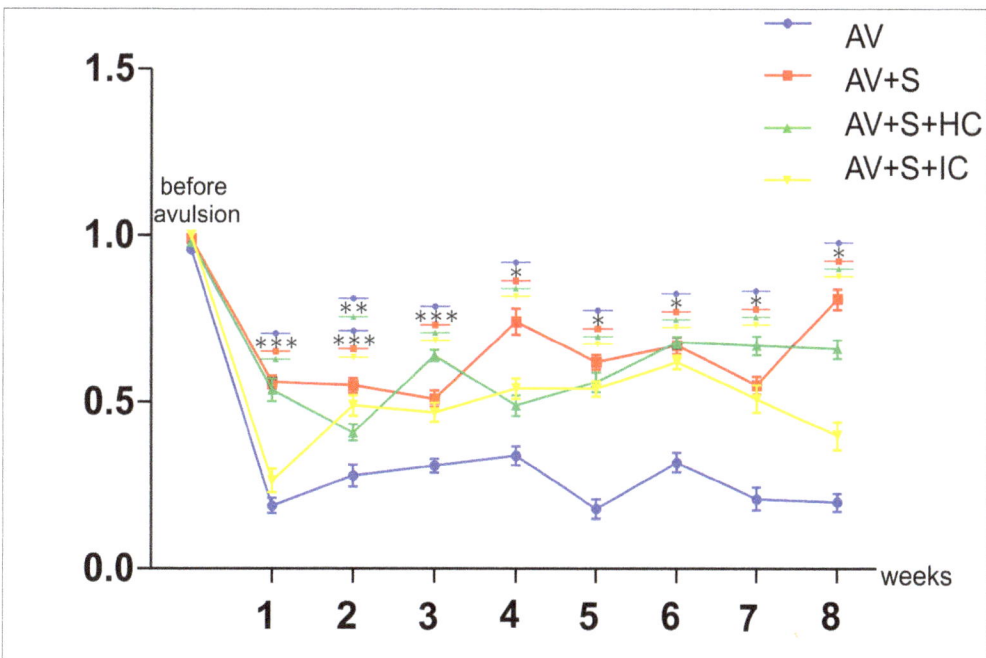

Figure 7. Motor function recovery after ventral root treatment. (A) Graph of the peroneal nerve functional index up to 8 weeks after avulsion. There is a significantly better performance of the three implanted groups compared to AV from the first week post lesion until the eighth week (***p<0.001, **p<0.01 and *p<0.05 n=10). (B) Restoration of weight-bearing capacity following avulsion. There is also a restoration of weight-bearing capacity following avulsion in implanted groups with or without cells from the first up to the eight week after injury. Values are expressed as the ratio of ipsi-/contralateral pressure exerted by the paw on the catwalk platform (***p<0.001 and *p<0.05, n=10).

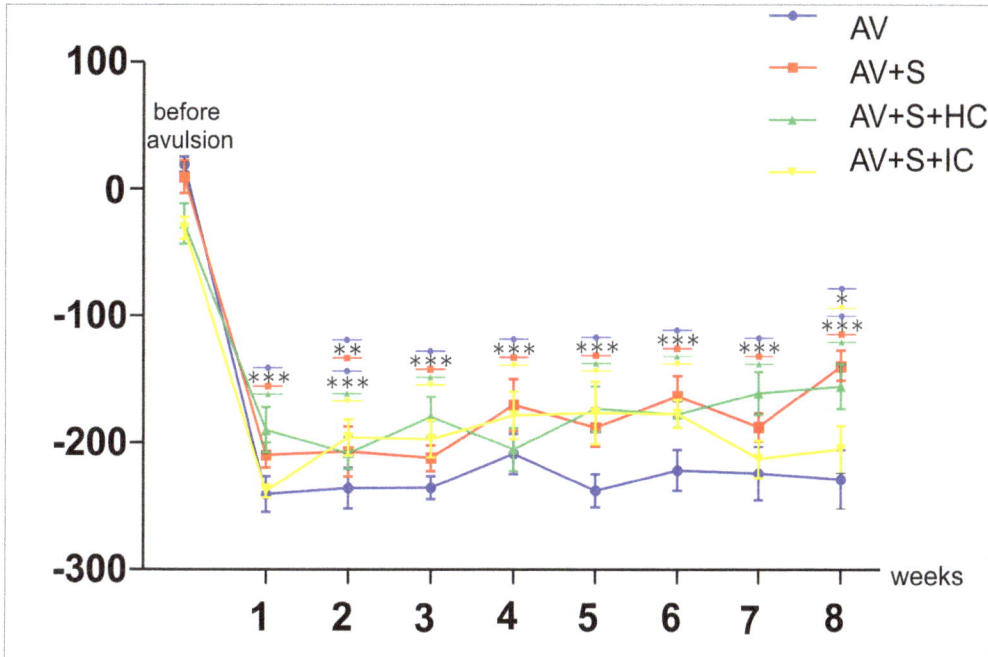

injury [17,18]. Nevertheless, the production of extracellular matrix molecules has also been suggested as neuroprotective [34]. Neuronal survival decreased at 8 weeks post injury, indicating that the therapeutic window for MC is relatively short and further cell treatments may be necessary to maintain the axotomized neurons.

Cell injection to the spinal cord gave similar results to the reimplantation alone, 4 weeks post injury. However, neuronal degeneration increased up to 8 weeks, reaching the level of avulsion only. We believe that the injection into the CNS/PNS interface result in a late inflammatory response that cause delayed cell death. In this sense, using a similar reimplantation approach, followed by mesenchymal stem cell injection, neuron preservation has been shown without significant functional recovery [35]. Overall, the neuronal survival results indicate that fibrin sealant homogenized MC result in acutely better results as compared to intraspinal engrafting.

According to prior studies, MC express BDNF and GDNF [3] in the PNS following sciatic nerve injury. BDNF is also produced by MCs in the CNS, 3 and 7 days after MC therapy [4]. In line with this, several studies have demonstrated neuroprotective effects of such neurotrophic factors [7,32,36], especially after spinal cord injury [37]. Neuroprotection is also achieved in neonatal animals [38], where the effects of axotomy are more drastic than in adults. The results herein are in line with the literature and show BDNF and GDNF production by the MC, 1 week post injury.

Interestingly, BDNF, which is exacerbated in the implant group, promotes axonal sprouting and elongation after peripheral nerve injury and during development [39]. This is in line with the motor recovery observed in all root reimplanted groups, suggesting regeneration of axons after avulsion.

Functional analysis of the peroneal nerve, as well as the pressure exerted by the ipsilateral paw, provides reliable data on functional recovery of animals with motor problems [40,41]. The motor improvement observed herein is noteworthy because gait restoration is necessarily related to motor units recovery, together with cerebral cortex control [42]. Importantly, the preservation of pre-synaptic inputs to the injured motoneurons after implantation, observed by immunohistochemistry, indicates preservation of supraspinal contacts.

An important occurrence following VRA is the reduction of pre-synaptic terminals to motoneurons [42,43]. This synaptic decrease become irreversible if the regrowing axons within the root do not reach their target muscles [43]. Importantly, the groups subjected to root reimplantation showed a significant preservation of synapses as compared to the avulsion only group.

In this case, cell treatment gave no further benefit, indicating that the restoration of CNS/PNS connection is sufficient to preserve spinal synaptic networks. Coupled with such synaptic changes, glial cells became reactive following VRA. Such reactive gliosis is characterized by hypertrophy of the cell body and processes of astrocytes and microglial hyperplasia [44–46].

Although the microglial reaction was morphologically decreased by MC treatment four weeks post lesion, at one week, an enhancement of Iba-1 gene transcripts was obtained. One possibility is that MCs increased or accelerated acute microglial response [47]. Regarding the astrogliosis, no differences were perceived between groups by immunohistochemical analysis. qPCR data, on the other hand, indicated a decreased number of GFAP gene transcripts following root reimplantation alone. This is in line with what has been observed 12 weeks after root reimplantation [10].

Conclusions

Taken together, the results of the present study indicate that MCs therapy further preserves injured motoneurons up to 4 weeks after implantation, in comparison to root reimplantation alone. Such fact is possibly related to the production of neurotrophic factors, such as BDNF and GDNF. Nonetheless, such difference was not seen at 4 weeks post injury. This may in turn indicate that restoration of the CNS/PNS connection must be carried out in a short period of time after avulsion. Importantly, the present data indicate that cell injection to the spinal cord does not result in long lasting neuroprotection. On the other hand, engrafting of MC at the site of injury with the aid of a fibrin scaffold is effective and may represent a more practical approach, with regard to translational medicine.

Acknowledgments

The authors are thankful to Prof. Dr. Alfredo M. Goes for providing the EGFP transgenic rats used in the present study. To Prof. Dr. Antonio C. Rodrigues for the fruitful discussions and to Prof. Dr. Dawidson A. Gomes and Prof. Dr. Ana Leda Longhini for expert flow cytometry analysis and comments.

Author Contributions

Conceived and designed the experiments: ALRO. Performed the experiments: ALRO MVC RB. Analyzed the data: ALRO MVC RB BB RSF. Contributed reagents/materials/analysis tools: ALRO BB RSF. Contributed to the writing of the manuscript: ALRO MVC RB BB RSF.

References

1. Goel RK, Suri V, Suri A, Sarkar C, Mohanty S, et al. (2009) Effect of bone marrow-derived mononuclear cells on nerve regeneration in the transection model of the rat sciatic nerve. J Clin Neurosci 16: 1211–1217.

2. de Freitas HT, da Silva VG, Giraldi-Guimaraes A (2012) Comparative study between bone marrow mononuclear fraction and mesenchymal stem cells treatment in sensorimotor recovery after focal cortical ablation in rats. Behav Brain Funct 8: 58.

3. Lopes-Filho JD, Caldas HC, Santos FC, Mazzer N, Simoes GF, et al. (2011) Microscopic evidences that bone marrow mononuclear cell treatment improves sciatic nerve regeneration after neurorrhaphy. Microsc Res Tech 74: 355–363.

4. Gubert F, Zaverucha-do-Valle C, Figueiredo FR, Bargas-Rega M, Paredes BD, et al. (2013) Bone-marrow cell therapy induces differentiation of radial glia-like cells and rescues the number of oligodendrocyte progenitors in the subventricular zone after global cerebral ischemia. Stem Cell Res 10: 241–256.

5. Thatte MR, Babhulkar S, Hiremath A (2013) Brachial plexus injury in adults: Diagnosis and surgical treatment strategies. Ann Indian Acad Neurol 16: 26–33.

6. Carlstedt T (2009) Nerve root replantation. Neurosurg Clin N Am 20: 39–50, vi.

7. Koliatsos VE, Price WL, Pardo CA, Price DL (1994) Ventral root avulsion: an experimental model of death of adult motor neurons. J Comp Neurol 342: 35–44.

8. Li L, Houenou LJ, Wu W, Lei M, Prevette DM, et al. (1998) Characterization of spinal motoneuron degeneration following different types of peripheral nerve injury in neonatal and adult mice. J Comp Neurol 396: 158–168.

9. Penas C, Casas C, Robert I, Fores J, Navarro X (2009) Cytoskeletal and activity-related changes in spinal motoneurons after root avulsion. J Neurotrauma 26: 763–779.

10. Barbizan R, Castro MV, Rodrigues AC, Barraviera B, Ferreira RS, et al. (2013) Motor recovery and synaptic preservation after ventral root avulsion and repair with a fibrin sealant derived from snake venom. PLoS One 8: e63260.

11. Cullheim S, Carlstedt T, Linda H, Risling M, Ulfhake B (1989) Motoneurons reinnervate skeletal muscle after ventral root implantation into the spinal cord of the cat. Neuroscience 29: 725–733.

12. Hoang TX, Nieto JH, Dobkin BH, Tillakaratne NJ, Havton LA (2006) Acute implantation of an avulsed lumbosacral ventral root into the rat conus medullaris promotes neuroprotection and graft reinnervation by autonomic and motor neurons. Neuroscience 138: 1149–1160.

13. Chang HY, Havton LA (2008) Surgical implantation of avulsed lumbosacral ventral roots promotes restoration of bladder morphology in rats. Exp Neurol 214: 117–124.

14. Carlstedt T (2008) Root repair review: basic science background and clinical outcome. Restor Neurol Neurosci 26: 225–241.

15. Eggers R, Tannemaat MR, Ehlert EM, Verhaagen J (2010) A spatio-temporal analysis of motoneuron survival, axonal regeneration and neurotrophic factor expression after lumbar ventral root avulsion and implantation. Exp Neurol 223: 207–220.

16. Giuffre JL, Kakar S, Bishop AT, Spinner RJ, Shin AY (2010) Current concepts of the treatment of adult brachial plexus injuries. J Hand Surg Am 35: 678–688; quiz 688.

17. Lang EM, Asan E, Plesnila N, Hofmann GO, Sendtner M (2005) Motoneuron survival after C7 nerve root avulsion and replantation in the adult rabbit: effects of local ciliary neurotrophic factor and brain-derived neurotrophic factor application. Plast Reconstr Surg 115: 2042–2050.

18. Rodrigues Hell RC, Silva Costa MM, Goes AM, Oliveira AL (2009) Local injection of BDNF producing mesenchymal stem cells increases neuronal survival and synaptic stability following ventral root avulsion. Neurobiol Dis 33: 290–300.

19. Oliveira AL, Thams S, Lidman O, Piehl F, Hokfelt T, et al. (2004) A role for MHC class I molecules in synaptic plasticity and regeneration of neurons after axotomy. Proc Natl Acad Sci U S A 101: 17843–17848.

20. Gasparotto VP, Landim-Alvarenga FC, Oliveira AL, Simoes GF, Lima-Neto JF, et al. (2014) A new fibrin sealant as a three-dimensional scaffold candidate for mesenchymal stem cells. Stem Cell Res Ther 5: 78.

21. Barros LC, Soares AM, Costa FL, Rodrigues VM, Fuly AL, et al. (2011) Biochemical and biological evaluation of gyroxin isolated from Crotalus durissus terrificus venom. The Journal of Venomous Animals and Toxins including Tropical Diseases 17: 23–33.

22. Barros LC, Ferreira RS, Jr., Barraviera SR, Stolf HO, Thomazini-Santos IA, et al. (2009) A new fibrin sealant from Crotalus durissus terrificus venom: applications in medicine. J Toxicol Environ Health B Crit Rev 12: 553–571.

23. Abercrombie M, Johnson ML (1946) Quantitative histology of Wallerian degeneration; nuclear population in rabbit sciatic nerve. J Anat 80: 37–50.

24. Freria CM, Velloso LA, Oliveira AL (2012) Opposing effects of Toll-like receptors 2 and 4 on synaptic stability in the spinal cord after peripheral nerve injury. J Neuroinflammation 9: 240.

25. Livak KJ, Schmittgen TD (2001) Analysis of relative gene expression data using real-time quantitative PCR and the 2(-Delta Delta C(T)) Method. Methods 25: 402–408.

26. Yao L, Chen X, Tian Y, Lu H, Zhang P, et al. (2012) Selection of housekeeping genes for normalization of RT-PCR in hypoxic neural stem cells of rat in vitro. Mol Biol Rep 39: 569–576.

27. Bain JR, Mackinnon SE, Hunter DA (1989) Functional evaluation of complete sciatic, peroneal, and posterior tibial nerve lesions in the rat. Plast Reconstr Surg 83: 129–138.

28. Yoshihara T, Ohta M, Itokazu Y, Matsumoto N, Dezawa M, et al. (2007) Neuroprotective effect of bone marrow-derived mononuclear cells promoting functional recovery from spinal cord injury. J Neurotrauma 24: 1026–1036.

29. Fernandes M, Valente SG, Fernandes MJ, Felix EP, Mazzacoratti Mda G, et al. (2008) Bone marrow cells are able to increase vessels number during repair of sciatic nerve lesion. J Neurosci Methods 170: 16–24.

30. Okada S, Ishii K, Yamane J, Iwanami A, Ikegami T, et al. (2005) In vivo imaging of engrafted neural stem cells: its application in evaluating the optimal timing of transplantation for spinal cord injury. FASEB J 19: 1839–1841.

31. Novikov L, Novikova L, Kellerth JO (1995) Brain-derived neurotrophic factor promotes survival and blocks nitric oxide synthase expression in adult rat spinal motoneurons after ventral root avulsion. Neurosci Lett 200: 45–48.

32. Kishino A, Ishige Y, Tatsuno T, Nakayama C, Noguchi H (1997) BDNF prevents and reverses adult rat motor neuron degeneration and induces axonal outgrowth. Exp Neurol 144: 273–286.

33. Oliveira AL, Langone F (2000) GM-1 ganglioside treatment reduces motoneuron death after ventral root avulsion in adult rats. Neurosci Lett 293: 131–134.

34. Ide C (1996) Peripheral nerve regeneration. Neurosci Res 25: 101–121.

35. Torres-Espin A, Corona-Quintanilla DL, Fores J, Allodi I, Gonzalez F, et al. (2013) Neuroprotection and axonal regeneration after lumbar ventral root avulsion by re-implantation and mesenchymal stem cells transplant combined therapy. Neurotherapeutics 10: 354–368.

36. Yan Q, Elliott J, Snider WD (1992) Brain-derived neurotrophic factor rescues spinal motor neurons from axotomy-induced cell death. Nature 360: 753–755.

37. Bregman BS, Coumans JV, Dai HN, Kuhn PL, Lynskey J, et al. (2002) Transplants and neurotrophic factors increase regeneration and recovery of function after spinal cord injury. Prog Brain Res 137: 257–273.

38. Sendtner M, Holtmann B, Kolbeck R, Thoenen H, Barde YA (1992) Brain-derived neurotrophic factor prevents the death of motoneurons in newborn rats after nerve section. Nature 360: 757–759.

39. Mendell LM, Munson JB, Arvanian VL (2001) Neurotrophins and synaptic plasticity in the mammalian spinal cord. J Physiol 533: 91–97.

40. Dijkstra JR, Meek MF, Robinson PH, Gramsbergen A (2000) Methods to evaluate functional nerve recovery in adult rats: walking track analysis, video analysis and the withdrawal reflex. J Neurosci Methods 96: 89–96.

41. Varejao AS, Meek MF, Ferreira AJ, Patricio JA, Cabrita AM (2001) Functional evaluation of peripheral nerve regeneration in the rat: walking track analysis. J Neurosci Methods 108: 1–9.

42. Purves D, Lichtman JW (1978) Formation and maintenance of synaptic connections in autonomic ganglia. Physiol Rev 58: 821–862.

43. Brannstrom T, Kellerth JO (1998) Changes in synaptology of adult cat spinal alpha-motoneurons after axotomy. Exp Brain Res 118: 1–13.

44. Privat A, Valat J, Fulcrand J (1981) Proliferation of neuroglial cell lines in the degenerating optic nerve of young rats. A radioautographic study. J Neuropathol Exp Neurol 40: 46–60.

45. Norton WT, Aquino DA, Hozumi I, Chiu FC, Brosnan CF (1992) Quantitative aspects of reactive gliosis: a review. Neurochem Res 17: 877–885.

46. Eng LF, Ghirnikar RS, Lee YL (2000) Glial fibrillary acidic protein: GFAP-thirty-one years (1969–2000). Neurochem Res 25: 1439–1451.

47. Grove JE, Bruscia E, Krause DS (2004) Plasticity of bone marrow-derived stem cells. Stem Cells 22: 487–500.

14

Interleukin-6 Secretion by Astrocytes Is Dynamically Regulated by PI3K-mTOR-Calcium Signaling

Simone Codeluppi[1]*, Teresa Fernandez-Zafra[1], Katalin Sandor[2], Jacob Kjell[3], Qingsong Liu[4,5¤a], Mathew Abrams[3¤b], Lars Olson[3], Nathanael S. Gray[4,5], Camilla I. Svensson[2], Per Uhlén[1]

1 Laboratory of Molecular Neurobiology, Department of Medical Biochemistry and Biophysics, Karolinska Institutet, Stockholm, Sweden, 2 Department of Physiology and Pharmacology, Karolinska Institutet, Stockholm, Sweden, 3 Department of Neuroscience, Karolinska Institutet, Stockholm, Sweden, 4 Department of Cancer Biology, Dana-Farber Cancer Institute, Boston, Massachusetts, United States of America, 5 Department of Biological Chemistry and Molecular Pharmacology, Harvard Medical School, Boston, Massachusetts, United States of America

Abstract

After contusion spinal cord injury (SCI), astrocytes become reactive and form a glial scar. While this reduces spreading of the damage by containing the area of injury, it inhibits regeneration. One strategy to improve the recovery after SCI is therefore to reduce the inhibitory effect of the scar, once the acute phase of the injury has passed. The pleiotropic cytokine interleukin-6 (IL-6) is secreted immediately after injury and regulates scar formation; however, little is known about the role of IL-6 in the sub-acute phases of SCI. Interestingly, IL-6 also promotes axon regeneration, and therefore its induction in reactive astrocytes may improve regeneration after SCI. We found that IL-6 is expressed by astrocytes and neurons one week post-injury and then declines. Using primary cultures of rat astrocytes we delineated the molecular mechanisms that regulate IL-6 expression and secretion. IL-6 expression requires activation of p38 and depends on NF-κB transcriptional activity. Activation of these pathways in astrocytes occurs when the PI3K-mTOR-AKT pathway is inhibited. Furthermore, we found that an increase in cytosolic calcium concentration was necessary for IL-6 secretion. To induce IL-6 secretion in astrocytes, we used torin2 and rapamycin to block the PI3K-mTOR pathway and increase cytosolic calcium, respectively. Treating injured animals with torin2 and rapamycin for two weeks, starting two weeks after injury when the scar has been formed, lead to a modest effect on mechanical hypersensitivity, limited to the period of treatment. These data, taken together, suggest that treatment with torin2 and rapamycin induces IL-6 secretion by astrocytes and may contribute to the reduction of mechanical hypersensitivity after SCI.

Editor: Simone Di Giovanni, Hertie Institute for Clinical Brain Research, University of Tuebingen, Germany

Funding: This work was supported by: Wenner-Gren foundation (SC, KS), Svenska Sällskapet för Medicinsk Forskning (SC), Becas Talentia (TFZ), Hjärnfonden (SC, PU), Swedish Research Council (CS, PU, LO), Linnaeus Center in Developmental Biology for Regenerative Medicine (PU), the Knut and Alice Wallenberg Foundation Grant to Center of Live Imaging of Cells at Karolinska Institutet (PU), the Royal Swedish Academy of Sciences (PU), Wings for Life (LO, MA), Vinnova (LO), Karolinska Distinguished Professor Award (LO), Karolinska StratNeuro program (LO). The funders had no role in study design, data collection and analysis, decision to publish, or preparation of the manuscript.

Competing Interests: The authors have declared that no competing interests exist.

* E-mail: simone.codeluppi@ki.se

¤a Current address: High Magnetic Field Laboratory, Chinese Academy of Sciences, Hefei, Anhui, P. R. China
¤b Current address: International Neuroinformatics Coordinating Facility, Karolinska Institutet, Stockholm, Sweden

Introduction

The physiological outcome after spinal cord injury (SCI) is the result of a coordinated response of many cell types. Astrocytes play a key role in the scar formation that follows SCI [1]. During this process, astrocytes interact with microglia and immune cells to isolate and clear damaged tissue and to reestablish normal homeostasis of the spinal cord [2,3]. In order to communicate with each other and regulate the surrounding environment these cells secrete cytokines [4]. Interestingly, the same signaling molecules can be secreted by different cell types at different time points after injury [5].

Interleukin-6 (IL-6) is a pleiotropic cytokine and its effects on SCI depend mostly on the temporal expression and the balance between survival-promoting and pro-inflammatory effects. Following SCI, microglia and macrophages secrete IL-6, which is thought to play a negative role in regeneration by recruiting immune cells to the site of injury and by promoting glial scar formation [6]. However, IL-6 expression also has positive roles in regeneration by promoting synaptic rearrangements, axon sprouting, and reducing tissue loss [7,8].

In order to implement its function, IL-6 needs to be released into the extracellular space; hence, regulation of transcription-translation as well as of secretion are important for IL-6 mediated responses [9]. The Nuclear Factor-κB (NF-κB) is a strong inducer of IL-6 mRNA [10]. Various signaling cascades intersect with NF-κB to tightly regulate its activity [11] For example, the mitogen activated protein kinase (MAPK) p38, the phosphoinositide-3-kinase (PI3K) and the mechanistic target of rapamycin (mTOR) pathways. While activation of p38 promotes IL-6 expression, both PI3K and mTOR can exert inhibitory effects, depending on the cell type examined [12,13].

After synthesis, IL-6 accumulates in secretory vesicles that upon stimulation fuse with the plasma membrane, releasing IL-6 into the extracellular space [9]. Increased intracellular calcium (Ca^{2+}) is required for exocytosis. In cells, the endoplasmic reticulum (ER) is the main storage of intracellular Ca^{2+}, which can be released into the cytoplasm through inositol-1,2,5-tris-phosphate receptors ($InsP_3R$) or ryanodine receptors (RyR) [14]. Both receptor types are regulated by accessory proteins, such as the FK506-binding proteins (FKBP)-12 [15]. FKBP12 inhibits RyR mediated Ca^{2+} release while its effect on $InsP_3Rs$ is cell dependent and can either be to promote or inhibit Ca^{2+} release [16–18]. Interestingly, patients harboring mutations that increase the leakiness of RyRs show increased IL-6 secretion [19].

Although it has been shown that astrocytes secrete IL-6 [20], the signaling pathways involved are not well characterized. Hence, this study aims to understand which signaling pathways are important in the regulation of IL-6 in astrocytes in order to identify or develop drugs that can be used to up-regulate and/or down-regulate its secretion *in vivo*.

Experimental Procedures

Antibodies and other Reagents

Antibodies. The following commercially available antibodies (Cell Signaling Technologies) were used: pERK (#9101), pAKT-S473 (#9271), pAKT-T308 (#2965), AKT (#9272), Cleaved caspase-3 (#9661), GAPDH (#2118), pS6(S235/236) (#4858), p-p38(#8690), pJNK (#4668), IL-6 (Abcam, ab6672), Aldh1L1 (NeuroMab, N103/31), Vimentin (V6630) and GFAP (G-3893) (Sigma), ED1 (MCA341R) and OX42 (MCA275R) (Serotec), and NeuN (Chemicon MAB377). Secondary antibodies for immuno-histochemistry and fluorescent western blotting (Life Technology), and HRP-conjugated secondaries (Sigma) were used.

Drugs. Rapamycin was commercially available (LC laboratories) as was LY294002 and FK506 (Tocris), the AKT inhibitor (Calbiochem) and Bapta-AM (Life Technology). Torin1 and torin2 were synthesized by Dr. Liu (Department of Cancer Biology, Dana-Farber Cancer Institute, Boston, MA).

Reagents. These included Complete mini (protease inhibitor) and phosphostop (phosphatase inhibitor) (Roche). All other reagents were from Sigma.

Plasmids

pTK-RL (Stratagene), p1168huIL6P-Luc+ (wt IL-6 promoter, LMBP 4495) and p1168hIL6mNFκB-Luc+ (NFκB mutated promoter, LMBP 4496) (Belgian Coordinated Collections of Microorganisms (BCCM/LMBP)), and pRIL6C.94 (ATCC, ATCC-37681) were used.

Astrocyte Cultures

Astrocyte cultures were prepared from spinal cords of adult male Sprague-Dawley rats (P65 to P70, weighing 200–250 grams Scanbur) using a method previously described [21]. For western blotting and real-time PCR, the cells were trypsinized and replated in 6-well plates (40,000 cells/well). The cultures were used for experiments when confluent (typically within 4–6 days). For mesoscale experiments, the cells were replated in 24-well plates (20,000 cells/well) and used when confluent (typically 2 days after plating). Before drug treatment the cells were incubated for 48 hours in growth-factor-free Dulbecco's modified Eagle's medium (GF Free DMEM), supplemented with 1% penicillin-streptomycin and 1% sodium pyruvate (Life Technologies).

Spinal Cord Contusion Injury

Animal work was approved by the North Stockholm Animal Ethics Committee (permit # N429/09 and N479/11). Female rats

(220 g, Scanbur, Sweden) were group-housed 4 animals per cage, and kept on a 12-hour light/dark cycle with food and water *ad libitum*. Spinal cord injury was done as previously described [22] with the Keck Center for Neurosciences impactor (NYU impactor) using a 10 g weight dropped from a height of 25 mm onto the dorsal surface of the exposed spinal cord. After recording BBB scores (see below), withdrawal thresholds evoked by touch stimulus, and body weights for the first week post-injury, animals were divided into 5 treatment groups: naïve (N = 4), sham (N = 6), vehicle (N = 6), torin2 (N = 6), and torin2+rapamycin (N = 8). Torin2 alone (4 mg/kg) or in combination with rapamycin (1.5 mg/kg) was administered orally by gavage once a day starting at day 15 after injury and ending at day 29. In sham operated rats only the laminectomy was performed. For all of the following experimental procedures and analyses, including behavioral testing and histological analyses, experimenters were blinded to the treatment groups.

Locomotor Evaluation

The Basso, Beattie, Bresnahan (BBB) locomotor rating scale [23] was used to evaluate hindlimb locomotor function in an open field on a weekly basis for 6 weeks. All experimenters involved with BBB evaluation were blinded to treatment group identity.

Assessment of Mechanical Hypersensitivity

Rats were habituated to the testing enclosure twice before the experiment started. Mechanical hypersensitivity was assessed three times prior to the surgery, once two weeks post-surgery to confirm the decrease in hind paw withdrawal threshold, and six times during the drug-treatment period on weeks 3–6 post-injury. Rats were placed in individual Plexiglas chambers on top of a wire mesh surface and allowed to acclimatize for 30 minutes prior to testing. Hind paw withdrawal thresholds were assessed by using calibrated von Frey filaments (Stoelting) with logarithmically incremental force of 0.4, 1, 2, 4, 6, 8, 10 and 15 g. A cut-off of 15 g was applied in order to avoid tissue damage, thus supra-threshold responses were not registered. Each filament was pressed perpendicularly against the plantar surface of the hind paw and held on for approximately 3 seconds. A positive response was recorded if the paw was withdrawn. The filaments were used according to the "up-down" method [24] and the 50% probability of withdrawal threshold described by Chaplan and co-workers [25] was calculated in grams for each hind paw and averaged. Mechanical hypersensitivity, the percent change from the average of the baseline values was also calculated.

Tissue Processing

Naïve and injured rats at 6 hours, 1, 2, and 3 weeks after SCI (N = 4 for each condition) were anaesthetized with 50 mg/kg pentobarbital and perfused with 50 ml of calcium free Tyrode's solution containing 0.1 ml heparin (5000 IE/ml) followed by 50 ml of 4% formaldehyde in PBS (PFA). For in situ hybridization and immunohistochemistry, spinal cords were dissected and post-fixed in 4% PFA at RT for 1 h and stored in 10% sucrose in PBS at 4°C. Spinal cords were then cut in 7 mm segments.

In situ Hybridization

RNA probes for rat IL-6 mRNA were prepared as previously described [26]. IL-6 mRNA *in situ* hybridization was performed in spinal cord sections of naïve and injured animals at 6 hours, 1, and 2 weeks after SCI. Briefly, sections were permeabilized in PBST (PBS, 0.3% Tween-20), followed by overnight hybridization at 45°C with 10 ng/μl of riboprobe in hybridization solution (4 mM

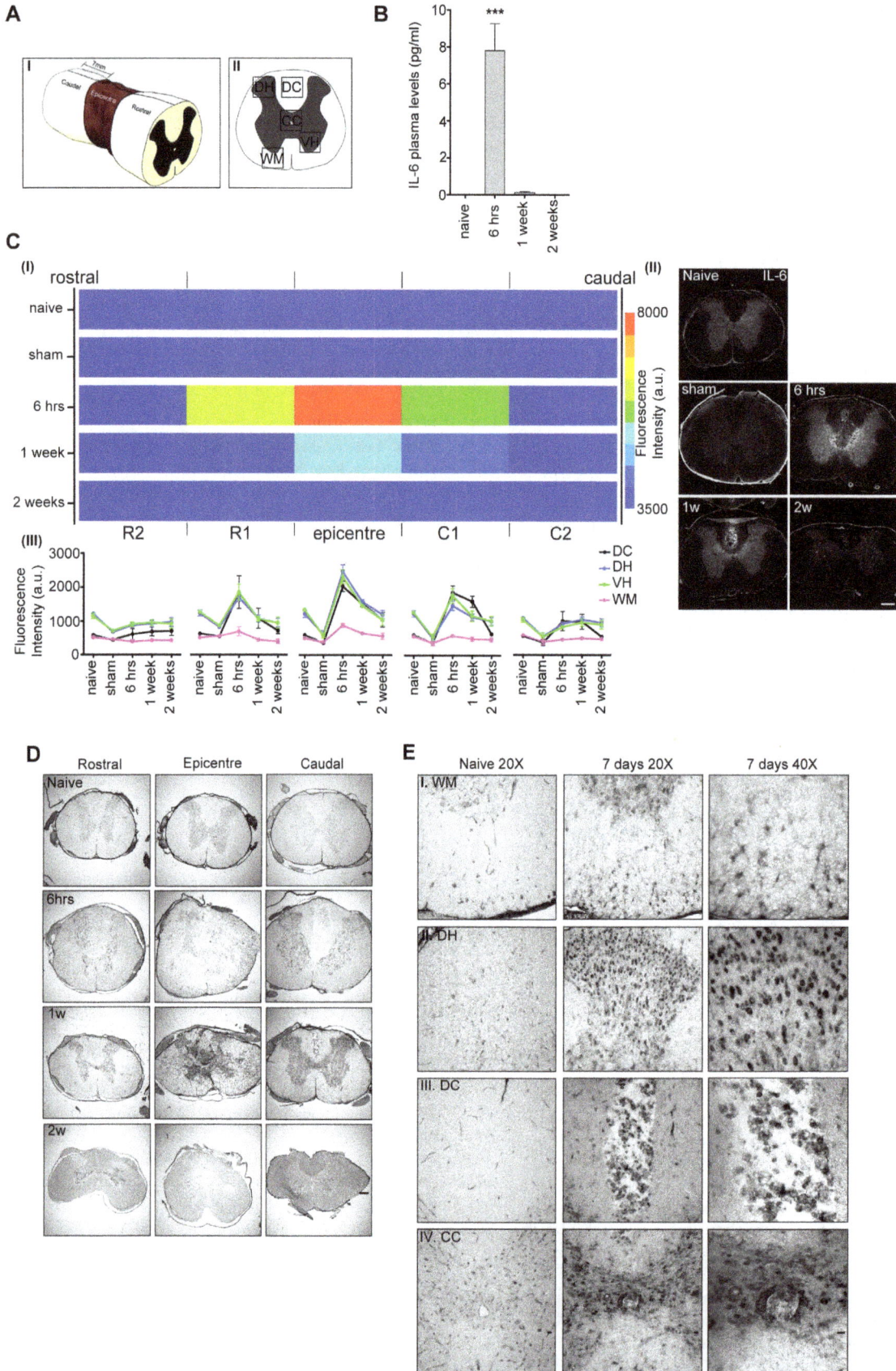

Figure 1. IL-6 is expressed in the spinal cord after contusion injury. After spinal cord contusion injury, IL-6 is upregulated in cells of the spinal cord. **A**, Cartoon depicting: (I) the 7 mm long segments (rostral, caudal, epicenter) in which the injured spinal cord is dissected for analysis. (II)

Regions of the spinal cord sections imaged. Dorsal horn (DH), dorsal column (DC), central canal (CC), white matter (WM) and ventral horn (VH). **B**, IL-6 levels in plasma of animals used for *in situ* hybridization and immunohistochemistry. Data are presented as mean ± SEM. ***p<0.001 for the comparison between naive and injured animals by one-way ANOVA with Bonferroni's *post hoc* test (N = 4 per group). **C**, (I) Representation of the IL-6 protein distribution quantified by immunohistochemistry in spinal cord segments at different time points after injury. Blue indicates the lowest and red the highest intensity of IL-6 immunofluorescence (arbitrary units, a.u.). R, rostral and C, caudal. (II) Representative images of IL-6 labeled sections from the C1 region of naïve, sham (1 week after injury) and injured animals. Scale bar = 20 μm. (III) Quantification of IL-6 immunoreactivity in different regions of the spinal cord at different time points after injury. N = 3 animals for each condition. For each spinal cord segment three sections have been imaged and fluorescence signal in the regions defined in A(II) was quantified and averaged in each section. **D**, *In situ* hybridization with an antisense IL-6 mRNA probe on sections from rostral, epicenter and caudal segments of spinal cord from naive and injured animals 6 hours, 1, and 2 weeks post-injury. Scale bar = 200 μm. **E**, High magnification images from sections of the caudal segment shown in D from naïve (20X) and 1 week injured spinal cord animals (20X and 40X). Scale bar = 20 μm for 20X and 40X. (N = 3 in each group).

Tris-HCl pH 7.5, Poly-A 0.5 mg/ml, salmon sperm 0.5 mg/ml, 50% formamide, 20% dextran sulphate, 0.1 M DTT, 0.3 M NaCl, 1X Denhardt's solution, 1 mM EDTA pH 8.0). Next, sections were washed twice for 15 min in 2X SSC at 45°C, 4×15 min with 0.1X SSC at 55°C, once for 10 min at RT in 5X MAB (2.5 M maleic acid; 3.75 M NaCl; pH 7.5), and three times for 10 min at RT in 1X MABT (0.5 M maleic acid; 0.75 M NaCl; 0.1% Tween-20; pH 7.5). Sections were then incubated with blocking solution (1X MAB, 20% donkey serum, 2% blocking agent; 0.1% Tween-20) for 1 h at RT followed by overnight incubation at RT with anti-digoxigenin antibody conjugated to alkaline phosphatase (Roche) (1:2000) in blocking solution. After washing 4×20 min in 1X MABT and 3×10 min in B3 (0.1 M Tris-HCl, pH 9.5; 0.1 M NaCl; 50 mM MgCl2; 0.1% Tween-20), sections were developed for 4 h with NBT/BCIP (Roche) (1:50) in B3 solution, and images were acquired (Olympus FV1000 CLSM Olympus).

Immunohistochemistry

Spinal cord sections were permeabilized twice for 5 min with TBST (TBS, 0.2% Tween-20), blocked for 1 h at RT in blocking solution (TBST with 5% goat serum), incubated overnight at 4°C with primary antibodies in blocking solution, and finally incubated for 1 h at RT with Alexa-conjugated secondary antibodies (Life Technologies) in blocking solution. DAPI staining was applied for 30 min in blocking solution. Images were acquired using confocal microscopy (Olympus FV1000 or Zeiss LSM700). Imaris 7.3.0 (Bitplane) was used to quantify the intensity of IL-6, pS6 and pS6/IL-6 colocalization in GFAP positive cells. In order to identify GFAP positive cells we first rendered the image stack in 3 D. The GFAP channel was then selected and the pixels above a minimal threshold were used to build a 3 D surface. This 3 D surface isolated the GFAP positive cells. IL-6 and pS6 intensity and pS6/IL-6 colocalization were quantified inside this GFAP positive surface. The settings used in the image processing were the same for all images analyzed. The figures were prepared using appropriate image handling software (Adobe Illustrator CS5, Adobe Systems). IL-6 immunofluorescence in the different regions and segments of the spinal cord was quantified by measuring the integrated intensity of ROIs selected (Fiji) [27]. The heat map in Figure 1C was generated using a custom script in python/matplotlib.

Real-time PCR

All reagents used were commercially available (Life Technologies). Probe and primer for IL-6 mRNA were "assay-on-demand" gene expression products (TaqMan Probe and primer ID Rn00561420_m1). After stimulation with drugs (8 hrs), astrocytes were washed with PBS and lysate using Trizol. Total RNA was purified using phenol-chloroform and reversed transcribed using random hexanucleotide primers. PCR amplification reactions were carried out in 25 μl containing 50 ng of cDNA

(MicroAmp Optical Plates with MicroAmp Optical Caps and the TaqMan Universal Master Mix). Incubations at 50°C for 2 min and at 95°C for 10 min were carried out to activate the polymerase (AmpliTaq polymerase), followed by 40 cycles at 95°C for 15 s and 60°C for 1 min. GAPDH was used as a loading control for each sample and the standard curve method was used for quantification [28].

Immunoblotting

Astrocyte cultures were lysed in RIPA buffer (Sigma) containing protease inhibitors and phosphatase inhibitor cocktails. Samples were analyzed by SDS-PAGE followed by immunoblotting. Membranes were incubated with primary antibodies followed by horseradish peroxidase-conjugated secondary antibodies and ECL prime chemiluminescence detection reagent (GE). Chemiluminescent signal was detected using a Biorad ChemiDocXRS+ (Biorad). For detection using near-infrared, membranes were incubated with secondary antibodies (Alexa-680 and Alexa-790) and scanned (Odyssey scanner, LICOR). Membranes were stripped (ReBlot Western Blot Recycling Kit, Millipore) before re-probing with a different antibody.

Transfection and Luciferase Gene Reporter Assay

In reporter gene assays, 10^6 cells were transiently transfected (Amaxa nucleofection, VPI-1006, electroporation program T-020) according to the manufacturer's instructions. Astrocytes were transfected with 400 ng of the pRL-TK-Luc plasmid together with 3600 ng of p1168huIL6P-Luc+ or p1168hIL6mNFkB-Luc+ plasmid and plated in complete media for 24 hrs. After 24 hours, the media was replaced with GF-free media for an additional 24 hours. Drugs were then applied and after 24 hours the cells were lysed in reporter lysis buffer (Promega). Reporter activity was determined (Promega dual luciferase assay system) according to manufacturer's instructions. Firefly and Renilla activities were detected (Victor^2 reader, Wallac). Firefly luciferase values were normalized for transfection efficiency by means of the Renilla luciferase activity that is constitutively expressed by pRL-TK.

Cytokine Detection

High sensitivity detection of rat IL-6 was carried out using a commercially available kit (KC153AKC-1 rat IL-6 ultra-sensitive kit, Mesoscale discovery, MSD). For cytokine detection in cell culture supernatant, 20,000 cells/well were plated in 24-well plates and incubated 2 days until confluent. Culture media was then replaced with GF-free media. After 48 hours, the GF-free media was replaced with GF-free media containing drugs. After 24 hours, the supernatant was collected and centrifuged at 4°C 10,000 rpm for 5 minutes to remove cell debris. The supernatant was collected without disturbing the pellet, aliquoted and frozen on dry ice. For analysis of cytokines in plasma, blood was collected by cardiac puncture before (naive), 6 hours, 7 days, and 14 days after injury. The blood was collected in micro container SSB tubes (BD) and

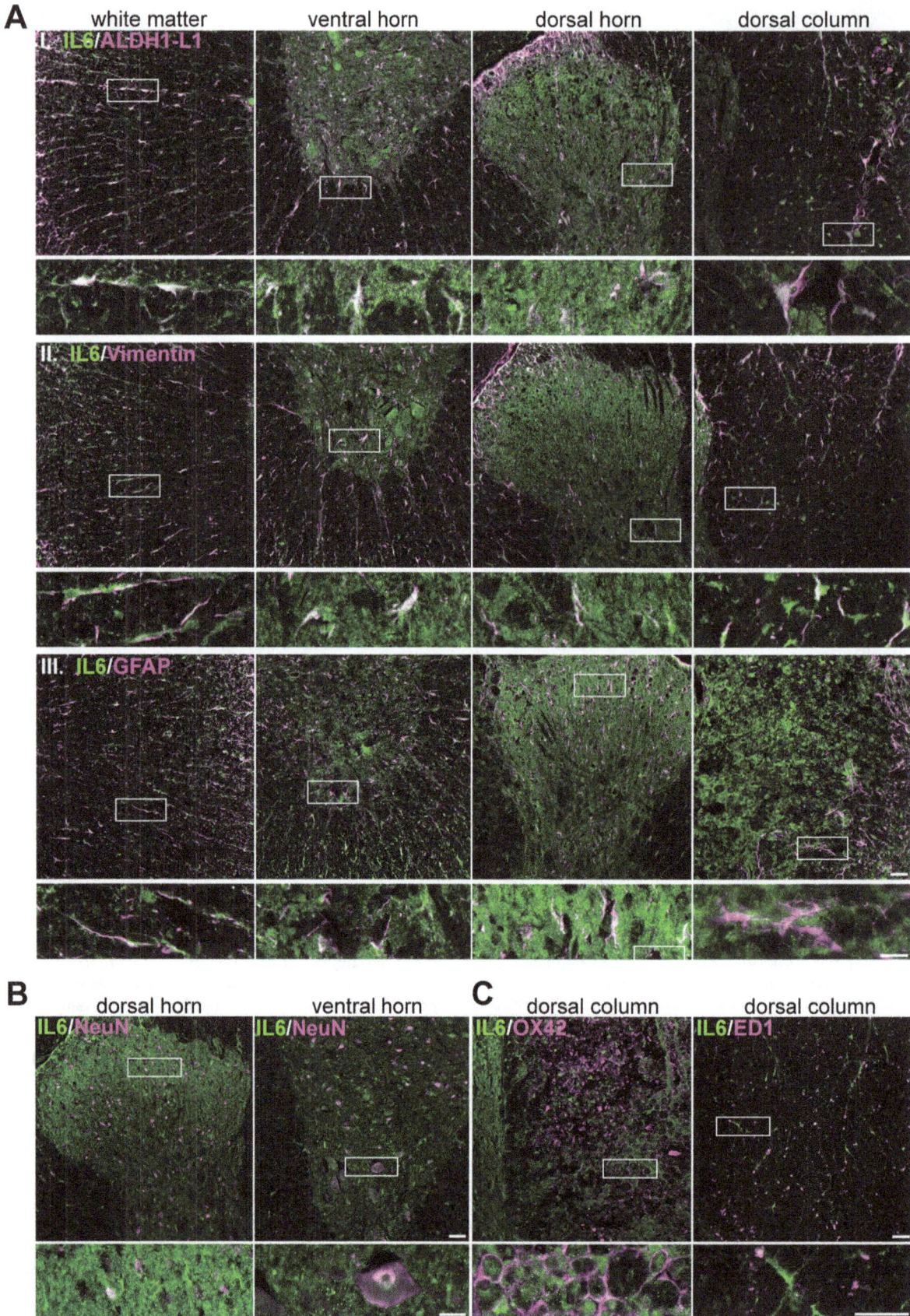

Figure 2. Astrocytes express IL-6 1 week after contusion injury. Reactive astrocytes express IL-6 after contusion injury as well as neurons and microglia/macrophages. **A**, Immunolabeling of IL-6 (green) and astrocyte markers (magenta) ALDH1L1 (I), vimentin (II) and GFAP (III) in different

regions of the caudal segment from spinal cords 1 week after injury. Scale bar = 20 µm. **B**, Immunolabeling of IL-6 (green) and the neuronal marker NeuN (magenta) in dorsal and ventral horns of caudal segments from spinal cords 1 week after injury. Scale bar = 20 µm. **C**, Immunolabeling for IL-6 (green) and the microglia and macrophage markers OX-42 and ED-1 (magenta) in the dorsal column of the caudal segment from spinal cords 1 week after injury. Scale bar = 20 µm. N = 3 for all conditions.

the plasma was separated by centrifugation at 6000 rcf for 90 seconds. After isolation, the plasma was frozen on dry ice.

For cytokine detections in supernatant and plasma samples, we followed the manufacturer's instructions with minor modification. The 96-well plates were incubated with diluent solution with 2% BSA (25 µl) for 30 minutes at RT on an orbital shaker. Samples and standards were added (25 µl) and the plate was incubated over night at 4°C on an orbital shaker. The wells were then washed three times using 200 µl PBS +0.05% Tween-20. The detection antibody was added and the plate was incubated for 2 hrs at room temperature on an orbital shaker. At the end of the incubation the plate was washed three times using 200 µl PBS +0.05% Tween-20. Read Buffer (150 µl, MSD) was then added to each well and IL-6 was measured (MSD Sector Imager 2400 plate reader). Raw data were analyzed using MSD software (Discovery Workbench 3.0). A 4-parameter logistic fit curve was generated using the standards and the concentration of each sample calculated.

Calcium Measurements

After 48 h starvation and 24 h treatment with torin2 and/or rapamycin, spinal cord astrocytes were loaded with 5 µM Fura2-AM and 0.1% Pluronic Acid (F-127 Life Technologies) for 30 min at 37°C in starving media, rinsed twice, and imaged in Ca^{2+}-free KREBS-Ringer's solution (119 mM NaCl, 2.5 mM KCl, 1 mM NaH2PO4, 2 mM EGTA, 1.3 mM MgCl2, 20 mM HEPES, 11 mM D-glucose) at 37°C. After baseline readings, 3 mM of 4-chloro-methylphenol (4-cmc) was bath-applied to the cells. mTOR inhibitors were present during loading and throughout the duration of the experiment. Images were acquired at 340 nm and 380 nm at a frequency of 0.5 Hz using an upright widefield microscope (Zeiss) equipped with a 20x water immersion objective. Image analysis was done using custom Python scripts.

In situ Detection of Fragmented DNA (TUNEL Assay)

Astrocytes were plated in poly-lysine-coated plates with transparent bottom for high content screening (BD). After 24 hours, the cells were incubated in GF-free media and 48 hours later the cells were incubated with GF-free media containing the drugs. After 24 hours incubation, fragmented DNA was detected using a commercially available kit (Click-iT TUNEL Alexa Fluor Imaging Assay, Life Technology) as indicated by the manufacturer. The plate was imaged using a cell observer (Zeiss) and the percentage of TUNEL-positive cells was quantified with a custom pipeline generated in CellProfiler [29].

Results

Reactive Astrocytes Express IL-6 after Contusion Spinal Cord Injury

In order to examine IL-6 expression in the spinal cord after injury, we used a contusion injury model. The corticospinal tract and other dorsal parts of the spinal cord were damaged by dropping a weight on the exposed dura using the NYU impactor [23,30]. We collected spinal cords and plasma from animals at 6 hours, 1, 2, and 3 weeks after injury, control cords were obtained from sham operated and naïve rats. It has been shown that strong astrocyte activation is detectable 1 week after contusion injury; however, the astrocyte scar is fully formed 2–3 weeks post-injury

[31]. Interestingly, IL-6 levels in plasma were already high 6 hours after injury, but returned to basal by week one (Figure 1B). We next examined spinal cord sections from the same animals by *in situ* hybridization and immunohistochemistry. In order to determine if IL-6 expression in the spinal cord correlated with the plasma levels, we divided the spinal cords in 7 mm-long segments and quantified IL-6 expression by immunohistochemistry (Figure 1A,C). We found that the IL-6 level was highest at 6 hours after injury and returned to baseline by week two (Figure 1C (I,II)). Noteworthy, sham surgery (1 week) did not cause an increase of IL-6 levels in the spinal cord compared to levels in naïve animals (Figure 1C). Moreover, IL-6 protein was not homogenously expressed along the spinal cord length; IL-6 was higher in the epicenter segment while levels were lower rostrally and caudally (Figure 1C (I)). Interestingly, when the different regions in the spinal cord sections were examined, IL-6 expression increased in the gray matter (dorsal and ventral horn) and in the dorsal column, but no changes were detectable in other regions (Figure 1C (III)).

In order to determine if cells of the injured spinal cord produce IL-6, we used *in situ* hybridization to detect IL-6 mRNA in tissue sections (Figure 1D–E). An increase of IL-6 mRNA was detectable in the injury epicenter, both dorsal and caudal to the injury site at 6 hours, 1, and 2 weeks after injury. These areas showed a marked upregulation of IL-6 mRNA in cells of gray and white matter of the injured spinal cord as compared to naïve animals (Figure 1D–E). An IL-6 sense *in situ* probe was used as a control and specificity was indicated by lack of signal in naïve tissue and in tissue harvested 1 and 2 weeks after injury (Figure S1). High magnification images of spinal cord sections showed that IL-6 mRNA was expressed in different cell types (Figure 1E).

To determine if astrocytes express IL-6, we assessed the colocalization of IL-6 immunoreactivity with the pan-astrocytic marker aldehyde dehydrogenase 1 family member L1 (ALDH1L1) and markers of reactive astrocytes, such as vimentin and glial fibrillary acidic protein (GFAP). We found that IL-6 protein expression colocalized with all three astrocyte markers in all regions of the spinal cord examined (Figure 2A). However, our *in situ* data showed that at 1 week post-injury, IL-6 mRNA was present in multiple cell types (Figure 1E). Hence, to investigate if IL-6 was also produced by neurons and/or microglia and macrophages, we determined the degree of colocalization between IL-6 and the neuronal marker NeuN and between IL-6 and the microglia/macrophage markers OX42, and ED1. We found that IL-6 was not only expressed by reactive astrocytes but also by neurons of the dorsal and ventral horn (Figure 2B) as well as by macrophages and microglia in the dorsal column (Figure 2C). However, at 1 week after injury, macrophages or microglia did not express IL-6 in the white matter or in any of the other regions of the spinal cord analyzed (Figure S2).

Because astrocyte properties change during the different phases of SCI [32], we examined if IL-6 immunoreactivity in astrocytes 1 and 3 weeks after injury (Figure 3A). We found that IL-6 expression in GFAP+ cells was significantly increased at 1 week (1.1±0.1 a.u.) and returned to sham levels (0.38±0.01 a.u.) at 3 weeks post-injury (0.59±0.04 a.u.), indicating that IL-6 was expressed at the beginning of the astrocyte response but returned to baseline when the scar was fully formed (Figure 3B).

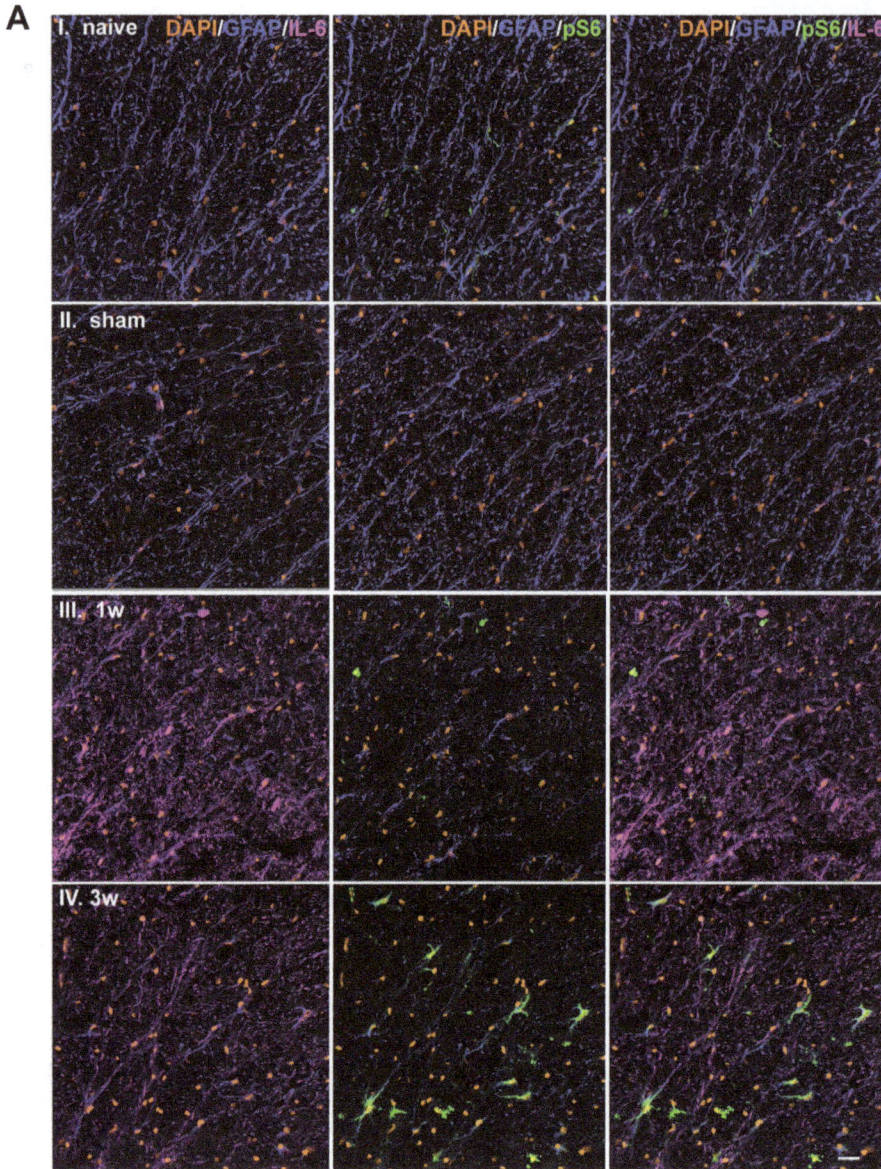

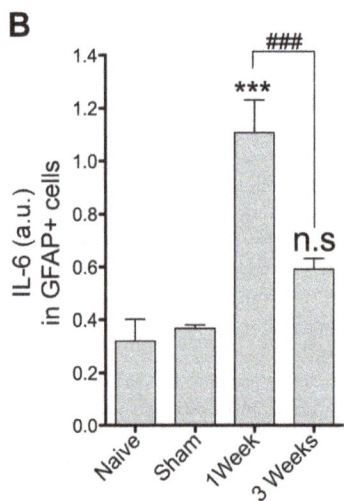

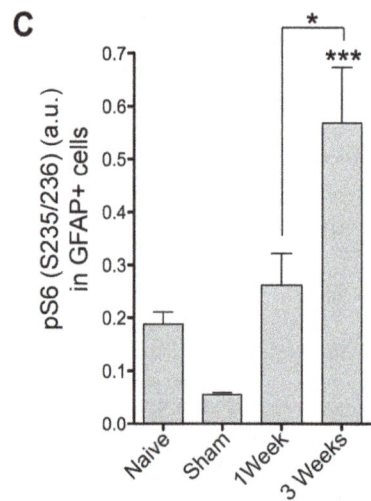

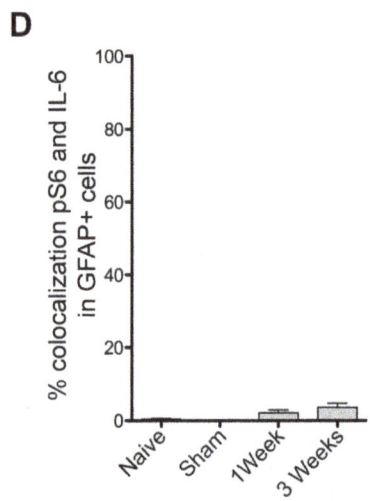

Figure 3. mTORC1 activity and IL-6 expression are negatively correlated in SCI. IL-6 expression in reactive astrocytes of the white matter returns to baseline three weeks after injury, at a time when mTORC1 activation peaks. **A**, Immunolabeling for pS6 (235/236) (green), IL-6 (magenta),

GFAP (blue), and DAPI (orange) in white matter of the caudal segment of spinal cords from naïve (I), sham (II) and injured animals 1 (III) and 3 (IV) weeks after injury. For all images, colocalization between IL-6 and pS6 is depicted in white. Scale bar=20 μM. **B**, Quantification of IL-6 immunofluorescence in GFAP+ astrocytes in white matter of the caudal segment of the spinal cord from naïve and sham animals and animals 1 and 3 weeks after injury. In each section IL-6 immunofluorescence is normalized to the total GFAP fluorescence signal. Data presented as mean ± SEM. ***p<0.001 and n.s. (not significant) for the comparison between sham and injured animals and ### p<0.01 for the comparison between 1 week and 3 weeks after injury by one-way ANOVA and Bonferroni's *post hoc* test (N=3 in each group). **C**, Quantification of pS6 immunofluorescence in GFAP+ astrocytes from the white matter of sections from the caudal segment of the spinal cord from naïve and sham animals and animals 1 and 3 weeks after injury. In each section, IL-6 immunofluorescence is normalized for the total GFAP fluorescence signal. Data are presented as mean ± SEM (N=3 in each group). ***p<0.001 for the comparison between sham and injured animals and * p<0.05 for the comparison between 1 week and 3 weeks injured animals by one-way ANOVA with Bonferroni's *post hoc* test. **D**, Quantification of IL-6 and pS6 colocalization in GFAP+ astrocytes from the white matter of sections from the caudal segment of the spinal cord from naïve, and sham and animals, and animals 1 and 3 weeks after injury.

mTORC1 Activity and IL-6 Expression are Negatively Correlated in SCI

Recent reports showed that PI3K and mTOR inhibition regulate IL-6 expression in immune cells [13,33]. Since mTORC1 is the main regulator of protein translation, we decided to examine if mTORC1 can regulate IL-6 expression in astrocytes following injury. As the mTORC1 activity readout, we measured the phosphorylation level of the downstream target ribosomal protein S6 by immunofluorescence in GFAP+ cells in tissue sections from spinal cord collected at 1 and 3 weeks after injury (Figure 3C). Interestingly, pS6 immunoreactivity negatively correlated with IL-6 expression in reactive astrocytes of the white matter. pS6 was low in astrocytes 1 week post-injury (0.26±0.06 a.u.), when IL-6 level was the highest (1.1±0.1 a.u.), and high at 3 weeks (0.57±0.1 a.u.), when IL-6 expression in astrocytes had returned to baseline (0.59±0.04 a.u.) (Figure 3B,C), suggesting that, *in vivo*, mTORC1 activity inhibits IL-6 expression. Moreover, no colocalization was detected between IL-6 and pS6 in GFAP+ astrocytes at any of the time points analyzed (Figure 3D).

The PI3K-mTOR Pathway Regulates IL-6 Expression in Cultured Spinal Cord Astrocytes

To increase understanding of the mechanisms that regulate IL-6 production in astrocytes, we used cultured astrocytes from adult rat spinal cord. More than 99% of these cells express astrocytic markers [21]. To avoid IL-6 induction, all experiments were performed with cultures incubated in growth factor free media (GF free). Noteworthy, the amino acids present in the media were sufficient to activate PI3K and both mTORC1 and mTORC2 (Figure 4C–D, GF free condition) [34].

We stimulated primary astrocytes with rapamycin for 8 hours and measured IL-6 mRNA by qPCR in order to determine if mTORC1 inhibition can also promote IL-6 expression. We found that rapamycin had no effect on IL-6 mRNA levels (Figure 4A–B). Even though rapamycin inhibits mTORC1, in astrocytes it also induces activation of mTORC2 as well as the PI3K downstream target pyruvate dehydrogenase kinase, isozyme 1 (PDK1), as shown by an increased phosphorylation of AKT at serine 473 (mTORC2 dependent) and threonine 308 (PDK1 dependent) (Figure 4C–D). Therefore, in order to inhibit both mTORC1 and mTORC2, we treated astrocytes with torin1 and torin2, two analogues that block the ATP binding site of mTOR [35,36]. Interestingly, both torin1 and torin2, at the concentration used (1 μM), inhibited mTORC1 and mTORC2, as well as AKT phosphorylation at threonine 300, suggesting inhibition of the PI3K-PDK1 pathway (Figure 4C–D and data now shown). Torin1 and torin2 treatment increased IL-6 mRNA, suggesting that the PI3K-mTOR pathway is a negative regulator of IL-6 expression in astrocytes (Figure 4A–B). Importantly, torin2 treatment did not show any cell toxicity, as no signs of cell death were observed by TUNEL assay or by detection of cleaved-caspase 3 by western blotting (Figure 4E–G).

NF-κB and p38 Mediate the Effect of PI3K-mTOR on IL-6 Expression

The transcription factor NF-κB is a strong inducer of IL-6 [10]; therefore, to determine if PI3K-mTOR inhibition induces IL-6 mRNA through NF-κB regulation, we transfected astrocytes with a plasmid containing the firefly luciferase gene under the control of either the wild type hIL-6 promoter (wt) or a hIL-6 promoter in which the binding site for NF-κB is mutated in order to prevent the binding of the transcription factor. It has been previously reported that both promoters are able to drive luciferase expression in the same way when stimulated by an NF-κB-independent stimulus [3,37]. The plasmids were co-transfected with the co-reporter vector pRL-TK. Astrocytes transfected with the wt hIL-6 promoter showed a strong induction of luciferase signal after torin2 treatment (472.9±97.1%), confirming that inhibition of PI3K-mTOR regulates IL-6 mRNA transcription (Figure 5A gray bars). The mutation of the NF-κB binding site reduced the luciferase signal to baseline (119.2±17.8%), indicating that NF-κB regulates IL-6 transcription (Figure 5A). These data indicate that the PI3K-mTOR pathway can regulate IL-6 transcription through modulation of NF-κB activity in astrocytes.

Previous work has shown that NF-κB activation requires phosphorylation and degradation of the inhibitory subunit IκB by the IκB kinase (IKK). MAPKs can regulate IL-6 mRNA expression via phosphorylation and activation of IKK. Once active, IKK acts by phosphorylating and degrading NF-κB inhibitory subunit IκB, resulting in NF-κB activation [11]. In order to examine if MAPKs activation is increased after PI3K-mTOR inhibition, we treated primary cultures of astrocytes with torin2 and blotted for the activated form of p38, ERK1/2, and JNK (Figure 5B). Astrocytes maintained in GF free media have a basal level of p38, ERK1/2, and JNK activation, and torin2 treatment increased p38 phosphorylation (355±40%) (Figure 5C), suggesting that NF-κB activation may result from increased p38 activation. In order to assess if p38 mediates the effect of PI3K-mTOR on IL-6 expression, we treated primary cultures with the p38 inhibitor SB203580 (Figure 5D), and found that SB203580 treatment blocked the IL-6 mRNA induction produced by torin2 treatment, suggesting that p38 can regulate IL-6 mRNA expression in astrocytes (Figure 5D).

PI3K-mTOR Inhibition and Increased Cytosolic Calcium are Necessary for IL-6 Secretion

We hypothesized that in order to induce IL-6 secretion in primary cultures of astrocytes, more than one of the molecular steps involved in regulation of cytokine production would have to be manipulated. Our data indicate that IL-6 expression in astrocytes can be induced by PI3K-mTOR inhibition by torin2 (Figure 4B). It has been previously reported that increased cytosolic Ca^{2+} through leaky RyRs in the ER promotes IL-6 secretion [19]. Interestingly, even though rapamycin is commonly used as an mTORC1 inhibitor, it functions by binding FKBP12, a

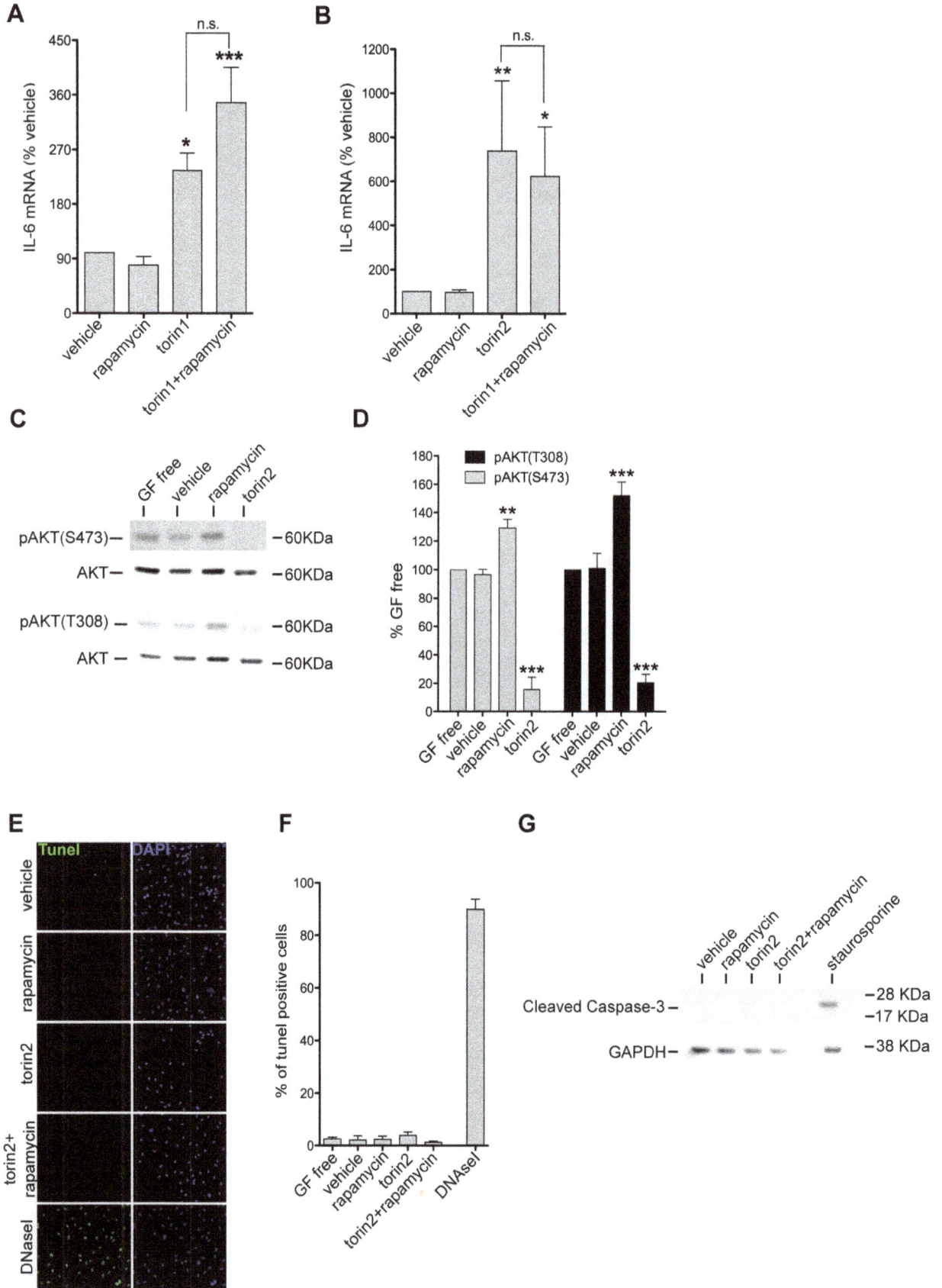

Figure 4. The PI3K-mTOR pathway regulates IL-6 expression in cultured spinal cord astrocytes. PI3K-mTOR inhibition with the ATP-competitive drugs, torin1 and torin2, inhibits AKT and induces IL-6 expression without increasing cell death in primary cultures of adult spinal cord

astrocytes. **A,** Torin1 and rapamycin effects on IL-6 mRNA expression quantified by qPCR and expressed as percentage of vehicle treated cells. Data presented as mean ± SEM. *p<0.05 and ***p<0.001 for the comparison between vehicle and torin1 or torin1+rapamycin treated cells and n.s. (not significant) for the comparison between torin1 and torin1+rapamycin treated cells by one-way ANOVA with Bonferroni's *post hoc* test (N = 4–5 per treatement). **B,** Torin2 and rapamycin effects on IL-6 mRNA expression quantified by qPCR and expressed as percentage of vehicle treated cells. Data presented as mean ± SEM. *p<0.05 and **p<0.01 for the comparison between vehicle and torin2 or torin2+rapamycin treated cells and n.s. (not significant) for the comparison between torin2 and torin2+rapamycin treated cells by one-way ANOVA with Bonferroni's *post hoc* test (N = 4–5 per treatement). **C,** Lysates from untreated cells (GF free) and cell treated with vehicle, rapamycin, and torin2 were probed by immunoblotting with the indicated antibodies. **D,** Optical densities of phospho-AKT serine 473 and threonine 308 bands normalized to levels of AKT in the lysates. Average levels of phospho-AKT serine 473 and phospho-AKT threonine 308 shown as percentage of GF free condition. Data are presented as mean ± SEM. ***p<0.001 and **p<0.01 for the comparison between vehicle and drug treated cells by one-way ANOVA with Bonferroni's *post hoc* test (N = 4–5 per treatement). **E,** Fragmented DNA labelled (tunel, green) in astrocytes treated with the indicated drugs or DNAseI as positive control. Astrocyte nuclei were visualized by DAPI (blue) staining. **F,** Numbers of tunel positive cells. **G,** Lysates from vehicle and cells treated with rapamycin, torin2, torin2+ rapamycin, and staurosporine probed by immunoblotting with cleaved caspase-3 antibody and GAPDH.

regulator of RyRs gating. Binding of rapamycin to FKBP12 results in increased open probability of RyRs and increased cytosolic Ca^{2+} concentration [15]. Hence, we induced IL-6 expression and affected RyRs by using a combined treatment of torin2 and rapamycin. We found that when astrocytes were treated with torin2/1+rapamycin, IL-6 was detected in the supernatant, but only when torin2 was used at 1 μM, the concentration at which also PI3K and PDK1-AKT pathways were inhibited (Figure 6A,C, 4B–C). Moreover, neither torin2 or rapamycin treatment alone was able to induce IL-6 protein secretion in the supernatant (Figure 6A), suggesting that in astrocytes an increase in gene expression and protein secretion are both necessary for IL-6 production. Noteworthy, IL-6 mRNA levels in torin1/2+rapamycin treated astrocytes were not statistically different from the increase caused by torin1/2 treatment alone, suggesting that the effect of rapamycin on IL-6 secretion is not caused by an enhanced IL-6 expression in the combined treatment (Fig. 4A–B).

To confirm that PI3K-mTOR inhibition is necessary for IL-6 secretion, we treated astrocytes with rapamycin together with the PI3K inhibitor LY294002 at a concentration of 30 μM, which is known to also inhibit mTOR [38]. Interestingly, LY294002+ rapamycin induced IL-6 secretion (1355±703%) at a level comparable to torin2+rapamycin treatment (1399±234%) (Figure 6B). Since torin2 treatment caused AKT inhibition in astrocytes (Figure 4C–D), we examined if AKT could be mediating the effect of PI3K-mTOR in IL-6 secretion. While the AKT inhibitor alone had no effect on IL-6 secretion, the combination with rapamycin strongly induced IL-6 in the supernatant (2576±1001%), indicating that AKT mediates the PI3K-mTOR effect on IL-6 secretion (Figure 6B). To confirm that the effect of rapamycin on IL-6 secretion was independent from its inhibitory function on mTORC1, but depended on its regulation of RyRs permeability and cytosolic Ca^{2+} concentration, we treated cells with FK506 (Figure 6C). FK506 is a potent immunosuppressant that forms a drug-immunophilin complex with FKBP12, displacing it from the RyRs [15]. However, the FK506-FKBP12 complex is not able to interact and inhibit mTOR, and thus is often used as a control to monitor mTOR-independent rapamycin effects [39]. IL-6 secretion in astrocytes was not affected by treatment with FK506 (Figure 6C); however, FK506 in combination with torin2 caused a strong secretion of IL-6 (Figure 6C), confirming that IL-6 secretion depends on RyRs. In order to determine whether IL-6 secretion caused by torin2+rapamycin treatment was Ca^{2+} dependent, we pre-treated cell cultures for 30 minutes with the Ca^{2+} chelator BAPTA-AM before incubation with torin2+rapamycin. Pre-treatment with BAPTA-AM inhibited IL-6 secretion, indicating that Ca^{2+} is required for IL-6 secretion (torin2+rapamycin 1975±472% and bapta+torin2+rapamycin 484±137%) (Figure 6D). To assess if the torin2+rapamycin treatment could affect ER Ca^{2+}, we performed Ca^{2+} imaging of

drug-treated primary cultures loaded with the ratiometric dye Fura-2. To evaluate ER Ca^{2+} content, we treated primary cultures of astrocytes with the RyRs agonist 4-chloro-*m*-cresol (4-cmc) in Ca^{2+}-free conditions, to avoid Ca^{2+} influx from the media [40]. Bath application of 4-cmc resulted in a rapid transient Ca^{2+} increase (peak 0.80±0.01 a.u., AUC 72±2 a.u.), followed by elevated intracellular Ca^{2+} levels (Figure 6D,E). The amplitude of this Ca^{2+} response is a measure of the Ca^{2+} stored in the ER. Stimulation with rapamycin increased the transient response (Figure 6D,E(I)) (peak 0.86±0.01 a.u.), in agreement with previous data reporting that rapamycin increases RyRs open probability without affecting the amount of Ca^{2+} stored in the ER (AUC 79±3 a.u.) [41]. Importantly, torin2 treatment caused a reduction of the peak induced by 4-cmc (Figure 6D,E(I)) (peak 0.765±0.008 a.u.), suggesting a depletion of Ca^{2+} in the ER. Stimulation of torin2+rapamycin treated astrocytes resulted in a significantly smaller peak delayed in time (peak 0.63±0.01 a.u.) (Figure 6D,E(I)). Moreover, both torin2 (AUC 53±4 a.u.) and torin2+rapamycin (AUC 36±2 a.u.) treatment also caused a decrease of the area under the curve suggesting a decrease in ER Ca^{2+} content or RyR expression (Figure 6D,E(II)).

Combined Treatment with Torin2 and Rapamycin has a Small Temporary Effect on Mechanical Hypersensitivity

In order to examine if torin2+rapamycin treatment has a positive effect on recovery from SCI, we treated injured animals daily from day 15 to day 29 after injury with torin2 alone or in combination with rapamycin. At this post-injury period the glia scar was already mature and the endogenous IL-6 expression of IL-6 was the same as sham animals. Even though both torin1 and torin2 strongly inhibit mTOR, we decided to use torin2 because it has a lower EC50, better bioavailability, and because we could develop a special formulation designed to enable oral administration of the drug [36]. Torin2 treatment alone did not have any effect on mechanical hypersensitivity or locomotion (Figure 7A,B). In contrast, dual treatment with torin2 and rapamycin had a small temporary effect on mechanical hypersensitivity during the treatment window (Figure 7A), thus indicating a beneficial role of the treatment.

Discussion

Spinal cord astrocytes respond to injury by forming a scar that protects the healthy tissue and inhibits regeneration. Therefore, the induction of regeneration promoting factors, such as IL-6 in reactive astrocytes, may be beneficial for recovery after injury. We found that SCI induces IL-6 in reactive astrocytes and that IL-6 levels decrease concomitantly with maturation of the glial scar. We show that IL-6 production by astrocytes requires inhibition of the PI3K-mTOR pathway, together with increased cytosolic Ca^{2+}

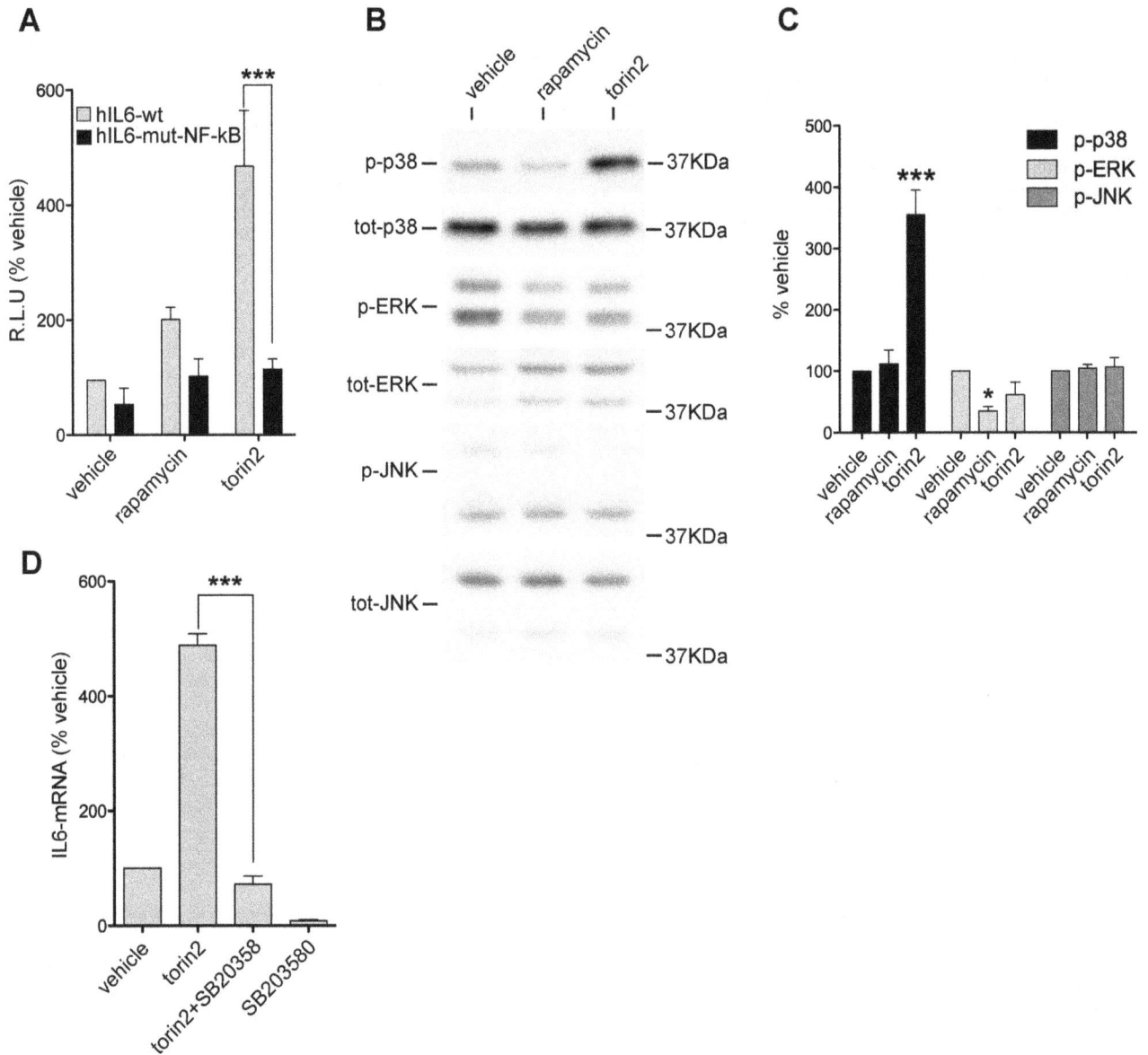

Figure 5. NF-κB and MAPKs mediate the effect of PI3K-mTOR on IL-6 expression. Astrocytes treated with torin2 have elevated MAPK signaling and express IL-6 in a NF-κB dependent manner. **A,** Bar graph showing luciferase activity (relative luciferase units R.L.U) expressed as percentage of luciferase activity in vehicle treated cells. The grey bars represent astrocytes transfected with a plasmid in which wild type hIL-6 promoter (hIL6-wt) drives luciferase expression. The black bars represent cells transfected with a plasmid in which a hIL-6 promoter with a mutated NF-κB binding site drives luciferase expression (hIL6-mut-NF-κB). Data are presented as mean ± SEM. ***p<0.001 for the comparison between wt and mut-NF-κB transfected astrocytes by two-way ANOVA with Bonferroni's *post hoc* test (N = 3 per treatement). **B,** Lysates from vehicle, rapamycin, and torin2 treated cells probed by immunoblotting with antibodies for phosphorylated and not phosphorylated forms of p38, ERK, and JNK. **C,** Optical densities of the phospho-protein bands were normalized to the levels of the corresponding not phosphorylated proteins in the lysates and expressed as percentage of vehicle treated cells. Average levels of phospho-ERK, phospho-JNK, and phospho-p38 shown as mean ± SEM. ***p<0.001 and *p<0.05 for the comparison between vehicle and drug treated cells by one-way ANOVA with Bonferroni's *post hoc* test (N = 3 per treatement). **D,** IL-6 mRNA expression quantified by real-time quantitative PCR and expressed as a percentage of expression in vehicle treated cells. Data are presented as mean ± SEM. ***p<0.001, for the comparison between torin2 and torin2+SB20358 treated cells by one-way ANOVA with Bonferroni's *post hoc* test (N = 4–5 per treatement).

concentration. Regulation of these pathways is achieved by treating astrocytes with the PI3K-mTOR inhibitor torin2 together with the RyRs opening facilitator, rapamycin. To determine if torin2+rapamycin treatment is beneficial for recovery, we treated injured animals when the scar had already been formed. Treated animals showed a temporary improvement of mechanical hypersensitivity limited to the drug treatment period.

In order to determine the time course of IL-6 induction after SCI, we measured cytokine levels in plasma and spinal cords from injured rats. In agreement with previous reports [42], we detected increased IL-6 levels in both plasma and spinal cord parenchyma. Interestingly, even though plasma levels returned to baseline one week after injury, spinal cord IL-6 levels remained elevated. Using *in situ* hybridization, we found that astrocytes, neurons and

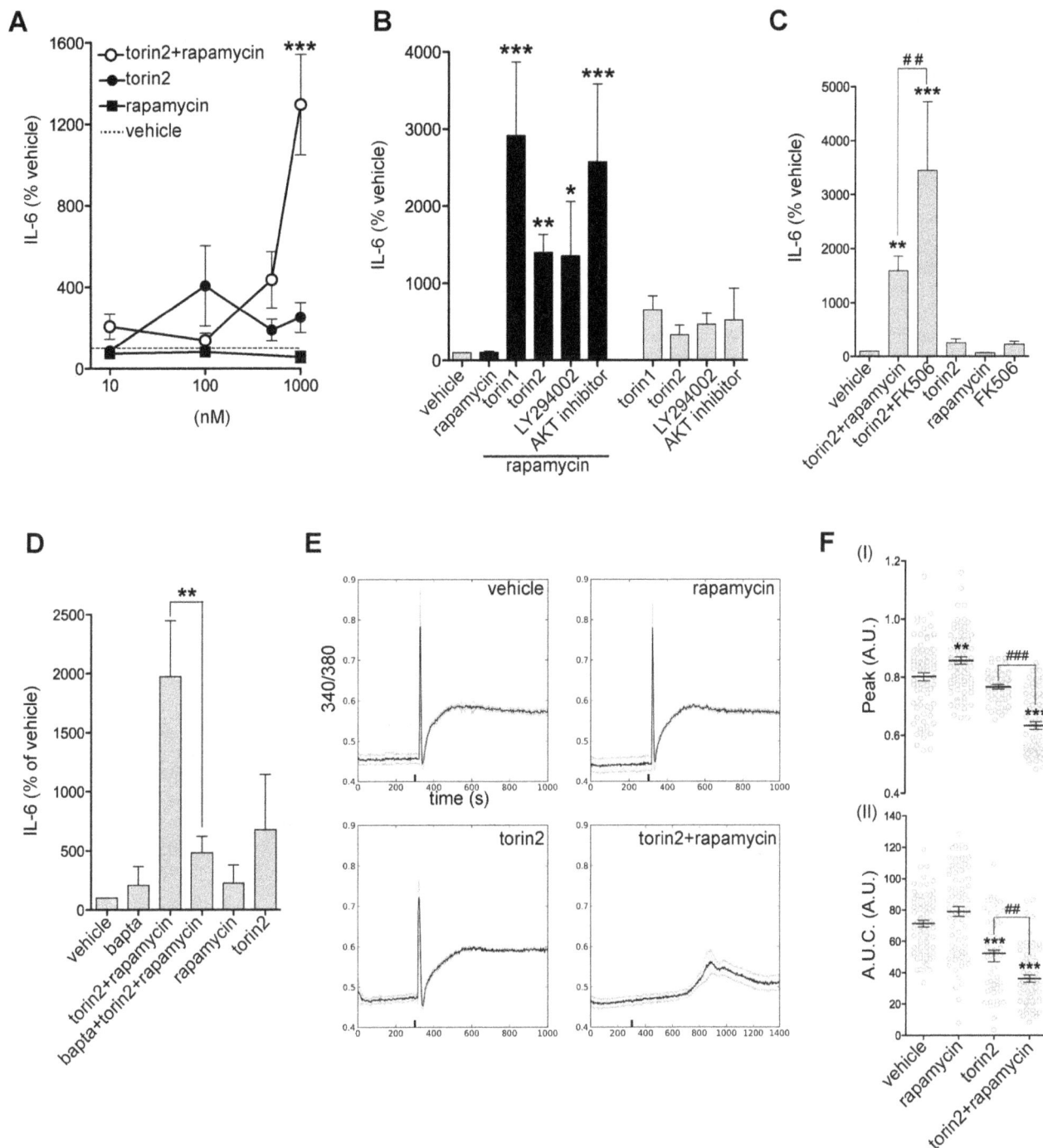

Figure 6. PI3K-mTOR inhibition and increased cytosolic calcium are necessary for IL-6 secretion. Combined treatment with torin2 and rapamycin induces IL-6 secretion by astrocytes as a result of PI3K-mTOR-AKT inhibition and increased intracellular calcium. **A**, Dose-response curve for rapamycin, torin2, and torin2+rapamycin treatments. IL-6 protein secretion in the supernatant was measured from cultures of astrocytes incubated with increasing concentrations (10 nM-1 μM) of torin2 or rapamycin alone or torin2 in combination with rapamycin (100 nM) (N = 3–7). ***p<0.001 for the comparison between torin2 (1 μM) and torin2 (1 μM)+rapamycin (100 nM) by one-way ANOVA with Bonferroni's *post hoc* test. **B**, IL-6 protein levels in the supernatant of astrocyte cultures treated for 24 hours with vehicle, rapamycin, torin1, torin2, LY294002, and AKT inhibitor alone or in combination with rapamycin. Mean and SEM (N = 4 12 per treatement). *p<0.05, **p<0.01 and ***p<0.001 for the comparison between drug treated cells by one-way ANOVA with Bonferroni's *post hoc* tests. **C**, IL-6 levels in the supernatant for cells treated with torin2, torin2+ rapamycin, torin2+ FK506, rapamycin, and FK506 (N = 3). **p<0.01 and ***p<0.001 for comparison between drug treated cells and vehicle and ##p<0.01 for the comparison torin2+rapamycin and torin2+FK506 by one-way ANOVA with Bonferroni's *post hoc* tests. **D**, IL-6 protein levels in the supernatant of astrocyte cultures treated for 24 hours with vehicle, rapamycin, torin2, and rapamycin+torin2 with or without bapta-1am pre-treatment, expressed as percentage of levels in vehicle treated cells (N = 4 per treatement). **p<0.01 comparison between torin2+rapamycin and torin2+rapamycin+bapta treated cells by one-way ANOVA with Bonferroni's *post hoc* tests. **E**, Representative Fura-2 calcium traces of 4-cmc treated cultures. Before stimulation cells were incubated 24 hours with vehicle, rapamycin, torin2, or torin2+rapamycin. The black bar at 300 (s) indicates the time of 4-cmc stimulation. Grey traces show the SEM of the response of all the cells analyzed in the experiment and the black trace corresponds to the average response. The

torin2+rapamycin graph shows a longer time scale to highlight the delay in the response (n = 49–78 cells per condition in a total of N = 3 experiments). **F**, Quantification of response (I) and area under the curve (A.U.C) (II) after stimulation with 4-cmc (n = 49–78 cells per condition in N = 3 experiments). **p<0.01 and ***p<0.001 for the comparison between torin2 and torin2+rapamycin with vehicle treated astrocytes. ###p<0.001 and ##p<0.01 for the comparison between torin2 and torin2+rapamycin treated cells by one-way ANOVA with Bonferroni's *post hoc* tests.

microglia/macrophages are positive for IL-6 mRNA even though there is no circulating IL-6, indicating that these cells are the local producers of IL-6 in the phase following the first reaction to injury. Thus, given that IL-6 can be produced by different cells at different time points and the levels can be elevated either systemically or only locally, it is plausible that IL-6 plays different roles in pathology and repair depending on the time frame and localization of expression. Importantly, spinal cord expression of IL-6 returns to baseline once the scar is mature three weeks after injury, and thus any positive effect of IL-6 on axonal regeneration would no longer be in place. Hence, one strategy to promote recovery after SCI even after the formation of a glial scar would be to drive continued release of IL-6 to enhance IL-6-mediated positive effect on regeneration. However, this requires an understanding of the molecular mechanisms that regulate expression and release of IL-6 by astrocytes.

The PI3K-mTOR pathway is one regulatory element for expression of inflammatory cytokines in immune cells [43], and here we showed that it inhibits IL-6 expression in astrocytes. PI3K-mTOR signaling converges on AKT, and it has been demonstrated that active AKT has an inhibitory impact on inflammatory genes in immune cells [44]. The negative impact on cytokine production by AKT is mediated by inhibition of p38 and/or NF-κB activity [45,46]. Astrocytes treated with the PI3K-mTOR inhibitor, torin2, have decreased AKT activity and increased MAPKs and NF-κB activities. Interestingly, it has been reported that p38 not only drives transcription of IL-6 by promoting NF-κB activity, but also stabilizes IL-6 mRNA [47]. Our data show that in astrocytes the IL-6 mRNA level is regulated by p38 and NF-κB activities with a molecular mechanism similar to what has been previously reported for immune cells. Even though PI3K-mTOR inhibition with torin2 increases IL-6 mRNA in astrocytes, we show that IL-6 protein is not secreted in drug-treated cultures. The lack of IL-6 in the supernatant may result

from inhibition of mRNA translation or lack of activation of secretory pathways. It has recently been shown that soluble cytokines like IL-6 are synthesized in the ER, transferred to the Golgi, and then collected in small secretory vesicles that release their cargo upon stimulation by fusing with the plasma membrane [9]. Though not studied in astrocytes, Ca^{2+} buffering in mast cells completely blocks IL-6 secretion [48]. Interestingly, when we stimulated astrocytes with rapamycin or FK506, compounds, which normally increase open probability and leakage from RYRs on the ER, no increase in IL-6 secretion was found. However, when the treatment was combined with PI3K-mTOR inhibitors, IL-6 levels were readily detectable in the supernatant of astrocyte cultures. This finding demonstrates that IL-6 secretion in astrocytes requires both mRNA production and increased intracellular Ca^{2+}. Additionally, comparing FK506 and rapamycin showed that FK506, in combination with torin2, is a stronger inducer of IL-6. This may be explained by the ability of FK506 to interact with calcineurin, releasing the inhibition of $InsP_3R$ in the ER, which can result in higher intracellular Ca^{2+} and therefore a stronger promotion of IL-6 secretion [16,17].

When astrocytes are stimulated with the RyRs agonist 4-cmc, they release Ca^{2+} from the ER. We found that 4-cmc stimulation of rapamycin-treated astrocytes induced a greater response, compared to vehicle treated cells, thus confirming that rapamycin can potentiate the effects of 4-cmc by increasing the open probability of RyRs. Furthermore, 4-cmc stimulation of torin2 treated astrocytes induced a smaller response compared to vehicle. We hypothesize that torin2 treatment caused a depletion of Ca^{2+} stored in the ER, and therefore not only reduced the response to 4-cmc but also increased the cytosolic Ca^{2+} concentration. However, we suggest that the increased cytosolic Ca^{2+} concentration was not enough to induce RyRs opening via a Ca^{2+}-induced Ca^{2+}-release mechanism, because torin2-treated cells still responded to 4-cmc stimulation. Additionally, the torin2-induced increase in cytosolic

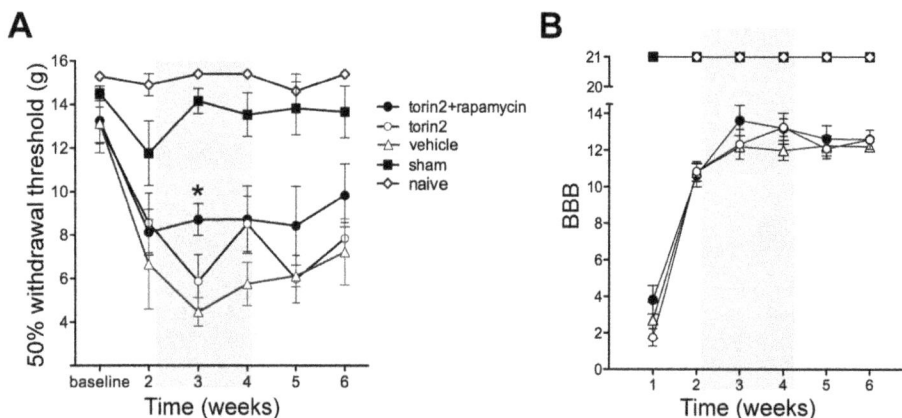

Figure 7. Combined treatment with torin2 and rapamycin improves mechanical hypersensitivity during treatment. Mechanical hypersensitivity and locomotion of injured animals assessed for 6 weeks after contusion using von Frey filaments and the BBB scale, respectively. The gray highlighted region represents the treatment period. **A,** Mechanical hypersensitivity expressed as changes in 50% withdrawal threshold (g) over time. Repeated measures two way-anova show a significant effect of torin2+rapamycin (p<0.05) in the treatment window. Using bonferroni post-test correction for multiple comparisons showed that torin2+rapamycin significantly reversed SCI-induced mechanical hypersensitivity at week three. (*p<0.05). **B,** Hindlimb locomotor function assessed by the BBB locomotor rating scale. (Naïve = 4, sham N = 6, pbs N = 6, torin2 N = 6, torin2+rapamycin N = 8).

Ca^{2+} concentration is not enough to induce IL-6 secretion. However, when rapamycin is added to torin2, the leakiness of RyRs is increased and the cells do not respond to 4-cmc stimulation. We suggest that the increase in cytosolic Ca^{2+} concentrations induced by torin2, in presence of rapamycin, is sufficient to cause the opening of the RyRs, thus depleting the ER from Ca^{2+} and inducing fusion of the IL-6 containing vesicles with the plasma membrane (hypothesis depicted in Figure S3). However, additional work is required in order to verify this hypothesis.

Our data show that IL-6 secretion from astrocytes requires PI3K-mTOR inhibition, and suggests that IL-6 mRNA is translated even when mTOR, the master controller of protein synthesis, is inhibited. mTOR has been shown to regulate CAP-dependent translation of transcripts with oligopyrimidine (TOP/TOP-like) motifs in the 5′-untranslated region (5′-UTR) [49]. The IL-6 5′-UTR does not match the characteristics of TOP/TOP-like mRNAs, when the classification criteria illustrated by Thoreen and co-workers are applied [50], suggesting CAP-independent translation. Interestingly, translation of stress-related proteins is also inhibited by the PI3K-mTOR pathway and is regulated through a non-well characterized CAP-independent mechanism [51].

Our data show that reactive astrocytes expressing IL-6 have a low mTOR activity, and three weeks after injury, when IL-6 level return to baseline, there is a concomitant increase in mTOR activity. An important implication of our findings is that by using torin2 and rapamycin, which block the PI3K-mTOR pathway and increases intracellular Ca^{2+} concentrations, it is possible to induce IL-6 release in reactive astrocytes. In light of the ability of IL-6 to promote axonal regeneration [52,53], these drugs have the potential to contribute to recovery after SCI. We tested this hypothesis by treating rats subjected to SCI with torin2+rapamycin for two weeks starting two weeks after injury. The role of IL-6 in pain transmission is somewhat controversial and there are only a few reports on the role of IL-6 in pain induced by SCI [54]. We found a transient reversal in hypersensitivity during the period of drug administration. However, because the drugs were administered systemically we cannot exclude that the positive effect of treatment was mediated through regulation of other factors or cell types. Further studies are required in order to determine this in detail. However, the positive effect noted during the treatment window suggests that a prolonged or chronic treatment might be more beneficial after SCI. However, recent studies suggest that chronic treatment with mTOR inhibitors like rapamycin may lead to insulin resistance [55,56]. However, a longer period of treatment may be enough to promote a more sustained reversal of mechanical hypersensitivity. Additional studies are necessary in order to determine the optimal treatment regiment.

In summary, we identified the PI3K-mTOR-Ca^{2+} pathway as the molecular mechanism that regulates IL-6 expression and secretion by astrocytes. We also identified that the combination of torin2 and rapamycin may have beneficial effects on sensory recovery after spinal cord injury, opening new possibilities for the development of a therapy.

Supporting Information

Figure S1 Control *in situ* hybridization with IL-6 sense mRNA probe. A, Cartoon depicting: (I) the 7 mm long segments (rostral, caudal, epicenter) in which the injured spinal cord is dissected for analysis. (II) Regions of the spinal cord sections imaged. Dorsal horn (DH), dorsal column (DC), central canal (CC), white matter (WM) and ventral horn (VH). **B**, IL-6 *in situ* hybridization with sense IL-6 mRNA probe on sections from rostral, caudal, and epicenter segments from spinal cord of naive and injured animals 6 hours, 1, and 2 weeks post-injury. Scale bar = 200 μm. **C**, High magnification images from sections of the caudal segment shown in B from naive (20X) and 1 week injured spinal cord animals (20X and 40X). Scale bar = 20 μm for 20X and 40X. (N = 3 in each group)

Figure S2 IL-6 is not expressed by immune cells in white and gray matter. A, Immunolabeling of IL-6 (green) and the microglia/macrophage marker OX-42 (magenta) of the white matter of the caudal segment from spinal cords 1 week after injury. **B**, Immunolabeling of IL-6 (green) and the microglia/macrophage ED1 (magenta) of the white matter of the caudal segment from spinal cords 1 week after injury. Scale bar = 20 μm. (N = 3 in each group)

Figure S3 Cartoon depicting the mechanism that regulates IL-6 secretion in astrocytes. A, An astrocyte in naïve condition where PI3K-mTOR-AKT pathway is activated and inhibits IL-6 expression. **B**, Inhibition of the PI3K-mTOR-AKT pathway results in p38 activation and NF-κB-mediated transcription of IL-6. Torin2 treatment also decreases ER Ca^{2+} content suggesting an increase of Ca^{2+} concentration in the cytosol. However, the increase is not sufficient to cause IL-6 secretion. **C**, A torin2 induced increase in cytosolic Ca^{2+} concentration is sufficient to cause opening of the RyR2 when rapamycin is also present in the cell. This causes a higher increase in Ca^{2+} concentration in the cytoplasm that is sufficient to induce IL-6 secretion.

Acknowledgments

The authors thank D. M. Sabatini, M. Laplante and G. Coppotelli for helpful comments on the manuscript.

Author Contributions

Conceived and designed the experiments: SC CIS. Performed the experiments: SC TFZ JK MA KS. Analyzed the data: SC CIS MA KS JK TFZ. Contributed reagents/materials/analysis tools: QL NSG LO PU. Wrote the paper: SC.

References

1. Silver J, Miller JII (2004) Regeneration beyond the glial scar. Nature Reviews Neuroscience 5: 146–156.
2. Schwartz M, Moalem G, Leibowitz-Amit R, Cohen I (1999) Innate and adaptive immune responses can be beneficial for CNS repair. Trends in Neurosciences 22: 295–299.
3. Rolls A, Shechter R, Schwartz M (2009) The bright side of the glial scar in CNS repair. Nature Reviews Neuroscience 10: 235–241.
4. Stammers AT, Liu J, Kwon BK (2011) Expression of inflammatory cytokines following acute spinal cord injury in a rodent model. Journal of Neuroscience Research 90: 782–790.
5. Pineau I, Lacroix S (2006) Proinflammatory cytokine synthesis in the injured mouse spinal cord: Multiphasic expression pattern and identification of the cell types involved. The Journal of Comparative Neurology 500: 267–285.
6. Okada S, Nakamura M, Renault-Mihara F, Mukaino M, Saiwai H, et al. (2008) The role of cytokine signaling in pathophysiology for spinal cord injury. Inflammation and Regeneration 28: 440–446.
7. Yang P, Wen H, Ou S, Cui J, Fan D (2012) IL-6 promotes regeneration and functional recovery after cortical spinal tract injury by reactivating intrinsic growth program of neurons and enhancing synapse formation. Experimental Neurology 236: 19–27.

8. Klusman I, Schwab ME (1997) Effects of pro-inflammatory cytokines in experimental spinal cord injury. Brain Research 762: 173–184.

9. Stanley AC, Lacy P (2010) Pathways for Cytokine Secretion. Physiology 25: 218–229.

10. Keller ET, Wanagat J, Ershler WB (1996) Molecular and cellular biology of interleukin-6 and its receptor. Frontiers in bioscience: a journal and virtual library 1: d340–357.

11. Oeckinghaus A, Hayden MS, Ghosh S (2011) Crosstalk in NF-κB signaling pathways. Nature Immunology 12: 695–708.

12. Craig R (2000) p38 MAPK and NF-kappa B Collaborate to Induce Interleukin-6 Gene Expression and Release. Evidence for a cytoprotective autocrine signaling pathway in a cardiac myocyte model system. Journal of Biological Chemistry 275: 23814–23824.

13. Powell JD, Pollizzi KN, Heikamp EB, Horton MR (2012) Regulation of Immune Responses by mTOR. Annual Review of Immunology 30: 39–68.

14. Parpura V, Baker BJ, Jeras M, Zorec R (2010) Regulated exocytosis in astrocytic signal integration. Neurochemistry International 57: 451–459.

15. Snyder SH, Lai MM, Burnett PE (1998) Immunophilins in the nervous system. Neuron 21: 283–294.

16. Cameron AM, Steiner JP, Sabatini DM, Kaplin AI, Walensky LD, et al. (1995) Immunophilin FK506 binding protein associated with inositol 1,4,5-trisphosphate receptor modulates calcium flux. Proceedings of the National Academy of Sciences of the United States of America 92: 1784–1788.

17. MacMillan D, Currie S, Bradley KN, Muir TC, McCarron JG (2005) In smooth muscle, FK506-binding protein modulates IP3 receptor-evoked Ca2+ release by mTOR and calcineurin. Journal of Cell Science 118: 5443–5451.

18. Kang CB, Hong Y, Dhe-Paganon S, Yoon HS (2008) FKBP Family Proteins: Immunophilins with Versatile Biological Functions. Neurosignals 16: 318–325.

19. Ducreux S (2004) Effect of Ryanodine Receptor Mutations on Interleukin-6 Release and Intracellular Calcium Homeostasis in Human Myotubes from Malignant Hyperthermia-susceptible Individuals and Patients Affected by Central Core Disease. Journal of Biological Chemistry 279: 43838–43846.

20. Benveniste EN, Sparacio SM, Norris JG, Grenett HE, Fuller GM (1990) Induction and regulation of interleukin-6 gene expression in rat astrocytes. Journal of neuroimmunology 30: 201–212.

21. Codeluppi S, Gregory EN, Kjell J, Wigerblad G, Olson L, et al. (2011) Influence of rat substrain and growth conditions on the characteristics of primary cultures of adult rat spinal cord astrocytes. Journal of neuroscience methods 197: 118–127.

22. Widenfalk J, Lundströmer K, Jubran M, Brene S, Olson L (2001) Neurotrophic factors and receptors in the immature and adult spinal cord after mechanical injury or kainic acid. The Journal of neuroscience : the official journal of the Society for Neuroscience 21: 3457–3475.

23. Basso DM, Beattie MS, Bresnahan JC (1996) Graded histological and locomotor outcomes after spinal cord contusion using the NYU weight-drop device versus transection. Experimental Neurology 139: 244–256.

24. Dixon WJ (1980) Efficient analysis of experimental observations. Annual review of pharmacology and toxicology 20: 441–462.

25. Chaplan SR, Bach FW, Pogrel JW, Chung JM, Yaksh TL (1994) Quantitative assessment of tactile allodynia in the rat paw. Journal of neuroscience methods 53: 55–63.

26. Zhu XL, Pacheco ND, Dick EJ, Rollwagen FM (1999) Differentially increased IL-6 mRNA expression in liver and spleen following injection of liposome-encapsulated haemoglobin. CYTOKINE 11: 696–703.

27. Schindelin J, Arganda-Carreras I, Frise E, Kaynig V, Longair M, et al. (2012) Fiji: an open-source platform for biological-image analysis. Nature Methods 9: 676–682.

28. Boyle DL, Rosengren S, Bugbee W, Kavanaugh A, Firestein GS (2003) Quantitative biomarker analysis of synovial gene expression by real-time PCR. Arthritis research & therapy 5: R352–360.

29. Ljosa V, Carpenter AE (2009) Introduction to the quantitative analysis of two-dimensional fluorescence microscopy images for cell-based screening. PLoS computational biology 5: e1000603.

30. Onifer SM, Rabchevsky AG, Scheff SW (2007) Rat models of traumatic spinal cord injury to assess motor recovery. ILAR journal/National Research Council, Institute of Laboratory Animal Resources 48: 385–395.

31. Renault-Mihara F, Okada S, Shibata S, Nakamura M, Toyama Y, et al. (2008) Spinal cord injury: Emerging beneficial role of reactive astrocytes' migration. The International Journal of Biochemistry & Cell Biology 40: 1649–1653.

32. Okada S, Nakamura M, Saiwai H, Kumamaru H, Toyama Y, et al. (2009) Physiological significance of astrogliosis after CNS injury. Inflammation and Regeneration: 1–5.

33. Luyendyk JP, Schabbauer GA, Tencati M, Holscher T, Pawlinski R, et al. (2008) Genetic analysis of the role of the PI3K-Akt pathway in lipopolysaccharide-induced cytokine and tissue factor gene expression in monocytes/macrophages. Journal of immunology (Baltimore, Md : 1950) 180: 4218–4226.

34. Tato I, Bartrons R, Ventura F, Rosa JL (2011) Amino Acids Activate Mammalian Target of Rapamycin Complex 2 (mTORC2) via PI3K/Akt Signaling. Journal of Biological Chemistry 286: 6128–6142.

35. Thoreen CC, Kang SA, Chang JW, Liu Q, Zhang J, et al. (2009) An ATP-competitive mammalian target of rapamycin inhibitor reveals rapamycin-resistant functions of mTORC1. The Journal of biological chemistry 284: 8023–8032.

36. Liu Q, Wang J, Kang SA, Thoreen CC, Hur W, et al. (2011) Discovery of 9-(6-Aminopyridin-3-yl)-1-(3-(trifluoromethyl)phenyl)benzo[h][1,6]naphthyridin-2(1 H)-one (Torin2) as a Potent, Selective, and Orally Available Mammalian Target of Rapamycin (mTOR) Inhibitor for Treatment of Cancer. Journal of Medicinal Chemistry 54: 1473–1480.

37. Vanden Berghe W, De Bosscher K, Boone E, Plaisance S, Haegeman G (1999) The nuclear factor-kappaB engages CBP/p300 and histone acetyltransferase activity for transcriptional activation of the interleukin-6 gene promoter. The Journal of biological chemistry 274: 32091–32098.

38. Brunn GJ, Williams J, Sabers C, Wiederrecht G, Lawrence JC, et al. (1996) Direct inhibition of the signaling functions of the mammalian target of rapamycin by the phosphoinositide 3-kinase inhibitors, wortmannin and LY294002. The EMBO Journal 15: 5256–5267.

39. Sabatini DM, Erdjument-Bromage H, Lui M, Tempst P, Snyder SH (1994) RAFT1: a mammalian protein that binds to FKBP12 in a rapamycin-dependent fashion and is homologous to yeast TORs. Cell 78: 35–43.

40. Matyash M (2001) Requirement of functional ryanodine receptor type 3 for astrocyte migration. The FASEB Journal.

41. MacMillan D, McCarron JG (2009) Regulation by FK506 and rapamycin of Ca2+ release from the sarcoplasmic reticulum in vascular smooth muscle: the role of FK506 binding proteins and mTOR. British journal of pharmacology 158: 1112–1120.

42. David S, Kroner A (2011) Repertoire of microglial and macrophage responses after spinal cord injury. Nature Reviews Neuroscience 12: 388–399.

43. Weichhart T, Haidinger M, Katholnig K, Kopecky C, Poglitsch M, et al. (2011) Inhibition of mTOR blocks the anti-inflammatory effects of glucocorticoids in myeloid immune cells. Blood 117: 4273–4283.

44. Guha M, Mackman N (2002) The PI3K-Akt pathway limits LPS activation of signaling pathways and expression of inflammatory mediators in human monocytic cells. The Journal of biological chemistry.

45. Blum S, Issbrüker K, Willuweit A, Hehlgans S, Lucerna M, et al. (2001) An inhibitory role of the phosphatidylinositol 3-kinase-signaling pathway in vascular endothelial growth factor-induced tissue factor expression. The Journal of biological chemistry 276: 33428–33434.

46. Gratton JP, Morales-Ruiz M, Kureishi Y, Fulton D, Walsh K, et al. (2001) Akt down-regulation of p38 signaling provides a novel mechanism of vascular endothelial growth factor-mediated cytoprotection in endothelial cells. The Journal of biological chemistry 276: 30359–30365.

47. Zhao W, Liu M, Kirkwood KL (2008) p38alpha stabilizes interleukin-6 mRNA via multiple AU-rich elements. The Journal of biological chemistry 283: 1778–1785.

48. Jeong H-J, Hong S-H, Lee D-J, Park J-H, Kim K-S, et al. (2002) Role of Ca(2+) on TNF-alpha and IL-6 secretion from RBL-2H3 mast cells. Cellular Signalling 14: 633–639.

49. Ma XM, Blenis J (2009) Molecular mechanisms of mTOR-mediated translational control. Nature Reviews Molecular Cell Biology 10: 307–318.

50. Thoreen CC, Chantranupong L, Keys HR, Wang T, Gray NS, et al. (2012) A unifying model for mTORC1-mediated regulation of mRNA translation. Nature 485: 109–113.

51. Sun J, Conn CS, Han Y, Yeung V, Qian S-B (2011) PI3K-mTORC1 attenuates stress response by inhibiting cap-independent Hsp70 translation. Journal of Biological Chemistry 286: 6791–6800.

52. Hirota H, Kiyama H, Kishimoto T, Taga T (1996) Accelerated Nerve Regeneration in Mice by upregulated expression of interleukin (IL) 6 and IL-6 receptor after trauma. The Journal of experimental medicine 183: 2627–2634.

53. Cafferty WBJ (2004) Conditioning Injury-Induced Spinal Axon Regeneration Fails in Interleukin-6 Knock-Out Mice. The Journal of neuroscience : the official journal of the Society for Neuroscience 24: 4432–4443.

54. Guptarak J, Wanchoo S, Durham-Lee J, Wu Y, Zivadinovic D, et al. (2013) Inhibition of IL-6 signaling: A novel therapeutic approach to treating spinal cord injury pain. PAIN.

55. Cunningham JT, Rodgers JT, Arlow DH, Vazquez F, Mootha VK, et al. (2007) mTOR controls mitochondrial oxidative function through a YY1-PGC-1α transcriptional complex. Nature 450: 736–740.

56. Lamming DW, Ye L, Katajisto P, Goncalves MD, Saitoh M, et al. (2012) Rapamycin-induced insulin resistance is mediated by mTORC2 loss and uncoupled from longevity. Science 335: 1638–1643.

15

Persistent At-Level Thermal Hyperalgesia and Tactile Allodynia Accompany Chronic Neuronal and Astrocyte Activation in Superficial Dorsal Horn following Mouse Cervical Contusion Spinal Cord Injury

Jaime L. Watson, Tamara J. Hala, Rajarshi Putatunda, Daniel Sannie, Angelo C. Lepore*

Department of Neuroscience, Farber Institute for Neurosciences, Sidney Kimmel Medical College at Thomas Jefferson University, Philadelphia, Pennsylvania, United States of America

Abstract

In humans, sensory abnormalities, including neuropathic pain, often result from traumatic spinal cord injury (SCI). SCI can induce cellular changes in the CNS, termed central sensitization, that alter excitability of spinal cord neurons, including those in the dorsal horn involved in pain transmission. Persistently elevated levels of neuronal activity, glial activation, and glutamatergic transmission are thought to contribute to the hyperexcitability of these dorsal horn neurons, which can lead to maladaptive circuitry, aberrant pain processing and, ultimately, chronic neuropathic pain. Here we present a mouse model of SCI-induced neuropathic pain that exhibits a persistent pain phenotype accompanied by chronic neuronal hyperexcitability and glial activation in the spinal cord dorsal horn. We generated a unilateral cervical contusion injury at the C5 or C6 level of the adult mouse spinal cord. Following injury, an increase in the number of neurons expressing ΔFosB (a marker of chronic neuronal activation), persistent astrocyte activation and proliferation (as measured by GFAP and Ki67 expression), and a decrease in the expression of the astrocyte glutamate transporter GLT1 are observed in the ipsilateral superficial dorsal horn of cervical spinal cord. These changes have previously been associated with neuronal hyperexcitability and may contribute to altered pain transmission and chronic neuropathic pain. In our model, they are accompanied by robust at-level hyperalgesia in the ipsilateral forepaw and allodynia in both forepaws that are evident within two weeks following injury and persist for at least six weeks. Furthermore, the pain phenotype occurs in the absence of alterations in forelimb grip strength, suggesting that it represents sensory and not motor abnormalities. Given the importance of transgenic mouse technology, this clinically-relevant model provides a resource that can be used to study the molecular mechanisms contributing to neuropathic pain following SCI and to identify potential therapeutic targets for the treatment of chronic pathological pain.

Editor: Guglielmo Foffani, Hospital Nacional de Parapléjicos, Spain

Funding: This work was funded by the NIH (1R01NS079702 to A.C.L.) and the Craig H. Neilsen Foundation (#190140 to A.C.L.). The funders had no role in study design, data collection and analysis, decision to publish, or preparation of the manuscript.

Competing Interests: The authors have declared that no competing interests exist.

* Email: Angelo.Lepore@jefferson.edu

Introduction

Spinal cord injury (SCI) is a debilitating condition with widespread symptoms that affect patient quality of life. As many as 327,000 SCI patients are currently living in the United States, and approximately 12,000 new cases are reported each year [1]. Clinical studies propose that 64–82% of SCI patients experience some form of pathological pain following injury, and this pain has been associated with mood changes as well as difficulty with work and social activities [2]. Neuropathic pain constitutes a significant percentage of pain resulting from SCI; 41% of patients encounter at-level and 34% experience below-level neuropathic pain [3] following injury. Although SCI most often involves an acute injury to the spinal cord, the resulting pathological pain is often chronic and can increase in severity over time [4]. Thus, SCI-related neuropathic pain and its treatment is an important focus of spinal cord research.

In this study, we wanted to identify the molecular changes accompanying the alterations of at-level pain sensitivity in a mouse model of cervical contusion SCI. We induced SCI in the mouse and measured changes in pain behavior, specifically thermal hyperalgesia and tactile allodynia. Additionally, we studied the expression of various proteins in the dorsal horn of the spinal cord that may contribute to neuropathic pain and the cell types expressing these proteins. Importantly, we chose to utilize a mouse model of SCI that is clinically relevant but has not previously been used to study neuropathic pain.

Currently, mouse models of SCI-induced neuropathic pain are available, but do not address cervical contusion injury. According to the National Spinal Cord Injury Statistical Center, the majority of SCI patients in the United States experience injury to the cervical regions of the spinal cord [1], but most rodent SCI models involve injury to thoracic regions. Therefore, we chose to target our SCI to the cervical region of the spinal cord.

Additionally, contusion-type injury is most common in human patients [5] and is a popular model of SCI in rodents [6]. The respiratory and other dysfunctions that commonly accompany cervical contusion injuries make this model difficult to study [7]. To date, our group [8], [9], [10] and others [11] have used models of cervical contusion SCI in the mouse and rat to study motor deficits following injury. In the study of neuropathic pain, however, contusive injury to the cervical regions of the spinal cord has not been utilized in mice. Instead, transection, compression, contusion and other procedures are used primarily at thoracic levels to induce SCI in mice for studying neuropathic pain [6]. Here, we designed a model of moderate hemicontusive injury to the cervical spinal cord in the mouse that does not develop significant respiratory or other life-threatening complications for the study of neuropathic pain.

The development of neuropathic pain following SCI involves the disruption of neurons involved in nociception in the dorsal horn of the spinal cord. Under normal circumstances, neurons in the superficial laminae of the dorsal horn are responsible for pain transmission from peripheral nociceptors to the thalamus and, ultimately, the sensory cortex. Upon injury to the spinal cord, however, local changes can occur that alter how nociceptive neurons respond to peripheral stimuli [12]. These changes, termed central sensitization, can underlie pathological pain behaviors such as allodynia and hyperalgesia [12], [13].

One mechanism involved in central sensitization is the hyperexcitability of pain transmission neurons. Neuronal hyperexcitability results in an increase in the response of neurons to electrical input or even the firing of neurons in the absence of input. Hyperexcitability is characterized by spontaneous neuronal activity, aberrant responses to subthreshold stimuli, and increased transmission of suprathreshold input [12], [13]. In SCI, pain projection neurons in the dorsal horn can become more easily excited by noxious as well as non-noxious stimuli, resulting in pathological pain transmission. Changes to the neuron itself, as well as to its extracellular environment, can alter the neuron's electrophysiological profile, increasing its resting membrane potential and/or decreasing its action potential threshold. As one example of a mechanism underlying central sensitization, increased activity of transcription factors can trigger changes in gene expression that lead to long-term alterations in neuronal function and excitability. For instance, ΔfosB, a commonly used marker of persistent neuronal activation, has been associated with plasticity of pain transmission circuits in inflammatory pain, possibly through downstream targets such as CDK5 [14], [15].

Underlying hyperexcitability and central sensitization in SCI are changes in glial activation and glutamate transporter function. Astrocytes play an essential role in the central nervous system, providing support to neurons, regulating the uptake of glutamate and other factors from the extracellular space, and modulating synapse formation and function [13], [16]. Soon after insult, astrocytes can become activated (marked by glial fibrillary acidic protein (GFAP)) and possibly even proliferative and act to minimize the effects of the injury by reestablishing the blood brain barrier, releasing antioxidants, and protecting the lesion site from detrimental molecules. Activation of astrocytes, however, can also be harmful to neighboring neurons; when persistently active, astrocytes can contribute to neuronal hyperexcitability through the release of factors such as proinflammatory molecules, nitric oxide, and ATP [13], [17], [18].

The loss of glutamate transporters by activated astrocytes and the resulting imbalance in glutamate homeostasis may also contribute to the development of post-SCI neuropathic pain. Under normal conditions, glutamate is cleared from the synapse via glutamate transporters, such as GLT1 and GLAST, located in the plasma membrane of neurons and, more often, astrocytes. However, elevated release of glutamate from presynaptic neurons and/or injured neurons and glia or from damage to the glutamate transporter system can cause an excess of glutamate to linger in synaptic and extra-synaptic locations [13]. This disruption in glutamate homeostasis leads to overactivation of glutamate receptors, which can in some instances result in increased Ca^{2+} concentrations in the postsynaptic neuron. These changes can have negative impacts on cell health and function and alter the activation state of the neuron [19], [20], [21]. In SCI, glutamate excitotoxic damage to inhibitory interneurons can also indirectly boost the excitability of nociceptive neurons in the dorsal horn [18]. In this way, the loss of GLT1 in astrocytes observed following injury by our group [22], [23], [24] and others [25], [26] may contribute to central sensitization and neuropathic pain.

Recently published data from our group showed changes in neuronal and astrocyte activation as well as GLT1 expression in the superficial dorsal horn following cervical contusion SCI-induced hyperalgesia in the rat [24]. The study characterized a moderate hemicontusion injury to cervical regions of the rat spinal cord, which resulted in ipsilateral hyperalgesic behavior. Accompanying hyperalgesia were chronic increases in ΔfosB expression in neurons, astrocyte activation and proliferation in addition to a loss of GLT1 both at the site of the injury and in intact spinal cord caudal to the contusion site [24].

In the current study we characterize increases in pain sensitivity in a mouse model of cervical contusion SCI and the accompanying molecular alterations in the dorsal horn of the spinal cord. Our model exhibits at-level thermal hyperalgesia and tactile allodynia in addition to increases in neuronal and astrocyte activation and a decrease in astrocyte glutamate transporter expression in the superficial dorsal horn. Alterations in pain behavior, as well as neuronal and glial activation and glutamate transport expression in the dorsal horn, have not previously been characterized in mice receiving cervical contusion SCI. Thus, this study provides an observation of the molecular and behavioral changes that occur following cervical SCI in the mouse that can be used to further study the mechanisms underlying neuropathic pain in SCI.

Methods

Animal Studies

Ethics Statement. All animal care and treatment were conducted in strict accordance with the *European Communities Council Directive* (2010/63/EU, 86/609/EEC and 87-848/EEC) and the *NIH Guide for the Care and Use of Laboratory Animals*. Experimental protocols were approved by the Thomas Jefferson University Institutional Animal Care and Use Committee.

Animals. Fifty-six male C57BL/6 mice (25–30 g; The Jackson Laboratory, USA) and 26 transgenic BAC-GLT1-eGFP reporter mice [27] were used. The BAC-GLT1-eGFP reporter mice were created by Regan et al. [27]. The transgene in these mice involves cDNA for eGFP inserted into the start codon of a mouse BAC encompassing the entire GLT-1 gene. Thus, in these mice, eGFP expression is driven by the GLT1 promoter. Mice were housed 5 per cage in a controlled light-dark environment in the Thomas Jefferson University Animal Facility and were given food and water *ad libitum*. To prevent suffering, a combination of ketamine/xylazine and isofluorane was used to anesthetize animals during surgical procedures.

SCI Models. We chose to utilize two models in the C57BL/6 mice in this study; one with injury at the C5 level and another with injury at the C6 level. We did this to show that contusion injury to various levels of the cervical spinal cord has the potential to produce at-level neuropathic pain. Mice were anesthetized initially with ketamine (100 mg/kg) and xylazine (5 mg/kg) injected intraperitoneally, and the anesthetic plane was maintained with 1% isoflurane for the duration of the surgery. The body was immobilized by taping the forelegs to a fixation plate, and the head was immobilized by the isoflurane nose cone. The skin and muscle overlying the spinal column were retracted from levels C3 to T1, and spinal cord was exposed by unilateral laminectomy from the midline blood vessel to the lateral edge of the vertebral lamina at the level of C5 or C6. The spinal column was stabilized at the C3 and T1 spinous processes by microforceps attached to the fixation plate and the far right and left corners. C57BL/6 mice received unilateral contusion injuries at the exposed portion of the spinal cord using the Infinite Horizon Impactor (Precision Systems and Instrumentation; Lexington, KY) with an impactor tip of 0.7 mm in diameter, a force of 40 kilodynes, two seconds of dwell time, and an approximately perpendicular impact angle, parameters similar to our previously published cervical contusion SCI paradigms [8], [9], [10]. Injury parameters for BAC-GLT1-eGFP mice included a 1.0 mm diameter tip, 50 kilodyne force, and no dwell time at the C5 level. Control animals received unilateral laminectomy but not contusion injury to the spinal cord. Following injury, the forceps were removed and the muscle layers were secured with a sterile 4-0 silk suture. Sterile wound clips were used to close the skin, and 1 ml of lactated Ringers solution and 0.1 mg/kg of buprenorphine-HCl were administered subcutaneously.

Unilateral Hargreaves Thermal Test. A modified version of the Hargreaves test for thermal hyperalgesia, based on previously established methods [28], was conducted for the forepaws of each animal. This test detects sensitivity to thermal nociceptive stimuli by determining the latency to withdrawal of the paw from an infrared stimulus of a particular intensity. Prior to surgery, baseline measures were collected once weekly for two weeks. Following contusion SCI or laminectomy, each animal was tested weekly for six weeks. Before the first baseline test, the animals were acclimated to the testing room for an hour each day for five days. Prior to each session, mice were also acclimated to the testing room for an hour. Individually, the mice were restrained manually by the scruff only and placed on a thin glass pane, with one of the forepaws directly above the source of the infrared stimulus (UgoBasile; Comerio, VA). The animals continued to be restrained, but movement of the forepaw was unimpeded. The stimulus was initiated, and a fiber optic sensor on the movable infrared heat source measured the time to forepaw withdrawal. Forepaw withdrawal was defined as a quick movement of the paw away from the infrared stimulus often accompanied by licking of the forepaw. Spontaneous movements of the forepaw were not considered forepaw withdrawal and resulted in discarding the data and repeating the trial. Three trials were conducted for each forepaw of each animal, alternating the left and right forepaws, with an inter-trial interval of 120 seconds.

von Frey Filament Test. Semmes-Weinstein monofilaments (Stoelting Company; Dale, IL) ranging from 1.65 grams to 4.56 grams of force were utilized to measure tactile allodynia using the up-down method. Testing occurred twice prior to surgery to obtain baseline data and once weekly for six weeks after injury. Acclimation procedures were the same as those used for the Hargreaves test. Each mouse experienced ten trials per testing day with an inter-trial interval of 120 seconds. The first trial of each testing day utilized a filament of 3.84 grams. A single trial involved directing a monofilament at the center of the plantar surface of the forepaw of interest and application until the filament buckled.

Mice were not restrained for this testing. The response of the mouse was then recorded as a positive or negative withdrawal response. The filament application was considered to produce a positive response if the mouse rapidly withdrew its forepaw, which was mostly accompanied by vocalization and/or licking of the forepaw. If the response was positive, the filament used in the next trial would be the next smaller filament. If instead the response was negative, the next larger filament would be used in the next trial. Withdraw threshold was determined as the lowest filament/force that evoked a positive withdrawal response in greater than 50% of the trials with that particular filament.

Grip Strength Testing. Grip strength was measured by the DFIS-2 Series Digital Force Gauge (Columbus Instruments, OH) [26], used previously by our group [8]. Attached to the force gauge is a triangular metal pull bar that allows for the transduction of force from the mouse to the gauge. The Digital Force Gauge measures the strength with which the mouse is able to grasp and hold onto a thin metal bar. Three baseline measures spread across two weeks were obtained prior to surgery, and mice were tested once weekly for six weeks following injury. In each trial, the mouse was allowed to grab the bar with one forepaw and was then quickly pulled away from the gauge so its grip was released, providing a measurement of the force with which the mouse gripped the bar. During each testing session, three trials for each forepaw were performed with an inter-trial interval of at least 60 seconds.

Histological Analyses

Tissue Processing. Mice were sacrificed at two days or two or six weeks following injury or laminectomy by anesthetic overdose and transcardial perfusion with 0.9% saline followed by 4% paraformaldehyde. The spinal cord was harvested following perfusion, fixed in 4% paraformaldehyde at room temperature for 24 hours, washed in 0.1M phosphate buffer at 4°C for 24 hours and then cryoprotected in 30% sucrose in 0.1M phosphate buffer at 4°C for three days. The cervical/rostral thoracic spinal cord was dissected from the rest of the cord, embedded in freezing medium, and flash-frozen with dry ice. Embedded tissue was cut transversely by cryostat at a thickness of 30 μm and mounted directly onto slides. Slides were stored at −20°C.

Motor Neuron Counts. A representative sample (i.e. every fifth section) of spinal cord tissue was used to locate the injury epicenter. Slides were thawed at room temperature for an hour and stained with 0.5% Cresyl violet acetate/Eriochrome cyanine. For each section, large motor neurons ventral to the central canal in the grey matter were counted for the ipsilateral and contralateral sides [9]. The motor neuron cell bodies were identified by their size and characteristic morphology. The injury epicenter was defined as the section with the fewest large motor neurons in the ipsilateral ventral grey matter.

Immunohistochemistry. Immunohistochemical analysis was performed both ipsilaterally and contralaterally to the unilateral injury at the injury epicenter as well as 1.05 mm caudal to the epicenter (Figure 1A–B). Sectioned tissue was thawed and dried at room temperature for an hour and then washed in TBS. Sections were blocked in 10% normal goat serum/0.2% Triton/TBS at room temperature for one hour followed by primary antibody incubation in 2% goat serum/0.5% Triton/TBS at 4°C overnight. Secondary antibody was incubated in 2% goat serum/0.5% Triton/TBS at room temperature for two hours. Primary and secondary antibodies used were rabbit polyclonal ΔfosB (IHC 1:100; Santa Cruz, USA) [30], rabbit polyclonal Ki67 (IHC 1:200; Abcam, USA) [31], mouse monoclonal GFAP (IHC 1:400, Sigma Aldrich, USA) [32], rabbit polyclonal GLT1 (IHC 1:800, kindly

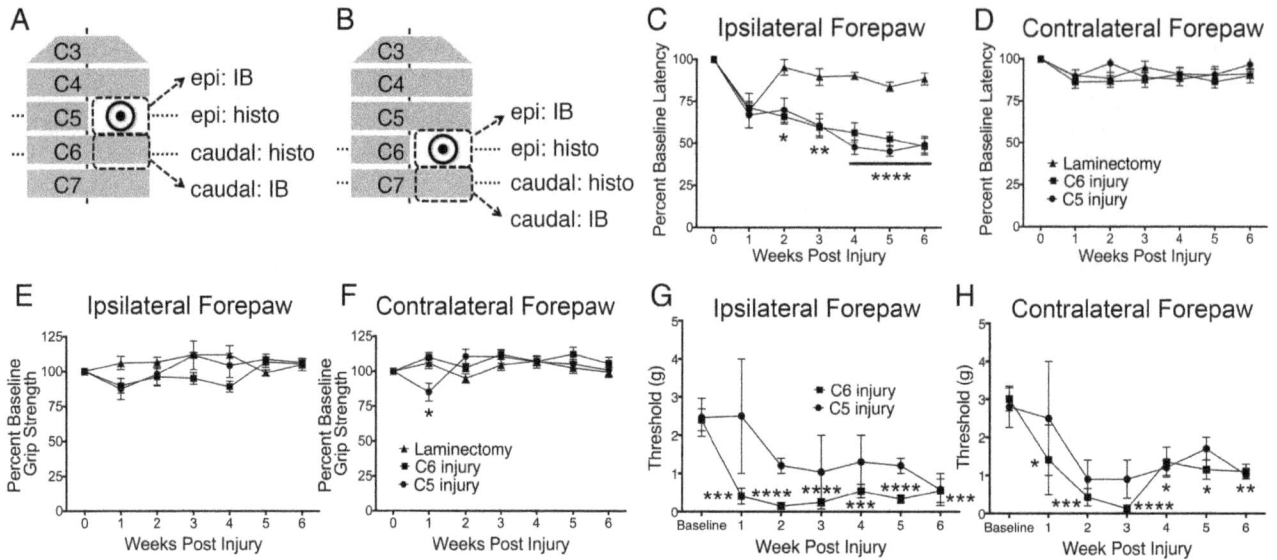

Figure 1. Animals receiving unilateral cervical contusion SCI exhibited persistent thermal hyperalgesia and tactile allodynia in the forepaw. Cervical contusion SCI was administered at the C5 or C6 level of the spinal cord while uninjured control animals received only laminectomy at the C6 level. Tissue from the level of laminectomy or epicenter of the injury and from the region immediately caudal was harvested for either immunoblotting or histology (A–B). Thermal hyperalgesia was measured using a modified version of the Hargreaves test. Animals receiving contusion injury showed a decrease in latency to withdrawal in the ipsilateral forepaw, measured as a percentage of baseline latency, compared to control animals (C). This difference was first observed at two weeks after injury and persisted until the animals were sacrificed at six weeks after injury. No change in withdrawal latency was seen in injured vs. uninjured animals in the contralateral forepaw (D). Animals receiving SCI were also tested for tactile allodynia using von Frey filament testing. In animals receiving C6 injury, but not C5 injury, a significant decrease compared to pre-injury baseline in the force threshold required to elicit a withdrawal response was evident both ipsilaterally (E) and contralaterally (F) for each of the six weeks following injury. The decrease in ipsilateral forepaw withdrawal latency and bilateral force threshold in injured animals occurred in the absence of changes in grip strength in either forepaw (G–H). Epi = epicenter; IB = immunoblotting; histo = histology; * = p<0.05; ** = p<0.01; **** = p<0.0001.

provided by Jeffrey Rothstein's lab at Johns Hopkins University) [29],, mouse monoclonal CD11b (IHC 1:4,000, AbD Serotec, USA), rhodamine-conjugated goat-anti-rabbit IgG (1:100; Jackson Immuno, USA) and FITC-conjugated goat-anti-mouse IgG (1:100; Jackson Immuno, USA).

Fluorescence Imaging and Quantification. Imaging and quantification of fluorescence immunostaining and BAC-GLT1-eGFP tissue were performed using a Zeiss Imager M2 upright fluorescence microscope [23]. Images were taken and analyses performed on saved PNG images for analyses. All immunostaining was quantified in the most superficial laminae (I–II) or lamina III of the spinal cord dorsal horn (Figure 2F–G). Laminae I–III were delineated by beginning at the most lateral portion of the dorsal horn, drawing a horizontal line across the gray matter, and following the outline of the gray matter back to the lateral extension of the dorsal horn. The border between laminae I–II and lamina III was identified by the change in tissue morphology represented by darker tissue in laminae I–II and lighter tissue in lamina III. Quantification analyses were performed using Metamorph software (Molecule Devices; Sunnyvale, CA). ΔfosB- and Ki67-positive cells were quantified by counting the stained nuclei in the superficial laminae. GFAP and GLT1 staining was more diffusely distributed and was therefore quantified in laminae I–II as an integrated intensity, or the sum of the intensity of pixels over a region, at constant exposure, brightness, and contrast. In BAC-GLT1-eGFP tissue, quantification was performed for laminae I–II and lamina III. eGFP-positive cells were counted separately for these regions [23].

Biochemical Analyses

Tissue Harvesting. Sacrifice occurred at two or six weeks after injury or laminectomy. Following anesthetic overdose, animals were perfused with 0.9% saline and the cervical spinal cord removed, dissected, and flash-frozen in dimethylbutane. The spinal cord was sub-dissected to collect the ipsilateral cord at the level of the injury and the segment directly caudal to the injury (Fig. 1A–B). To identify the regions of interest, the muscles were first removed to expose the spinal column. The laminectomy area was located, and the contralateral vertebral lamina was removed. Microdissection scissors were used to cut the spinal cord along the midline, and a 1.0 mm piece of tissue between the remaining laminae was collected. Flash-frozen tissue was stored at −80°C.

Western Blotting. Tissue samples were homogenized on ice in 50 μl of RIPA buffer containing 50 mM TRIS-HCl pH 7.6, 150 mM NaCl, 2 mM EDTA, 0.1% SDS, 0.01% NP-40, and Protease Inhibitor Cocktail (Roche Diagnostics, Indianapolis, IN). Protein concentration was determined by the Bradford assay, and equal amounts of protein were run on 4–12% Bis-Tris gels and transferred to nitrocellulose membranes. Odyssey blocking buffer (Li-Cor; Lincoln, NE) was used to block the membranes at room temperature for one hour. Primary antibodies for GLT1 (1:2,000) and actin (1:2,000; Abcam) were diluted in Odyssey blocking buffer and membranes were incubated at 4°C overnight. The membranes were then probed with IRDye-conjugated goat anti-rabbit or goat anti-mouse IgG (1:20,000; Li-Cor) at room temperature for one hour. Imaging was performed by the Li-Cor Odyssey infrared imaging system, and GLT1 band intensity was measured and normalized to actin band intensity using ImageJ software [22].

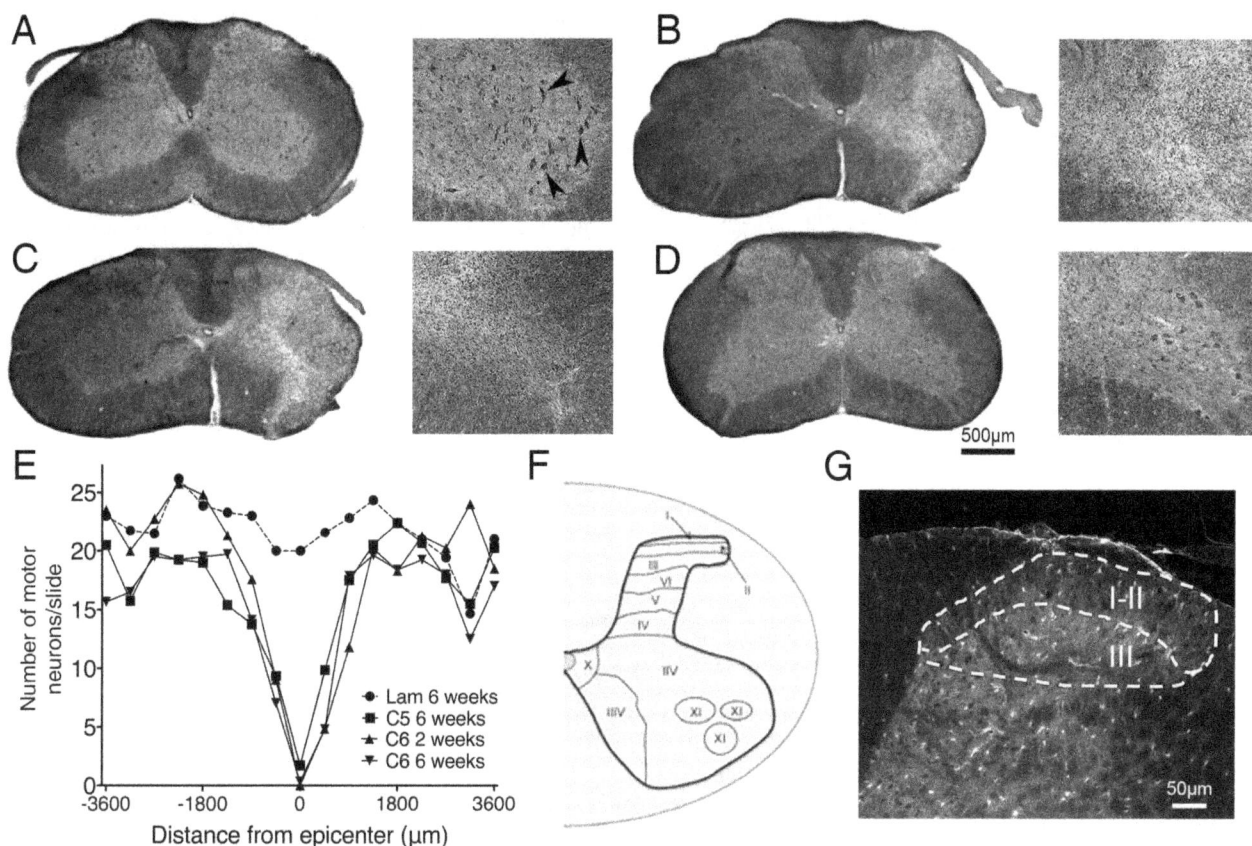

Figure 2. Unilateral contusion SCI induced a loss of ventral horn motor neurons at the injury epicenter. Harvested tissue was stained with Cresyl violet and Eriochrome cyanine. At the level of the laminectomy, uninjured control animals (A) exhibited large motor neurons in the ventral horn (arrowheads). At six weeks post-injury, animals receiving unilateral C5 (B) or C6 (C) contusion SCI showed a loss of these motor neurons at the injury epicenter but not 1.0 mm caudal to the injury (D). The spread of ventral horn motor neuron loss was approximately 1.0 mm rostrally and 1.0 mm caudally (2.0 mm total) from the epicenter (E). Immunohistochemical analyses of the injury models were performed in laminae I–II and lamina III of the cervical spinal cord dorsal horn (F–G). Lam = laminectomy.

Statistical Analyses

All data are presented as mean ± SEM. Statistical analyses were performed using GraphPad Prism (GraphPad Software, Inc.; La Jolla, CA). Bar graphs are presented as averages with error bars representing standard error. The Hargreaves test and von Frey threshold data were analyzed using a two-way ANOVA with repeated measured to compare the means within each group (laminectomy, C5 injury, or C6 injury) at each time point. The immunohistochemical and biochemical data were assessed with one-way ANOVA, comparing each group (laminectomy, C6 2 weeks, or C6 6 weeks) to one another. Statistical significance is defined as $p < 0.05$ for all analyses.

Results

Robust and persistent forepaw thermal hyperalgesia and tactile allodynia were observed following unilateral cervical contusion SCI

Here we present a model of unilateral cervical contusion SCI in the mouse that exhibits persistent changes in pain behavior in the absence of motor deficits. Following baseline behavior testing, animals received unilateral laminectomy and contusion injury of 40 kilodyne of force with two seconds of dwell time at either the C5 (Fig. 1A) or C6 (Fig. 1B) level of the spinal cord. Control animals underwent laminectomy without injury. In both injury models, no grossly observable deficits in respiratory or other vital functions were present.

Beginning one week after injury, thermal hyperalgesia, tactile allodynia and grip strength were measured in laminectomy (n = 8) and injured animals (C5: n = 8; C6: n = 10) for six weeks. A modified version of the Hargreaves test was utilized to measure sensitivity to noxious thermal stimuli in the ipsilateral and contralateral forepaws. In both injured and uninjured animals, forepaw withdrawal upon noxious thermal stimulation was deliberate and was often accompanied by licking or scratching of the paw. Two-way ANOVA was used to compare withdrawal latency between animals with C5 injury, C6 injury, and laminectomy only at each time point. Post-injury measurements of latency to forepaw withdrawal are reported as a percentage of the baseline average for each animal. In laminectomy-only animals, withdrawal latency non-significantly decreased in the ipsilateral forepaw at one week post-injury but returned to and persisted at baseline levels until six weeks after injury (Fig. 1C). Beginning two weeks after injury and persisting for the length of testing, ipsilateral forepaw withdrawal latencies for animals receiving unilateral contusion SCI at the C5 or C6 level were significantly reduced compared to uninjured laminectomy animals (Fig. 1C). In the contralateral forepaw, no significant changes amongst the three experimental groups were seen (Fig. 1D).

In addition, tactile allodynia was assessed in C5 injured and C6 injured animals. The threshold force required to elicit a withdrawal response in each of the forepaws was measured by the von Frey test. In the C6 injury group, but not as robustly in the C5 injury group, tactile allodynia was evident (Fig. 1E–F). Animals were tested prior to injury to obtain baseline data and were then assessed for six weeks following injury. When values for each testing week were compared to pre-injury baseline data, animals receiving C6 injury exhibited a significant decrease in threshold force both ipsilaterally (Fig. 1E) and contralaterally (Fig. 1F). Although the data were not significant for animals receiving C5 injury, there was a similar trend in decreased response threshold.

While thermal and mechanical sensitivity increased in injured animals, this was not associated with changes in grip strength. Grip strength results were analyzed by two-way ANOVA to identify significance between each group at each time point. For the ipsilateral forepaw, no changes were observed between injured and uninjured animals for the six weeks following surgery (Fig. 1G). A significant decrease in contralateral grip strength for animals receiving injury at the C5 level was seen one week after injury compared to laminectomy or C6 injury (Fig. 1H). However, because the change occurred so soon after surgery and grip strength recovered to baseline levels by the next testing session, a spinal shock mechanism may be responsible for this unexpected change.

Together, the Hargreaves, von Frey, and grip strength data suggest hypersensitivity to noxious thermal and tactile stimuli in the absence of altered grip strength, indicating that the observed changes in forepaw withdrawal resulted from aberrant pain processing rather than motor deficits.

Unilateral cervical contusion SCI produced an injury characterized by a focal loss of ventral horn motor neurons

The animals that received unilateral contusion SCI exhibited loss of large motor neurons in the ventral grey matter as well as a disruption of lateral grey matter, dorsolateral funiculus, and ventrolateral funiculus of the ipsilateral hemicord (Fig. 2B–C). In laminectomy-only animals (n = 8), large motor neurons of distinct morphology were present throughout the ipsilateral ventral horn (Fig. 2A). These motor neurons were absent or their numbers were greatly reduced, however, at the injury site in animals receiving C5 (Fig. 2B; n = 8) or C6 (Fig. 2C; 2 weeks: n = 8; 6 weeks: n = 10) injury. This effect was limited to the injury site, as motor neuron populations and white matter were intact in regions rostral and caudal to the injury (Fig. 2D). Additionally, no loss of motor neurons was observed on the contralateral side of the spinal cord at any point along the rostral-caudal axis (data not shown). Thus, the anatomical disruption sustained by injured animals was restricted to the injury site ipsilaterally.

In order to quantify the contusion injury sustained by the animals and identify the injury epicenter along the rostral-caudal axis, sections were stained with Cresyl violet acetate/Eriochrome cyanine and motor neurons in the ventral horn were counted. The epicenter of the injury was determined by the extent of motor neuron loss, and the motor neuron counts were plotted by distance from this site (Fig. 2E). Significance was determined using one-way ANOVA to compare motor neuron counts between each group. Compared to laminectomy animals, a significant decrease in ventral horn motor neurons was observed for animals receiving injury at either cervical level and at both time points. The spread of both C5 and C6 injuries was approximately 2.0 mm (1.0 mm rostrally and 1.0 mm caudally from the epicenter) with a gradual decrease in motor neurons immediately rostral and caudal to the

epicenter. The epicenter identified by this method was used for further immunohistochemical analyses of the neuronal and glial populations of the spinal cord dorsal horn, which were performed in laminae I–II and laminae III (Fig. 2F–G).

Chronic neuronal activation in the superficial laminae of the dorsal horn resulted from contusion SCI

Because injury at either the C5 or C6 level produced thermal hyperalgesia and tissue damage to a similar extent, we chose to move forward with a single model, the C6 injury, for further analyses. ΔfosB, a truncated splice version of the immediate early gene c-fos, is a transcription factor and marker of persistent neuronal activation. Chronic upregulation of this gene has been implicated in plasticity and inflammatory pain [14], [15] and has the potential to contribute to neuropathic pain. To study the extent of ΔfosB expression in our SCI model, we sacrificed animals at two weeks and six weeks after injury (n = 7–10) or six weeks after laminectomy (n = 8). Immunohistochemistry for ΔfosB was performed at the injury epicenter and 1.0 mm caudal to the injury in laminae I–II.

We found that ΔfosB-positive cells exhibited a defined pattern of nuclear staining in the superficial laminae. In our SCI model, we observed a persistent increase in the number of Δfos-expressing cells, suggesting chronic neuronal activation following cervical contusion injury. One-way ANOVA was used to compare the number of ΔfosB-positive cells between each group. Following laminectomy, limited-to-no ΔfosB expression was seen in the dorsal horn (Fig. 3A). Two weeks after injury (Fig. 3B), there was an increase in ΔfosB-positive cells on the ipsilateral side at and caudal to the injury epicenter. At six weeks (Fig. 3C), ΔfosB was upregulated bilaterally in the superficial laminae at the injury epicenter and 1.0 mm caudal. These changes are quantified in Figure 3D. The greatest increase in ΔfosB expression was observed at six weeks, suggesting that its expression was persistent and cumulative over time. Additionally, the expression of ΔfosB in the injured animals was specific to the dorsal horn of the spinal cord. There were few to no ΔfosB-positive cells in other regions of the spinal cord, including the ventral horn. This suggests that the effects of our injury paradigm on chronic neuronal activation were focal to the dorsal horn, an important region of the spinal cord for pain transmission and modulation.

Astrocytes were activated and proliferated in the dorsal horn of the spinal cord following cervical contusion SCI

Astrocytes play important protective and homeostatic roles in both the immediate and delayed response to CNS injury. Chronic activation in the spinal cord, however, can contribute to neuronal hyperexcitability of pain transmission neurons that underlies neuropathic pain [12], [13]. When astrocytes become activated, they express distinct proteins and in some cases proliferate [21]. In order to measure the spatial and temporal change in astrocyte activation in our model of SCI, we used immunohistochemistry to stain for GFAP, expressed by activated astrocytes, and Ki67, a marker of cellular proliferation. As in the previous immunohistochemical analyses, animals were studied two or six weeks after injury (n = 7–10) or six weeks after laminectomy (n = 8). For each analysis, one-way ANOVA was utilized to identify significance between the three groups.

Figure 4B shows the distinct morphology of activated astrocytes observed following injury compared to uninjured control (Fig. 4A). We found that injury induced diffuse GFAP expression throughout the gray matter of the spinal cord; therefore, we quantified astrocyte expression in laminae I–II by measuring GFAP intensity.

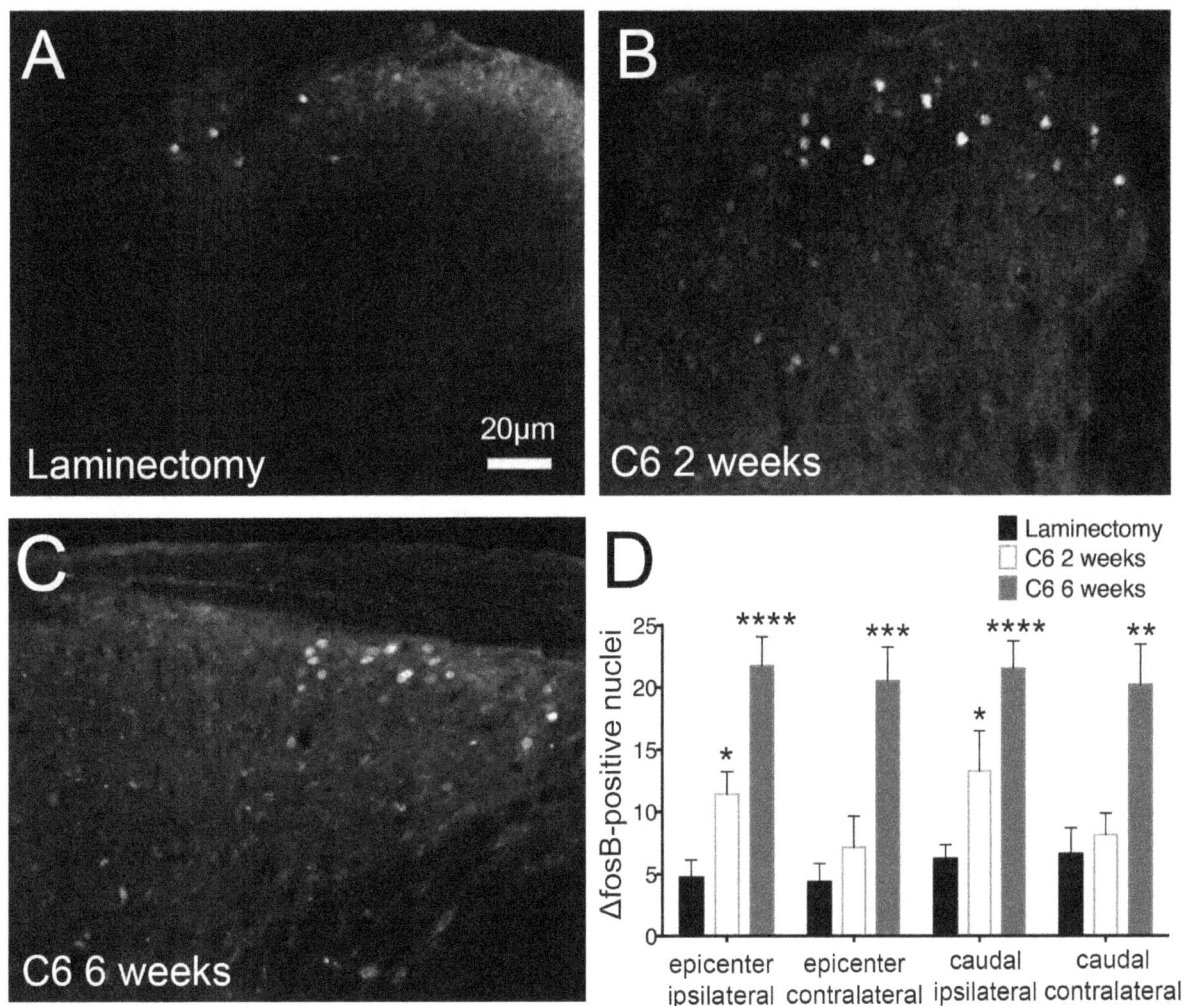

Figure 3. Chronic neuronal activation in the dorsal horn resulted from cervical contusion SCI. ΔfosB staining was used to measure the extent of persistent neuronal activation in the spinal cord. Following injury, ΔfosB-positive nuclei (arrowheads) were evident in laminae I–II (A–C). At all regions, laminectomy control animals (A) showed little-to-no ΔfosB expression (D). Two weeks after C6 injury (B), a significant increase in numbers of ΔfosB expressing cells in the superficial laminae of the ipsilateral dorsal horn was observed at the injury epicenter and caudal to the injury (D). ΔfosB levels were further increased at all regions in animals sacrificed six weeks post-injury (C, D). * = p<0.05; ** = p<0.01; *** = p 0.001; **** = p< 0.0001.

Compared to laminectomy (Fig. 4C), GFAP intensity was significantly greater at both time points in animals receiving contusion SCI (Fig. 4D–E). These changes were observed ipsilaterally at the injury epicenter, with no alterations in GFAP expression at the other regions analyzed (Fig. 4F). GFAP expression was highest two weeks after injury, which suggests that, while post-injury astrocyte activation is chronic, it may lessen over time.

We next sought to study the extent of astrocyte proliferation in the dorsal horn to further support our assertion that astrocytes respond to the spinal cord insult we induced. We confirmed using confocal microscopy that, after injury, the majority of Ki67-expresing cells in the superficial were GFAP-positive astrocytes (Fig. 5A). Basally, proliferating cell numbers, and thus Ki67 expression, in the spinal cord were low (Fig. 5B). Two weeks following injury (Fig. 5C), the superficial laminae expressed a robust increase in bilateral Ki67 that was also seen in the ipsilateral dorsal horn caudal to the injury (Fig. 5E). At six weeks

(Fig. 5D), an increase in Ki67 was also observed but did not reach the levels seen at two weeks.

We identified the phenotypes of these Ki67-positive proliferative cells. First, we quantified microglial activation in the superficial dorsal horn by immunostaining for CD11b (Fig. 5G–I). Like astrocytes, microglia play a role in both immediate and delayed responses to injury to the spinal cord and may contribute to the development of pathological pain (13). Compared to laminectomy (Fig. 5G), the intensity of CD11b expression was greater in animals with C6 SCI at both two (Fig. 5H–I) and six (Fig. 5I) weeks after injury. This increase was significant at the injury site both ipsilaterally and contralaterally, as well as caudal to the injury on the ipsilateral side (Fig. 5I).

We also quantified the percentage of Ki67-positive cells that were either GFAP-positive or CD11b-positive. This allowed us to determine if the proliferative cells are, in fact, astrocytes (GFAP-positive) or microglia (CD11b-positive). One-way ANOVA was used to identify significance in Ki67 and GFAP or CD11b colocalization. In laminectomy animals, the percentage of cells

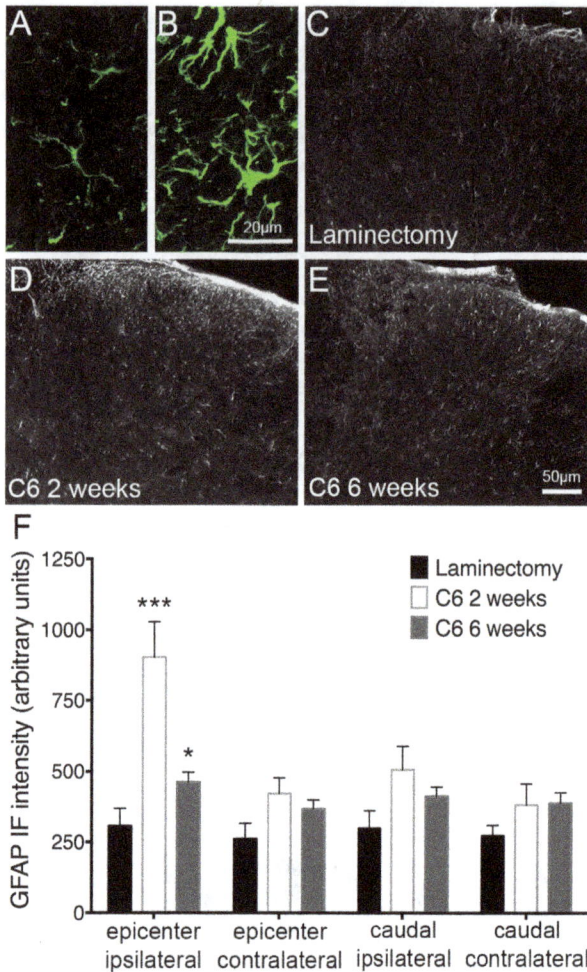

Figure 4. Astrocytes were activated and proliferated in the dorsal horn following cervical contusion SCI. Astrocyte activation in the superficial dorsal horn was characterized by quantification of GFAP expression in laminae I–II. (A) and (B) show representative images of dorsal horn GFAP expression at high magnification in laminectomy and injured animals, respectively. At the injury epicenter, compared to uninjured control animals (C), an increase in GFAP expression in the ipsilateral dorsal horn was evident at two (D) and six weeks (E) following injury. No significant changes in GFAP expression were observed at the other regions studied (F). IF = immunofluorescence; * = p<0.05; *** = p<0.001.

that are positive for both Ki67 and GFAP or CD11b is zero because there are no Ki67-positive cells present (Fig. 5F). At both two weeks and six weeks after C6 injury, there is a significant increase in the percentage of Ki67-positive cells that are also GFAP-positive or CD11b-positive (Fig. 5F). No significant difference exists between the percentage of Ki67-positive cells that are GFAP-positive or those that are CD11b-positive (Fig. 5F). Thus, both astrocytes and microglia are proliferative following cervical contusion SCI. These data further support the notion that activated astrocytes are present in the spinal cord following injury but retreat over time and/or that proliferation is mostly an early process of astrocyte activation post-SCI. The effects of astrocyte activation can be lasting, however, through the release of factors, for example, that can contribute to hyperexcitability.

Cervical contusion SCI led to reduced expression of GLT1 in the superficial dorsal horn of the spinal cord

The most abundant glutamate transporter in the CNS is GLT1, and its greatest expression is in astrocytes [33]. Through GLT1 and other glutamate transporters, astrocytes clear excitatory amino acids from the synapse after they are released, regulating glutamate's duration of action, controlling normal synaptic communication, and protecting cells from excitotoxic effects [33]. After SCI, we and others [23], [24], [25], [26] have reported a loss in astrocyte GLT1 expression. In this study, we utilized two animal models to study localized decreases in GLT1 in the context of neuropathic pain in the superficial dorsal horn.

In BAC-GLT1-eGFP reporter mice, the GLT1 promoter drives expression of eGFP [27]. Following injury, we sacrificed animals at two days (n = 7), two weeks (n = 9), and six weeks (n = 8) and quantified eGFP-positive cells separately in laminae I–II and lamina III. We used one-way ANOVA to compare the number of eGFP-positive cells at each time point. In uninjured animals (Fig. 6D; n = 6), eGFP expression was robust and widespread throughout the grey and white matter. Furthermore, almost all of the GFAP-expressing astrocytes in these regions co-localized with eGFP-positive cells (Fig. 6A–B). eGFP-positive cells were decreased, however, at two days, two weeks, and six weeks (Fig. 6E) at various regions in the spinal cord. Despite the increase in GFAP expression after injury, there were few cells co-expressing eGFP and GFAP, suggesting a loss of GLT1 expression in activated astrocytes (Fig. 6C). At the injury epicenter, eGFP expression was downregulated at two days ipsilaterally (Fig. 6F) and at all time points contralaterally in laminae I–II (Fig. 6G). In lamina III, a decrease in eGFP-positive cells was observed bilaterally at the injury epicenter (Fig. 6F–G). Caudal to the injury, we report a decrease in eGFP at all time points in laminae I–II and at two days and six weeks in lamina III (Fig. 6H). No changes in the contralateral dorsal horn caudal to the injury were observed (Fig. 6I).

In wild-type C57BL/6 animals, we employed immunohistochemical staining for GLT1 after C6 injury (n = 7–10) or laminectomy (n = 8). One-way ANOVA was used to identify significant differences in GLT1 staining between laminectomy, injured animals at 2 weeks, and injured animals at six weeks. Compared to laminectomy-only animals (Fig. 7A), animals receiving injury two weeks (Fig. 7B) or six weeks (Fig. 7C) prior to analysis showed a decrease in diffuse GLT1 protein expression in laminae I–II. These changes were seen at all regions analyzed (Fig. 7D). We further quantified the extent of GLT1 protein expression in injured (n = 7–8) and uninjured animals (n = 7) using immunoblotting techniques. At the injury epicenter, we observed a decrease in GLT1 protein in the ipsilateral hemicord at both time points after injury (Fig. 7E). Caudal to the injury, however, this glutamate transporter loss was not observed (Fig. 7F).

These data seem to contradict the immunohistochemical results we reported above. Thus, we performed immunohistochemical quantifications in regions outside of the superficial dorsal horn to try to identify the source of these contradictory results. At six weeks after injury, there is a significant loss of GLT1 expression in the ventral horn ipsilaterally at the epicenter compared to laminectomy animals (Fig. 7G). No significant change is seen in the ventral horn or white matter ipsilaterally caudal to the injury (Fig. 7G). These data suggest that, focally at the injury site, GLT1 loss occurs in multiple anatomical regions. However, caudal to the injury, the decrease in GLT1 expression may be more specific to the superficial dorsal horn (Fig. 7G). The changes in GLT1 from the immunoblotting data may not be evident due to the lack of anatomical specificity.

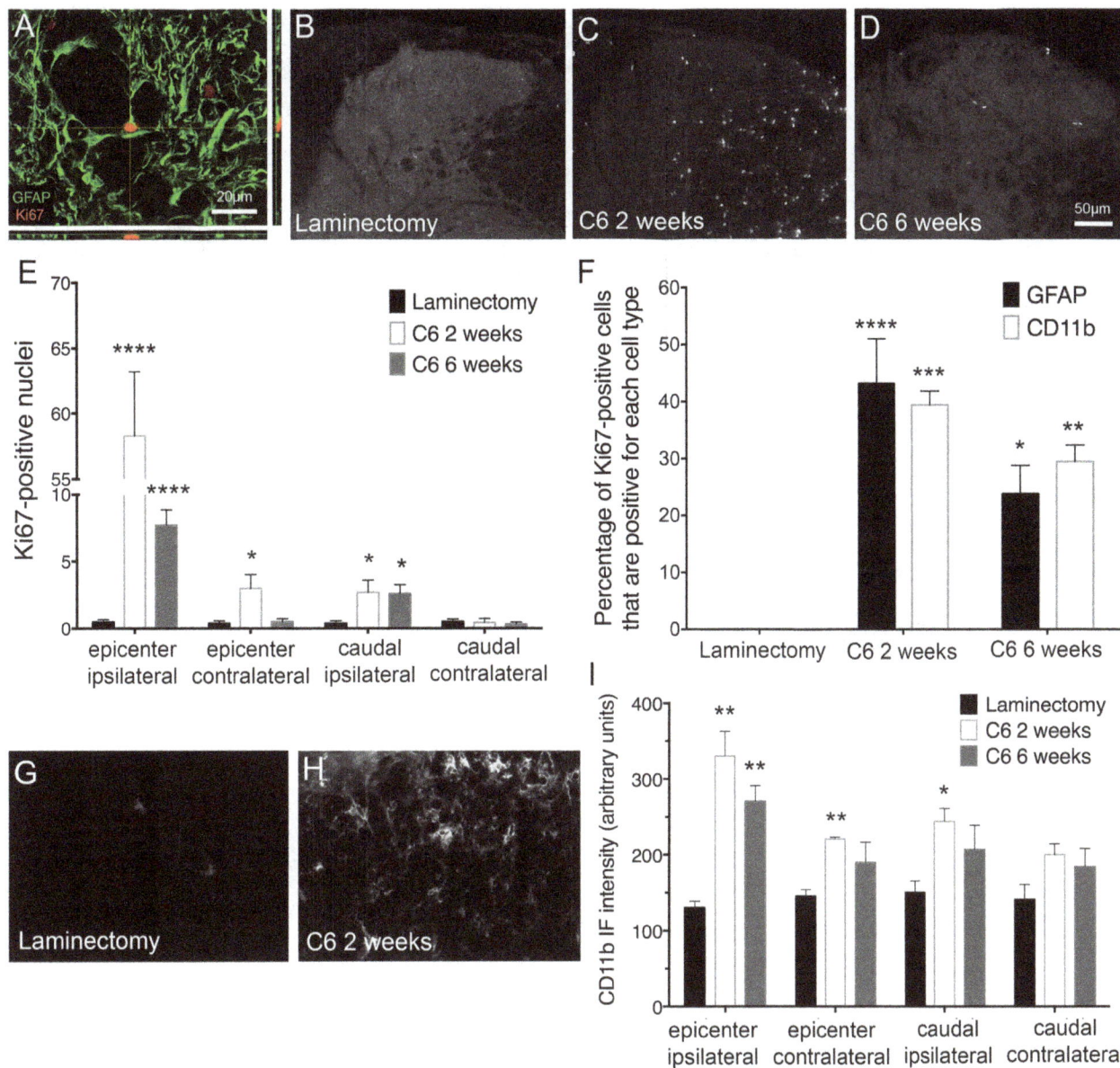

Figure 5. Enhanced cell proliferation, including proliferation of astrocytes, was evident after cervical contusion SCI. In the superficial laminae of the injured ipsilateral dorsal horn, we observed cells co-expressing GFAP and Ki67 (A), representing activated and proliferating astrocytes. In laminectomy control animals, little to no cell proliferation was evident (B). However, the number of Ki67-positive cells was significantly increased at two weeks (C) and six weeks (D) after injury on the ipsilateral side both at the level of and caudal to the injury (E). Additionally, at two weeks, there was a significant increase in proliferating cells contralaterally at the injury site (E). At both two and six weeks, a significant percentage of Ki67-positive cells were also either GFAP-positive or CD11b-positive (F). Compared to laminectomy (G), the intensity of CD11b expression in the superficial dorsal horn was greater in animals with C6 SCI at both two (H–I) and six (I) weeks after injury. This increase was significant at the injury site both ipsilaterally and contralaterally, as well as caudal to the injury on the contralateral side (I). * = p<0.05; ** = p<0.01; **** = p<0.0001.

Discussion

Here we describe changes in neuronal, astrocyte and microglial activation and GLT1 expression accompanying at-level thermal hyperalgesia in a cervical contusion SCI mouse model. In our model, robust and persistent thermal hyperalgesia and tactile allodynia are evident beginning one-two weeks after injury. Additionally, cervical contusion SCI induces an upregulation of ΔfosB, a marker of neuronal activity, in the superficial laminae of the dorsal horn. Astrocyte and microglial activation and proliferation, as measured by increases in GFAP, CD11b and Ki67

immunostaining, are also increased in these regions. We also observe a decrease in GLT1 expression and the number of GLT1-expressing cells in this model. These molecular changes that accompany hyperalgesia and allodynia in this study may contribute to the development of this aberrant pain response and represent important targets for better understanding the development of and treating neuropathic pain in SCI.

Hyperalgesia, defined as an increase in sensitivity to noxious stimuli, whether due to a decrease in pain threshold or an increase in response to stimuli above the pain threshold [36], is common in humans and is associated with sensory changes resulting from

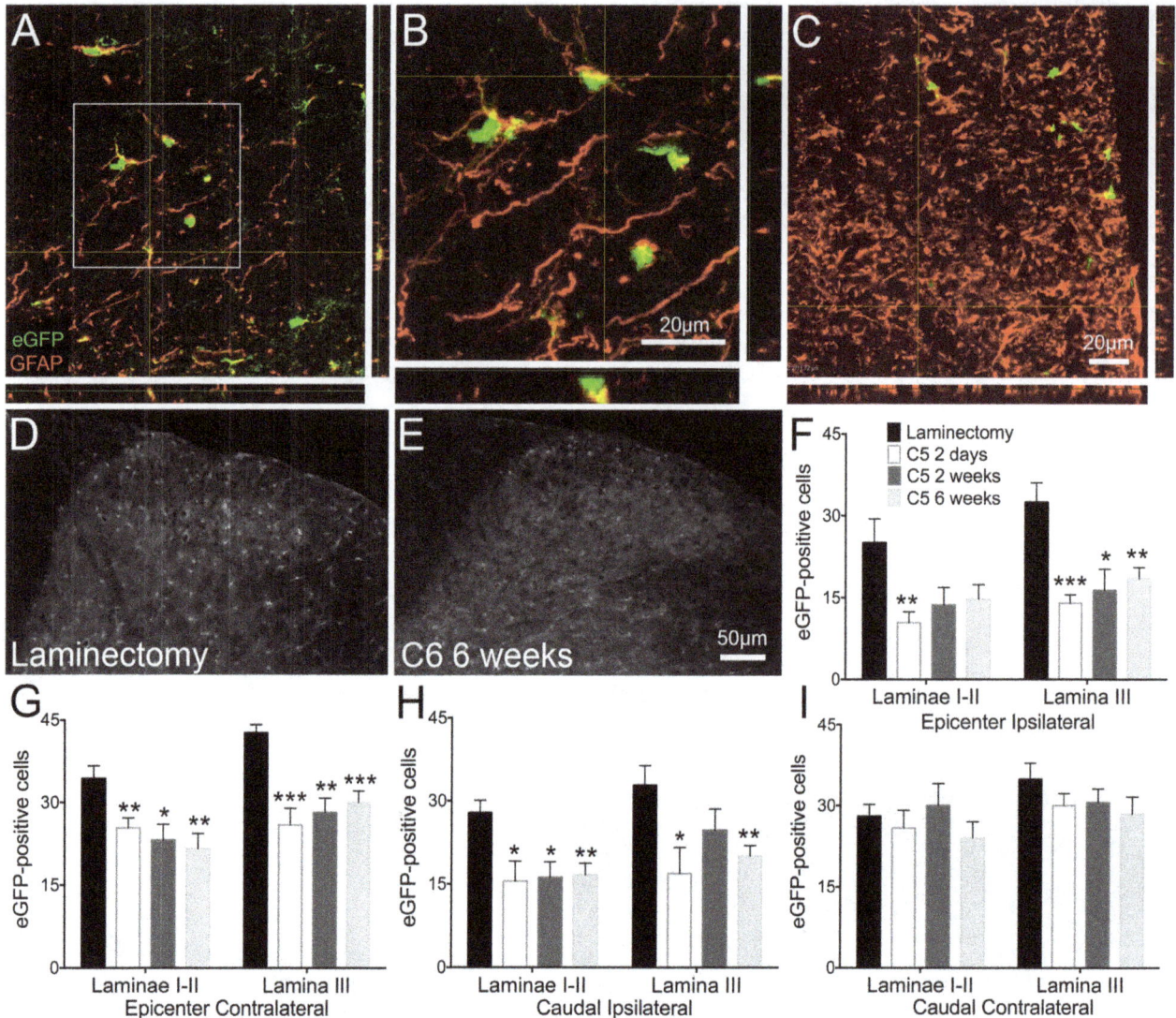

Figure 6. Astrocyte GLT1 promoter activity was reduced in injured BAC-GLT1-eGFP transgenic reporter mice. Following cervical contusion SCI, GLT1 expression/promoter activity, represented by eGFP-positive cells, was decreased in the superficial dorsal horn. In laminectomy animals, there were low levels of GFAP, although many of the cells that were GFAP-positive also expressed GLT1 (A–B). Following injury, however, an increase in GFAP was observed, but fewer of these activated astrocytes co-expressed GLT1 (C). Laminectomy control animals (D) had greater numbers of eGFP-positive cells compared to animals that received contusion injury two days, two weeks, or six weeks (E) prior to analysis. This decrease in GLT1 expression was observed at the injury epicenter in both the ipsilateral (F) and contralateral (G) superficial laminae as well as caudal to the injury on the ipsilateral side (H). No change in the number of eGFP-positive cells was found caudal to the injury on the contralateral side (I). $* = p < 0.05$; $** = p < 0.01$; $*** = p\ 0.001$.

neuronal hyperexcitability [34], [35]. In mice, hyperalgesia in response to thermal stimuli can be measured using the Hargreaves test, in which a noxious infrared heat stimulus is placed under the paw and the paw withdrawal is recorded. In the models presented here, we observe thermal hyperalgesia in the ipsilateral forepaw beginning two weeks following cervical contusion SCI and persisting for the duration of the experiment. This is consistent with data from other groups, which report the development of hyperalgesia between two and three weeks after contusion SCI at various spinal levels in the mouse [37], [38] [39]. In the rat, our group and others observed thermal hyperalgesia as early as one week after cervical contusion injury [24], [40].

Like injured animals, laminectomy control animals show a decrease in withdrawal latency one week after surgery in the ipsilateral forepaw. This finding was unexpected, but not previously unreported. The development of post-laminectomy pain has been studied in the context of the extent of laminectomy, spinal deformation, and the loss of spinal stability following surgery [41], [42]. Researchers also showed that minimal laminectomy can induce transient hyperalgesic behavior at about one week after surgery [41]. While the cause of this pain behavior is unknown, it could reflect peripheral changes or spinal deformity rather than central sensitization or only transient central sensitization.

The ipsilateral development of thermal hyperalgesia in the mouse after SCI is consistent with the injury we see histologically. At the site of the injury, we observe a loss of ventral horn motor neurons and a disruption of normal tissue anatomy on the ipsilateral but not contralateral side. This suggests a disruption of

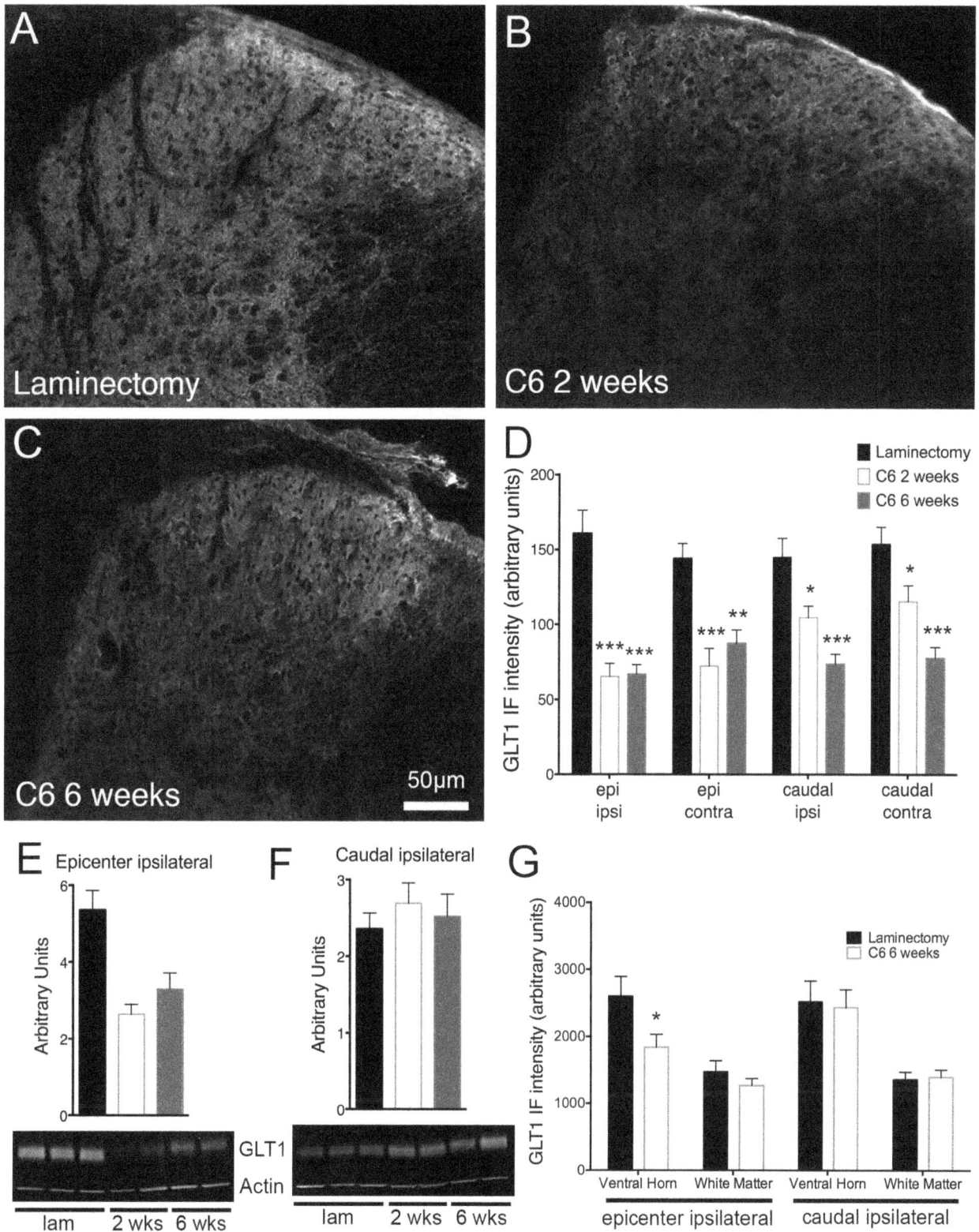

Figure 7. Cervical contusion SCI resulted in decreased astrocyte GLT1 expression in the dorsal horn. Immunohistochemical analysis revealed a decrease in GLT1 protein expression two (B) and six weeks (C) after cervical contusion SCI compared to laminectomy (A). This downregulation of the glutamate transporter was seen in the superficial dorsal horn on both sides of the spinal cord both at the injury site and caudal to the injury (D). Immunoblots of spinal cord tissue also showed a significant loss of GLT1 expression on the ipsilateral side at both time points following injury. However, this difference was seen only at the epicenter (E) and not caudal to the injury (F). Representative immunoblots are shown for each region (E–F). Analysis of GLT1 levels in regions of the spinal cord other than the superficial laminae at six weeks after injury reveal a loss of GLT1 expression in the ventral horn at the epicenter with no changes caudal to the injury (G). IF = immunofluorescence; epi = epicenter; ipsi = ipsilateral; contra = contralateral; lam = laminectomy; * = p<0.05; ** = p<0.01; *** = p 0.001.

pain transmission circuitry on the side of the injury, which may contribute to the hyperalgesia in the ipsilateral forepaw displayed by injured animals. The unilateral extent of the injury is also consistent with previous findings from our group; we previously reported damage to the ipsilateral dorsolateral and ventrolateral funiculi that did not extend bilaterally following moderate unilateral cervical SCI [10].

Unlike other studies [40], [44], we observe thermal hyperalgesia ipsilaterally but not contralaterally to the site of the injury. This discrepancy may reflect the modified version of the Hargreaves test that we utilized compared to these other groups. The Hargreaves test is most often used to measure thermal hyperalgesia in the hindpaw rather than the forepaw. Despite attempts to perform the Hargreaves test without restraint, including changes to the environment and longer acclimation times, we were unable to obtain reliable results. To overcome these difficulties, we restrained the mice in a way that did not impede forepaw movement but ensured that the mice remained still long enough to respond to the thermal stimulus. This method was introduced previously by Menendez, Lastra, Hidalgo, and Baamonde [28] for the study of hyperalgesia in the mouse forepaw. While the restraint improved the reliability of our thermal hyperalgesia measures, however, it may have affected the sensitivity of the mice to pain, which could have influenced the results we observed contralaterally.

Interestingly, while the hyperalgesia behavior changes we see are limited to the injured side of the spinal cord, we observe some molecular changes both ipsilaterally and contralaterally. ΔfosB and Ki67 expression is increased and GLT1 levels are decreased contralaterally after injury. The one alteration that is present ipsilaterally but not contralaterally is the activation of astrocytes. One possible explanation for the lack of hyperalgesic behavior in the contralateral forepaw is that the molecular changes we see are all required to elicit changes in pain behavior. There may be some interaction between activated neurons and glia that can disrupt pain transmission in the superficial laminae of the spinal cord following injury. Without activation of glia, pain transmission may continue normally.

Using von Frey filament testing, we assessed tactile allodynia following SCI. Allodynia, defined as a pain response to a previously non-noxious stimulus, is a common form of neuropathic pain [34]. In our model, we were able to identify allodynia following injury compared to baseline in the C6 injury group, but a similar significant effect was not observed in animals receiving C5 injury. We observed persistent tactile allodynia in both forepaws, which unlike the thermal testing results coincides with the anatomy of the histological findings.

Both hyperalgesia and allodynia are evoked pain behaviors in that they require a stimulus, whether noxious or non-noxious. We did not, however, study spontaneous pain, meaning pain that occurs in the absence of an external stimulus [43]. Spontaneous pain could potentially result, for example, from spontaneous activity in dorsal horn nociceptive neurons. Furthermore, while we measured at-level pain in the forepaw, we did not investigate below-level pain, which describes pain in dermatomes caudal to the level of injury and has been observed in the hindpaws of rats receiving cervical contusion SCI [40].

In this study, changes in pain behavior are exhibited in the absence of changes in motor behavior, as measured by grip strength. Because measures of evoked pain, such as the Hargreaves test and von Frey test, rely on motor activity (i.e. forepaw withdrawal) as a response, any dysfunction in motor behavior could affect test outcomes. The decrease in grip strength seen in the contralateral forepaw of C5 injury animals at one-week post

injury was unexpected and could reflect transient local changes to the cervical spinal cord rather than a global alteration of pain transmission circuitry. Importantly, grip strength returns to baseline levels after this first week, at which point hyperalgesia and allodynia have developed.

Despite the maintenance of forepaw grip strength, we observed a significant loss of ventral horn motor neurons at the injury epicenter on the ipsilateral side following injury. One likely explanation for this disconnect is that our current injury model is milder and results in less motor neuron loss compared to our previous unilateral cervical contusion model in the mouse [9], which did produce persistent forelimb motor dysfunction. There is presumably some level of motor neuron loss necessary to result in quantifiable motor deficits.

At the molecular level, changes in ΔfosB and GLT1 were observed in the superficial dorsal horn of the injured spinal cord of our SCI model. Alterations in the expression of these proteins may contribute to central sensitization of pain transmission neurons in the cervical spinal cord. Central sensitization, including post-translational and transcriptional changes to dorsal horn neurons, affects the output of nociceptive neurons and the way in which peripheral stimuli are perceived. Thus, the observed changes may contribute to the hyperalgesic and allodynic phenotypes seen in our cervical contusion SCI.

C-fos is a member of the Fos family of transcription factors, which are induced quickly and transiently by a variety of stimuli. Because its expression is stimulated by an influx of calcium into neurons, c-fos acts as a marker of neuronal activity [45]. Previously, researchers have shown an induction of c-fos expression in the dorsal horn of the spinal cord following exposure to noxious stimuli in various forms [46],[47], [48], [49], [50]. ΔfosB is a truncated splice variant of the Fos family member, FosB. Unlike c-fos, which is expressed quickly but returns to basal levels within hours after stimulation, ΔfosB is induced gradually and is stable, so it accumulates over time and persists on the order of weeks or months [50]. ΔfosB has been implicated in a number of processes in the nervous system, including addiction, plasticity, and stress [45], [50] but may also play a role in neuronal changes associated with pain [14], [15].

In our SCI model, we see long-term elevation in the levels of ΔfosB in the superficial dorsal horn of the spinal cord, suggesting persistently increased activation of these neurons. These results are in accordance with another study that reported an increase in ΔfosB expression following pain induction, specifically carrageenan-induced inflammation [14]. Additionally, we previously reported an increase in ΔfosB expression in the rat following cervical contusion SCI [24]. While ΔfosB expression is significantly increased ipsilaterally at two weeks after injury, there is an even greater increase that spreads bilaterally at the six-week time point. This is consistent with the protein's stability and tendency to accumulate over time [46]. Furthermore, this persistent expression of the protein in the dorsal horn suggests an increase in the activity of these nociceptive neurons, possibly due to an increase in spontaneous firing and/or synaptic input, which may contribute to central sensitization. Thus the expression of ΔfosB that we see in our injury model is likely in accordance with its role in pain and plasticity.

In the nucleus accumbens and cortex, identified targets of ΔfosB include GluA2 and GluN1. In these regions, ΔfosB has been shown to upregulate these two proteins [50]. These targets are subunits of the glutamate receptors AMPAR and NMDAR, and their upregulation may contribute to increased glutamatergic transmission. Excessive stimulation of glutamate receptors can lead to hyperexcitability directly by increased activation of dorsal horn neurons and indirectly via glutamate excitotoxic loss of inhibitory interneurons [18]. It is unknown whether ΔfosB also targets these AMPAR and NMDAR subunits in the spinal cord following SCI. However, researchers have reported changes in GluA1 trafficking and expression in spinal neurons following central and peripheral injury and pain [51], [52], [53] as well as an upregulation of GluN1 and GluN2A in the ventral horn as a result of contusion SCI [54]. Despite this potential connection between ΔfosB and glutamate receptor subunits, ΔfosB does not definitively measure hyperexcitability. Instead, a continuation of this experiment to provide more conclusive evidence of the hyperexcitability could include electrophysiological measures of dorsal horn neurons.

Also following injury, we observe an increase in GFAP, a protein upregulated in activated astrocytes, in the dorsal horn of the spinal cord. We see this change at both time points, but it is more pronounced two weeks after injury. These data are in accordance with our group and others who have shown localized increases in markers of astrocyte activation following SCI [23], [24], [55], [56]. The observed increase in GFAP is seen only at the injury epicenter on the ipsilateral side, suggesting that this change is region-specific and may not play a role in potential above- or below-level changes, at least in our model.

The increase in activated astrocytes in our model of SCI could potentially have negative effects on the injured spinal cord and pain transmission circuitry. Often, activated astrocytes in the context of SCI and other injuries are considered detrimental because of their role in the formation of the glial scar, which can inhibit axon regeneration and plasticity, and the release of pro-inflammatory and other harmful molecules that can alter the excitability of neurons. Astrocytes, however, play many beneficial roles in the CNS, such as maintaining extracellular ion and neurotransmitter homeostasis, providing neurotrophic factor support, aiding in metabolic functions, and regulating the formation and maintenance of synapses [57].

Interestingly, while at-level thermal hyperalgesia is maintained through six weeks after injury, GFAP levels decrease slightly by this time point. Activated astrocytes play a significant role in the structural and molecular maintenance of the injury site [13], [17], [18], [57], [58]. The repair process following spinal cord injury, however, occurs in various phases, including acute, sub-acute, and chronic. While the effects of the glial scar and other repair processes can last months or years, not all of the molecules contributing to post-injury repair may be present at all stages. Thus, some astrocytes may return to the basal state in the days or weeks following injury, explaining the decrease in GFAP we see at six weeks compared to two weeks. Another explanation for the persistence of thermal hyperalgesia and tactile allodynia despite GFAP levels decreasing is that the loss of GLT1 also persists and contributes more strongly to the development of neuropathic pain after SCI. Alternatively, there may be irreversible damage to the spinal cord at this point that the inactivation of astrocytes may have no effect on.

Considering the various roles that astrocytes play following injury, it is important not only to study the reactive state of astrocytes in our model but also the effects of our injury on important homeostatic and protective functions of astrocytes. In light of this, we decided to investigate how our injury paradigm alters a centrally important function of astrocytes in the CNS, the uptake of glutamate through GLT1. Several groups have reported decreases in GLT1 levels following SCI [22], [23], [24], [25], [26], but the role of such changes has not been studied extensively in the context of neuropathic pain. To study GLT1 expression, we utilized both C57BL/6 wild-type and BAC-GLT1-eGFP reporter mice as well as both immunohistochemistry and western blotting.

In our mouse cervical contusion SCI model, GLT1 levels are diminished in the dorsal horn at both time points at the epicenter and caudally on the ipsilateral side, suggesting a significant compromise in glutamate clearance in the injured spinal cord. Unlike with wild-type mice, in BAC-GLT1-eGFP mice, we see no change in the caudal contralateral region of the dorsal horn. This is likely due to a slightly different injury used in these two mouse paradigms.

Western blotting reveals that GLT1 protein levels are decreased ipsilaterally at the epicenter. However, no change in GLT1 levels is observed at the caudal ipsilateral region, which is contrary to the results we report using immunohistochemistry. This discrepancy likely reflects the difference in spatial resolution between these two techniques. Using immunohistochemistry, analyses of very specific regions, such as the superficial dorsal horn, are possible. For western blotting, however, we use a piece of tissue that encompasses an entire spinal cord level, including both the dorsal and ventral horn and surrounding white matter tracts. For our immunohistochemical analyses of the injured spinal cord, we examined the most superficial laminae of the dorsal horn, laminae I–II, as well as laminae III.

Importantly, co-localization analyses of GFAP and GLT1-eGFP at high-magnification reveal that, in control animals, most of the GLT1-positive cells are also GFAP-positive astrocytes. However, after injury, while the number of GFAP-positive cells is increased, the number and percentage of these astrocytes also expressing GLT1 is greatly reduced. This suggests that the loss of GLT1 that is observed in our animals occurs mostly in astrocytes, supporting our proposal that astrocytes activated after injury are deficient in glutamate clearance.

Like astrocytes, microglia play a major role in both immediate and delayed responses to injury to the spinal cord and may contribute to the development of pathological pain [13]. We also noted significant microglial activation in the superficial dorsal horn following cervical contusion SCI. Unlike astrocyte reactivity, we observed microglial activation not just at the ipsilateral epicenter region, but also at contralateral epicenter and caudal ipsilateral locations. Though we focused mostly on astrocyte changes, including down-regulation of GLT1 expression, it is likely that microglial activation also played a significant role in the persistent neuropathic pain phenotype observed in this study.

Here we present a model of unilateral cervical contusion SCI in the mouse that is representative of typical injury seen clinically in humans [1], [5]. The model exhibits at-level neuropathic pain accompanied by relevant molecular changes in the superficial dorsal horn. The protein expression changes suggest the presence of activated and proliferating astrocytes and a loss of GLT1 function, which may contribute to central sensitization, and underlie the development of neuropathic pain. We have identified a number of proteins that are altered by SCI and accompany thermal hyperalgesia and tactile allodynia, but their roles in the development of neuropathic pain have yet to be fully elucidated. Further research with the model may include identifying the factors and processes underlying the formation and maintenance of neuropathic pain in the spinal cord as well as recognizing targets for the treatment of chronic pathological pain resulting from SCI and similar injuries. Importantly, the availability of this model in the mouse allow for the use of valuable transgenic tools.

Acknowledgments

We would like to thank Drs. Luis Menéndez and Ana Baamonde for their assistance in the thermal testing procedures. We would also like to thank Dr. Jeannie Chin, Dr. Anupam Hazra and Brain Corbett for their advice and technical help with ΔFosB immunohistochemistry. Additionally, J.W.

would like to thank the members of her thesis committee, Dr. Piera Pasinelli and Dr. Lorraine Iacovitti, for their guidance and support.

Author Contributions

Conceived and designed the experiments: JLW ACL. Performed the experiments: JLW TJH RP DS ACL. Analyzed the data: JLW TJH RP DS ACL. Wrote the paper: JLW ACL.

References

1. National Spinal Cord Injury Statistical Center, University of Birmingham, Alabama (2013) Spinal cord injury facts and figures at a glance. Available: https://www.nscisc.uab.edu/PublicDocuments/fact_figures_docs/Facts%202013.pdf.

2. de Miguel M, Kraychete DC (2009) Pain in patients with spinal cord injury: A review. Rev Bras Anestheiol 59: 350–357.

3. Siddall PJ, McClelland JM, Rutkowski SB, Cousins MJ (2003) A longitudinal study of the prevalence and characteristics of pain in the first 5 years following spinal cord injury. Pain 103: 249–257.

4. Ravenscroft A, Ahmed YS, Burnside IG (2000) Chronic pain after SCI: A patient survey. Spinal Cord 38: 611–614.

5. McDonald JW, Becker D (2003) Spinal cord injury: Promising interventions and realistic goals. Am J Phys Med Rehabil 82: S38–S49.

6. Nakae A, Nakai K, Yano K, Hosokawa K, Shibata M, et al. (2011) The animal model of spinal cord injury as an experimental pain model. J Biomed Biotechnol 2011: 939023.

7. Kundi S, Bicknell R, Ahmed Z (2013) Spinal cord injury: Current mammalian models. Am J Neurosci 4: 1–12.

8. Nicaise C, Hala TJ, Frank DM, Parker JL, Authelet M, et al. (2012) Phrenic motor neuron degeneration compromises phrenic axonal circuitry and diaphragm activity in a unilateral cervical contusion model of spinal cord injury. Exp Neurol 235: 539–552.

9. Nicaise C, Putatunda R, Hala TJ, Regan KA, Frank DM, et al. (2012) Degeneration of phrenic motor neurons induces long-term diaphragm deficits following mid-cervical spinal contusion in mice. J Neurotrauma 29: 2748–2760.

10. Nicaise C, Frank DM, Hala TJ, Authelet M, Pochet R, et al. (2013) Early phrenic motor neuron loss and transient respiratory abnormalities after unilateral cervical spinal cord contusion. J Neurotrauma 30: 1092–1099.

11. Streijger F, Beernink TM, Lee JH, Bhatnagar T, Park S, et al. (2013) Characterization of a cervical spinal cord hemicontusion injury in mice using the infinite horizon impactor. J Neurotrauma 30: 869–883.

12. Latremoliere A, Woolf CJ (2009) Central sensitization: A generator of pain hypersensitivity by central neural plasticity. J Pain 10: 895–926.

13. Hulsebosch CE, Hains BC, Crown ED, Carlton SM (2009) Mechanisms of chronic central neuropathic pain after spinal cord injury. Brain Res Rev 60: 202–213.

14. Luis-Delgado OE, Barrot M, Rodeau JL, Ulery PG, Freund-Mercier MJ, et al. (2006) The transcription factor deltafosB is recruited by inflammatory pain. J Neurochem 98: 1423–1431.

15. Pareek TK, Kulkarni AB (2006) Cdk5: A new player in pain signaling. Cell Cycle 5: 585–588.

16. Clarke LE, Barres BA (2013) Emerging roles of astrocytes in neural circuit development. Nat Rev Neurosci 14: 311–321.

17. Karimi-Abdolrezaee S, Billakanti R (2012) Reactive astrogliosis after spinal cord injury: Beneficial and detrimental effects. Mol Neurobiol 46: 251–264.

18. Nakagawa T, Kaneko S (2010) Spinal astrocytes as therapeutic targets for pathological pain. J Pharmacol Sci

19. Chen CJ, Liao SL, Kuo JS (2000) Gliotoxic action of glutamate on cultured astrocytes. J Neurochem 74: 1557–1565.

20. Mark LP, Prost RW, Ulmer JL, Smith MM, Daniels DL, et al. (2001) Pictorial review of glutamate excitotoxicity: Fundamental concepts for neuroimaging. AJNR Am J Neuroradiol 22: 1813–1824.

21. Doble A (1999) The role of excitotoxicity in neurodegenerative disease: Implications for therapy. Pharmacol Ther 81: 163–221.

22. Lepore AC, O'Donnell J, Kim AS, Yang EJ, Tuteja A, et al. (2011) Reduction in expression of the astrocyte glutamate transporter, GLT1, worsens functional and histological outcomes following traumatic spinal cord injury. Glia 59: 1996–2005.

23. Lepore AC, O'Donnell J, Bonner JF, Paul C, Miller ME, et al. (2011) Spatial and temporal changes in promoter activity of the astrocyte glutamate transporter GLT1 following traumatic spinal cord injury. J Neurosci Res 89: 1001–1017.

24. Putatunda R, Hala TJ, Chin J, Lepore AC (2014) Chronic at-level thermal hyperalgesia following rat cervical contusion spinal cord injury is accompanied by neuronal and astrocyte activation and loss of the astrocyte glutamate transporter, GLT1, in superficial dorsal horn. Brain Res: in press.

25. Vera-Portocarrero LP, Mills CD, Ye Z, Fullwood SD, McAdoo DJ, et al. (2002) Rapid changes in expression of glutamate transporters after spinal cord injury. Brain Res 927: 104–110.

26. Olsen ML, Campbell SC, McFerrin MB, Floyd CL, Sontheimer H (2010) Spinal cord injury causes a wide-spread, persistent loss of Kir4.1 and glutamate transporter 1: Benefit of 17 beta-oestradiol treatment. Brain 133: 1013–1025.

27. Regan MR, Huang YH, Kim YS, Dykes-Hoberg ML, Jin L, et al. (2007) Variations in promoter activity reveal a differential expression and physiology of glutamate transporters by glia in the developing and mature CNS. J Neurosci 27: 6607–6619.

28. Menendez L, Lastra A, Hidalgo A, Baamonde A (2002) Unilateral hot plate test: a simple and sensitive method for detecting central and peripheral hyperalgesia in mice. J Neurosci Methods 113: 91–97.

29. Lepore AC, Rauck B, Dejea C, Pardo AC, Rao MS, et al. (2008) Focal transplantation-based astrocyte replacement is neuroprotective in a model of motor neuron disease. Nat Neurosci 11: 1294–1301.

30. Perrotti LI, Weaver RR, Robison B, Renthal W, Maze I, et al. (2008) Distinct patterns of DeltaFosB induction in brain by drugs of abuse. Synapse 62: 358–369.

31. Lepore AC, Dejea C, Carmen J, Rauck B, Kerr DA, et al. (2008). Selective ablation of proliferating astrocytes does not affect disease outcome in either acute or chronic models of motor neuron degeneration. Exp Neurol 211: 423–432.

32. Lepore AC, Fischer I. (2005) Lineage-restricted neural precursors survive, migrate, and differentiate following transplantation into the injured adult spinal cord. Exp Neurol 194: 230–242.

33. Maragakis NJ, Rothstein JD (2001) Glutamate transporters in neurologic disease. Arch Neurol 58: 365–370.

34. Jorum E, Warncke T, Stubhaug A (2003) Cold allodynia and hyperalgesia in neuropathic pain: The effect of N-methyl-D-aspartate (NMDA) receptor antagonist ketamine–double-blind, cross-over comparison with alfentanil and placebo. Pain 101: 229–235.

35. Gwak YS, Hulsebosch CE (2011) Neuronal hyperexcitability: A substrate for central neuropathic pain after spinal cord injury. Curr Pain Headache Rep 15: 215–222.

36. Sandkuhler J (2009) Models and mechanisms of hyperalgesia and allodynia. Physiol Rev 89: 707–758.

37. Hoschouer EL, Basso DM, Jakeman LB (2010) Aberrant sensory responses are dependent on lesion severity after spinal cord contusion injury in mice. Pain 148: 328–342.

38. Meisner JG, Marsh AD, Marsh DR (2010) Loss of GABAergic interneurons in laminae I–III of the spinal cord dorsal horn contributes to reduced GABAergic tone and neuropathic pain after spinal cord injury. J Neurotrauma 27: 729–737.

39. Hoschouer EL, Yin FQ, Jakeman LB (2009) L1 cell adhesion molecule is essential for the maintenance of hyperalgesia after spinal cord injury. Exp Neurol 216: 22–34.

40. Detloff MR, Wade ER Jr, Houle JD (2013) Chronic at- and below-level pain after moderate unilateral cervical spinal cord contusion in rats. J Neurotrauma 30: 884–890.

41. Kosta V, Kojundzic SL, Sapunar LC, Sapunar D (2012) The extent of laminectomy affects pain-related behavior in a rat model of neuropathic pain. Eur J Pain 13: 243–248.

42. Busic Z, Kostic S, Kosta V, Carija R, Puljak L, et al. (2012) Postlaminectomy stabilization of the spine in a rat model of neuropathic pain reduces pain-related behavior. Spine 15: 1874–1882.

43. Djouhri L, Koutsikou S, Fang X, McMullan S, Lawson SN (2006) Spontaneous pain, both neuropathic and inflammatory, is related to frequency of spontaneous firing in intact C-fiber nociceptors. J Neurosci 26:1281–1292.

44. Christensen MD, Everhart AQ, Pickelman JT, Hulsebosch CE (1996) Mechanical and thermal allodynia in chronic central pain following spinal cord injury. Pain 68: 97–107.

45. Bullitt E (1990) Expression of c-fos-like protein as a marker for neuronal activity following noxious stimulation in the rat. J Comp Neurol 296: 517–530.

46. Abbadie C, Honore P, Besson JM (1994) Intense cold noxious stimulation of the rat hindpaw induces c-fos expression in lumbar spinal cord neurons. Neuroscience 59: 457–468.

47. Jinks SL, Simons CT, Dessirier JM, Carstens MI, Antognini JF, et al. (2002) C-fos induction in rat superficial dorsal horn following cutaneous application of noxious chemical or mechanical stimuli. Exp Brain Res 145: 261–269.

48. Yi DK, Barr GA (1995) The induction of Fos-like immunoreactivity by noxious thermal, mechanical and chemical stimuli in the lumbar spinal cord of infant rats. Pain 60: 257–265.

49. Bester H, Beggs S, Woolf CJ (2000) Changes in tactile stimuli-induced behavior and c-Fos expression in the superficial dorsal horn and in parabrachial nuclei after sciatic nerve crush. J Comp Neurol 428: 45–61.

50. McClung CA, Ulery PG, Perrotti L, Zachariou V, Berton O, et al. (2004) DeltaFosB: A molecular switch for long-term adaptation in the brain. Brain Res Mol Brain Res 132: 146–154.

51. Galan A, Laird JM, Cervero F (2004) In vivo recruitment by painful stimuli of AMPA receptor subunits to the plasma membrane of spinal cord neurons. Pain 112: 315–323.

52. Katano T, Furue H, Okuda-Ashitaka E, Tagaya M, Watanabe M, et al. (2008) N-ethylmaleimide-sensitive fusion protein (NSF) is involved in central sensitization in the spinal cord through GluR2 subunit composition switch after inflammation. Eur J Neurosci 27: 3161–3170.

53. Larsson M, Broman J (2008) Translocation of GluR1-containing AMPA receptors to a spinal nociceptive synapse during acute noxious stimulation. J Neurosci 28: 7084–7090.

54. Grossman SD, Wolfe BB, Yasuda RP, Wrathall JR (2000) Changes in NMDA receptor subunit expression in response to contusive spinal cord injury. J Neurochem 75: 174–184.

55. Iwasaki R, Matsuura Y, Ohtori S, Suzuki T, Kuniyoshi K, et al. (2013) Activation of astrocytes and microglia in the C3-T4 dorsal horn by lower trunk avulsion in a rat model of neuropathic pain. J Hand Surg Am 38: 841–846.

56. Cho DC, Cheong JH, Yang MS, Hwang SJ, Kim JM, et al. (2011) The effect of minocycline on motor neuron recovery and neuropathic pain in a rat model of spinal cord injury. J Korean Neurosurg Soc 49: 83–91.

57. Pekny M, Nilsson M (2005) Astrocyte activation and reactive gliosis. Glia 50: 427–434.

58. Rolls A, Schechter R, Schwartz M (2009) The bright side of the glial scar in CNS repair. Nat Rev Neurosci 10: 235–241.

16

Fatty Acid Amide Hydrolase (FAAH) Inhibitors Exert Pharmacological Effects, but Lack Antinociceptive Efficacy in Rats with Neuropathic Spinal Cord Injury Pain

Aldric T. Hama[1]*, Peter Germano[2], Matthew S. Varghese[1], Benjamin F. Cravatt[3], G. Todd Milne[2], James P. Pearson[2], Jacqueline Sagen[1]

1 Miami Project to Cure Paralysis, University of Miami Miller School of Medicine, Miami, Florida, United States of America, 2 Ironwood Pharmaceuticals, Inc., Cambridge, Massachusetts, United States of America, 3 Department of Chemical Physiology, The Skaggs Institute for Chemical Biology, The Scripps Research Institute, La Jolla, California, United States of America

Abstract

Amelioration of neuropathic spinal cord injury (SCI) pain is a clinical challenge. Increasing the endocannabinoid anandamide and other fatty acid amides (FAA) by blocking fatty acid amide hydrolase (FAAH) has been shown to be antinociceptive in a number of animal models of chronic pain. However, an antinociceptive effect of blocking FAAH has yet to be demonstrated in a rat model of neuropathic SCI pain. Four weeks following a SCI, rats developed significantly decreased hind paw withdrawal thresholds, indicative of below-level cutaneous hypersensitivity. A group of SCI rats were systemically treated (i.p.) with either the selective FAAH inhibitor URB597 or vehicle twice daily for seven days. A separate group of SCI rats received a single dose (p.o.) of either the selective FAAH inhibitor PF-3845 or vehicle. Following behavioral testing, levels of the FAA N-arachidonoylethanolamide, N-oleoyl ethanolamide and N-palmitoyl ethanolamide were quantified in brain and spinal cord from SCI rats. Four weeks following SCI, FAA levels were markedly reduced in spinal cord tissue. Although systemic treatment with URB597 significantly increased CNS FAA levels, no antinociceptive effect was observed. A significant elevation of CNS FAA levels was also observed following oral PF-3845 treatment, but only a modest antinociceptive effect was observed. Increasing CNS FAA levels alone does not lead to robust amelioration of below-level neuropathic SCI pain. Perhaps utilizing FAAH inhibition in conjunction with other analgesic mechanisms could be an effective analgesic therapy.

Editor: Vinod K. Yaragudri, Nathan Kline Institute for Psychiatric Research and New York School of Medicine, United States of America

Funding: This work supported in part by Ironwood Pharmaceuticals, Inc. and by the National Institutes of Health Neurological Disorders & Stroke NS61172 (to JS). The funder provided support in the form of salaries for authors PG, GTM and JPP, and research materials but did not have any additional role in the study design, data collection and analysis, decision to publish, or preparation of the manuscript. The specific roles of these authors are articulated in the 'author contributions' section.

Competing Interests: The current work was supported in part by Ironwood Pharmaceuticals, Inc. Co-authors Peter Germano, James P. Pearson and G. Todd Milne are stockholders, Peter Germano and G. Todd Milne are employees, and James P. Pearson is a paid consultant of Ironwood Pharmaceuticals which has a FAAH inhibitor program. The specific roles of these authors are articulated in the 'author contributions' section. Ironwood provided research materials required per the study design. There are no patents, products in development or marketed products to declare that would represent a conflict of interest.

* E-mail: ahama@miami.edu

Introduction

In addition to motor and visceral dysfunction, a serious consequence of spinal cord injury (SCI) is chronic pain. It is estimated that 65% of SCI patients suffer from chronic pain, with about one-third of these patients rating their pain as severe [1]. Although pain can occur above and at the level of the spinal lesion, symptoms with similarity to peripheral neuropathic pain can occur below the spinal lesion [2]. Also, below-level neuropathic pain is particularly challenging to treat in that adverse side effects of commonly prescribed neuropathic pain analgesics may exacerbate existing dysfunctions, such as urinary retention with antidepressants and constipation with opioids. Thus, it is crucial that novel therapeutics be developed for this particular patient population.

A number of studies have shown that activation of the cannabinoid (CB) receptor leads to a robust antinociception in a variety of preclinical pain models [3]. The antinociceptive effects

of nonselective CB receptor agonists in rats are blocked with either cannabinoid receptor type-1 (CB_1) or cannabinoid receptor type-2 (CB_2) receptor antagonists. Limited clinical evidence and SCI patient survey suggests that CB receptor activation with CB ligands derived from *Cannabis sativa* reduces SCI pain [4,5]. In humans, the psychological and physiological effects of CB agonists are blocked by treatment with the CB_1 receptor antagonist rimonabant (SR141719A) indicating the importance of CB_1 receptors in mediating the effects of CB [6].

Intrathecal administrations of fatty acid amide (FAA) endocannabinoids, such as N-arachidonoylethanolamide (AEA), demonstrate robust antinociception in models of tissue injury-induced cutaneous hypersensitivity [7,8]. One method of enhancing CNS levels of endocannabinoids and other antinociceptive non-cannabinoid FAA, such as N-oleoyl ethanolamide (OEA) and N-palmitoyl ethanolamide (PEA), is by blocking one of their catabolic enzymes, fatty acid amide hydrolase (FAAH) [9,10]. Systemic as well as intrathecal administration of selective FAAH inhibitors have demonstrated significant antinociception in preclinical models of peripheral neuropathic pain [3,9,11]. The antinociceptive effects positively correlated with increased CNS endocannabinoid levels and were blocked with administration of either CB_1 or CB_2 receptor antagonist [12,13]. Even though the antinociceptive effect is mediated by CB_1 receptors, there is a lack of side effects with FAAH inhibition commonly associated with CB_1 receptor agonists, including hypothermia, catalepsy and decreased locomotor activity [14]. It is possible that a part of the antinociceptive effect of increased CNS FAA is due to a non-CB receptor mediated mechanism, such activity at the transient receptor potential vanilloid receptor (TRPV1) channel [11].

Acute SCI in rats can lead to persistent neuropathic pain-like symptoms [15–17]. Robust cutaneous hypersensitivity of the hind paws to both noxious and innocuous stimuli is obtained following spinal compression [18]. A number of clinical analgesics do not display efficacy in SCI rats despite demonstrating efficacy in other neuropathic pain models [17,18]. However, treatment with a non-subtype selective CB receptor agonist WIN 55,212-2 led to a significant antinociception which was reversed by treatment with rimonabant indicating that therapeutic efficacy was mediated by CB_1 receptors [19]. Furthermore, no tolerance to the antinociceptive effect of WIN 55,212-2 was observed over a seven-day treatment period, whereas morphine efficacy gradually diminished during the same treatment period [20]. While exogenous CB_1 receptor agonists may hold promise as analgesics for neuropathic SCI pain, in addition to target-mediated side effects, their current legal status and difficulty in "blinding" the psychotropic effects of cannabinoids make clinical development controversial [21]. Although antinociceptive efficacy of FAAH inhibitors has been observed in various models of peripheral tissue injury-induced pain, efficacy has yet to be demonstrated in neuropathic SCI pain.

The goal of the current study is to evaluate the effect of blocking FAAH with the inhibitors URB597 and PF-3845 on below-level cutaneous hypersensitivity SCI rats. URB597 is a phenyl carbamate inhibitor and PF-3845 is a piperidine urea FAAH inhibitor [9] which irreversibly bind to FAAH. Most previous studies of URB597 demonstrated antinociception following a single dose, but one study showed that repeated dosing over time was needed to attain significant efficacy [22]. Thus, in the current study, SCI rats were systemically treated with URB597 over a seven-day period. Following the treatment and testing period, brain and spinal cord were collected for measurement of FAA by liquid chromatography-tandem mass spectrometry (LC-MS/MS) analysis. As a comparator, WIN 55,212-2 was tested in parallel with FAAH inhibitors in SCI rats. Whereas treatment with WIN 55,212-2 resulted in marked antinociception, there was a lack of comparable antinociception following FAAH treatment in SCI rats.

Materials and Methods

Animals

All procedures were reviewed and approved by the University of Miami Animal Care and Use Committee (Protocol No. 07-134) and followed the recommendations within the *Guide for the Care and Use of Laboratory Animals* (National Research Council). Every effort was made to use the least possible number of animals and to minimize pain and distress. Male Sprague-Dawley rats (130–150 g at the time of surgery; Harlan, Indianapolis, IN) were housed two per cage and allowed free access to food and water before and after surgery. Lighting was on a 12 hr light/dark cycle. Temperature and humidity were controlled to $22 \pm 1^\circ C$ and

$50 \pm 10\%$, respectively. Rats were acclimated to the animal facility for at least 5 days prior to use.

General experimental plan

Baseline hind paw withdrawal thresholds and locomotor function were assessed before and 4 weeks following SCI surgery. Spinal cord injured rats were dosed beginning 4 weeks after surgery for seven days. Although SCI rats were dosed daily, withdrawal thresholds were measured only on the first, third and seventh day of dosing (i.e. 28, 30 and 35 days post-SCI surgery). To assess a possible effect of daily compound treatment on locomotor function, locomotor rating scores were obtained from SCI rats 4 weeks after surgery, prior to compound administration, and on the sixth day of compound treatment (i.e. 34 days post-SCI surgery).

Spinal cord injury in the rat

Aseptic surgical technique and sterile instruments were used. The procedure to induce an acute SCI has been previously described [18]. Rats were anesthetized and maintained with isoflurane in O_2 for the duration of the surgery. The back was shaved and the skin cleaned with chlorhexadine. A laminectomy was performed to expose spinal segment T6-T7. A microvascular clip (20 g compressive force, Harvard Apparatus, Hollister, MA) was placed vertically on the exposed thoracic spinal cord, such that clip compressed the entire segment, and then left in place for 60 seconds. Care was taken not to cut the dura or disturb nearby spinal nerve roots. Following spinal compression, the clip was removed, the muscles sutured shut and the skin closed with wound clips. Urinary bladders were expressed twice daily until voiding was regained. Spontaneous voiding returned about 1 or 2 days following spinal compression.

Hind paw withdrawal threshold

Prior to spinal compression surgery, hind paw withdrawal thresholds were measured. The up-down method was used to quantify hind paw responsiveness to innocuous tactile stimulation [23]. Rats were placed in clear Plexiglas containers resting on an elevated wire mesh floor and allowed to acclimate to the chamber for at least 30 min. Eight specific calibrated von Frey filaments were used to determine the withdrawal threshold (0.4, 0.6, 1, 2, 4, 6, 8, 15 grams; Stoelting Co., Woodale, IL). The filament was applied perpendicularly the plantar skin of the hind paw, bowed slightly and held in place for six seconds. A hind paw withdrawal from the filament led to testing with a lower force filament. A lack of response led to the use of the next higher force filament. From the pattern of responses to the filaments, a withdrawal threshold was calculated. Both hind paws were tested and about 5 min separated testing of the opposite paw. An upper withdrawal threshold of 15 g was used. Prior to surgery, rat withdrawal thresholds were 15 g. In order for SCI rats to be included in the study, withdrawal thresholds of one paw needed to be 4 g or less.

Locomotor function: Basso, Beattie, and Bresnahan Score

Following threshold measurement, below-level motor functionality was assessed using a standardized "Locomotor Rating Scale" devised by Basso, Beattie, and Bresnahan (BBB) [24]. The scale ranges from 0, no hind limb function, to 21, normal, coordinated movement of the hind limbs as observed in uninjured rats. Rats were placed in a 1.2 m diameter arena and allowed to continuously move within a four minute observation period. Two observers rated hind limb function, such as movement at joints, hind paw stepping and fore paw-hind paw coordination.

Following the observation period, the scores from both hind limbs were averaged to give a final BBB score. Prior to surgery, BBB scores of naive rats are 21. Spinal cord injured-rats were rated one day prior to the beginning of the treatment period and reassessed on the sixth day of treatment following determination of withdrawal thresholds.

Pharmacological treatments

Following baseline behavioral assessment in SCI rats, rats were divided into four treatment groups. Spinal cord-injured rats were injected with either URB597 (i.p.), WIN 55,212-2 (s.c.) or vehicle (i.p.) twice daily (at approximately 900 and 1700) for 7 days. Withdrawal thresholds were measured following the first daily injection. Following injection, rats were tested once every 30 minutes for up to four hours post-injection. On the sixth day of treatment, following final determination of withdrawal threshold, BBB scores were determined. On the seventh day, immediately following testing at four hours post-injection, rats were deeply anesthetized with isoflurane, decapitated and brain and spinal cord tissues were collected.

In a separate group of SCI rats, either PF-3845 or vehicle was orally administered and rats were tested once every hour up to four hours post-administration. Because of stress associated with p.o. dosing in SCI rats, rats were dosed only once and not treated over a seven-day period. At the last testing time point, rats were deeply anesthetized with isoflurane, decapitated and brain and spinal tissues were collected. Uninjured age-matched rats were also treated with either PF-3845 or vehicle (p.o.) and tissues were collected at the same time as the SCI rats. At the same time, age-matched uninjured rats were treated with either URB597 (i.p.), WIN 55,212-2 (s.c.), or vehicle (i.p.), were deeply anesthetized, decapitated and tissues were collected four hours post-treatment to determine baseline FAA levels and to determine the acute effects of the compounds on FAA levels in uninjured rats. An additional group of uninjured rats were treated with URB597 (i.p.) or vehicle (i.p.), euthanized and brain and spinal cord tissues were collected two hours after treatment.

The spinal cord was divided into four segments: lumbar (L4/L5), a 1 cm segment rostral to the compression epicenter, a 1 cm segment of the epicenter and a 1 cm segment caudal to the epicenter. Tissues were flash frozen on dry ice and stored at $-80°C$ until assay.

Assessment of brain and spinal cord levels of fatty acid amides by liquid chromatography-tandem mass spectrometry

Brain samples were prepared using a method adapted from previously published methods [25]. Briefly, brain samples were removed from $-80°C$ freezer and placed on dry ice. Individual brains were transferred to a clean, tared 50 ml capacity polypropylene conical tube and weights were recorded. A solution of ethyl acetate:hexanes (9:1) was immediately added to each conical tube along with a FAA standard molecule (Palmitoyl Propanolamide, Ironwood Pharmaceuticals, Inc., Cambridge, MA). Samples were homogenized for 15 seconds using an electric-powered mechanical tissue disrupter (Omni Prep Multi-Sample Homogenizer Part Number: 06-021, Omni International, Kennesaw, GA) fitted with stainless steel probe (10 mm×110 mm Stainless Steel Omni Prep/THQ Homogenizer Probe, Omni International, Kennesaw, GA) washed with approximately 30% water, and homogenized for another 15 seconds. Samples were vortexed and centrifuged (2,000×g for 30 minutes at 10°C). After centrifugation, the upper organic layer was recovered and the

samples were evaporated to dryness under nitrogen gas. Samples were not subjected to solid phase extraction. After reconstitution in 1 ml chloroform:methanol (1:3), samples were centrifuged (16,000×g for 3 minutes at room temperature) to sediment any particulates. A 100 μl aliquot of each sample supernatant was transferred to individual wells on a 96 well plate. Each sample was diluted 1:1 with methanol containing the internal standard d4-AEA (arachidonoyl-ethanolamide) labeled with 4 deuterium atoms replacing the 4 H's on the methylenes of ethanolamine moiety, Cayman Chemical, Ann Arbor, MI) Waters Acquity/TQD system in positive ion (ES+) mode. Samples were maintained at 6°C.

The procedure for FAA extraction from spinal cord tissue segments was similar to brain FAA extraction procedure listed above with the following change. After evaporation of organic solvents from tissue homogenates the residue from extraction was dissolved in 0.25 ml chloroform:methanol (1:3) instead of 1 ml volume used for brain extracts.

Liquid chromatography-tandem mass spectrometry conditions

Liquid chromatography was conducted using a Higgins Clipeus HPLC column [C8 reverse phase, dimensions 2.1×30 mm, particle size 5 micron (Mountain View, CA)] and samples were eluted using a gradient employing 2 mobile phases A and B from 30%–95% B [HPLC mobile phases A (5 mM ammonium acetate in water) and HPLC mobile phase B (5 mM ammonium acetate in 85:10:5 acetonitrile: isopropanol: water)] using a flow rate of 0.4 ml/min. MS/MS. The following mass transitions were monitored AEA: 348.2>62 m/z, OEA: 326.2>62 m/z, PEA: 300.2>62 m/z, Palmitoyl Propanolamide: 314.2>75.9 m/z, D4-AEA: 352.2>66 m/z (last two are internal standards for fatty acid amides). Chromatograms were integrated and quantified by response to the internal standard peak area using Quanlynx software V4.0 SP4 (Micromass, Ltd).

Compound treatments

URB597 (3 mg/kg, Cayman Chemicals, Ann Arbor, MI) was dissolved in 10% dimethyl sulfoxide (DMSO): 10% Cremophor EL: 80% saline and administered i.p. in a volume of 1.5 ml/kg. URB597 was prepared daily, prior to dosing. WIN 55,212-2 mesylate (3 mg/kg, Sigma-Aldrich Co., St. Louis, MO) was dissolved in 45% (2-Hydroxypropyl)-β-cyclodextrin (Sigma-Aldrich, Co.) in saline and administered s.c. in a volume of 2 ml/kg. PF-3845 (3, 10 mg/kg, synthesized as described by Ahn et al., 2009 b was dissolved in 10% DMSO: 10% Cremophor EL: 80% saline and administered p.o. in a volume of 5 ml/kg.

Statistical analysis

Analyses of LC-MS/MS data were conducted using GraphPad Prism software. For FAA, statistical comparisons between treatment groups were made using an unpaired, two-tailed Student's t-test. To determine fold-change in levels of FAA, the levels were normalized to the respective vehicle-treated group. p values less than 0.05 were considered significant. To assess the effect of treatment over time on behaviors, a two-way repeated measures analysis of variance (ANOVA) was performed with Student-Newman-Keuls for post hoc analysis. Fatty acid amide levels from each rat were plotted (Fig. 1–5) and the mean ± S.E.M. were calculated. Behavioral data are presented as mean ± S.E.M.

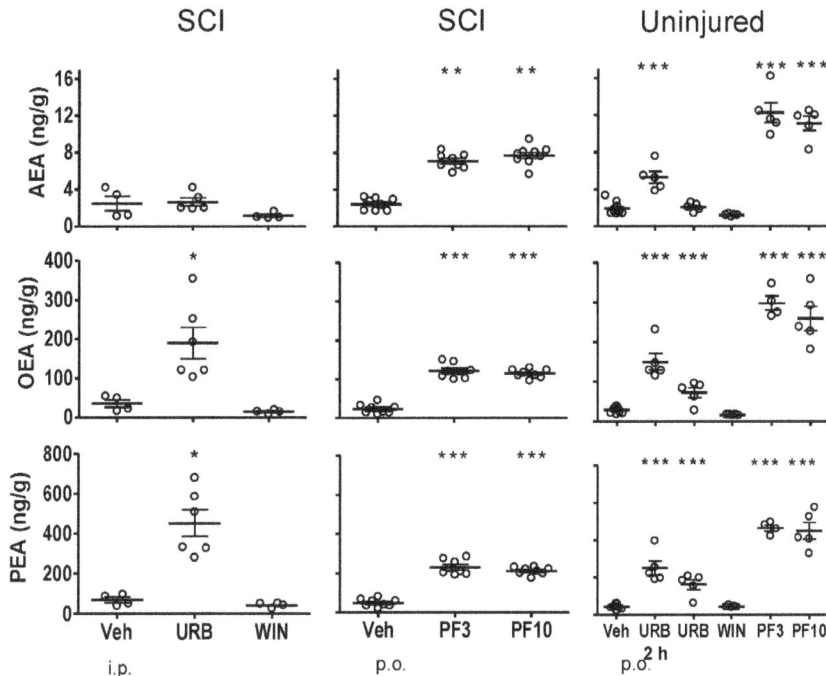

Figure 1. Fatty acid amide concentrations in brain following treatment with FAAH inhibitors, WIN 55,212-2 and vehicle in SCI and uninjured rats. Rats were treated with either URB597 (URB; 3 mg/kg, i.p.), WIN 55,212-2 (WIN; 3 mg/kg, s.c.) or vehicle (Veh; 1.5 ml/kg, i.p.) for seven days and euthanized four hours following the last treatment. One group of URB597 rats were euthanized two hours (2 h) following a single treatment. Rats that received PF-3845 (PF3, PF10; 3, 10 mg/kg, p.o) or vehicle (Veh, p.o.) were treated once and euthanized four hours following dosing. Levels of AEA, OEA and PEA from each rat are shown, the thick horizontal line is the mean and the thin horizontal lines are the S.E.M. n = 4–10/group. * $p < 0.05$, **$p < 0.01$, ***$p < 0.001$ vs. vehicle (Student's t-test).

Results

Effect of spinal cord injury on CNS FAA levels

Table 1 summarizes changes in CNS FAA levels four weeks after SCI. The most apparent changes in SCI tissue, compared to uninjured tissues, are of decreased levels of OEA and PEA of thoracic spinal cord at and near the epicenter.

Whole Brain. In untreated, uninjured rats, the mean brain levels of AEA, OEA and PEA were 2.2±0.51, 33.7±3.8 and 67.7±5.0 ng/g tissue, respectively (Fig. 1). In SCI vehicle-treated rats, the mean brain levels of AEA, OEA and PEA were 2.5±0.8, 35.6±9.3 and 69.4±13.6 ng/g tissue, respectively. Brain FAA levels from vehicle-treated SCI rats were not significantly different from brain levels from uninjured rats ($p > 0.05$).

Thoracic Spinal Cord. Spinal cord injury led to marked decreases in OEA and PEA content in spinal tissues. The mean level of OEA in thoracic spinal cord from uninjured rats was 652.1±99.1 ng/g tissue. The mean levels of OEA in tissue rostral to the epicenter, the epicenter and caudal to the epicenter from SCI rats were 318.6±44.1, 188.8±17.9 and 275.3±22.3 ng/g tissue, respectively ($p < 0.05$, rostral, epicenter and caudal vs. uninjured OEA; Fig. 2–4). The mean level of PEA in thoracic spinal cord from uninjured rats was 1108.0±148.7 ng/g tissue. The mean level of PEA in tissue rostral to the epicenter, the epicenter and caudal to the epicenter from SCI rats were 941.4±122.3, 351.5±56.5 and 740.2±53.2 ng/g tissue (e.g. Fig. 3; $p < 0.05$, epicenter and caudal vs. uninjured PEA).

By contrast, mean levels of AEA in spinal tissues from SCI rats were not significantly changed from that of uninjured rats. Levels of AEA in the rostral, epicenter and caudal spinal segments from SCI rats were 5.1±1.1, 4.6±1.3 and 5.4±1.0 ng/g tissue,

respectively. Levels of AEA in comparable spinal segments from uninjured rats were 6.0±1.3, 8.0±1.9 and 6.2±0.4 ng/g tissue, respectively. While there was a trend of decreased levels of AEA in spinal tissues from SCI rats, this was not statistically significant from that of uninjured rats ($p > 0.05$).

Lumbar Spinal Cord. In lumbar spinal cord from untreated, uninjured rats, the mean levels of AEA, OEA and PEA were 3.8±0.4, 241.0±32.8 and 493.4±61.5 ng/g tissue, respectively. In lumbar spinal cord from SCI rats, the mean levels of AEA, OEA and PEA were 2.6±0.1, 224.1±30.0 and 344.7±53.8 ng/g tissue, respectively. The levels of FAA in lumbar spinal cord from SCI rats, while slightly decreased, were not significantly different from that of uninjured rats ($p > 0.05$; Fig. 5).

Effect of FAAH inhibitors and WIN 55,212-2 on CNS FAA levels

URB597. Four hours post-treatment with URB597, levels of AEA, OEA and PEA were significantly increased in spinal segments rostral (Fig. 2) and caudal (Fig. 4) to the injury and lumbar segment (Fig. 5) of spinal cord from SCI rats ($p < 0.05$ vs. vehicle treatment). Levels of AEA were unchanged in brains from both uninjured and SCI rats, despite clear increases in OEA and PEA (Fig. 1). To confirm that the dose of URB597 was effective in blocking brain FAAH, uninjured rats were euthanized two hours following URB597 treatment; FAA were significantly increased ($p < 0.05$ vs. vehicle; Fig. 1). In contrast to the increases in FAA rostral and caudal to the spinal injury, there was a lack of effect of URB597 treatment at the epicenter four hours after treatment ($p > 0.05$ vs. vehicle treatment, Fig. 3).

Table 2 summaries changes in CNS FAA content following URB597 treatment in SCI and uninjured rats. The effects of

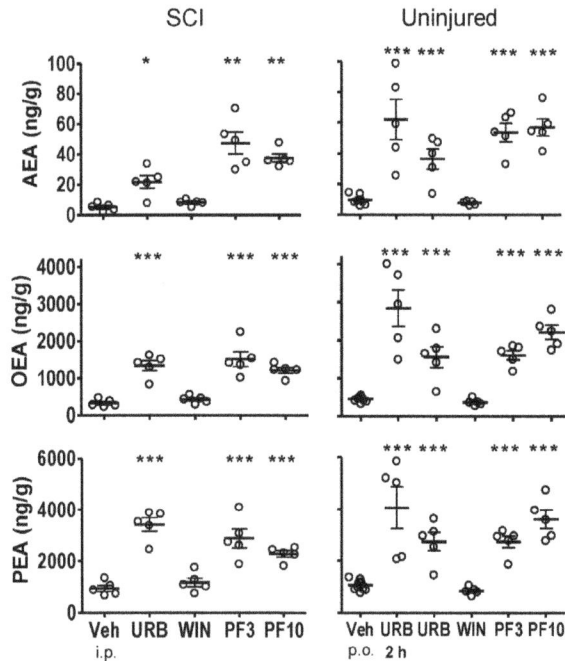

Figure 2. Fatty acid amide concentrations in thoracic spinal cord segments rostral to the spinal injury from SCI rats or comparable thoracic spinal cord segments from uninjured rats following treatment with FAAH inhibitors, WIN 55,212-2 and vehicle. Both SCI and uninjured rats were treated with either URB597 (URB; 3 mg/kg, i.p.), WIN 55,212-2 (WIN; 3 mg/kg, s.c.) or vehicle (Veh; 1.5 ml/kg, i.p.) for seven days and euthanized four hours following the last treatment. Rats that received PF-3845 (PF3, PF10) were treated once (3, 10 mg/kg, p.o.) and euthanized four hours following dosing. One group of uninjured rats was treated once with URB597 and euthanized two hours (2 h) following treatment. The FAA levels of thoracic spinal cord of uninjured rats from this figure are repeated for Figures 3 and 4. Levels of AEA, OEA and PEA from each rat are shown, the thick horizontal line is the mean and the thin horizontal lines are the S.E.M. n = 4–10/group. * $p<0.05$, **$p<0.01$, ***$p<0.001$ vs. vehicle (Student's t-test).

URB597 treatment, as fold-change over vehicle-treatment, on CNS FAA are summarized following a seven day treatment schedule and following a single treatment.

PF-3845. PF-3845 also consistently increased CNS FAA levels in both uninjured and SCI rats. However, unlike URB597, PF-3845 also elevated FAAs at the epicenter in this experiment, at both doses, four hours after treatment ($p<0.05$ vs. vehicle; Fig. 1–5). Overall, the effect of PF-3845 at 3 mg/kg and 10 mg/kg on tissue FAA appeared to be similar with the potential exception of effects at the epicenter.

Table 3 summaries CNS FAA content, as fold-change over vehicle treatment, following PF-3845 treatment in SCI and uninjured rats.

WIN 55,212-2. Interestingly, there were trends towards changes in FAA concentrations following treatment with the nonselective CB receptor agonist WIN 55,212-2 in both uninjured (single treatment) and SCI rats (seven-day treatment). In brain and thoracic spinal cord from uninjured rats, there were tendencies for reduced FAA (Fig. 1–5; Table 2). However, a trend towards an increase in AEA in lumbar spinal cord in uninjured rats was observed following a single treatment of WIN 55,212-2 ($p>0.05$ vs. vehicle treatment).

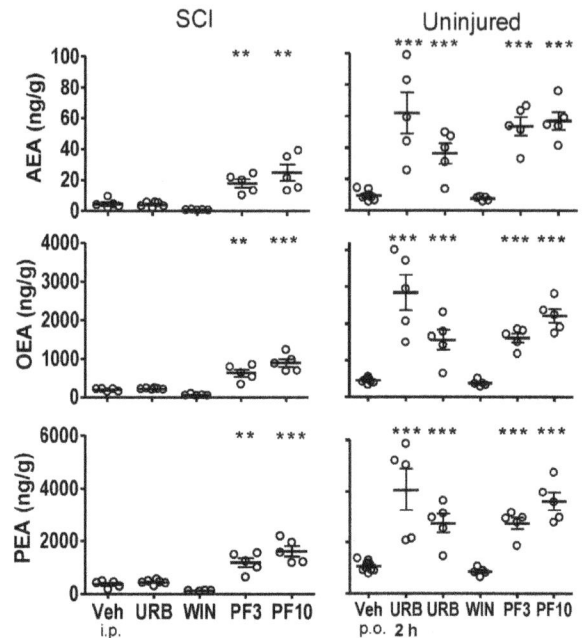

Figure 3. Fatty acid amide concentrations in thoracic spinal cord segments from the epicenter of injury from SCI rats or comparable spinal cord segments from uninjured rats following treatment with FAAH inhibitors, WIN 55,212-2 and vehicle. Both SCI and uninjured rats were treated with either URB597 (URB; 3 mg/kg, i.p.), WIN 55,212-2 (WIN; 3 mg/kg, s.c.) or vehicle (Veh; 1 ml/kg, i.p.) for seven days and euthanized four hours following the last treatment. One group of uninjured rats was treated once with URB597 and euthanized two hours (2 hr) following treatment. Rats that received PF-3845 (PF3, PF10) were treated once (3, 10 mg/kg, p.o.) and euthanized four hours following dosing. Levels of AEA, OEA and PEA from each rat are shown, the thick horizontal line is the mean and the thin horizontal lines are the S.E.M. n = 4–10/group. * $p<0.05$, **$p<0.01$, ***$p<0.001$ vs. vehicle (Student's t-test).

In SCI rats, there were trends towards both decreased and increased tissue FAA content following WIN 55,212-2 treatment. A trend towards decreased FAA was observed in brain from SCI rats following seven days WIN 55,212-2 treatment ($p>0.05$ vs. vehicle treatment; Table 2). At the same time, spinal cord rostral and caudal to the epicenter showed increased levels of FAA ($p>0.05$ vs. vehicle treatment; Table 2).

Antinociceptive effect of FAAH inhibitors and WIN 55,212-2 in SCI rats

Prior to seven day dosing, the mean hind paw withdrawal threshold of all SCI rats was 3.9 ± 0.6 g (Fig. 6). The mean baseline withdrawal thresholds, within each treatment group, prior to the morning treatment, did not significantly change over the seven day treatment period ($p>0.05$). Significant increases in withdrawal thresholds were observed 30 min following treatment with WIN 55,212-2 on each day of behavioral testing. In fact, on each day of testing, WIN 55,212-2 fully ameliorated hind paw cutaneous hypersensitivity ($p<0.05$ vs. vehicle treatment and vs. baseline; two-way repeated measures-ANOVA). Furthermore, on each of the testing days the effect persisted for the duration of the four hour testing period. By contrast, URB597 did not significantly increase withdrawal thresholds at any time post-treatment ($p>0.05$ vs. vehicle treatment). Likewise, vehicle treatment did not significantly alter withdrawal thresholds.

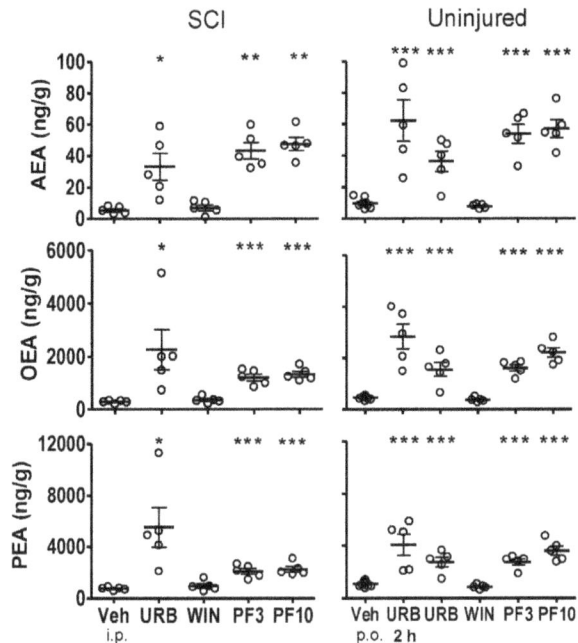

Figure 4. Fatty acid amide concentrations in thoracic spinal cord segments caudal to the spinal injury from SCI rats or comparable spinal cord segments from uninjured rats following treatment with FAAH inhibitors, WIN 55,212-2 and vehicle. Rats were treated with either URB597 (URB; 3 mg/kg, i.p.), WIN 55,212-2 (WIN; 3 mg/kg, s.c.) or vehicle (Veh; 1 ml/kg, i.p.) for seven days and euthanized four hours following the last treatment. One group of uninjured rats was treated once with URB597 and euthanized two hours (2 h) following treatment. Rats that received PF-3845 (PF3, PF10) were treated once (3, 10 mg/kg, p.o.) and euthanized four hours following dosing. Levels of AEA, OEA and PEA from each rat are shown, the dark horizontal line is the mean and the light horizontal lines are the S.E.M. n = 4–10/group. * $p < 0.05$, **$p < 0.01$, ***$p < 0.001$ vs. vehicle (Student's t-test).

A separate group of SCI rats was dosed once with PF-3845 (Fig. 7). Four weeks following SCI, the mean withdrawal threshold of all rats was 2.3±0.2 g. Increases in withdrawal thresholds were observed with PF-3845 (10 mg/kg) at one and three hours post-treatment ($p < 0.05$ vs. vehicle treatment). The increase in withdrawal threshold at one and three hours post-treatment is about a 40% maximum possible effect (100% effect = 15 g). No significant effects on withdrawal threshold were observed with either 3 mg/kg or vehicle ($p > 0.05$).

Effect of URB597 and WIN 55,212-2 on below-level motor function in SCI rats

Prior to treatment, the mean BBB Locomotor Scores of all SCI rats was significantly decreased from 21 to 9.8±0.4 ($p < 0.05$; Fig. 8). This score means frequent stepping with the dorsal rather than the plantar hind paw and no fore limb-hind limb coordination. After six days of treatment with either URB597, WIN 55,212-2 or vehicle, BBB Locomotor Scores were 9.9±0.6, 10.2±1.3, 10.6±0.5, respectively ($p > 0.05$ vs. vehicle treatment). Compared with BBB Scores before treatment, BBB Scores were not significantly changed after six days of treatment in SCI rats ($p > 0.05$; Fig. 8). The effect of a single dose of PF-3845 on BBB Locomotor Scores was not assessed.

Discussion

Despite significantly increasing brain and spinal cord tissue levels of FAA in SCI rats, seven day systemic administration of the FAAH inhibitor URB597 did not demonstrate antinociception. Acute treatment with the FAAH inhibitor PF-3845, which also significantly increased CNS levels of FAA, led to a moderate, non-dose dependent antinociception in SCI rats. By contrast, WIN 55,212-2 robustly ameliorated below-level cutaneous hypersensitivity in SCI rats for the duration of the seven-day treatment period. Markedly decreased tissue levels of OEA and PEA were observed at the epicenter and tissue caudal to the epicenter in SCI rats. While both FAAH inhibitors increased tissue FAA in SCI rats, only PF-3845 increased AEA, OEA and PEA at the epicenter, which in part could underlie PF-3845's modest antinociceptive effect. Neither FAAH inhibition nor CB receptor activation over seven days improved hind limb motor function. While direct activation of CB receptors leads to a significant and sustained antinociception, the current data indicate that increasing CNS FAA levels alone may not be sufficient for ameliorating below-level neuropathic SCI pain.

Changes in FAA levels in spinal tissue segments that may be crucial in the initiation and maintenance of neuropathic pain following a SCI were reported in the current study. The current study confirmed a previous finding of no change in levels of AEA and PEA in spinal tissue rostral to the epicenter and at the epicenter four weeks after a SCI [26]. However, the current study observed that PEA was decreased caudal to the epicenter and that OEA was decreased both rostrally and caudally to the epicenter as well as within the epicenter. It is speculated that the loss of tonic FAA-mediated inhibition following SCI could contribute to enhanced excitability of spinal dorsal horn neurons either rostral or caudal to the epicenter [2,27]. In the current study, slight decreases ($p > 0.05$; Table 1) in FAA were observed in the lumbar spinal cord, which receives primary afferents that innervate the hind paw. The mechanism that leads to an apparent decrease of FAA in lumbar segment, several segments from the epicenter, has yet to be elucidated, but a consequence could be dorsal horn neuron hyperexcitability. However, lumbar spinal cord FAA were significantly increased following URB597 treatment without being accompanied by significant antinociception. Likewise, FAA levels in lumbar spinal cord were increased following PF-3845, but only a slight antinociceptive effect was obtained. Convincing evidence that the loss of CB_1 receptor-mediated tonic inhibition alone can lead to hyperexcitable lumbar dorsal horn neurons is lacking, but perhaps it is a fusion of diminished functioning of several neurotransmitter systems (e.g. GABA) that leads to the neuropathic pain state following SCI [28,29].

Changes in supraspinal function could also be crucial in the maintenance of neuropathic SCI pain [16,19]. The current study found no significant change in whole brain FAA levels following SCI, but perhaps there are changes in specific pain-related brain nuclei following SCI. It is further speculated that processes involved in cellular function and intercellular signaling could be altered in the brain as well as in the spinal cord following injury [30,31]. Changes in the brain opioid system have been suggested to underlie reduced efficacy of supraspinal injection of morphine in SCI rats [32,33]. By contrast, supraspinal injection of WIN 55,212-2 is fully efficacious in SCI rats [19]. Changes in either brain CB receptors or FAA level have yet to be identified following SCI. Nonetheless, despite a robust increase in whole brain FAA following FAAH inhibition, there was a lack of robust antinociception; a role for brain FAA in SCI pain will need further elucidation.

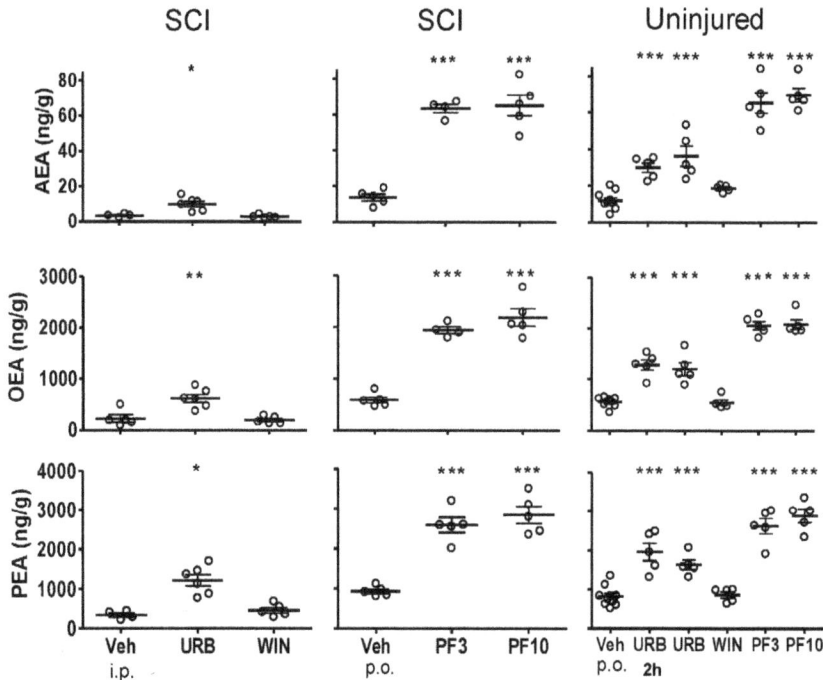

Figure 5. Fatty acid amide concentrations in lumbar spinal cord from SCI rats or uninjured rats following treatment with FAAH inhibitors, WIN 55,212-2 and vehicle. Rats were treated with either URB597 (URB; 3 mg/kg, i.p.), WIN 55,212-2 (WIN; 3 mg/kg, s.c.) or vehicle (Veh; 1.5 ml/kg, i.p.) for seven days and euthanized four hours following the last treatment. One group of uninjured rats was treated once with URB597 and euthanized two hours (2 h) following treatment. Rats that received PF-3845 (PF3, PF10) were treated once (3, 10 mg/kg, p.o.) and euthanized four hours following dosing. Levels of AEA, OEA and PEA from each rat are shown, the thick horizontal line is the mean and the thin horizontal lines are the S.E.M. n = 4–10/group. * $p < 0.05$, **$p < 0.01$, ***$p < 0.001$ vs. vehicle (Student's t-test).

A number of preclinical neuropathic pain studies have demonstrated marked antinociception following both acute and repeated activation of CB receptors, which appears to be in part mediated through the CB_1 receptor [3,20,34–38]. It is possible that attenuation of specific symptoms, such as hypersensitivity to noxious stimulation (hyperalgesia), could be ameliorated through other CB receptors or non-CB receptors [11,39].

The current study confirms previous findings in neuropathic pain models of a lack tolerance to the antinociceptive effect following repeated treatment with a CB receptor agonist [20,35,36]. By contrast, a loss of efficacy following repeated treatment with morphine in SCI rats has been observed [20]. Thus, a potential advantage of CB1 receptor agonists over, for

example, opioid receptor agonists is sustained efficacy over the course of the treatment period. Tolerance to CB receptor agonists does appear however, under specific circumstances. In the case of an acute pain state, as modeled by the hot plate test in uninjured animals, tolerance to the antinociceptive effect appears within five days of daily treatment [20,40]. The mechanism by which CB receptor agonists retain efficacy in some pain states and not in others is currently unknown. While it is possible that the injury state could underlie the development of antinociceptive tolerance, the test stimulus could also influence whether or not tolerance is obtained.

One issue raised by CB receptor agonists is the presence of motoric effects at or near antinociceptive doses. In the case of

Table 1. Summary of Changes in Fatty Acid Amides Four Weeks Following a Spinal Cord Injury in Rats.

	AEA	OEA	PEA
Brain	n.c.	n.c.	n.c.
Spinal cord			
Rostral to epicenter	↓ n.s.	↓ *	↓ *
Epicenter	↓ n.s.	↓ *	↓ *
Caudal to epicenter	↓ n.s.	↓ *	↓ *
Lumbar spinal cord	↓ n.s.	↓ n.s.	↓ n.s.

Changes in fatty acid amides (AEA, N-arachidonoylethanolamide; OEA, N-oleoyl ethanolamide; PEA, N-palmitoyl ethanolamide) four weeks following spinal cord injury compared to that of uninjured rats.
↓, decrease; n.c., no change; n.s., not statistically significant; *$p < 0.05$ (Student's t-test).

Table 2. Fold-change of tissue fatty acid amide levels following treatment with URB597 or WIN 55,212-2 relative to vehicle treatment.

Rats	Treatment	AEA Brain	Rostral	Epicenter	Caudal	Lumbar	OEA Brain	Rostral	Epicenter	Caudal	Lumbar	PEA Brain	Rostral	Epicenter	Caudal	Lumbar
Seven days																
SCI	Vehicle	1	1	1	1	1	1	1	1	1	1	1	1	1	1	1
SCI	URB	1.6 (*)	4.3 (**)	0.9 (n.s.)	6.1 (*)	2.9 (*)	5.3 (*)	4.2 (***)	1.2 (n.s.)	8.2 (*)	2.8 (**)	6.5 (***)	3.6 (***)	1.2 (n.s.)	7.5 (*)	3.5 (*)
SCI	WIN	0.5 (n.s.)	1.6 (n.s.)	0.2 (n.s)	1.3 (n.s.)	0.9 (n.s.)	0.4 (n.s.)	1.3 (n.s.)	0.3 (n.s.)	1.2 (n.s.)	0.9 (n.s.)	0.6 (n.s.)	1.3 (n.s.)	0.3 (n.s.)	1.3 (n.s.)	1.3 (n.s.)
One day																
N.I.	Vehicle	1	—	1	—	1	1	—	1	—	1	1	—	1	—	1
N.I.	URB (2 h)	2.7 (*)	—	6.5 (***)	—	2.5 (***)	5.1 (***)	—	6.3 (***)	—	2.3 (***)	5.7 (***)	—	3.8 (***)	—	2.3 (***)
N.I.	URB	1. (n.s.)	—	3.8 (***)	—	3.0 (***)	2.5 (***)	—	3.5 (***)	—	2.2 (***)	3.6 (***)	—	2.6 (***)	—	2.0 (***)
N.I.	WIN	0.6 (n.s.)	—	0.8 (n.s.)	—	1.6 (n.s)	0.6 (n.s.)	—	0.8 (n.s.)	—	1 (n.s.)	1 (n.s.)	—	0.8 (n.s.)	—	1 (n.s.)

Values are fold-changes compared to vehicle treatment levels in spinal cord injured (SCI) and non-injured (N.I.) rats. On the seventh day of treatment, tissues were collected 4 hours post-administration with either vehicle, URB597 (URB, 3 mg/kg, i.p.) or WIN 55,212-2 (WIN, 3 mg/kg, s.c.) from SCI rats. Non-injured rats were treated once and tissues collected four hours post-treatment. In one set of non-injured rats (n = 5), tissues were collected two hours (2 h) post-treatment with URB597.

"Epicenter" refers to thoracic spinal cord tissue either from the site of injury from SCI rats or comparable spinal cord tissue from non-injured rats.

n.s., not significant.

$*p<0.05$, $**p<0.01$, $***p<0.001$ vs. vehicle-treated (Student's t-test).

Table 3. Fold-change of tissue fatty acid amide levels following a single oral treatment with PF-3845 compared to oral vehicle treatment.

Rats	Treatment	AEA Brain	Rostral	Epicenter	Caudal	Lumbar	OEA Brain	Rostral	Epicenter	Caudal	Lumbar	PEA Brain	Rostral	Epicenter	Caudal	Lumbar
SCI	Vehicle	1	1	1	1	1	1	1	1	1	1	1	1	1	1	1
SCI	PF, 3	2.5 (**)	9.8 (***)	4.3 (***)	5.7 (***)	4.6 (***)	5.2 (***)	4.1 (***)	2.7 (**)	3.4 (***)	3.3 (***)	4.5 (***)	3.3 (***)	2.0 (**)	2.6 (***)	2.8 (***)
SCI	PF, 10	3.2 (**)	7.7 (***)	5.9 (***)	6.2 (***)	4.7 (***)	4.9 (***)	3.3 (***)	3.9 (***)	3.8 (***)	3.8 (***)	4.2 (***)	2.6 (***)	2.8 (***)	2.8 (***)	3.1 (***)
N.I.	Vehicle	1	—	1	—	1	1	—	1	—	1	1	—	1	—	1
N.I.	PF, 3	6.4 (***)	—	5.6 (***)	—	5.5 (***)	10.2 (***)	—	3.6 (***)	—	3.7 (***)	10.4 (***)	—	2.6 (***)	—	3.1 (***)
N.I.	PF, 10	5.8 (***)	—	6.0 (***)	—	5.8 (***)	8.9 (***)	—	4.9 (***)	—	5.8 (***)	10.1 (***)	—	3.4 (***)	—	3.5 (***)

Values are fold-changes compared to vehicle treatment levels in spinal cord injured (SCI) and non-injured (NJ) rats. Tissues were collected 4 hours post-oral administration of either PF-3845 (3, 10 mg/kg) or vehicle.

"Epicenter" refers to thoracic spinal cord tissue either from the site of injury from SCI rats or comparable spinal cord tissue from non-injured rats.

$*p<0.05$, $**p<0.01$, $***p<0.001$ vs. vehicle-treated (Student's t-test).

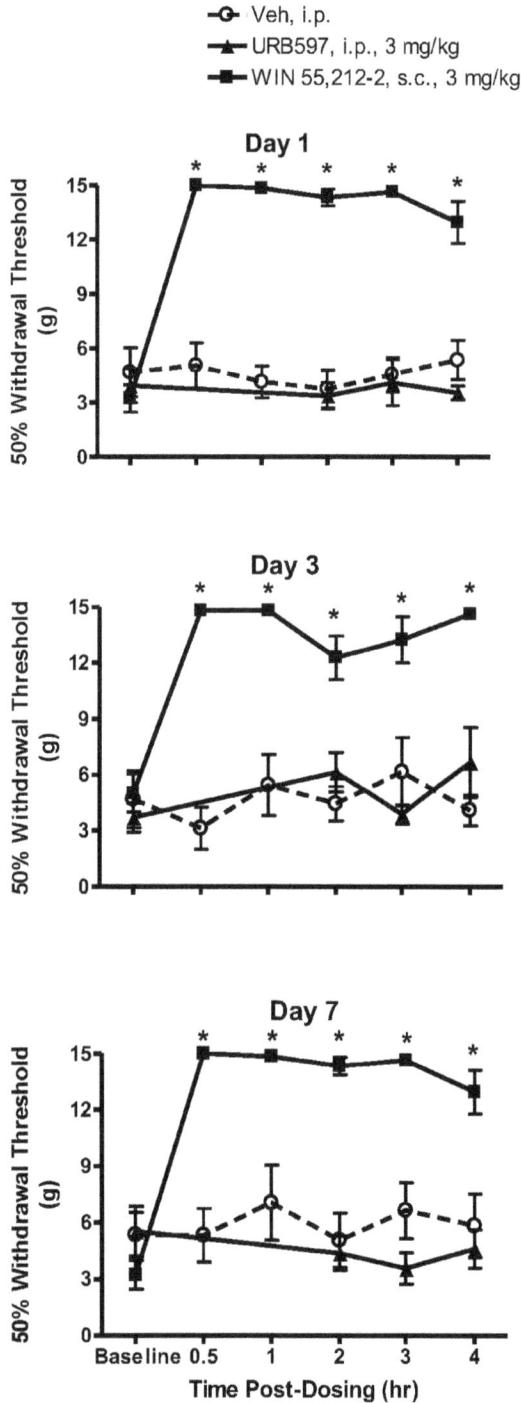

Figure 6. Effects of URB597 and WIN 55,212-2 treatment over seven days on below-level cutaneous hypersensitivity in rats with neuropathic SCI pain. Baseline hind paw withdrawal thresholds were measured prior to treatment with either URB597 (3 mg/kg, i.p.), WIN 55,212-2 (3 mg/kg, s.c.) or vehicle (Veh, 1.5 ml/kg, i.p.). Rats were treated twice daily and tested following the first daily injection. On the first day of testing, a robust antinociception was observed beginning 30 min post-injection of WIN 55,212-2, which was observed also on days 3 and 7. By contrast, no antinociceptive effects were observed following treatment with either URB597 or vehicle. Data presented as mean ± S.E.M. n = 8–10/group. * $p<0.05$ vs. vehicle (Two-way repeated measures ANOVA, Student-Newman-Keuls test).

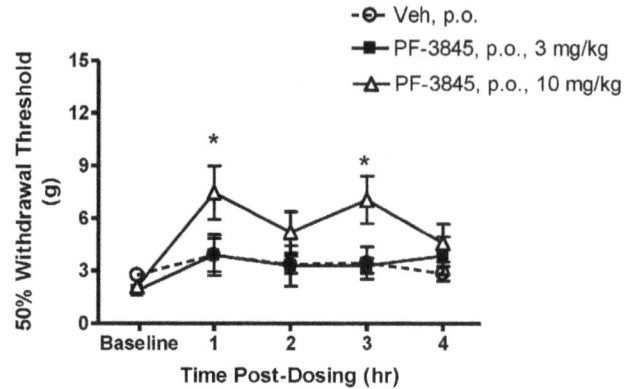

Figure 7. Effect of PF-3845 treatment on below-level cutaneous hypersensitivity in rats with neuropathic SCI pain. Following baseline hind paw withdrawal threshold measurement, SCI rats were treated with either PF-3845 (3, 10 mg/kg, p.o.) or vehicle (Veh; 5 ml/kg, p.o.). An antinociceptive effect was observed 1 and 3 hours following administration of 10 mg/kg, but not 3 mg/kg. Data presented as mean ± S.E.M. n = 8–9/group. * $p<0.05$ vs. vehicle (Two-way repeated measures ANOVA, Student-Newman-Keuls test).

WIN 55,212-2, the 50% antinociceptive dose is 0.9 mg/kg (s.c., 30 min post-dosing) whereas the dose needed to produce 50% disruption on the rotarod test (s.c., 3 hrs. post-dosing) is about the same [14,20]. In a previous study, a sedating dose of the anxiolytic drug diazepam, did not increase hind paw withdrawal thresholds in SCI rats, indicating that the behavioral endpoint is sensitive to antinociceptive treatment rather than to a treatment that merely disrupt motor function [18]. Thus, the increase in withdrawal thresholds observed with WIN 55,212-2 in the current study cannot be entirely attributed to catalepsy or motor dysfunction.

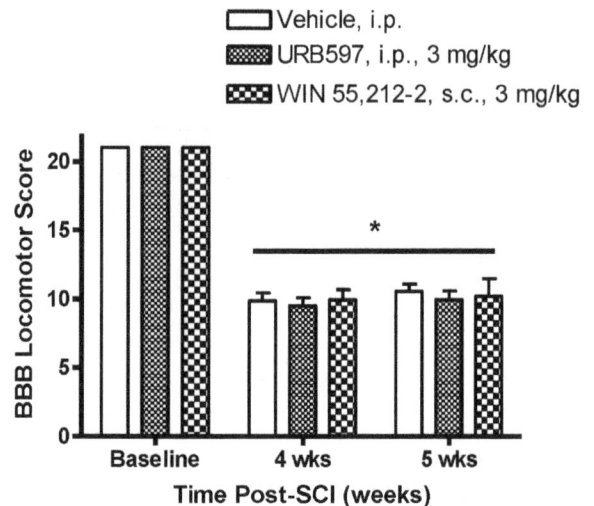

Figure 8. Effects of URB597 and WIN 55,212-2 on BBB Locomotor Scores in SCI rats. Prior to spinal compression surgery ("Baseline"), BBB Locomotor Scores were 21, indicating normal hind limb function. (A Score of "0" indicates no hind limb function.) The mean BBB Locomotor Score obtained the day before initiation of the seven-day treatment procedure ("4 wks" post-SCI) was 9.8±0.4. Spinal cord-injured rats were evaluated again on the sixth day of treatment ("5 wks" post-SCI) and there were no significant changes in BBB Scores. Data presented as mean ± S.E.M. n = 8–10/group. * $p<0.05$ vs. pre-SCI (Two-way repeated measures ANOVA, Student-Newman-Keuls test).

While targeting CB_1 receptors is a promising therapeutic strategy for ameliorating neuropathic SCI pain, prominent psychomotor side effects are associated with CB_1 receptor activation [14,20]. Alternatively, elevating synaptic levels of FAA is antinociceptive and does not appear to induce adverse side effects as the antinociception appears to be mediated through the CB_2 receptor, and possibly through other non-CB mediated mechanisms, such as through activation of the TRPV1 channel, as well as through the CB_1 receptor [9–11,41]. URB597 is a potent FAAH inhibitor—50% of brain FAAH activity is inhibited at a dose of 0.15 mg/kg (i.p.) [10]. At doses higher than 0.3 mg/kg, 1 and 3 mg/kg (i.p.), levels of FAA do not appear to be greatly increased, thus a FAAH inhibition plateau is reached at about 1 mg/kg [42]. In vivo, URB597 inhibits the degradation of AEA within 15 min of injection and significant inhibition of FAAH activity is observed up to 12 hours post-injection [10]. Importantly, no deleterious effect on motor function, as assessed in the rotarod test, was observed at doses of up to 5 mg/kg of URB597 and robust behavioral effects (e.g. antinociception, anxiolytic-like effects) were observed at very low doses (0.1–0.5 mg/kg, i.p.) [13,43]. In the current study, significant spinal tissue levels of FAA were obtained with 3 mg/kg URB597 in both SCI and uninjured rats. Similarly, both doses of PF-3845 significantly raised FAA levels in spinal tissues, including the epicenter of spinal cord from SCI rats as well as spinal tissue from uninjured rats. Thus, the current study demonstrates that it is possible to increase FAA in injured spinal tissue.

Despite significantly increasing CNS FAA levels, no antinociceptive effect was observed with URB597 in SCI rats, following either a single dose (day 1) or multiple doses (at either day 3 or day 7). A single dose of URB597 in peripheral nerve-injured mice resulted in a small antinociceptive effect, but four days of treatment, however, led to an even greater antinociceptive effect [22]. One significant difference between the previous studies showing efficacy with URB597 and the current study is that previous studies utilized models of peripheral neuropathy whereas the current study utilized a model of central pain following a SCI. There are a number of drugs that are efficacious in peripheral neuropathic pain models but are not efficacious in neuropathic SCI models [17,18]. Why this is so is not entirely clear, but the differential pharmacology between peripheral and central neuropathic pain states highly suggests that there are meaningful differences in the substrates that mediate the symptoms presented by these pain states. The differential substrates hypothesized to exist in preclinical models is indirectly supported by clinical findings, as a similar pharmacological divergence also exists between clinical neuropathic SCI and peripheral neuropathic pains [2].

Whereas URB597 lacked efficacy, PF-3845 led to a partial, non-dose dependent amelioration of neuropathic SCI pain. In addition to inhibitory effects on neurons, FAA concurrently suppress the release of pro-inflammatory mediators from immune cells and facilitate the release of anti-inflammatory substances [26]. It is possible that PF-3845 is more potent than URB597 on FAAH expressed in microglia and macrophage or that PF-3845 better penetrates damaged tissue as found at the epicenter to reach these cell types. In fact, 3 mg/kg (p.o.) PF-3845 led to a greater increase of AEA in CNS tissues, including the epicenter, compared to 3 mg/kg (i.p.) URB597. It has been reported elsewhere that FAA levels in mice treated with PF-3845 were higher compared to mice treated with URB597, despite the same dose and route [12]. Following PF-3845 treatment, FAA and anti-inflammatory substances from the epicenter could diffuse to nearby spinal dorsal horn neurons that are hyperexcited following SCI [44]. Perhaps it

is the increase in anti-inflammatory substances within and adjacent to the epicenter that is crucial in suppressing hyperexcited central neurons. The antinociceptive effect observed with PF-3845 in neuropathic SCI rats could be partially mediated through a combination of CB receptor-dependent and CB receptor-independent mechanisms [45,46].

While no robust effect was observed on below-level pain in the current study, it is possible that above-level and at-level SCI pain could be attenuated by FAAH inhibition. In addition to significant hyperexcitation of central neurons, there appears to be significant primary afferent hyperexcitation following SCI, which could underlie cutaneous hypersensitivity and spontaneous pain at and above the SCI [44,47,48]. These afferents could be sensitive to FAA through CB receptor or non-CB receptor mediated mechanisms or both. Increased sodium channel expression has been observed in injured peripheral nerves following injury— perhaps a similar increase in sodium channel expression in peripheral nerves following a SCI, as reported in the CNS, underlies at-level pain [49,50]. Indeed, SCI patients have reported relief from at-level pain following application of either capsaicin, a TRPV1 agonist, or lidocaine, a sodium channel blocking local anesthetic [51,52]. Perhaps the slight increase in FAA obtained with PF-3845 would have been sufficient to reduce at-level neuropathic pain. Further studies, however, are needed to characterize the extent of the involvement of primary afferent neurons in SCI pain.

A closer examination of studies that tested FAAH inhibitors on peripheral neuropathic cutaneous hypersensitivity indicates weak to no efficacy. As mentioned earlier, a single treatment of URB597 (10 mg/kg, p.o.) in mice with a chronic constriction injury of the sciatic nerve led to a small antinociceptive effect [22]. In rats with a spinal nerve ligation, URB597 (0.3 mg/kg, i.p.) treatment led to a 42% reversal of hind paw tactile hypersensitivity [42]. It is possible that higher doses of URB597 could yield greater antinociception, even though Karbarz et al. (2009) reported no further increases in FAA with higher doses. In rats with a partial sciatic nerve ligation, no effect was obtained with URB597 (0.3 mg/kg, i.p.), but the same dose was significantly efficacious in rats with a peripheral inflammation [13]. Likewise, significant antinociception and brain FAA levels were obtained in rats with a hind paw inflammation at 3 mg/kg PF-3845 (p.o.) [12]. In FAAH deficient mice, brain AEA levels were about 10-fold higher than that of wild-type mice [53]. Following a sciatic nerve injury, FAAH knockout mice demonstrated marked ipsilateral hind paw hypersensitivity, indicating that increased CNS AEA did not prevent the onset of nerve injury-induced nociception. However, the degree of hind paw carrageenan-induced hypersensitivity in FAAH deficient mice was not as severe as that seen in wild-type mice. While the findings indicate some antinociception following increased CNS FAA in the neuropathic state, the antinociception is not as robust as compared to that obtained in the painful inflammatory state. It is speculated that a SCI that is accompanied by significant inflammation could be sensitive to the effect of FAAH inhibition. Perhaps early treatment, around the time of injury or soon thereafter, will be efficacious.

A potential limitation of the current study is the dose of URB597 used. Perhaps a much greater dose of URB597 would have shown efficacy, even though it appears that there is no further gain in FAA levels in the CNS [42]. In mice with a peripheral nerve injury antinociceptive effects of URB597 were observed at 10 mg/kg (i.p.) and at 50 mg/kg (p.o.) [22,54]. The antinociceptive effects were attenuated with CB_1 receptor antagonist, indicating mediation through CB_1 receptors. Interestingly, Russo et al. (2007) saw only partial attenuation of the effect of

URB597 with CB$_2$ receptor antagonist treatment whereas Kinsey et al. (2009) observed full attenuation. The different behavioral endpoints and potential off-target activity of a high dose could in part explain the differences between the two findings. Nonetheless, perhaps much higher doses of URB597 in the SCI rats could lead to robust antinociception.

A recent clinical study of the FAAH inhibitor PF-04457845 in osteoarthritis pain [55] showed a lack of analgesic efficacy despite demonstration of significant elevation of FAA in patients' plasma and significant efficacy in preclinical studies in rodent models of non-neuropathic pain [56]. The disconnection between the preclinical findings and clinical outcomes raises issues of translatability, of whether clinical experimental methods in fact parallel preclinical experimental methods and whether preclinical models accurately model the clinical state. On one hand, it is not entirely clear if peripherally measured levels of the biomarker of interest are adequate in order to make predictions on behaviors that are CNS mediated. On the other hand, there may be a tenuous relationship of some preclinical animal models (e.g. the rat hind paw formalin test) to long-standing pathologies such as osteoarthritis. The current study utilized a rat model of neuropathic SCI pain, in which analgesics used for clinical neuropathic SCI pain appear antinociceptive [18]. The current findings suggest that increasing FAA alone may not be an efficacious treatment specifically for below-level SCI neuropathic pain.

While the current study suggests at most a weak antinociceptive effect of FAAH inhibition alone, greater antinociceptive effects could be obtained by combining an FAAH inhibitor with a known analgesic drug, thereby enhancing the efficacy of the analgesic drug [57]. The combination of opioids with AEA leads to a synergistic antinociception [58,59]. A metabolite of acetaminophen has been shown to enhance synaptic AEA by blocking its transporter [60]. Although acetaminophen alone is not antinociceptive in SCI rats, adding it to analgesic drugs led to synergistic antinociception which was CB$_1$ receptor-mediated [61]. Combination drug therapy, with FAAH inhibitors at the core, could be of great value for neuropathic SCI pain, for which few effective analgesic treatments exist [9,62].

Acknowledgments

We are highly grateful for the technical assistance of Ironwood scientists Rob Busby, Ada Silos-Santiago, Alex Bryant, Gerhard Hannig, Galen Carey and Mark Currie and of University of Miami scientists Maria Collado, Shyam Gajavelli, Stanislava Jergova, and Lyudmila Rusakova. We also thank Kay Ahn and Doug Johnson (Pfizer, Inc.) for the precursor to PF-3845.

Author Contributions

Conceived and designed the experiments: ATH PG GTM JPP JS. Performed the experiments: ATH PG MV. Analyzed the data: MV ATH JPP GTM JS. Contributed reagents/materials/analysis tools: BFC. Wrote the paper: JS ATH GTM JPP.

References

1. Siddall PJ (2009) Management of neuropathic pain following spinal cord injury: now and in the future. Spinal Cord 47: 352–359.
2. Finnerup NB and Jensen TS (2004) Spinal cord injury pain—mechanisms and treatment. Eur J Neurol 11: 73–82.
3. Rahn EJ and Hohmann AG (2009) Cannabinoids as pharmacotherapies for neuropathic pain: from the bench to the bedside. Neurotherapeutics 6: 713–737.
4. Cardenas DD and Jensen MP (2006) Treatments for chronic pain in persons with spinal cord injury: A survey study. J Spinal Cord Med 29: 109–117.
5. Russo EB (2008) Cannabinoids in the management of difficult to treat pain. Ther Clin Risk Mang 4: 245–259.
6. Huestis MA, Gorelick DA, Heishman SJ, Preston KL, Nelson RA, et al. (2001) Blockade of effects of smoked marijuana by the CB1-selective cannabinoid receptor antagonist SR141716. Arch Gen Psychiatry 58: 322–328.
7. Richardson JD, Aanonsen L and Hargreaves KM (1998) Antihyperalgesic effects of spinal cannabinoids. Eur J Pharmacol 345: 145–153.
8. Helyes Z, Nemeth J, Than M, Bolcskei K, Pinter E, et al. (2003) Inhibitory effect of anandamide on resiniferatoxin-induced sensory neuropeptide release in vivo and neuropathic hyperalgesia in the rat. Life Sci 73: 2345–2353.
9. Ahn K, Johnson DS and Cravatt BF (2009) Fatty acid amide hydrolase as a potential therapeutic target for the treatment of pain and CNS disorders. Expert Opin Drug Discov 4: 763–784.
10. Piomelli D, Tarzia G, Duranti A, Tontini A, Mor M, et al. (2006) Pharmacological profile of the selective FAAH inhibitor KDS-4103 (URB597). CNS Drug Reviews 12: 21–38.
11. Starowicz K, Makuch W, Korostynski M, Malek N, Slezak M, et al. (2013) Full inhibition of spinal FAAH leads to TRPV1-mediated analgesic effects in neuropathic rats and possible lipoxygenase-mediated remodeling of anandamide metabolism. PLoS One 8: e60040.
12. Ahn K, Johnson DS, Mileni M, Beidler D, Long JZ, et al. (2009) Discovery and characterization of a highly selective FAAH inhibitor that reduces inflammatory pain. Chem Biol 16: 411–420.
13. Jayamanne A, Greenwood R, Mitchell VA, Aslan S, Piomelli D, et al. (2006) Actions of the FAAH inhibitor URB597 in neuropathic and inflammatory chronic pain models. Br J Pharmacol 147: 281–288.
14. Fox A, Kesingland A, Gentry C, McNair K, Patel S, et al. (2001) The role of central and peripheral Cannabinoid1 receptors in the antihyperalgesic activity of cannabinoids in a model of neuropathic pain. Pain 92: 91–100.
15. Christensen MD and Hulsebosch CE (1997) Chronic central pain after spinal cord injury. J Neurotrauma 14: 517–537.
16. Enomoto M and Hama AT (2012) Pain management following spinal cord injury: clinical and basic science perspectives. In: A. A Martin and J. E Jones, editors. Spinal Cord Injuries: Causes, Risk Factors and Management. Hauppauge, NY: Nova Science Publishers. pp. 49–88.
17. Xu XJ, Hao JX, Aldskogius H, Seiger A and Wiesenfeld-Hallin Z (1992) Chronic pain-related syndrome in rats after ischemic spinal cord lesion: a possible animal model for pain in patients with spinal cord injury. Pain 48: 279–290.
18. Hama A and Sagen J (2007) Behavioral characterization and effect of clinical drugs in a rat model of pain following spinal cord compression. Brain Res 1185: 117–128.
19. Hama A and Sagen J (2011) Activation of spinal and supraspinal cannabinoid-1 receptors leads to antinociception in a rat model of neuropathic spinal cord injury pain. Brain Res 1412: 44–54.
20. Hama A and Sagen J (2009) Sustained antinociceptive effect of cannabinoid receptor agonist WIN 55,212-2 over time in rat model of neuropathic spinal cord injury pain. J Rehabil Res Dev 46: 135–143.
21. Cohen PJ (2009) Medical marijuana: The conflict between scientific evidence and political ideology. Utah Law Review 2009: 35–104.
22. Russo R, Loverme J, La Rana G, Compton TR, Parrott J, et al. (2007) The fatty acid amide hydrolase inhibitor URB597 (cyclohexylcarbamic acid 3'-carbamoylbiphenyl-3-yl ester) reduces neuropathic pain after oral administration in mice. J Pharmacol Exp Ther 322: 236–242.
23. Chaplan SR, Bach FW, Pogrel JW, Chung JM and Yaksh TL (1994) Quantitative assessment of tactile allodynia in the rat paw. J Neurosci Methods 53: 55–63.
24. Basso DM, Beattie MS and Bresnahan JC (1995) A sensitive and reliable locomotor rating scale for open field testing in rats. J Neurotrauma 12: 1–21.
25. Richardson D, Ortori CA, Chapman V, Kendall DA and Barrett DA (2007) Quantitative profiling of endocannabinoids and related compounds in rat brain using liquid chromatography-tandem electrospray ionization mass spectrometry. Anal Biochem 360: 216–226.
26. Garcia-Ovejero D, Arevalo-Martin A, Petrosino S, Docagne F, Hagen C, et al. (2009) The endocannabinoid system is modulated in response to spinal cord injury in rats. Neurobiol Dis 33: 57–71.
27. Drew GM, Siddall PJ and Duggan AW (2004) Mechanical allodynia following contusion injury of the rat spinal cord is associated with loss of GABAergic inhibition in the dorsal horn. Pain 109: 379–388.
28. Gwak YS and Hulsebosch CE (2011) GABA and central neuropathic pain following spinal cord injury. Neuropharmacol 60: 799–808.
29. Liu C and Walker JM (2006) Effects of a cannabinoid agonist on spinal nociceptive neurons in a rodent model of neuropathic pain. J Neurophysiol 96: 2984–2994.
30. Aguilar J, Humanes-Valera D, Alonso-Calvino E, Yague JG, Moxon KA, et al. (2010) Spinal cord injury immediately changes the state of the brain. J Neurosci 30: 7528–7537.
31. Hains BC, Klein JP, Saab CY, Craner MJ, Black JA, et al. (2003) Upregulation of sodium channel Nav1.3 and functional involvement in neuronal hyperexcitability associated with central neuropathic pain after spinal cord injury. J Neurosci 23: 8881–8892.

32. Yu W, Hao JX, Xu XJ and Wiesenfeld-Hallin Z (1997) Comparison of the anti-allodynic and antinociceptive effects of systemic; intrathecal and intracerebroventricular morphine in a rat model of central neuropathic pain. Eur J Pain 1: 17–29.

33. Abraham KE, McGinty JF and Brewer KL (2001) Spinal and supraspinal changes in opioid mRNA expression are related to the onset of pain behaviors following excitotoxic spinal cord injury. Pain 90: 181–190.

34. Sain NM, Liang A, Kane SA and Urban MO (2009) Antinociceptive effects of the non-selective cannabinoid receptor agonist CP 55,940 are absent in CB1(−/−) and not CB2(−/−) mice in models of acute and persistent pain. Neuropharmacol 57: 235–241.

35. Costa B, Colleoni M, Conti S, Trovato AE, Bianchi M, et al. (2004) Repeated treatment with the synthetic cannabinoid WIN 55,212-2 reduces both hyperalgesia and production of pronociceptive mediators in a rat model of neuropathic pain. Br J Pharmacol 141: 4–8.

36. De Vry J, Denzer D, Reissmueller E, Eijckenboom M, Heil M, et al. (2004) 3-[2-cyano-3-(trifluoromethyl)phenoxy]phenyl-4,4,4-trifluoro-1-butanesulfo nate (BAY 59-3074): a novel cannabinoid Cb1/Cb2 receptor partial agonist with antihyperalgesic and antiallodynic effects. J Pharmacol Exp Ther 310: 620–632.

37. Bridges D, Ahmad K and Rice AS (2001) The synthetic cannabinoid WIN55,212-2 attenuates hyperalgesia and allodynia in a rat model of neuropathic pain. Br J Pharmacol 133: 586–594.

38. Chin CL, Tovcimak AE, Hradil VP, Seifert TR, Hollingsworth PR, et al. (2008) Differential effects of cannabinoid receptor agonists on regional brain activity using pharmacological MRI. Br J Pharmacol 153: 367–379.

39. Ahmed MM, Rajpal S, Sweeney C, Gerovac TA, Allcock B, et al. (2010) Cannabinoid subtype-2 receptors modulate the antihyperalgesic effect of WIN 55,212-2 in rats with neuropathic spinal cord injury pain. The Spine Journal: Official Journal of the North American Spine Society 10: 1049–1054.

40. De Vry J, Jentzsch KR, Kuhl E and Eckel G (2004) Behavioral effects of cannabinoids show differential sensitivity to cannabinoid receptor blockade and tolerance development. Behav Pharmacol 15: 1–12.

41. Niforatos W, Zhang XF, Lake MR, Walter KA, Neelands T, et al. (2007) Activation of TRPA1 channels by the fatty acid amide hydrolase inhibitor 3′-carbamoylbiphenyl-3-yl cyclohexylcarbamate (URB597). Mol Pharmacol 71: 1209–1216.

42. Karbarz MJ, Luo L, Chang L, Tham CS, Palmer JA, et al. (2009) Biochemical and biological properties of 4-(3-phenyl-[1,2,4] thiadiazol-5-yl)-piperazine-1-carboxylic acid phenylamide, a mechanism-based inhibitor of fatty acid amide hydrolase. Anesth Analg 108: 316–329.

43. Kathuria S, Gaetani S, Fegley D, Valino F, Duranti A, et al. (2003) Modulation of anxiety through blockade of anandamide hydrolysis. Nat Med 9: 76–81.

44. Drew GM, Siddall PJ and Duggan AW (2001) Responses of spinal neurones to cutaneous and dorsal root stimuli in rats with mechanical allodynia after contusive spinal cord injury. Brain Res 893: 59–69.

45. Brown AJ (2007) Novel cannabinoid receptors. Br J Pharmacol 152: 567–575.

46. Costa B, Comelli F, Bettoni I, Colleoni M and Giagnoni G (2008) The endogenous fatty acid amide, palmitoylethanolamide, has anti-allodynic and anti-hyperalgesic effects in a murine model of neuropathic pain: involvement of CB(1), TRPV1 and PPARgamma receptors and neurotrophic factors. Pain 139: 541–550.

47. Bedi SS, Yang Q, Crook RJ, Du J, Wu Z, et al. (2010) Chronic spontaneous activity generated in the somata of primary nociceptors is associated with pain-related behavior after spinal cord injury. Journal of Neuroscience 30: 14870–14882.

48. Lenz FA, Tasker RR, Dostrovsky JO, Kwan HC, Gorecki J, et al. (1987) Abnormal single-unit activity recorded in the somatosensory thalamus of a quadriplegic patient with central pain. Pain 31: 225–236.

49. Thakor DK, Lin A, Matsuka Y, Meyer EM, Ruangsri S, et al. (2009) Increased peripheral nerve excitability and local NaV1.8 mRNA up-regulation in painful neuropathy. Mol Pain 5: 14.

50. Hains BC, Saab CY and Waxman SG (2005) Changes in electrophysiological properties and sodium channel Nav1.3 expression in thalamic neurons after spinal cord injury. Brain 128: 2359–2371.

51. Wasner G, Naleschinski D and Baron R (2007) A role for peripheral afferents in the pathophysiology and treatment of at-level neuropathic pain in spinal cord injury? A case report. Pain 131: 219–225.

52. Sandford PR and Benes PS (2000) Use of capsaicin in the treatment of radicular pain in spinal cord injury. J Spinal Cord Med 23: 238–243.

53. Lichtman AH, Shelton CC, Advani T and Cravatt BF (2004) Mice lacking fatty acid amide hydrolase exhibit a cannabinoid receptor-mediated phenotypic hypoalgesia. Pain 109: 319–327.

54. Kinsey SG, Long JZ, O'Neal ST, Abdullah RA, Poklis JL, et al. (2009) Blockade of endocannabinoid-degrading enzymes attenuates neuropathic pain. Journal of Pharmacology and Experimental Therapeutics 330: 902–910.

55. Huggins JP, Smart TS, Langman S, Taylor L and Young T (2012) An efficient randomised, placebo-controlled clinical trial with the irreversible fatty acid amide hydrolase-1 inhibitor PF-04457845, which modulates endocannabinoids but fails to induce effective analgesia in patients with pain due to osteoarthritis of the knee. Pain 153: 1837–1846.

56. Ahn K, Smith SE, Liimatta MB, Beidler D, Sadagopan N, et al. (2011) Mechanistic and pharmacological characterization of PF-04457845: a highly potent and selective fatty acid amide hydrolase inhibitor that reduces inflammatory and noninflammatory pain. J Pharmacol Exp Ther 338: 114–124.

57. Tallarida RJ (2007) Interactions between drugs and occupied receptors. Pharmacol Ther 113: 197–209.

58. Tuboly G, Mecs L, Benedek G and Horvath G (2009) Antinociceptive interactions between anandamide and endomorphin-1 at the spinal level. Clin Exp Pharmacol Physiol 36: 400–405.

59. Haller VL, Stevens DL and Welch SP (2008) Modulation of opioids via protection of anandamide degradation by fatty acid amide hydrolase. Eur J Pharmacol 600: 50–58.

60. Hogestatt ED, Jonsson BA, Ermund A, Andersson DA, Bjork H, et al. (2005) Conversion of acetaminophen to the bioactive N-acylphenolamine AM404 via fatty acid amide hydrolase-dependent arachidonic acid conjugation in the nervous system. J Biol Chem 280: 31405–31412.

61. Hama AT and Sagen J (2010) Cannabinoid receptor-mediated antinociception with acetaminophen drug combinations in rats with neuropathic spinal cord injury pain. Neuropharmacol 58: 758–766.

62. Fowler CJ, Naidu PS, Lichtman A and Onnis V (2009) The case for the development of novel analgesic agents targeting both fatty acid amide hydrolase and either cyclooxygenase or TRPV1. Br J Pharmacol 156: 412–419.

17

Different Epigenetic Alterations Are Associated with Abnormal *IGF2/Igf2* Upregulation in Neural Tube Defects

Baoling Bai, Qin Zhang, Xiaozhen Liu, Chunyue Miao, Shaofang Shangguan, Yihua Bao, Jin Guo, Li Wang, Ting Zhang, Huili Li*

Beijing Municipal Key Laboratory of Child Development and Nutriomics, Capital Institute of Pediatrics, Beijing, 100020, China

Abstract

The methylation status of DNA methylation regions (DMRs) of the imprinted gene *IGF2/Igf2* is associated with neural tube defects (NTDs), which are caused by a failure of the neural tube to fold and close and are the second-most common birth defect; however, the characterization of the expression level of *IGF2/Igf2* in neural tissue from human fetuses affected with NTDs remains elusive. More importantly, whether abnormal chromatin structure also influences *IGF2/Igf2* expression in NTDs is unclear. Here, we investigated the transcriptional activity of *IGF2/Igf2* in normal and NTD spinal cord tissues, the methylation status of different DMRs, and the chromatin structure of the promoter. Our data indicated that in NTD samples from both human fetuses and retinoic acid (RA)-treated mouse fetuses, the expression level of *IGF2/Igf2* was upregulated 6.41-fold and 1.84-fold, respectively, compared to controls. *H19* DMR1, but not *IGF2* DMR0, was hypermethylated in human NTD samples. In NTD mice, *h19* DMR1 was stable, whereas the chromatin structure around the promoter of *Igf2* might be loosened, which was displayed by higher H3K4 acetylation and lower H3K27 trimethylation. Therefore, the data revealed that *IGF2/Igf2* expression can be ectopically up-regulated by dual epigenetic factors in NTDs. In detail, the upregulation of *IGF2/Igf2* is likely controlled by hypermethylation of *H19 DMR1* in human NTDs, however, in acute external RA-induced NTD mice it is potentially determined by more open chromatin structure.

Editor: Yong-hui Dang, Xi'an Jiaotong University School of Medicine, China

Funding: This study is supported by National Natural Science Foundation of China, Beijing, China (No. 81471163; No. 81300489) and National "973" project (2013CB945404). The funders had no role in study design, data collection and analysis, decision to publish, or preparation of the manuscript.

Competing Interests: The authors have declared that no competing interests exist.

* Email: lihuili2011@gmail.com

Introduction

Neural tube defects (NTDs; OMIM 182940) are early, severe and complicated congenital malformations, which result from the failure of the neural tube to close and include cranial NTDs, such as anencephaly; caudal NTDs, such as spina bifida or meningomyelocele; or neural tube closure failure over the entire body axis, called craniorachischisis. In 2003, an epidemiological study reported a high prevalence of 138.7 per 10,000 births in the Shanxi province of Northern China [1]; however, the multifactorial influences that determine the pathogenesis of this disease remain elusive. Importantly, several clues have indicated that the inheritance in NTDs can be shown by a parental-specific feature, suggesting that abnormal genomic imprinting might be a pathogenic factor for NTDs [2,3].

Insulin-like growth factor 2 (*IGF2*) plays a key role in cell division and differentiation and participates in fetal growth and metabolism regulation; its coding gene is a maternal imprinted gene located in the *IGF2/H19* imprinted cluster. The imprinted control region (ICR) of this cluster is the six CCCTC-binding factor (CTCF)-binding site in the DMRs upstream of *H19* (namely, *H19 DMR1*: GenBank accession numbers AF125183; Chr11: 2021103-2021304, UCSC database, Feb2009 (GRCh37/hg19)). With or without methylated CpG in the ICR influence

CTCF binding to the same enhancers, which regulates *H19* or *IGF2* expression (Fig. 1A) [4,5]. Except for the *H19* DMR1, human *IGF2* also harbors two DMRs, namely DMR0 (GenBank accession number Y13633; Chr11: 2169466-2169537, UCSC database, Feb2009 (GRCh37/hg19)) between exon2 and exon3 at the P0 promoter and DMR2 (Chr11: 2154682-2154973, UCSC database, Feb2009(GRCh37/hg19)) between exon8 and exon9. *IGF2* transcription can be primarily regulated by the *H19* DMR1 in the ICR and the *IGF2* DMR0 [3,6]. *H19* DMR1 is conserved in mice, but *Igf2* DMR0 is placenta-specific [3]. Several studies have indicated that *IGF2*-relevant DMRs are potentially associated with NTDs [7–10]. In our present NTD cohort, Wu et al. reported that hypermethylated *IGF2* DMR0 is associated with the NTD-affected cohort [10]. In contrast, Liu et al. reported that the *H19* DMR1 was hypermethylated, whereas the *IGF2* DMR0 had no significant differences in the NTD and control cohorts [8]. The previous evidence therefore implies that *IGF2* in human NTDs could be regulated by different factors. However, to date, the *IGF2* expression in NTD has not been explored.

Local chromatin structure can regulate a gene's active transcription. Loosely packaged chromatin is associated with active genes, while tightly packaged chromatin is associated with inactive genes. The histone modifications within a promoter region effectively alter local chromatin structures; for example,

A

IGF2/H19

B

KCNQ1/KCNQ1OT1

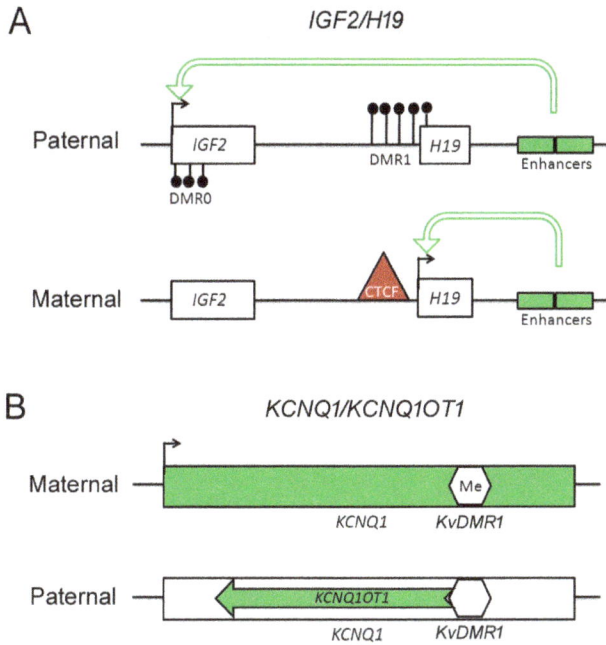

Figure 1. Schematic for the imprinting mechanism of *IGF2* and *KCNQ1*. In (A), the rectangle represents each gene, and the black circle is methylated DNA. In (B), the green arrow in the lower panel represents lncRNAs *KCNQ1OT1*, and the hexagon represents *KvDMR1* that is methylated or not.

H3K27 trimethylation (H3K27me3) is found on the inactive promoter, while histone acetylation enhances gene expression [11]. In addition, several H3K27me3 methyltransferase knockout mice or histone acetyltransferase knockout mice present NTD phenotypes [12], and the enrichment of H3K27me3 in the early developmental enhancers of ESC differentiation genes promotes the early step of neurulation in differentiated hESCs [13]. Therefore, evidence has demonstrated that the chromatin status determined by histone modifications is highly relevant with NTDs. Moreover, our previous data indicated direct associations between changes in histone modifications and DNA methylation with human NTDs [14,15].

In the present study, we investigated the status of the *IGF2*-relevant DMR methylation levels and chromatin status in the promoters in human NTD samples and confirmed the corresponding transcriptional activity of *IGF2*. To further understand the complex epigenetic mechanisms of this imprinting gene regulation, we also employed the same strategy to test the above epigenetic regulatory characteristics in a mouse model with a rapid retinoic acid (RA)-induced NTD.

Materials and Methods

Animals

C57BL/6J mice were used to obtain spinal cord tissue from mice with a spina bifida phenotype. All experimental procedures were reviewed and approved by the Animal Ethics Committee of the Capital Institute of Pediatrics (Permit Number: SYXK 2008–0011). Three doses of 20 mg/kg body weight of all-trans retinoic acid (Sigma, USA) suspended in olive oil were administered intraperitoneally into the mothers on GD8.0-0h, GD8.0-6h, GD8.0-12h when the neural tube and neuropore are fusing. The control consisted of olive oil administration. All surgery was performed under sodium pentobarbital anesthesia, and all efforts were made to minimize suffering. In the present study, under consideration of insufficient tissue for one assay, the spinal cords from twenty-one embryonic day18 fetuses with a spina bifida phenotype were collected and divided into three groups. Additionally, ten control fetuses were divided into three groups.

Human subjects

Stillborn NTD case subjects were obtained from Shanxi Province of Northern China [16]. The enrolled pregnant women were diagnosed by trained local clinicians using ultrasonography and then registered in a database. The surgical details were as previously described [14,17]. The Committee of Medical Ethics in the Capital Institute of Pediatrics (Beijing, China) approved this study (SHERLLM2014002). Written informed consent was obtained from the parents on behalf of the fetuses. Four NTD-affected fetuses and four age-matched controls were subjected, and the spinal cord tissues were used in the following experiments. To explore the *IGF2* mRNA level in brain, six NTD-affected fetuses and four controls were used (for details, see results).

RNA isolation and real-time qPCR

Spinal cord tissues of mouse fetuses were collected on dry ice, and then total RNA was isolated and purified. The concentration of each individual total RNA sample was standardized to 250 ng/μl. Equal volumes of this standardized total RNA from mice were pooled and used for cDNA synthesis. Two micrograms of total RNA was used as the starting template for first strand cDNA synthesis using the PCR cDNA Synthesis Kit (Promega, USA) according to the manufacturer's instructions. Real-time PCR was performed using Applied Biosystem's 7500Fast Real-Time PCR system and 2× PCR UltraSYBR Mixture (with ROX) Kit (CWBIO #CW0956, China) according to the manufacturer's protocol. The primers are listed in Table S1. The results were first normalized to the amount of target gene mRNA in relation to the amount of reference *Gapdh* gene. All data were collected in a blinded fashion.

Human mRNA detection

NanoString nCounter system was used to analyze the mRNA expression level of degradative spinal cords and brain tissues from human fetus samples. The spinal cords from four fetuses affected with NTDs or brains from six fetuses affected with NTDs and eight matched controls were disaggregated in lysis buffer (Ambion). Hybridizations were conducted according to the NanoString Gene Expression Assay Manual. Approximately 100 ng of each RNA sample was mixed with 20 μl of nCounter Reporter probes (Table S1) in hybridization buffer and 5 μl of nCounter Capture probes for a total reaction volume of 30 μl. The hybridizations were incubated at 65°C for approximately 16 hours. After washing, the purified target/probe complexes were eluted and immobilized in the cartridge for data collection, which was performed on the nCounter Digital Analyzer. The results were referenced to the *GAPDH*, *MTA2*, and *TBP* genes.

DNA methylation level analysis and bisulfite treatment

A total of 200 ng of genomic DNA from each sample was bisulfite-treated with the Methylamp DNA Modification Kit (Epigentek). The quality of the bisulfite conversion was controlled using PCR products that had no methyl group. The Sequenom MASSARRAY platform (CapitalBio, Beijing, China) uses matrix-assisted laser desorption/ionization time-of-flight (MALDI-TOF) mass spectrometry in combination with RNA base-specific cleavage (MassCLEAVE). A detectable pattern is then analyzed for its methylation status [15]. PCR primers were designed with Methprimer (http://epidesigner.com), and the primer sequence can be found in Table S1.

Chromatin immunoprecipitation (ChIP) assay

ChIP assays were performed on the spinal cord tissues from human and mouse fetuses using the MAGnify chromatin immunoprecipitation system (Invitrogen, California, USA) following the manufacturer's protocols. Chromatin was prepared, sonicated to DNA segments between 300 and 500 bp and then immunoprecipitated with anti-H3K4ac (ab113672, Abcam, Cambridge, UK), anti-H3K4me (ab106165, Abcam), anti-H3K27me3 (17-622, Millipore, Billerica, USA) and anti-H3K9me3 (ab8898, Abcam) antibodies. The immunoprecipitated DNA was eluted in a total volume of 150 μl, and 4 μl of each DNA sample was analyzed by real time PCR. The primer pairs used for ChIP assays are shown in Table S1. Amplification, data acquisition and analysis were performed using 7500Fast with SYBR Green detection. Three independent ChIP experiments were performed for each analysis. Mouse and rabbit IgG antibodies were used as negative controls in the immunoprecipitations. The following equation was used to calculate percent input $= \text{CT}^{\text{input}}\text{-CT}^{\text{ChIP}})$ × Fd ×100%, where CT^{ChIP} and CT^{input} are threshold cycle values obtained from the exponential phase of quantitative PCR, and Fd is a dilution factor for the input DNA to balance the difference in amounts of ChIP samples. The PCR primer sequences can be found in Table S1.

Statistical analyses

The DNA methylation data were added into the EPI 3.1 Database (EpiData Association, dense, Denmark) and analyzed with the SPSS-11.5 software package (McGraw-Hill Inc., New York, USA). An independent Student's t-test was performed to evaluate the significance of any differences between RA-treated mouse fetuses or human fetuses with NTDs and control groups. $P<0.05$ was considered statistically significant.

Results

Excessively active *IGF2* transcription in human fetuses with NTDs

We first examined the mRNA level of *IGF2* in spinal cord tissues from four NTD-affected and four normal control human fetuses. The clinical phenotypes of the four cases were one thoracic meningomyelocele (24-gestation week, female), one anencephaly and occipital encephalomeningocele (17-gestation week, female), and two thoracic and lumbar spina bifidas (20-gestation week, female and 26-gestation week, female). NanoString technology was used, and the original number of *IGF2* transcripts was detected. The results showed that in affected fetuses the level of *IGF2* mRNA was significantly increased 6.41-fold compared to control samples (Student's t-test: $P = 0.0001$) (Fig. 2A). Furthermore, we also assayed the level of *IGF2* in the brain tissues of six NTD-affected cases, of whom the clinical phenotypes were two occipital encephalomeningoceles (20-gestation week, female; 22-gestation week, male); one anencephaly and holorachischisis (20-gestation week, female); one anencephaly and parietal encephalomeningocele (22-gestation week, female); one occipital encephalomeningocele and cervical, thoracic spina bifida (37-gestation week, female); and one parietal encephalomeningocele (24-gestation week, male). The four controls (18-gestation week, female; 19-gestation week, male; 18-gestation week, male; 22-gestation week, male) were assayed in parallel. The results in the brain strongly supported the

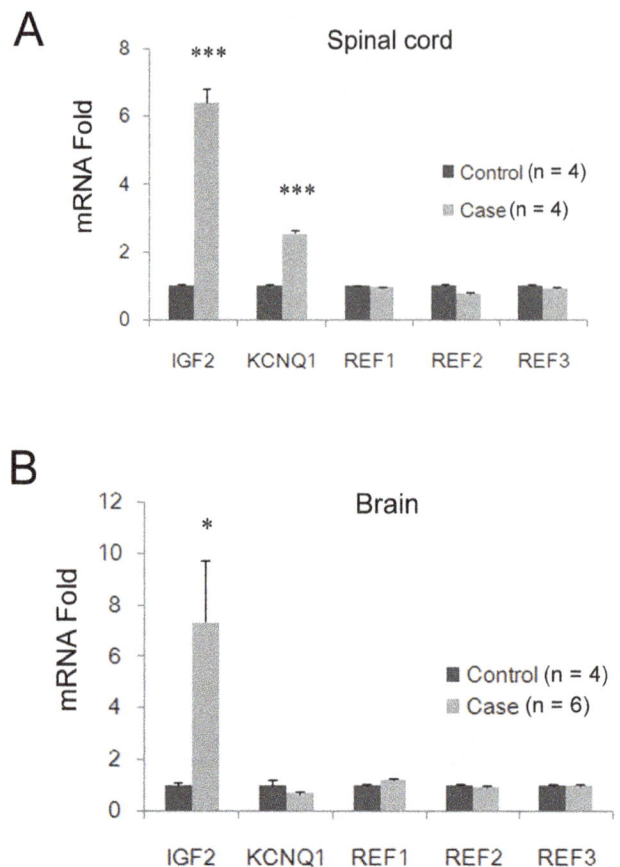

Figure 2. Enhanced mRNA levels of *IGF2* in the spinal cord and brains of human fetuses with NTDs. (A) In the spinal cord and (B) brains of human fetuses with NTDs, *IGF2* mRNA levels were dramatically upregulated. *: $P<0.05$; **: $P<0.01$; ***: $P<0.0001$ (Student's t-test).

data from the spinal cord (7.34-fold, Student's t-test: $P = 0.03$) (Fig. 2B). Thus, we conclude that in some human NTD cases *IGF2* transcription is abnormally enhanced.

Hypermethylation in *H19* DMR1 but no alteration in *IGF2* DMR0

To uncover the determinant for enhanced *IGF2* expression, we examined the DNA methylation levels of *H19* DMR1 and *IGF2* DMR0. The results revealed that the DNA methylation level of the CTCF-binding site in *H19* DMR1 in the Watson strand was stable in cases and controls; however, a CpG site 33bp away was dramatically hypermethylated from $30.86\pm1.19\%$ to $49.62\pm1.62\%$ ($P = 2.33\text{e-}07$, Student's t-test; Fig. 3A), suggesting that *H19* DMR1 is hypermethylated in NTD cases. To explore strand-specific DNA methylation level on transcription activity, we also detected DNA methylation on the Crick strand, and the data indicated that the DNA methylation levels of the sites corresponding to the CTCF-binding site and the hypermethylated site were not detected, but one CpG site was hypermethylated compared with the control ($36.25\pm1.19\%$ vs. $42.5\pm1.79\%$, $P = 0.015$; Student's t-test) (Fig. 3A). Thus, we identified that the DNA methylation levels on the Watson and Crick strands are different. We further evaluated the DNA methylation levels of CpGs in *IGF* DMR0 and did not find any significant alteration between the cases and controls (Fig. 3B). We think that in the present study the

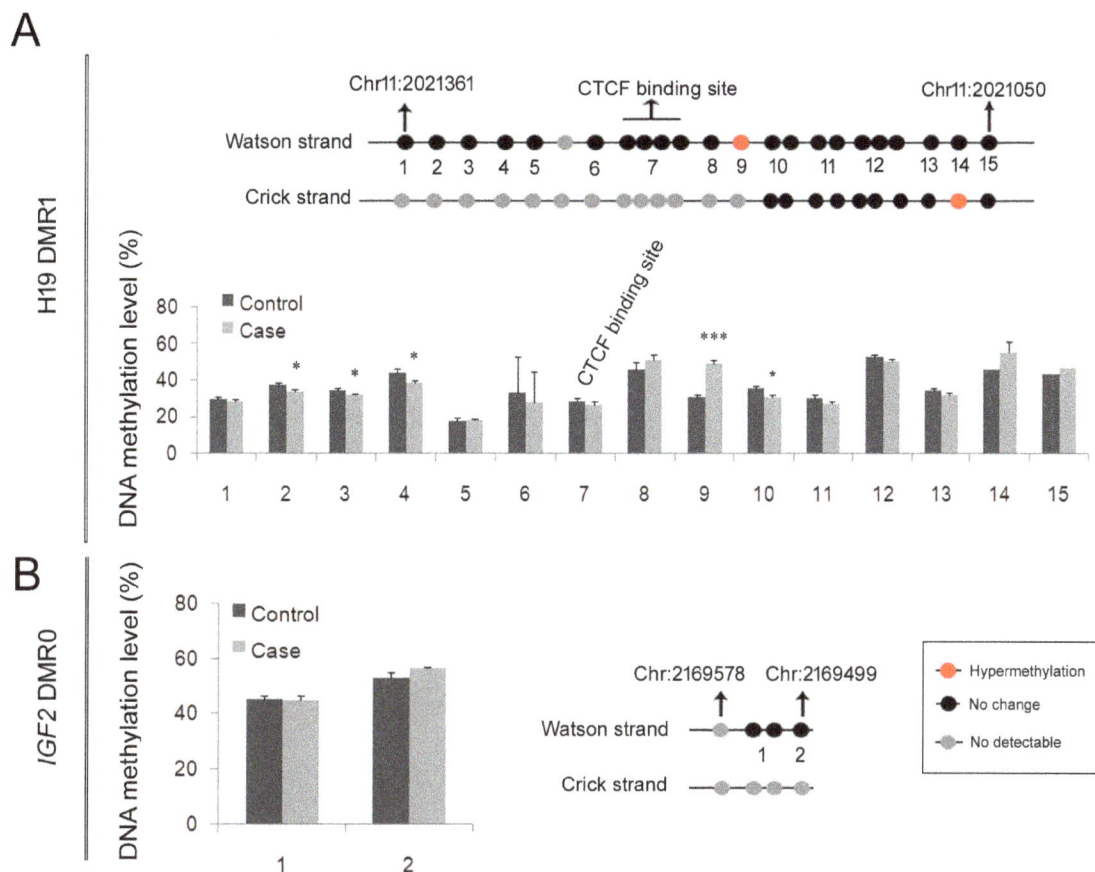

Figure 3. Hypermethylated *H19* DMR1 and stably methylated *IGF2* DMR0 in human fetuses with NTDs. The DNA methylation levels of the *H19* DMR1 (A) and *IGF2* DMR0 (B) were examined through matrix-assisted laser desorption/ionization time-of-flight (MALDI-TOF) mass spectrometry. In the upper panel in (A) and right panel in (B), the methylation status of all detected CpG sites was visualized. Each solid circle represents a "CG" site. (A)The number in upper panel refers to the CG site(s) in the lower histogram. (B) The number in the left panel refers to the site in the right histogram. ***: $P<0.0001$ (Student's *t*-test).

elevated *IGF2* expression in the cases might be not due to *IGF2* DMR0.

Altered chromatin status around the promoter is negatively associated with enhanced *IGF2* expression

To further specify the causes that are responsible for the increased *IGF2* transcription in NTDs, we investigated the chromatin status of the promoter region of this gene. From the ENCODE database, we know that the *IGF2* promoter enriches H3K27me3 and H3K4me2 in H1 ESCs (Fig. S1). However, the ChIP assay results indicated that active H3K4ac enrichment was decreased but repressive H3K27me3 enrichment was increased in the corresponding promoter regions (Fig. 4B), while the DNA methylation levels were significantly enhanced in NTDs (Fig. 4C). However, unlike the data from the ENCODE dataset, no H3K4 methylation enrichment was detected, suggesting a cell-specific feature of this histone modification. The alterations in chromatin structure are negatively associated with enhanced *IGF2* expression. So, combined with the data from the test of DNA methylation levels of *H19* DMR1 and *IGF2* DMR0, we deduced that in human NTDs, high *IGF2* expression might be an epigenetic regulatory outcome of the CpG hypermethylation of *H19* DMR1.

To further validate the above possibility, we tested the DNA methylation level of *KvDMR1* (chr11: 2721164-2721464; UCSC database, Feb2009 (GRCh37/hg19)), which is located in the ICR for the imprinted *KCNQ1/KCNQ1OT1* cluster on chromosome 11 distal regions near the *IGF2/H19* cluster (Fig. 1B). The data indicated that in the *KvDMR1* regions the CpG islands were diffusely hypermethylated (Fig. 4F). This result coincided with the up-regulated transcription of *KCNQ1* in the spinal cord of human NTDs (Fig. 2A), because hypermethylated *KvDMR1* is known to inhibit the expression of the lncRNA *Kcnq1ot1* gene, and loss function of *Kcnq1ot1* consequently promotes *KCNQ1* transcription (Fig. 1B) [18]. On the other hand, alterations of the chromatin status of the promoter region seemed to be poised because of the attenuated H3K4ac and H3K9me3 (Fig. 4E). These results agree with the alteration of *IGF2*, suggesting that in human NTDs, abnormal ICR methylation status might determine the transcriptional activities of the *IGF2* and *KCNQ1* imprinting genes.

Increased *Igf2* expression in overdose RA-induced NTD mice

We next questioned whether the imprinted *IGF2/Igf2* gene was only controlled by the ICR and independent of the chromatin status of the promoter regions in NTDs. Considering that our NTD cases are natural and the pathogenecity is possibly caused during a long period, we employed a rapid RA-induced NTD mouse model, in which an overdose RA was injected on

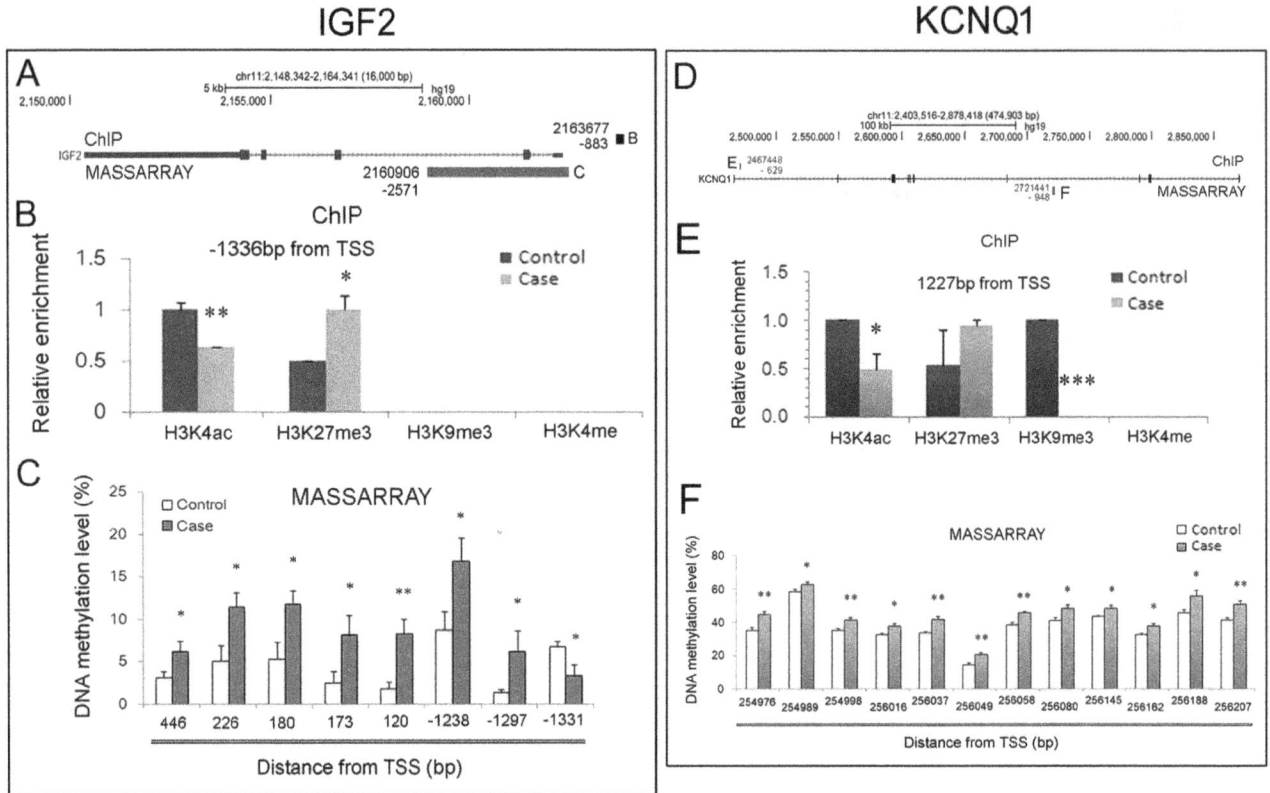

Figure 4. Chromatin status in the promoter region of the *IGF2* gene is negatively associated with gene expression. (A) and (D): The genomic profile of genes displayed in UCSC (hg19), the genomic locus of target regions in ChIP assay (black block on the gene schematic) and the CpG island (green block underneath the gene schematic) assayed by the MASSARRAY platform are shown. The capital letter beside the block indicates the corresponding panel below. The number beside the block indicates the genomic location that was targeted. In the ChIP assay results (B and E), the enrichment in the y-axis represents the relative enrichment fold in which the higher enrichment in case or in control is designated as 1. C) and F) indicate the DNA methylation level. Notably, in F, the DNA methylation status of *KvDMR1* is shown.*: $P<0.05$; **: $P<0.01$ (Student's *t*-test). TSS: transcription start site.

embryonic day 8 to induce a spina bifida phenotype. The real-time qPCR assays indicated that in the spinal cords of mice fetuses with spina bifida, the *Igf2* mRNA level was increased 1.84-fold compared to control ($P = 0.0057$, Student's *t*-test) (Fig. 5B), but in human NTDs, this increment fold was 6.41 (Fig. 2A). Meanwhile, the mRNA level of *h19* was not changed in mice with NTDs (Fig. 5B), implying that in NTD mouse fetuses the increased *Igf2* mRNA level might be not due to the change in the *h19* DMR1 methylation level. To further clarify the association between the changes in mRNA expression and the imprinting activities in mouse NTD samples, we checked the expression of other 60 imprinted genes located on ten chromosomes. The results revealed that among these genes, thirty-seven were upregulated and five were downregulated compared to the control (Fig. 5 and Fig. S2). Moreover, the altered genes were distributed on each targeted chromosome, and regardless of paternal or maternal imprinting, this result indicates that wide alterations in imprinted genes occur in NTDs, potentially which are not determined by the imprinting mechanism.

No alteration in *h19* DMR1 in mouse fetuses with NTDs compared to control

Concerning the conserved imprinted mechanism in mice and humans, we first examined the *h19* DMR1 methylation level. The MASSARRAY results indicated that in both the Watson and

Crick strands, the methylation level had no change except for a slight decrease in the Crick strand ($38.33\pm0.57\%$ vs. $36.33\pm1.32\%$, $P = 0.0132$; Student's *t*-test) (Fig. 6A). This result demonstrates that *h19* DMR1 does not answer for abnormal *Igf2* expression in the present mouse NTDs. Furthermore, the location of captured CpG islands were a slightly different in the two strands (Fig. 6A). This result further supports the notion that methylated CpG islands are distributed in different patterns on Crick and Watson strands.

Altered chromatin status in the promoter region is positively associated with excessive *Igf2* transcription

Given that the DNA methylation in the ICR of *Igf2/h19* did not change in mouse fetuses with NTDs, we then investigated the chromatin status of the promoter regions according to the public database (Fig. S3). The ChIP assay data uncovered increased enrichment of H3K4ac and attenuated enrichment of H3K27me3 on several regions of the promoter in NTDs (Fig. 6C and 6D). Meanwhile, one CG site was also hypomethylated (Fig. 6E). These lines of evidence agree with the enhanced *Igf2* expression. Similar to *Igf2*, *Kcnq1* mRNA was up-regulated (Fig. 5B), which was supported by increased H3K4ac enrichment (Fig. 6G and 6H) and hypomethylated CpG islands (Fig. 6I) in the promoter region, but not a stable methylation level of *KvDMR1* (data not shown). These results further assured us that in the RA-induced NTD

A

B

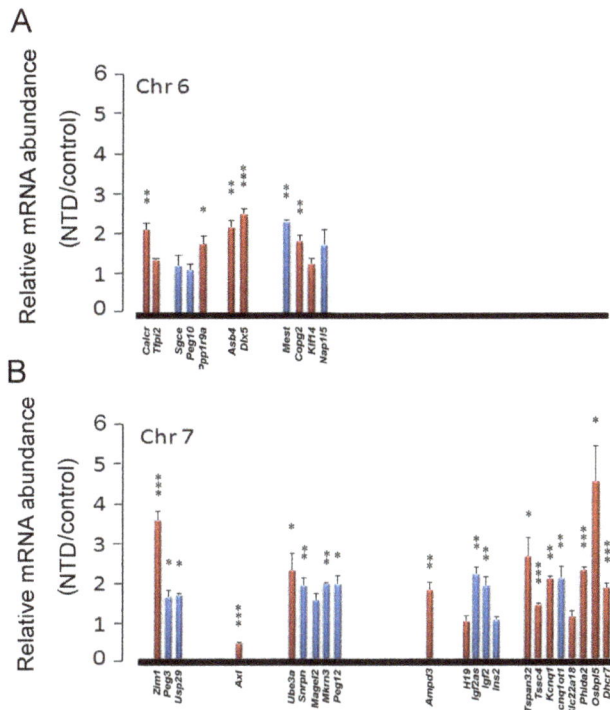

Figure 5. Wide ectopic mRNA levels of imprinted genes in mouse fetuses with RA-induced spina bifida. (A and B) The real-time qPCR assay results indicate the fold change in imprinted genes on each chromosome in the spinal cord tissue of E18 RA-induced mice with NTDs compared with control. The x-axis represents the chromosome and the relative genomic position of each gene. The y-axis represents the relative mRNA abundance in NTDs compared with the control. The red column indicates a maternally expressed gene, while the blue column indicates a paternally expressed gene. *: $P<0.05$; **: $P<0.01$; ***: $P<0.0001$ (Student's t-test).

mice, the abnormal expression of the Igf2 and Kcnq1 genes possibly result from changes of chromatin status in the promoter rather than changes in methylation of the ICRs.

Discussion

By investigating the mRNA level of imprinted genes and epigenetic regulation, we explored that in NTD cases of both humans and mice, IGF2/Igf2 expression was significantly enhanced, but the change in transcriptional activities might due to multifactorial etiology. In detail, for human NTDs, the change might be controlled by hypermethylated H19 DMR1, whereas in acute drug-induced mouse NTDs, the change seems to be determined by a more open chromatin structure in the promoter of the target gene.

Altered IGF2 expression occurs in multiple neurodevelopment diseases and cancer. In Bechwith-Wiedeman syndrome, both alleles of IGF2 were expressed [19], and similar cis genetic defects account for approximately 20% of cases [20]. High IGF2 expression is also strongly associated with ovarian cancer and stem cell-like neuroblastoma [21,22]. These studies support the result of enhanced IGF2 expression in NTDs. However, in prostate cancer, abolished IGF2 expression has also been observed [23]. These results demonstrate that IGF2 is positively or negatively associated with multiple human diseases. In mice,

Igf2 is down-regulated at E11.5 and E13.5 in the cranial neural tube and choroid plexus in maternal diabetic mice [24]; however, in2,3,7,8-Tetrachlorodibenzo-p-dioxin (TCDD)-induced rat, in which $21.79\pm17.71\%$ of fetuses display a spina bifida phenotype, the level of Igf2 is elevated in liver tissue, but not kidney, bones or skeletal muscle [25]. This result strongly suggests a possible complicated etiology induced by the overexpression or absence of IGF2 expression, even in the same disease. We hypothesized that the diversity in expression in NTDs is likely to attribute to different external causes; however, temporal factors should also be considered, although the IGF2 enhancement induced by TCDD continuously increased at 2 h, 6 h, and 24 h after TCDD treatment [25].

The enhanced IGF2 expression is potentially due to either hypermethylated H19 DMR1 or excessively open chromatin structure. Murrell et al. also refer to the distinct and multiple DMR methylation changes at the IGF2-H19 locus in Beckwith-Wiedemann and Silver-Russell syndromes and Wilms tumor [26]. This result demonstrates that indeed IGF2 can be regulated by different factors in one disease. The previous [8] and present data indicate that in the present NTD cohort, the H19 DMR1 is hypermethylated. Moreover, compared with the control, IGF2 mRNA expression in human NTDs was upregulated 6.41-fold, while in mice the expression was only upregulated approximately 2-fold. In humans, the dramatic increase should be controlled by the ICR in which the enhancer potentially binds to IGF2 because of H19 DMR1 hypermethylation. This notion is supported by Sparago's work in which a microdeletion in the H19 DMR1 cause both alleles to be expressed and H19 expression is 34 times lower than the proband's mother [19]. These results indicate that the reduction in CTCF binding exactly attenuates enhancer function by promoting H19 but enhances its role on IGF2 expression. Furthermore, in the present study, the change in chromatin structure in the promoter region is also a potential factor involved in the regulation of IGF2 expression; such fine tuning explains the two-fold increase in RA-induced NTDs. Consistently, in TCDD-induced NTD mice, the Igf2 expression is also altered at most by 2.6-fold. This result suggests that acute external stimuli mainly elicit changes in the open chromatin structure, but loss of imprinting might be established by a long period of environmental attack during gametogenesis or early development in NTDs.

The cause of loss of imprinting in NTDs has not been examined in the present study. However, a previous study in the present cohort indicated lower serum concentrations of 5-MeTHF, 5-FoTHF, total folate and vitamin B12 and remarkably higher concentrations of SAH in cases than in controls [27], and a recent report supports that in offspring a high level of methylation in IGF2 is detected after maternal folic acid use after 12 weeks of gestation. Unfortunately, we cannot know which DMR is hypermethylated in their study, although the selective DMRs are IGF2 DMR2 (AC132217) and H19 DMR1 (AF125183) [28]. However, another study provides evidence that compared to no folic acid intake before or during pregnancy, the methylation levels at the H19 DMR1, but not the IGF2 DMR0, decreased with increasing folic acid intake [7]. These results further reflect that a long period of folic acid intake can influence the relevant IGF2 DMR methylation level, and a low folic acid level is associated with a high methylation level at the H19 DMR1.

Recent studies have identified many epigenetic alterations in human or animal fetuses affected with NTDs, including H3K79me2, LINE-1 associated DNA methylation and micro-RNAs [10,14,15,29,30], demonstrating that multiple epigenetic regulations are involved in the etiology of NTDs. In the present study, the enhanced H3K4ac and depressed H3K27me3 are

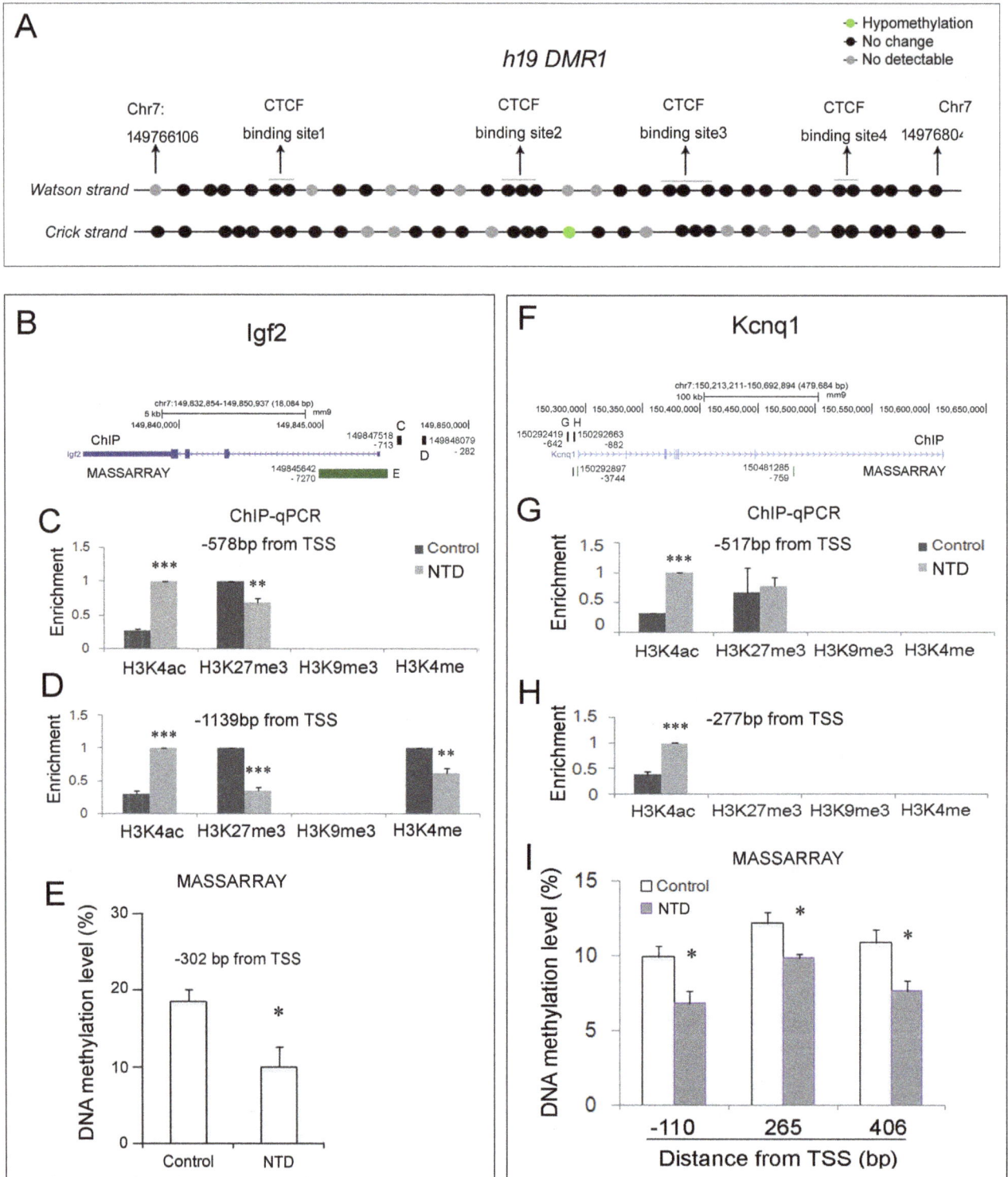

Figure 6. More open chromatin structure in mice fetuses with RA-induced spina bifida. (A) The methylation level of *H19* DMR1 is stable in RA-treated mice. For details, see the legend in Fig. 3. (B) and (F): The genomic profile of genes displayed in UCSC (mm9), the genomic locus of target regions in ChIP assay (black block in the gene schematic) (corresponding results shown in C and D or G and H), and the CpG island (green block underneath the gene schematic) (corresponding results shown in E and I) detected by MASSARRAY assay are shown. The number beside the block indicates the genomic location that was targeted. In the ChIP assay results (C and D or G and H), the enrichment in the y-axis represents the relative fold enrichment in which the higher enrichment in case or control is designated as 1. *: $P<0.05$; **: $P<0.01$; ***: $P<0.0001$ (Student's *t*-test). TSS: transcription start site.

associated with elevated *Igf2* expression in RA-induced NTD mice. Histone acetylation is an active chromatin mark, and H3K4ac is found enriched at active promoters [31]. The acetyltransferase CBP and EP300 complex can be recruited by the RA receptor RAR [32]; thus, we postulate that the RA-induced abnormal recruitment influences the H3K4 acetylation on the promoter of *Igf2*. In addition, RAR and its corepressor SMRT repress expression of the H3K27 demethylase JMJD3, which inhibits the capacity to activate specific components of the neurogenic program of neural stem cells [33]. Therefore, the depressed H3K27me3 on *Igf2* is likely to be associated with JMJD3 derepression.

Conclusion

Our present results indicate that the enhanced *IGF2* expression in NTDs as an early congenital defect and the changes of different epigenetic determinants occur in a context-specific manner. Our findings provide insight into the potential contributions of imprinted genes on early birth defects and its diverse pathogenecity. Future studies will elucidate the impact of changed imprinted genes expression to hopefully expand our understanding of a context-dependent individualization of prevention and therapy for NTDs.

Supporting Information

Figure S1 The referenced chromatin modification of two imprinted genes in humans. The histone modification and DNA methylation level status in H1 embryonic stem cells were referenced. The figures were download from the ENCODE database at UCSC GRCh37/hg19.

Figure S2 The mRNA levels of imprinted genes on eight other chromosomes. The figure shows the mRNA levels of the examined imprinted genes, except for chromosome 6 and 7,

which are shown in Fig. 5. For details, please see the legend for Fig. 5.

Figure S3 The referenced chromatin structure of two imprinted genes in mice. The histone modification and DNA methylation level status in Bruce embryonic stem cells were referenced. The figures were download from the ENCODE database at UCSC NCBI37/mm9.

Table S1 Primers or probes used in all kinds of assays. Sheet "mouse qPCR": The primers for realtime RT-PCR assays subjected on mouse spinal cord tissues with or without retinoic acid treatment. **Sheet "Nanostring probe":** The probes used in NanoString nCounter detections subjected on human fetuses' brain or spinal cord tissues **Sheet "mouse DNA methylation primer":** The primers for detection of DNA methylation level in mouse spinal cords by using MASSARRAY platform, in which "Watson" represents the primers are designed for Watson strand, "Crick" represents the primers are designed for Crick strand. **Sheet "Human DNA methylation primer":** The primers for detection of DNA methylation level in human fetuses spinal cords by using MASSARRAY platform, in which "Watson" represents the primers are designed for Watson strand, "Crick" represents the primers are designed for Crick strand. **Sheet "mouse ChIP-qPCR":** The primers for qPCR detection after ChIP assays in mouse spinal cord tissues. **Sheet "Human ChIP-qPCR":** The primers for qPCR detection after ChIP assays in human fetuses's spinal cord tissues.

Author Contributions

Conceived and designed the experiments: HL BB TZ. Performed the experiments: BB QZ XL CM SS. Analyzed the data: HL. Contributed reagents/materials/analysis tools: BB YB JG LW. Wrote the paper: BB HL TZ.

References

1. Li Z, Ren A, Zhang L, Ye R, Li S, et al. (2006) Extremely high prevalence of neural tube defects in a 4-county area in Shanxi Province, China. Birth Defects Res A Clin Mol Teratol 76: 237–240.
2. Byrne J, Cama A, Reilly M, Vigliarolo M, Levato L, et al. (1996) Multigeneration maternal transmission in Italian families with neural tube defects. Am J Med Genet 66: 303–310.
3. Moore T, Constancia M, Zubair M, Bailleul B, Feil R, et al. (1997) Multiple imprinted sense and antisense transcripts, differential methylation and tandem repeats in a putative imprinting control region upstream of mouse Igf2. Proc Natl Acad Sci U S A 94: 12509–12514.
4. Kurukuti S, Tiwari VK, Tavoosidana G, Pugacheva E, Murrell A, et al. (2006) CTCF binding at the H19 imprinting control region mediates maternally inherited higher-order chromatin conformation to restrict enhancer access to Igf2. Proc Natl Acad Sci U S A 103: 10684–10689.
5. Leighton PA, Saam JR, Ingram RS, Stewart CL, Tilghman SM (1995) An enhancer deletion affects both H19 and Igf2 expression. Genes Dev 9: 2079–2089.
6. Forne T, Oswald J, Dean W, Saam JR, Bailleul B, et al. (1997) Loss of the maternal H19 gene induces changes in Igf2 methylation in both cis and trans. Proc Natl Acad Sci U S A 94: 10243–10248.
7. Hoyo C, Murtha AP, Schildkraut JM, Jirtle RL, Demark-Wahnefried W, et al. (2011) Methylation variation at IGF2 differentially methylated regions and maternal folic acid use before and during pregnancy. Epigenetics 6: 928–936.
8. Liu Z, Wang L, Li Y, Ouyang S, Chang H, et al. (2012) Association of genomic instability, and the methylation status of imprinted genes and mismatch-repair genes, with neural tube defects. Eur J Hum Genet 20: 516–520.
9. Stolk L, Bouwland-Both MI, van Mill NH, Verbiest MM, Eilers PH, et al. (2013) Epigenetic profiles in children with a neural tube defect; a case-control study in two populations. PLoS One 8: e78462.
10. Wu L, Wang L, Shangguan S, Chang S, Wang Z, et al. (2013) Altered methylation of IGF2 DMR0 is associated with neural tube defects. Mol Cell Biochem 380: 33–42.
11. Zhou VW, Goren A, Bernstein BE (2011) Charting histone modifications and the functional organization of mammalian genomes. Nat Rev Genet 12: 7–18.
12. Copp AJ, Greene ND (2010) Genetics and development of neural tube defects. J Pathol 220: 217–230.
13. Rada-Iglesias A, Bajpai R, Swigut T, Brugmann SA, Flynn RA, et al. (2011) A unique chromatin signature uncovers early developmental enhancers in humans. Nature 470: 279–283.
14. Zhang Q, Xue P, Li H, Bao Y, Wu L, et al. (2013) Histone modification mapping in human brain reveals aberrant expression of histone H3 lysine 79 dimethylation in neural tube defects. Neurobiol Dis 54: 404–413.
15. Wang L, Wang F, Guan J, Le J, Wu L, et al. (2010) Relation between hypomethylation of long interspersed nucleotide elements and risk of neural tube defects. Am J Clin Nutr 91: 1359–1367.
16. Gu X, Lin L, Zheng X, Zhang T, Song X, et al. (2007) High prevalence of NTDs in Shanxi Province: a combined epidemiological approach. Birth Defects Res A Clin Mol Teratol 79: 702–707.
17. Chen X, Shen Y, Gao Y, Zhao H, Sheng X, et al. (2013) Detection of copy number variants reveals association of cilia genes with neural tube defects. PLoS One 8: e54492.
18. Koerner MV, Pauler FM, Huang R, Barlow DP (2009) The function of non-coding RNAs in genomic imprinting. Development 136: 1771–1783.
19. Sparago A, Cerrato F, Vernucci M, Ferrero GB, Silengo MC, et al. (2004) Microdeletions in the human H19 DMR result in loss of IGF2 imprinting and Beckwith-Wiedemann syndrome. Nat Genet 36: 958–960.
20. Abi Habib W, Azzi S, Brioude F, Steunou V, Thibaud N, et al. (2014) Extensive investigation of the IGF2/H19 imprinting control region reveals novel OCT4/SOX2 binding site defects associated with specific methylation patterns in Beckwith-Wiedemann syndrome. Hum Mol Genet.
21. Mohlin S, Hamidian A, Pahlman S (2013) HIF2A and IGF2 expression correlates in human neuroblastoma cells and normal immature sympathetic neuroblasts. Neoplasia 15: 328–334.

22. Brouwer-Visser J, Lee J, McCullagh K, Cossio MJ, Wang Y, et al. (2014) Insulin-like growth factor 2 silencing restores taxol sensitivity in drug resistant ovarian cancer. PLoS One 9: e100165.

23. Ribarska T, Goering W, Droop J, Bastian KM, Ingenwerth M, et al. (2014) Deregulation of an imprinted gene network in prostate cancer. Epigenetics 9: 704–717.

24. Jiang B, Kumar SD, Loh WT, Manikandan J, Ling EA, et al. (2008) Global gene expression analysis of cranial neural tubes in embryos of diabetic mice. J Neurosci Res 86: 3481–3493.

25. Wang J, Liu X, Li T, Liu C, Zhao Y (2011) Increased hepatic Igf2 gene expression involves C/EBPbeta in TCDD-induced teratogenesis in rats. Reprod Toxicol 32: 313–321.

26. Murrell A, Ito Y, Verde G, Huddleston J, Woodfine K, et al. (2008) Distinct methylation changes at the IGF2-H19 locus in congenital growth disorders and cancer. PLoS One 3: e1849.

27. Zhang HY, Luo GA, Liang QL, Wang Y, Yang HH, et al. (2008) Neural tube defects and disturbed maternal folate- and homocysteine-mediated one-carbon metabolism. Exp Neurol 212: 515–521.

28. Dupont JM, Tost J, Jammes H, Gut IG (2004) De novo quantitative bisulfite sequencing using the pyrosequencing technology. Anal Biochem 333: 119–127.

29. Wei X, Li H, Miao J, Liu B, Zhan Y, et al. (2013) miR-9*- and miR-124a-Mediated switching of chromatin remodelling complexes is altered in rat spina bifida aperta. Neurochem Res 38: 1605–1615.

30. Wang F, Wang J, Guo J, Chen X, Guan Z, et al. (2013) PCMT1 gene polymorphisms, maternal folate metabolism, and neural tube defects: a case-control study in a population with relatively low folate intake. Genes Nutr 8: 581–587.

31. Guillemette B, Drogaris P, Lin HH, Armstrong H, Hiragami-Hamada K, et al. (2011) H3 lysine 4 is acetylated at active gene promoters and is regulated by H3 lysine 4 methylation. PLoS Genet 7: e1001354.

32. Torchia J, Rose DW, Inostroza J, Kamei Y, Westin S, et al. (1997) The transcriptional co-activator p/CIP binds CBP and mediates nuclear-receptor function. Nature 387: 677–684.

33. Jepsen K, Solum D, Zhou T, McEvilly RJ, Kim HJ, et al. (2007) SMRT-mediated repression of an H3K27 demethylase in progression from neural stem cell to neuron. Nature 450: 415–419.

Permissions

The contributors of this book come from diverse backgrounds, making this book a truly international effort. This book will bring forth new frontiers with its revolutionizing research information and detailed analysis of the nascent developments around the world.

We would like to thank all the contributing authors for lending their expertise to make the book truly unique. They have played a crucial role in the development of this book. Without their invaluable contributions this book wouldn't have been possible. They have made vital efforts to compile up to date information on the varied aspects of this subject to make this book a valuable addition to the collection of many professionals and students.

This book was conceptualized with the vision of imparting up-to-date information and advanced data in this field. To ensure the same, a matchless editorial board was set up. Every individual on the board went through rigorous rounds of assessment to prove their worth. After which they invested a large part of their time researching and compiling the most relevant data for our readers.

The editorial board has been involved in producing this book since its inception. They have spent rigorous hours researching and exploring the diverse topics which have resulted in the successful publishing of this book. They have passed on their knowledge of decades through this book. To expedite this challenging task, the publisher supported the team at every step. A small team of assistant editors was also appointed to further simplify the editing procedure and attain best results for the readers.

Apart from the editorial board, the designing team has also invested a significant amount of their time in understanding the subject and creating the most relevant covers. They scrutinized every image to scout for the most suitable representation of the subject and create an appropriate cover for the book.

The publishing team has been an ardent support to the editorial, designing and production team. Their endless efforts to recruit the best for this project, has resulted in the accomplishment of this book. They are a veteran in the field of academics and their pool of knowledge is as vast as their experience in printing. Their expertise and guidance has proved useful at every step. Their uncompromising quality standards have made this book an exceptional effort. Their encouragement from time to time has been an inspiration for everyone.

The publisher and the editorial board hope that this book will prove to be a valuable piece of knowledge for researchers, students, practitioners and scholars across the globe.

List of Contributors

Sarah A. Figley and Spyridon K. Karadimas
Department of Genetics and Development, Toronto Western Research Institute, and Spinal Program, Krembil Neuroscience Centre, University Health Network, Toronto, Ontario, Canada
Institute of Medical Sciences, University of Toronto, Toronto, Ontario, Canada

Yang Liu, Kajana Satkunendrarajah and Peter Fettes
Department of Genetics and Development, Toronto Western Research Institute, and Spinal Program, Krembil Neuroscience Centre, University Health Network, Toronto, Ontario, Canada

S. Kaye Spratt, Gary Lee, Dale Ando and Richard Surosky
Department of Therapeutic Development, Sangamo BioSciences, Pt. Richmond, California, United States of America

Martin Giedlin
Institute of Medical Sciences, University of Toronto, Toronto, Ontario, Canada

Michael G. Fehlings
Department of Genetics and Development, Toronto Western Research Institute, and Spinal Program, Krembil Neuroscience Centre, University Health Network, Toronto, Ontario, Canada
Institute of Medical Sciences, University of Toronto, Toronto, Ontario, Canada
Department of Surgery, University of Toronto, Toronto, Ontario, Canada

Sujata Saraswat Ohri and Ashley Mullins
Kentucky Spinal Cord Injury Research Center, University of Louisville, Louisville, Kentucky, United States of America
Department of Neurological Surgery, University of Louisville, Louisville, Kentucky, United States of America

Michal Hetman
Kentucky Spinal Cord Injury Research Center, University of Louisville, Louisville, Kentucky, United States of America

Department of Neurological Surgery, University of Louisville, Louisville, Kentucky, United States of America
Department of Pharmacology & Toxicology, University of Louisville, Louisville, Kentucky, United States of America
Department of Anatomical Sciences & Neurobiology, University of Louisville, Louisville, Kentucky, United States of America

Scott R. Whittemore
Kentucky Spinal Cord Injury Research Center, University of Louisville, Louisville, Kentucky, United States of America
Department of Neurological Surgery, University of Louisville, Louisville, Kentucky, United States of America
Department of Anatomical Sciences & Neurobiology, University of Louisville, Louisville, Kentucky, United States of America

Jonathan M. Levine and Sharon C. Kerwin
Department of Small Animal Clinical Sciences, College of Veterinary Medicine and Biomedical Sciences, Texas A&M University, College Station, Texas, United States of America

Noah D. Cohen
Department of Large Animal Clinical Sciences, College of Veterinary Medicine and Biomedical Sciences, Texas A&M University, College Station, Texas, United States of America

Michael Heller and Augusta Modestino
Department of Bioengineering, University of California San Diego, San Diego, California, United States of America

Virginia R. Fajt
Department of Veterinary Physiology and Pharmacology, College of Veterinary Medicine and Biomedical Sciences, Texas A&M University, College Station, Texas, United States of America

Gwendolyn J. Levine
Department of Veterinary Pathobiology, College of Veterinary Medicine and Biomedical Sciences, Texas A&M University, College Station, Texas, United States of America

Alpa A. Trivedi and Thomas M. Fandel
Department of Neurological Surgery, University of California San Francisco, San Francisco, California, United States of America

Zena Werb
Department of Anatomy, University of California San Francisco, San Francisco, California, United States of America

Linda J. Noble-Haeusslein
Department of Neurological Surgery, University of California San Francisco, San Francisco, California, United States of America
Department of Physical Therapy and Rehabilitation, University of California San Francisco, San Francisco, California, United States of America

Katarina Vajn and Denis Suler
Department of Physical Medicine and Rehabilitation, University of Pittsburgh School of Medicine, Pittsburgh, Pennsylvania, United States of America

Jeffery A. Plunkett
School of Science Technology and Engineering Management, St. Thomas University, Miami Gardens, Florida, United States of America

Martin Oudega
Department of Physical Medicine and Rehabilitation, University of Pittsburgh School of Medicine, Pittsburgh, Pennsylvania, United States of America
Department of Bioengineering, University of Pittsburgh School of Medicine, Pittsburgh, Pennsylvania, United States of America
Department of Neurobiology, University of Pittsburgh School of Medicine, Pittsburgh, Pennsylvania, United States of America

Shuo Tang, Zeyu Huang and Fuxing Pei
Department of Orthopaedics, West China Hospital, Sichuan University, Chengdu, China

Xiang Liao
Department of Pain Medicine, Shenzhen Nanshan Hospital, Shenzhen, China

Bo Shi
Department of Orthopaedics, Mianyang Center Hospital, Mianyang, China

Yanzhen Qu and Xiaodong Guo
Department of Orthopaedics, Union Hospital, Tongji Medical College, Huazhong University of Science and Technology, Wuhan, China

Qiang Lin
Department of Orthopaedics, Guangdong hospital of traditional Chinese medicine, Guangzhou, China

Subhra Prakash Hui, Dhriti Sengupta, Sudip Kundu and Sukla Ghosh
Department of Biophysics, Molecular Biology and Bioinformatics, University of Calcutta, Kolkata, India

Serene Gek Ping Lee and Sinnakaruppan Mathavan
Genome Institute of Singapore, Singapore, Singapore

Triparna Sen
Chittaranjan National Cancer Research Institute, Kolkata, India

Hussain Al Dera
Department of Anatomy and Neuroscience, University of Melbourne, Victoria, Australia
Basic Medical Sciences, College of Medicine, King Saud bin Abdulaziz University for Health Sciences, Riyadh, Saudi Arabia

Brid P. Callaghan and James A. Brock
Department of Anatomy and Neuroscience, University of Melbourne, Victoria, Australia

Yuling Meng, Aaron An, Asim Mahmood, Ye Xiong and Yanlu Zhang
Department of Neurosurgery, Henry Ford Hospital, Detroit, Michigan, United States of America

Michael Chopp
Department of Neurology, Henry Ford Hospital, Detroit, Michigan, United States of America
Department of Physics, Oakland University, Rochester, Michigan, United States of America

Zhongwu Liu
Department of Neurology, Henry Ford Hospital, Detroit, Michigan, United States of America

Torge Rempe
Dept of Neuroradiology, University Hospital of Kiel, Arnold-Heller-Strasse 3, Haus 41, 24105 Kiel, Germany
Dept of Neurology, University Hospital of Kiel, Arnold-Heller-Strasse
3, Haus 41, 24105 Kiel, Germany

Stephan Wolff, Christian Riedel and Olav Jansen
Dept of Neuroradiology, University Hospital of Kiel, Arnold-Heller-Strasse 3, Haus 41, 24105 Kiel, Germany

Ralf Baron
Dept of Neurology, University Hospital of Kiel, Arnold-Heller-Strasse
3, Haus 41, 24105 Kiel, Germany
Division of Neurological Pain Research and Therapy, University Hospital of Kiel, Arnold-Heller-Strasse 3, Haus 41, 24105 Kiel, Germany

Patrick W. Stroman
Centre for Neuroscience Studies, Dept of Diagnostic Radiology, Dept of Physics, 228 Botterell Hall, Queen's University, Kingston, Ontario, Canada

Janne Gierthmühlen
Dept of Neuroradiology, University Hospital of Kiel, Arnold-Heller-Strasse 3, Haus 41, 24105 Kiel, Germany
Division of Neurological Pain Research and Therapy, University Hospital of Kiel, Arnold-Heller-Strasse 3, Haus 41, 24105 Kiel, Germany

Liuliu Pan, Hilary A. North, Vibhu Sahni, Su Ji Jeong, Tammy L. Mcguire and John A. Kessler
Department of Neurology, Northwestern University, Chicago, Illinois, United States of America

Eric J. Berns
Department of Biomedical Engineering, Northwestern University,
Evanston, Illinois, United States of America

Samuel I. Stupp
Department of Materials Science and Engineering, Northwestern University, Evanston, Illinois, United States of America
Department of Chemistry, Northwestern University, Evanston, Illinois, United States of America
Department of Medicine and Institute for BioNanotechnology in Medicine, Northwestern University, Chicago, Illinois, United States of America

Saïd M'Dahoma, Sylvie Bourgoin, Valérie Kayser, Sandrine Barthélémy, Caroline Chevarin and Michel Hamon
Centre de Psychiatrie et Neurosciences, Institut National de la Santé et de la Recherche Médicale, INSERM U894, Université Paris Descartes, Paris, France
Neuropsychopharmacologie, Faculté de Médecine Pierre et Marie Curie, site Pitié-Salpêtrière, Paris, France

Farah Chali and Didier Orsal
Laboratoire de Neurobiologie des Signaux Intercellulaires, Centre National de la Recherche Scientifique, CNRS UMR 7101, Université Pierre et Marie Curie, Paris, France

Hisayo Jin and Makiko Kashio
Department of Anesthesiology, Chiba University Graduate School of Medicine, Chiba City, Chiba, Japan

Naoya Mimura
Department of Medicine and Clinical Oncology, Chiba University Graduate School of Medicine, Chiba City, Chiba, Japan

Haruhiko Koseki
Laboratory for Developmental Genetics, RIKEN Research Center for Allergy and Immunology, Yokohama, Japan

Tomohiko Aoe
Department of Anesthesiology, Chiba University Graduate School of Medicine, Chiba City, Chiba, Japan
Department of Anesthesiology, Tokyo Women's Medical University, Yachiyo Medical, Center, Yachiyo, Chiba, Japan

Roberta Barbizan, Mateus V. Castro and Alexandre L. R. Oliveira
Laboratory of Nerve Regeneration, Department of Structural and Functional Biology, University of Campinas - UNICAMP, Campinas, São Paulo, Brazil

Benedito Barraviera and Rui S. Ferreira Jr.
Center for the Study of Venoms and Venomous Animals (CEVAP), São Paulo State University (UNESP – Univ Estadual Paulista), Botucatu, São Paulo, Brazil

Simone Codeluppi, Teresa Fernandez-Zafra and Per Uhlén
Laboratory of Molecular Neurobiology, Department of Medical Biochemistry and Biophysics, Karolinska Institutet, Stockholm, Sweden

Katalin Sandor and Camilla I. Svensson
Department of Physiology and Pharmacology, Karolinska Institutet, Stockholm, Sweden

Jacob Kjell, Mathew Abrams and Lars Olson
Department of Neuroscience, Karolinska Institutet, Stockholm, Sweden

Qingsong Liu and Nathanael S. Gray
Department of Cancer Biology, Dana- Farber Cancer Institute, Boston, Massachusetts, United States of America
Department of Biological Chemistry and Molecular Pharmacology, Harvard Medical School, Boston, Massachusetts, United States of America

Jaime L. Watson, Tamara J. Hala, Rajarshi Putatunda, Daniel Sannie and Angelo C. Lepore
Department of Neuroscience, Farber Institute for Neurosciences, Sidney Kimmel Medical College at Thomas Jefferson University, Philadelphia, Pennsylvania, United States of America

Aldric T. Hama, Matthew S. Varghese and Jacqueline Sagen
Miami Project to Cure Paralysis, University of Miami Miller School of Medicine, Miami, Florida, United States of America

Peter Germano, G. Todd Milne and James P. Pearson
Ironwood Pharmaceuticals, Inc., Cambridge, Massachusetts, United States of America

Benjamin F. Cravatt
Department of Chemical Physiology, The Skaggs Institute for Chemical Biology, The Scripps Research Institute, La Jolla, California, United States of America

Baoling Bai, Qin Zhang, Xiaozhen Liu, Chunyue Miao, Shaofang Shangguan, Yihua Bao, Jin Guo, Li Wang, Ting Zhang and Huili Li
Beijing Municipal Key Laboratory of Child Development and Nutriomics, Capital Institute of Pediatrics, Beijing, 100020, China

Index

www.ingramcontent.com/pod-product-compliance
Lightning Source LLC
Chambersburg PA
CBHW061240190326
41458CB00011B/3540